T0210340

THE MONT REID SURGICAL HANDBOOK

SEVENTH EDITION

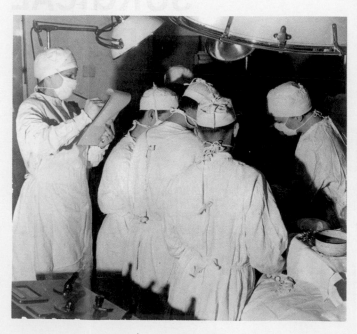

Miss Mary Maciel sketching an operative procedure beside the surgeons in an operating room -

THE MONT REID SURGICAL HANDBOOK

SEVENTH EDITION

The University of Cincinnati Residents
From the Department of Surgery
University of Cincinnati College of Medicine
Cincinnati, Ohio

EDITORS

Jeffrey M. Sutton, MD
M. Aaron Beckwith, MD
Bobby L. Johnson, MD
J. Leslie Knod, MD
Ashley Walther, MD
Carey L. Watson, MD
Gregory C. Wilson, MD

ELSEVIER

ELSEVIER

1600 John F. Kennedy Blvd.
Ste 1800
Philadelphia, PA 19103-2899

THE MONT REID SURGICAL HANDBOOK,
SEVENTH EDITION   ISBN: 978-0-323-52980-8

Previous editions copyrighted 2008, 2005, 1997, 1994, 1990, 1987 by Saunders, an imprint of Elsevier.

Library of Congress Cataloging-in-Publication Data
Names: Sutton, Jeffrey M., editor. | University of Cincinnati. Department of
    Surgery.
Title: The Mont Reid surgical handbook / the University of Cincinnati
    residents from the Department of Surgery, University of Cincinnati College
    of Medicine, Cincinnati, Ohio ; editors, Jeffrey M. Sutton [and 6 others].
Other titles: Surgical handbook
Description: Seventh edition. | Philadelphia, PA : Elsevier, [2018] |
    Includes bibliographical references and index.
Identifiers: LCCN 2017041248 | ISBN 9780323529808 (paperback : alk. paper)
Subjects: | MESH: Surgical Procedures, Operative | Handbooks
Classification: LCC RD49 | NLM WO 39 | DDC 617/.9—dc23 LC record available at
    https://lccn.loc.gov/2017041248

Executive Content Strategist: James Merritt
Content Development Specialist: Jennifer Ehlers
Publishing Services Manager: Patricia Tannian
Senior Project Manager: Claire Kramer
Designer: Bridget Hoette

Printed in India

Last digit is the print number: 9   8   7   6   5

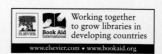

Working together to grow libraries in developing countries

www.elsevier.com • www.bookaid.org

FOREWORD

The mission of the Surgical Residency Training Program at the University of Cincinnati is to foster the development of the next generation of surgeons, scholars, and leaders. Vital to this charge is the continuous commitment to improve the care of our patients, as well as advancing the scientific basis for clinical practice. The seventh edition of *The Mont Reid Surgical Handbook* is written by our surgical residents under the supervision and leadership of our faculty. Our commitment to training and developing the next generation of surgical leaders is evident in the quality of each chapter, culminating in a comprehensive and practical document that represents our dedication to patient care and surgical practice.

As the Christian R. Holmes Professor and Chair of the Department of Surgery at the University of Cincinnati College of Medicine, I consider it a privilege to chair a department with such a great legacy. *The Mont Reid Surgical Handbook* is tangible evidence of our historic and ongoing commitment to excellence in the comprehensive missions of clinical service, education, and scholarship.

Michael J. Edwards, MD, FASC
Christian R. Holmes Professor of Surgery
and Chairman of the Department of Surgery
University of Cincinnati Medical Center
Cincinnati, Ohio

PREFACE

The Surgical Residency Training Program at the University of Cincinnati dates back to 1922 and was established by Dr. George J. Heuer and Dr. Mont R. Reid, students of Dr. William Halsted. As the second Christian R. Holmes Professor of Surgery, Dr. Reid expanded and matured the training program, building the solid foundation on which it relies today. The traditions and history initiated by Dr. Mont Reid remain at the core of our Department of Surgery and sustain our culture of excellence in patient care and surgical education.

The Mont Reid Surgical Handbook exemplifies the tradition and legacy of the University of Cincinnati. Initially published in 1987, the handbook embodies the hard work and dedication that is paramount to our residency. In addition to many updates and revisions, this seventh edition features artistic renderings from Miss Mary Maciel, our former surgical illustrator and medical artist. Mary Maciel established the School of Medical Illustration at the University of Cincinnati College of Medicine in 1947 and was its director for 25 years. She created a library of innumerable medical illustrations and selflessly donated her work to our Department of Surgery. One of her artistic renderings appears as the cover image, and others appear on the part opening pages. They represent an additional piece of the history of the Department of Surgery at the University of Cincinnati. A photograph of Mary Maciel at work also appears in the handbook's front matter.

Publication of *The Mont Reid Surgical Handbook* would not be possible without the support of our chairman, Dr. Michael J. Edwards, as well as the chairmen who have preceded him. The commitment and dedication of our chair to our residency training program at the University of Cincinnati fuel our drive to succeed and are an inspiration.

Our residency training program is focused on the development of the next generation of strong surgical leaders, and our pride in the residency is evident throughout the pages of this handbook. It is not meant to be an exhaustive representation of surgical information but will serve as a concise guide to common surgical conditions and treatment. Much of the information presented in this edition is influenced by our philosophy and tradition at the University of Cincinnati, but included as well in this revision are references to current literature and added online self-assessment questions to augment the text.

Finally, this handbook is and always will be written by surgical residents, for students and residents. We are proud to present the seventh edition of *The Mont Reid Surgical Handbook*.

The graduating Surgical Chief Resident Class of 2017:

Jeffrey M. Sutton, MD
M. Aaron Beckwith, MD
Bobby L. Johnson, MD
J. Leslie Knod, MD
Ashley Walther, MD
Carey L. Watson, MD
Gregory C. Wilson, MD

CHAPTER TITLE	RESIDENT	FACULTY ADVISOR
1. Surgical History and Physical Examination	Young Kim, MD, MS	Kenneth Davis Jr., MD
2. Fluids and Electrolytes	Joshua Kuethe, ND	D Millar, MD
3. Nutrition	Joshua Kuethe, MD	Joseph Lacy, MS, RD, LD
4. Wound Healing	Aaron Seitz, MD	Ryan Gobble, MD
5. Surgical Risk Assessment	Young Kim, MD, MS	D Millar, MD
6. Suture Types, Needle Types, and Instruments	Drew D. Jung, MD	Jason J. Schrager, MD
7. Local Anesthesia	Fernando Ovalle Jr., MD	Andrew Friedrich, MD
8. Conscious Sedation	Bobby L. Johnson, MD	Vanessa Nomellini, MD, PhD
9. General Anesthesia	Lauren M. Baumann, MD	Andrew Friedrich, MD
10. Surgical Infection	Aaron Seitz, MD	Betty Tsuei, MD
11. Hemorrhage and Coagulation	Peter L. Jernigan, MD	Michael Goodman, MD
12. Shock	Amanda M. Pugh, MD	Michael Goodman, MD
13. Cardiopulmonary Monitoring	Paul T. Kim, MD	Betty Tsuei, MD
14. Mechanical Ventilation	Paul T. Kim, MD	Richard Branson, RRT
15. Primary and Secondary Survey	Meghan C. Daly, MD	Joel Elterman, MD
16. Abdominal Trauma	Amanda M. Pugh, MD	Krishna Athota, MD
17. Thoracic Trauma	Nick Charles Levinsky Jr., MD	Jason J. Schrager, MD
18. Extremity Trauma	Ryan M. Boudreau, MD	Brian Gavitt, MD
19. Burn Care	Lauren M. Baumann, MD	Elizabeth Dale, MD
20. Neurosurgical Emergencies	Christopher P. Carroll, MD	Norberto O. Andaluz, MD
21. Acute Abdomen	Ben Huebner, MD	Jay Johannigman, MD
22. Abdominal Wall Hernias	Richard S. Hoehn, MD	Timothy A. Pritts, MD, PhD
23. Gastrointestinal Bleeding	Richard S. Hoehn, MD	Amy T. Makley, MD
24. Intestinal Obstruction	Drew D. Jung, MD	Timothy A. Pritts, MD, PhD

CONTENTS

THE MONT REID SURGICAL HANDBOOK

SEVENTH EDITION

PART I

Perioperative Care

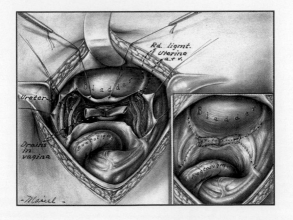

PART I

Perioperative Care

Surgical History and Physical Examination

Young Kim, MD, MS

The first principle is that of the necessity of making a serious and thorough attempt at diagnosis.

—W. Silen

I. INTRODUCTION AND INITIAL CONTACT

1. The history and physical examination are an integral aspect of patient care. Many diagnoses can be confirmed or refuted with a carefully obtained history. The physical examination can also direct further need for other diagnostic modalities such as imaging and serologic tests. During this initial encounter, the surgeon also establishes a patient-doctor relationship, which is essential to patient care. In the trauma patient, constant reevaluation must be performed to discover new findings, as well as to evaluate the course of previously noted findings.

2. *KISS mnemonic*: *k*nock, *i*ntroduce yourself, *s*crub your hands, *s*it down.

3. Ensure the patient is at ease. Close the door to protect patient privacy. Establish rapport with the patient and, if present, family and loved ones. Minimize any environmental distractions.

4. Start with open-ended questions and listen to the patient. They will often cover most of the relevant facts. Then transition to focused and close-ended questions to obtain smaller details. Ask the patient about his/her goals of care so that they may be addressed properly.

5. For non-English-speaking patients, a certified translator should be used. Focus your attention on the patient and not on the translator, if this is the case.

II. HISTORY

A. CHIEF COMPLAINT

1. The patient's reason for hospital or clinical visit, in his/her own words in quotations

B. HISTORY OF PRESENT ILLNESS

1. Relevant details surrounding the chief complaint

2. OLD CARTS mnemonic: *o*nset, *l*ocation/radiation, *d*uration, *c*haracter, *a*ggravating factors, *r*elieving factors, *t*iming, *s*everity.

   a. *Onset*: When did it start? Was it gradual or sudden onset? What were you doing when it began? Have you experienced any similar episodes in the past?

    b. *Location/radiation*: Where is it located? Is it focal or diffuse? Does it radiate? Has it migrated over time?

    c. *Duration*: How long has it been going on?

    d. *Character*: How would you describe your complaint?

    e. *Aggravating factors*: What makes it worse? Position? Movement? Eating?

    f. *Relieving factors*: What makes it better? Position? Movement? Eating?

    g. *Timing*: Has it changed over time? Does it come and go, or is it persistent? How frequently?

    h. *Severity*: How would you rate it on a scale of 1 to 10, with 10 being the worst? Is it always at that severity, or has it changed over time?

C. REVIEW OF SYSTEMS

1. Yes-or-no questions that further direct the history of present illness toward a specific diagnosis. Currently, 14 systems are recognized.
2. *Constitutional:* fevers, chills, weight loss, night sweats, fatigue
3. *Eyes*: visual changes, eye pain, diplopia, scotomas, floaters
4. *Ears, nose, mouth, throat*: epistaxis, ear pain, tinnitus, toothache, sore throat
5. *Cardiovascular:* chest pain, dyspnea, orthopnea, palpitations, claudication
6. *Respiratory:* wheezing, cough, dyspnea, hemoptysis
7. *Gastrointestinal*: abdominal pain, nausea, emesis, diarrhea, constipation/obstipation, hematemesis, hematochezia, melena, tenesmus
8. *Genitourinary*: dysuria, hematuria, urgency, nocturia, vaginal discharge, pain
9. *Musculoskeletal*: pain, stiffness, joint swelling, limited range of motion
10. *Integumentary*: rash, pruritus, lesions, wounds, erythema, tumors
11. *Neurologic*: headache, paresthesias, numbness, weakness, poor balance, changes in senses
12. *Psychiatric*: depression, changes in sleep patterns, anxiety, paranoia, mania, suicidal or homicidal ideation
13. *Endocrine*: lethargy, hyperactivity, palpitations, tremor, fatigue
14. *Hematologic/lymphatic*: anemia, petechiae, purpura
15. *Allergic/immunologic*: lymphadenopathy, allergic response to offending agents, anaphylaxis

D. ALLERGIES

1. Offending agents and medications
2. Specific reactions to these medications (e.g., rash/hives, stridor, anaphylaxis)

E. MEDICATION

1. Medication name, timing, and dosage
2. Duration if relevant (e.g., antibiotics)

F. PAST MEDICAL HISTORY

1. If possible, obtaining previous medical reports before a patient encounter can help direct questions toward pertinent details. Always try to obtain discharge summaries, prior operative reports, and imaging/laboratory studies through the medical record system.
2. Acute illnesses (e.g., pneumonia, diabetic ketoacidosis (DKA), biliary colic)
3. Chronic illnesses (e.g., diabetes mellitus, chronic obstructive pulmonary disease (COPD), malignancy)
4. Injuries or accidents (e.g., prior trauma)
5. Gynecologic history
   a. Last menstrual period
   b. Gravida, para, abortus
   c. History of sexually transmitted illnesses

G. PAST SURGICAL HISTORY

1. Again, obtaining previous operative reports can often be more accurate than relying on a patient's recollection of events
2. Type of operation, date, hospital, name of surgeon
3. Indications for surgery
   a. Elective vs. emergent
4. Previous difficulties with anesthesia
5. Perioperative complications

H. FAMILY HISTORY

1. Chronic illnesses
2. Malignancy
3. Bleeding or clotting disorders
4. Problems with anesthesia

I. SOCIAL HISTORY

1. Alcohol use/abuse
2. Tobacco use/abuse
3. Illicit drug abuse
4. Sexual history/orientation
5. Religion

III. PHYSICAL EXAMINATION

A. VITAL SIGNS

1. Vital signs are an integral part of the physical examination. They measure and quantify clinical variables into four numbers, which help assess the patient's overall condition in an objective fashion.
2. Temperature
   a. *Reference range*: 36°C (96.8°F) to 38°C (100.4°F)
      (1) Regulated by the hypothalamus
   b. *Fever*: greater than 38.6°C (101.5°F)

SURGICAL HISTORY AND PHYSICAL EXAMINATION

1

(1) Systemic inflammatory response syndrome (SIRS) indicates that an inflammatory process has spread from a diseased organ to the entire body. In the clinical setting, two of four criteria must be met to establish this diagnosis. These include white blood cell count ($<4000/mm^3$ or $>12,000/mm^3$), heart rate (>90 beats/min), respiratory rate (>20 breaths/min or $pCO_2 <32$ mm Hg), and temperature ($<36°C$ or $>38°C$). Note that blood pressure does not need to be altered in this condition.

c. *Hypothermia*: less than 35°C (95°F)
   (1) The triad of death—acidosis, coagulopathy, and hypothermia—indicates a rapidly deteriorating patient status.

3. Heart rate

a. *Reference range*: 60–100 beats/min (in adults)
b. *Tachycardia*: greater than 100 beats/min
   (1) Tachycardia is the most common vital sign change associated with early hypovolemic shock but may not present until greater than 15% of total blood volume has been lost.
   (2) Beta-blockers may blunt the physiologic response in heart rate to reflect the clinical situation.
c. *Bradycardia*: less than 60 beats/min
   (1) Symptomatic bradycardia should be treated with atropine.
   (2) Asymptomatic bradycardia may be present in athletes, elderly adults, and those taking beta-blockers.

4. Blood pressure

a. *Reference range*: systolic pressure 90–140 mm Hg, diastolic pressure 60–90 mm Hg (in adults)
   (1) Palpable carotid, femoral, and radial pulses indicate an estimated systolic pressure of at least 60, 70, and 80 mm Hg, respectively.
   (2) Bilateral measurements should be compared
   (3) Mean arterial pressure = ($\frac{1}{3}$ × systolic blood pressure [sBP]) + ($\frac{2}{3}$ × diastolic blood pressure [dBP])
      (a) *Reference range*: 80–90 mm Hg
      (b) More consistent indicator of peripheral perfusion compared with systolic blood pressure
b. *Hypertension*: greater than 140/90 mm Hg
   (1) *Hypertensive urgency*: greater than 180/110 without evidence of end-organ damage
   (2) *Hypertensive emergency*: greater than 180/110 with evidence of end-organ damage
   (3) An inappropriately sized blood pressure cuff is a common source of error in measuring blood pressure. The width of the cuff itself should encircle at least half of the patient's upper arm, or the blood pressure readings may be incorrectly elevated.
c. *Hypotension*: less than 90/40 mm Hg
   (1) *Orthostatic hypotension*: increase of heart rate by 30 beats/min, decrease in blood pressure by 20 mm Hg, or dizziness after standing

(2) Narrowed pulse pressure (sBP-dBP) of less than 30 mm Hg may be an early indicator of hypovolemic or cardiogenic shock.

5. Respiratory rate
   a. *Reference range*: 12–20 breaths/min (in adults)
   b. *Tachypnea*: greater than 20 breaths/min
      (1) May reflect pain or systemic acidosis
   c. *Bradypnea*: less than 12 breaths/min
      (1) May reflect oversedation with narcotic pain medications
6. Oxygen saturation
   a. *Reference range*: greater than 92%
      (1) Pulse oximeter should not be placed distal to the blood pressure cuff.
   b. *Hypoxemia*: less than 92%
      (1) Patients with COPD often have a lower resting SpO_2 fraction.
      (2) Measurement may be confounded by factors such as hypotension, vasoactive medications, hypothermia, poor lighting, or nail polish.
      (3) Carbon monoxide or cyanide poisoning (methemoglobinemia) can lead to erroneous values.

B. GENERAL APPEARANCE

1. The four tenets of a physical examination are inspection, auscultation, palpation, and percussion. Each of these techniques can be used in each organ system to varying degrees. Inspection should precede the other three techniques, as to guide the remainder of the physical examination and avoid further harm to the injured patient.
2. Inspection
   a. Level of consciousness, mental status
      (1) Glasgow Coma Scale (GCS) should be used to evaluate trauma patients; scores range from 3 to 15 (Table 1.1).
         (a) Eyes are scored from 1 to 4.
         (b) Verbal is scored from 1 to 5.
         (c) Motor is scored from 1 to 6.
            (i) Most useful predictor of long-term functional outcomes among severe TBI patients.

TABLE 1.1
GLASGOW COMA SCORE

Motor Response		Verbal Response		Eye-Opening Response	
Obeys commands	6	—		—	
Localizes pain	5	Oriented speech	5	—	
Withdraws from pain	4	Confused speech	4	Opens spontaneously	4
Flexion response	3	Inappropriate words	3	Opens to command	3
Extension response	2	Incomprehensible words	2	Opens to pain	2
No response	1	No verbal response	1	Does not open eyes	1

The Glasgow Coma Scale (GCS) scoring system is primarily used in trauma situations. The motor response is the most prognostic of the three subcategories. A GCS score of 8 is consistent with coma or severe brain injury.

1

SURGICAL HISTORY AND PHYSICAL EXAMINATION

     (2) Agitation or combativeness may be a sign of hypoxia.

     (3) *CO₂ narcosis*: hypercarbia, obtundation, and decreased respiratory rate secondary to narcotic overmedication

  b. Body habitus

     (1) Strong indicator of overall nutritional state, intubation risk, and surgical risk

     (2) Obesity

     (3) Abnormal facies, facial trauma

     (4) Muscle mass (e.g., temporal wasting)

C. HEAD AND NECK

1. Inspection

  a. Head

     (1) Lacerations

     (2) Contusions

     (3) Depressions/deformities

     (4) *Raccoon eyes*: periorbital ecchymoses; indicates basilar skull fracture

     (5) *Battle sign*: retroauricular ecchymoses; indicates basilar skull fracture

     (6) Airway burns

       (a) Singed nasal hairs

       (b) Carbonaceous sputum

       (c) Stridor

       (d) Signs of upper airway compromise

       (e) Erythematous, blistered, or leathery skin

  b. Eyes

     (1) Visual acuity

     (2) Pupil size and reactivity to light

       (a) If there is any possibility for neurologic compromise in the trauma patient, pupil-dilating medications should be withheld.

       (b) *Anisocoria*: Unequal pupil size may be an indicator of epidural hematoma with traumatic brain injury.

     (3) Globe position within the orbit

     (4) Ocular mobility

       (a) Limited mobility or pain on movement may indicate entrapment of the ocular muscles.

     (5) Conjunctival pallor or hemorrhage

     (6) Foreign bodies or contact lenses

  c. Ears

     (1) *Hemotympanum*: blood behind the tympanic membranes

  d. Nose

     (1) Otorrhea, rhinorrhea

     (2) Septal hematoma

(3) Nasal deviation
e. Throat
  (1) Foreign bodies
  (2) Presence/absence of teeth
  (3) Dental occlusion
    (a) Malocclusion may hint at facial fractures
  (4) Mucous membrane moisture
  (5) Mallampati scoring system
    (a) Predicts difficulty of intubation on the basis of physical examination findings
    (b) *Technique*: Patient should sit upright and open mouth widely. Then ask the patient to protrude tongue as far as possible without phonating. Identify visible posterior oropharyngeal structures in a well-lit environment.
    (c) Class I/II: soft palate, complete uvula
    (d) Class III: soft palate, partial uvula
    (e) Class IV: hard palate only
f. Neck
  (1) Tracheal deviation
  (2) *Jugular venous distention (JVD)*: Right internal jugular vein pulsations are normally visible with proper lighting and patient position. Have the patient relaxed and lying down at a 30-degree incline. The venous pulse differs from the arterial pulse with its double-wave and inspiratory collapse.

2. Auscultation
  a. Airway assessment
    (1) Clear speech indicates patent airway.
    (2) Gasping may indicate oropharyngeal obstruction.
    (3) Stridor is a sign of upper airway compromise.
  b. Carotid artery bruits

3. Palpation
  a. Head
    (1) Step-offs
    (2) Open fractures
  b. Face
    (1) Localized tenderness
    (2) Step-offs
    (3) Open fractures
    (4) Paresthesias
    (5) Fracture tests
      (a) *Generalized facial fracture*: Press on masseter muscles while patient is biting down; lack of pain hints at an absence of fracture.
      (b) *Midface stability test*: Grasp upper incisors and move anteriorly and posteriorly.

        (c) *Tongue blade test*: Ask the patient to bite down on a tongue blade; if you are able to break the wooden blade, then a mandibular fracture is highly unlikely (>95%).
  c. Neck
    (1) Crepitus
      (a) One-third of patients with palpable crepitus of the neck have upper airway or esophageal injury as the causative factor.
    (2) Tracheal deviation
    (3) Carotid artery pulses
    (4) Nuchal rigidity
    (5) Cervical spine tenderness or step-offs
    (6) Hematomas
    (7) Open wounds
      (a) Open wounds through platysma should never be probed because of the high risk for hemorrhage.
    (8) Thyroid examination
      (a) *Technique*: Palpate thyroid tissue on the anterior surface of the trachea. Locate the lateral lobes through the sternocleidomastoid muscles, with the patient's head facing the examined side to relax the muscles. Bilateral digital palpation is used to locate and characterize any nodules or deformities.

D. CHEST
1. Inspection
  a. Bilateral chest wall expansion during inspiration
  b. Respiratory rate and depth
  c. Use of accessory muscles indicates difficulty with ventilation (e.g., trapezius, upper neck muscles).
  d. Chest wall contusions or lacerations
  e. Breast examination
    (1) Symmetry
    (2) Erythema
    (3) Edema
    (4) Dimpling
    (5) Peau d'orange
    (6) Nipple deviation
    (7) Ulceration
    (8) Gynecomastia (males)
    (9) Surgical scars
2. Auscultation
  a. *Technique*: Ensure airway patency. Have the patient take a deep breath through the mouth. Listen at the anterior apices of the lungs; then move caudally, comparing both right and left sides. Repeat posteriorly.
  b. Absent or decreased breath sounds hint at pneumothorax, hemothorax, or other causes of pleural effusion.

    c. *Wheezing*: short inspiration, long expiration with polyphonic pitch

    d. *Crackles*: inspiratory Velcro-like sounds at bases of lungs

    e. *Hamman's sign*: subcutaneous crunching sounds with systolic beats due to pneumomediastinum; often associated with traumatic esophageal injury

3. Palpation

    a. *Technique*: Apply firm, steady pressure to chest. Avoid open wounds or fractures. Examine for crepitus, instability, step-offs, swelling, and point-tenderness.

      (1) Clavicles

      (2) Sternum

      (3) Sternoclavicular, acromioclavicular, and costosternal junctions

      (4) Intercostal spaces

      (5) Rib segments

    b. Breast examination

      (1) *Technique*: With patient in a sitting position, support the patient's arm on your shoulder and palpate the axilla to detect for lymphadenopathy. Have the patient lie in a supine position and place her hand behind her head. Palpate each breast in a radial motion, first examining the superficial tissue and then the deeper breast tissue with firmer movements. Palpate the nipple for discharge.

      (2) Examine masses for location, size, consistency, shape, mobility, and/or tenderness with palpation

4. Percussion

    a. *Technique*: Gently place the middle finger of the nondominant hand on the body surface. Strike the distal interphalangeal (DIP) joint of the nondominant hand with the middle finger of the dominant hand. Repeat across the chest surface, comparing left and right sides.

    b. Hyperresonance to percussion is consistent with pneumothorax.

    c. Dullness to percussion indicates mass lesion (e.g., lobar pneumonia), hemothorax, or other causes of pleural effusion

E. CARDIOVASCULAR

1. Inspection

    a. Cardiac

      (1) Precordial box: demarcated by the clavicles superiorly, costal margin inferiorly, and nipples laterally

      (2) Contusions or lacerations within the precordial box indicate further need to rule out traumatic cardiac injury.

    b. Vascular

      (1) Active hemorrhage

      (2) Acute arterial insufficiency

        (a) Pain

        (b) Pallor/cyanosis

(3) Chronic arterial insufficiency
    (a) Hair loss
    (b) Nail changes
    (c) Nonhealing wounds
    (d) Ischemic ulcers
        (i) Located frequently on digital tips, malleolus, heel, metatarsal head, and dorsal arch
(4) Acute venous stasis
    (a) Phlegmasia alba dolens: pain, swelling, and pallor secondary to impaired venous outflow from massive deep vein thrombosis (DVT)
    (b) Phlegmasia cerulea dolens: pain, swelling, and cyanosis secondary to impaired venous outflow and decreased arterial perfusion from massive DVT
(5) Chronic venous stasis
    (a) Brawny edema
    (b) Varicose veins
    (c) Hyperpigmentation
    (d) Indurated cellulitis
    (e) Painless ulceration
        (i) Located frequently on the superior and posterior aspect of the medial malleolus because of the location of the perforators of the great saphenous vein
(6) Extremity thrombosis
    (a) Swelling
    (b) Erythema

2. Auscultation
  a. Cardiac
    (1) Rate and rhythm
    (2) Murmurs indicate valvular stenosis or insufficiency.
    (3) Muffled heart sounds
  b. Vascular
    (1) Bruits indicate stenosis or arteriovenous fistulization.

3. Palpation
  a. Vascular
    (1) Temperature
      (a) Compare bilaterally
    (2) Pulse examination
      (a) Carotid
      (b) Upper extremity (axillary, brachial, radial)
      (c) Lower extremity (femoral, popliteal, posterior tibial, anterior tibial, dorsalis pedis)
      (d) Bypass grafts
    (3) Compare pulses bilaterally
    (4) Palpable/digital pulses
    (5) Doppler/signal pulses

(6) *Acute arterial insufficiency*: 6 Ps—pain (with passive movement), pallor, paresthesias, paralysis, poikilothermia, pulselessness

(7) Expanding or pulsatile hematoma

(8) Venous insufficiency

    (a) *Trendelenburg test*: The patient should lie down in a supine position. Have the patient raise his/her leg to drain the venous system. Apply a tourniquet over the femorosaphenous junction; then have the patient stand up. Rapid filling of varicose veins before tourniquet release is indicative of valvular insufficiency. Rapid filling after release is indicative of an incompetent femorosaphenous valve.

(9) Palpable cord hints at a superficial venous thrombosis

(10) *Homans' sign*: increased resistance or calf tenderness with passive ankle dorsiflexion

(11) *Ankle-brachial index (ABI)*: Measure blood pressure at bilateral upper and lower extremities. The highest ankle pressure divided by the highest brachial pressure on the ipsilateral side is the ABI. A normal ABI is slightly greater than 1. An ABI of less than 0.9 is 95% sensitive and 97% specific for a major vascular injury. Diabetics may have a falsely elevated ABI because of dystrophic calcification of the vessel walls.

F. ABDOMEN

1. Inspection

a. Examining the overall patient demeanor is the first aspect of the abdominal examination. Patients with diffuse peritonitis often lie still and try to resist any active or passive movement. They will also have their knees drawn up to decrease stretching of the irritated peritoneum. Patients with colic are restless, whereas those with a mesenteric vascular event will be writhing in pain (out of proportion to the examination).

b. Abdominal contour

    (1) Visible masses

    (2) Visible peristalsis

    (3) Engorged veins

    (4) Caput medusa

    (5) Bulging flanks

c. External signs of injury

    (1) Seat-belt sign

    (2) Scars (surgical, traumatic)

    (3) Abdominal striae

    (4) Ecchymoses

        (a) *Cullen sign*: periumbilical ecchymosis

        (b) *Fox sign*: inguinal ligament ecchymosis

        (c) *Grey-Turner sign*: flank ecchymosis

    (5) Rashes

   d. Distention
     (1) *Rule of 6 Fs*: *f*at, *f*luid, *f*latus, *f*eces, *f*atal growth (malignancy), *f*etus
     (2) The age of the fetus can be determined by fundal height. A 12-week fetus can be felt above the pubic symphysis, whereas a 20-week gestational age fetus has a fundal height at approximately the umbilicus. The fundus grows at approximately 1 cm/week at gestational age.
   e. Herniation
     (1) Inguinal hernias can be felt or expressed around the inguinal ligament.
     (2) Femoral hernias can be felt or expressed below the inguinal ligament, medial to the femoral arterial pulse.
     (3) Umbilical hernias are located around the umbilicus.
     (4) Ventral or incisional hernias are evident on the anterior abdominal wall, either midline or near a surgical scar.

2. Auscultation
   a. Hypoactive bowel signs indicate ileus or inflamed bowel but may take a long period of auscultation to confirm.
   b. Flatus is more indicative of bowel function, specifically large bowel function.
   c. Bruits
   d. Hiccups (singultus)
     (1) Can be a sign of gastric distention or diaphragmatic irritation (e.g., subphrenic abscess)
   e. Belching (eructation)

3. Palpation
   a. Inquire about the point of maximal tenderness. Then make sure to palpate this area of the abdomen last.
   b. *Technique*: Initially, the entire abdomen should be palpated lightly, observing the patient's facial expression. Minimize the abdominal wall resistance as much as possible. Flexion of the hips and knees will relax the abdominal musculature. Deeper palpation can be performed by pressing the fingers of the nondominant hand with the dominant hand. Examine all four quadrants in a systematic fashion.
   c. Pain on palpation
     (1) Guarding points toward an inflamed or irritated peritoneum
     (2) *Rebound tenderness*: painful response to gentle depression and quick release of the abdominal wall, indicative of peritoneal irritation
     (3) *Murphy's sign*: inspiratory arrest following deep palpation beneath the right costal margin, indicative of acute cholecystitis
     (4) *Carnett's sign*: Abdominal pain becomes more pronounced with tension of the abdominal wall, compared with a relaxed state, indicating that the origin of the pain is from the abdominal wall itself (e.g., abdominal wall hematoma).

d. Bulges and masses
   (1) Nearly all masses arise from previously normal organ tissue. A palpable liver tumor, for example, will likely be located in the right upper quadrant under the costal margin.
   (2) Spleen
      (a) *Technique*: With the patient supine, place the examining left hand underneath the patient's left rib cage, supporting upward, and use the right hand to palpate. With a light touch, depress the skin under the left costal margin. Splenomegaly can be felt as a round edge that slips under the examiner's fingers at the end of inspiration.
   (3) Liver
      (a) *Technique*: With the patient supine, place the left hand underneath the patient's right rib cage, supporting the floating ribs. Use the right hand to palpate. After inspiration, the liver should be palpable approximately 3 cm below the right costal margin in the midclavicular line. Make sure to note contour, nodularity, and any tenderness on palpation.
   (4) Male inguinal hernia
      (a) *Technique*: Have the patient stand up in a comfortable position. Place the fingertip at the most dependent part of the scrotum, and invaginate the scrotal wall to insert the finger into the external inguinal ring. If the ring is sufficiently relaxed, guide the finger gently cephalad and laterally through the inguinal canal. Have the patient turn his head and cough. A hernia will be evident at the end of the fingertip, if present.
   (5) Abdominal aortic aneurysm can be felt as a palpable pulsatile mass in the epigastric region, although an obese habitus may preclude the ability to palpate this finding.
e. Digital rectal examination
   (1) *Technique*: Inspect the perineal skin and perianal region for signs of local inflammation, abscesses, sinus tracts, fissures, fistulae, or bulges. Using lubricating jelly, press a gloved finger on the anus. Slowly increase pressure on the anal sphincter. When the external sphincter is relaxed, rotate the finger into the axis of the anal canal and insert gently.
   (2) Findings
      (a) Sphincter tone
      (b) Hemorrhoids
      (c) Masses
      (d) Feces
      (e) Blood
      (f) Signs of injury (bony fragments, bowel wall integrity)
      (g) Prostatic examination

4. Percussion
   a. Tympanic percussion indicates distended bowel lumen
   b. Dullness to percussion may reflect mass or fluid accumulation
   c. Liver span
      (1) *Reference range*: 6–12 cm in the right midclavicular line; 4–8 cm in the midsternal line
      (2) *Technique*: Measure vertical span of liver dullness in the right midclavicular line. Percuss upward from below the umbilicus and caudal from the right nipple.
   d. Bladder distention can be felt as a tender mass above the pubic symphysis.
   e. Ascites
      (1) Abnormal accumulation of splanchnic lymphatic fluid within the peritoneal cavity
      (2) *Technique*: With the patient supine, percuss the level of flank dullness, and mark on the skin. Then turn the patient to one side and percuss a second level of dullness. Approximately 1 L of free peritoneal fluid is required to appreciate this finding.
      (3) *Fluid wave test*: Press sharply with one hand while the other hand receives an impulse when placed against the opposite flank, with a perceptible time lag. Mesenteric fat produces a similar wave, so the fat must be blocked by having either the patient or another assistant press along the abdominal midline.
   f. Rebound tenderness can also be felt as pain on percussion, indicating peritoneal irritation.

G. GENITOURINARY

1. Inspection
   a. Signs of injury
      (1) Blood at the penile meatus or female urethra
      (2) Gross hematuria
      (3) Contusions
      (4) Lacerations
      (5) Perineal ecchymoses
      (6) Scrotal hematoma
2. Palpation
   a. Vaginal examination
      (1) Cervical discharge
      (2) Cervical motion tenderness
      (3) Palpation of uterine size/shape
      (4) Palpation of ovarian masses
      (5) Lacerations
      (6) Blood in vaginal vault
      (7) Malodorous scent

H. SKIN

1. Inspection
   a. Color
      (1) Pallor
         (a) Indicator of anemia or poor peripheral perfusion
      (2) Jaundice
         (a) Bilirubin reposition in peripheral tissue when total circulating serum bilirubin is greater than 2–3 mg/dL
         (b) Appears first on the frenulum of the tongue
      (3) Erythema
         (a) May indicate inflammation or infection
      (4) Cyanosis
         (a) Reflects hypoxemia or poor peripheral circulation
         (b) Digital pallor, cyanosis, and erythema are indicators of Raynaud phenomenon.
   b. Integrity
      (1) Burn wounds
         (a) Graded into four degrees on the basis of depth of injury
         (b) *First degree*: erythema, peeling of epidermis
         (c) *Second degree*: partial-thickness, blistering, mottled pink/white surface, painful
         (d) *Third degree*: full-thickness, leathery, firm, depressed, painless
         (e) *Fourth degree*: extends into underlying fascia, charred
      (2) Decubitus ulcers
         (a) Graded into four stages on the basis of depth of injury
         (b) Develops with persistent local pressure lasting over 2 hours
         (c) *Stage 1*: erythema
         (d) *Stage 2*: partial-thickness skin loss
         (e) *Stage 3*: full-thickness skin loss
         (f) *Stage 4*: extends into underlying fascia (e.g., muscle, bone)
      (3) Wounds
   c. Lesions
      (1) *Petechiae*: 1–3 mm deep red or purplish spots
      (2) *Purpura*: greater than 3 mm deep red or purplish spots
      (3) *Spider angiomata*: central arteriole surrounded by smaller vessels
         (a) Blanches with central pressure
         (b) Indicator of hyperestrinism (e.g., liver failure, pregnancy)
      (4) Catheter site erythema or drainage
      (5) Malignant lesions
         (a) Melanoma
            (i) *ABCDE rule*: *a*symmetry, *b*order irregularity, *c*olor variegation, *d*iameter (>6 mm), *e*volution over time
         (b) Basal cell carcinoma

        (i) Pink, ulcerated papule with rolled, "pearly borders"

        (ii) Commonly located on the upper lip and above

    (c) Squamous cell carcinoma

        (i) Ulcerated nodule with raised, hyperkeratotic papules

        (ii) Commonly located on the lower lip and below

  (6) Signs of injury

    (a) Contusions

    (b) Hemorrhage

    (c) Deformity

    (d) Lateralizing signs

2. Palpation

  a. Skin temperature

  b. Skin turgor

    (1) Poor turgor may indicate hypovolemic state.

    (2) Pinching the skin from the dorsal hand and releasing it is an easy way to assess turgor. Persistent fold reflects loss of turgor.

  c. Peripheral edema

    (1) Distribution of edema

    (2) Interstitial fluid may accumulate to 5 kg before pitting edema can be detected.

I. MUSCULOSKELETAL

1. Inspection

  a. Limb deformity

    (1) Shortening

    (2) Angulation

  b. Neuromuscular function

    (1) Disability

    (2) Abnormal motility

  c. Skeletal injury

    (1) Point tenderness

    (2) Deformity

  d. Ligamentous injury

2. Palpation

  a. Identify localized bone tenderness or crepitus

  b. *Pelvic fracture test*: Have the patient lie in supine position. Gentle anterior-to-posterior compression at the anterior iliac crests, pubic symphysis, or medial compression at hips can elicit pain and instability.

  c. Spine

    (1) Step-offs

    (2) Deformity

    (3) Tenderness

  d. Extremities

    (1) Pulse examination

      (a) Compare pulses bilaterally

      (2) Joint stability

      (3) Impaired sensation

      (4) Weakness/paralysis

      (5) Limb viability (muscle turgor)

        (a) Soft muscles are likely viable.

        (b) Doughy muscles may be ischemic.

        (c) Rigid muscles are likely nonviable.

      (6) Extremity compartment syndrome

        (a) Edematous and tense area of extremity

        (b) Tender musculature with pain on passive movement

        (c) Pain is often out of proportion to clinical findings.

        (d) Paresthesias are the first sign and precede pulselessness.

J. LYMPHATICS

1. Lymphadenopathy can be localized or generalized. When swollen lymph nodes are discovered on physical examination, it is important to evaluate other nodal basins to differentiate the two types. Furthermore, the etiology of lymphatic nodal enlargement can be due to malignancy or reactive to local inflammation. A careful history and physical examination are imperative to discern the cause.

2. Inspection

   a. Lymphadenopathy

      (1) Generalized

      (2) Localized

   b. Red streaks

   c. Lymphedema

   d. Lacerations or open wounds

3. Palpation

   a. Location

      (1) Cervical

      (2) Occipital

      (3) Epitrochlear

      (4) Submandibular

      (5) Axillary

      (6) Supraclavicular

        (a) The right supraclavicular node drains the lungs and esophagus, whereas the left (Virchow's) node drains the abdominal cavity.

      (7) Periumbilical

        (a) *Sister Mary Joseph node*: The Mayo brothers' head surgical nurse, whose name was Sister Mary Joseph, is credited with noticing periumbilical adenopathy in patients with metastatic gastric cancer.

      (8) Inguinal

      (9) Femoral

    b. Size
    c. Consistency
    d. Tenderness
    e. Mobility
        (1) Fixed nodes are more concerning than mobile ones.

K. NEUROLOGIC
1. Inspection
    a. Mental status
        (1) Person
        (2) Place
        (3) Time
        (4) Situation
    b. Pupillary examination
        (1) Size
        (2) Reactivity to light
        (3) Symmetry
    c. Motor response
        (1) *Technique*: If the patient is not paralyzed or sedated, ask the patient to hold up fingers and move toes. If the patient is unable to comply, check for a localization response to painful central stimulus (e.g., sternal rub).
           (a) Flexor response indicates a high brainstem injury.
           (b) Extensor response indicates a low brainstem injury.
           (c) Nonresponse indicates possible cervical spine injury or brain death.
        (2) If there is any asymmetry in the motor response, then use the best response in calculating the GCS score (see Table 1.1).
    d. Cranial nerve (CN) examination
        (1) Olfactory nerve (CN I): smell
        (2) Optic nerve (CN II): visual acuity
        (3) Oculomotor nerve (CN III): eyeball movement
        (4) Trochlear nerve (CN IV): eyeball movement
        (5) Trigeminal nerve (CN V): facial sensation
        (6) Abducens nerve (CN VI): eyeball movement
        (7) Facial nerve (CN VII): facial movement
        (8) Vestibulocochlear nerve (CN VIII): hearing, balance
        (9) Glossopharyngeal nerve (CN IX): gag reflex, normal swallow
     (10) Vagus nerve (CN X): gag reflex, normal swallow
     (11) Accessory nerve (CN XI): shoulder lift
     (12) Hypoglossal nerve (CN XII): midline position of protruded tongue
    e. Brachial plexus evaluation
        (1) Axillary nerve: arm abduction
        (2) Median nerve: ability to make a fist

      (3) Musculocutaneous nerve: forearm flexion, bicep flexion

      (4) Radial nerve: arm extension, wrist extension

      (5) Ulnar nerve: finger abduction/adduction

f. Brain death examination

   (1) The following criteria must be met and confirmed by a separate physician. These criteria are determined invalid in the presence of any of the following conditions:

      (a) Drug or metabolic intoxication

      (b) Electrolyte imbalances or hyperosmolar coma

      (c) Hypothermia

      (d) Hypotension

   (2) In addition, all sedating and paralyzing medications must be withheld, and note that the administration of Advanced Cardiac Life Support medications (e.g., atropine) may cause findings such as pupillary dilation. Patients who lack pupillary and corneal reflexes at 24 hours and/or have no motor response at 72 hours have a minuscule chance at meaningful neurologic recovery.

   (3) Brain death criteria

      (a) GCS score of 3 (lowest number possible)

      (b) Absent cerebral function

         (i) No response to stimuli above the neck

         (ii) Complete loss of responsiveness, vocalization, volitional activity

      (c) Absent brainstem function

         (i) *Pupillary light reflex*: Pupillary constriction occurs with direct and consensual light exposure.

         (ii) *Corneal reflex*: Corneal touching elicits a blinking response.

         (iii) *Doll's eye reflex:* Passive rotation of the head elicits ocular movement in a direction opposite to the direction of head movement.

           (*a*) Cervical spine must first be cleared of injury.

         (iv) *Vestibulo-ocular reflex*: With the patient in supine position and head elevated at 30 degrees, instilling 200 mL of cold water into the external ear canal elicits nystagmus.

         (v) *Oropharyngeal reflex*: Gag response occurs as a result of oropharyngeal touching.

      (d) No spontaneous respiratory effort

         (i) *Apnea*: Lack of ventilation causes an increase in serum $PaCO_2$. A $PaCO_2$ level of greater than 60 mm Hg for 30 seconds is defined as adequate stimulation for the respiratory drive.

      (e) No spontaneous, purposeful movement

RECOMMENDED READINGS

Cartwright SL, Knudson MP. Evaluation of acute abdominal pain in adults. *Am Fam Physician*. 2008;77:971–978.

DeGowin RL, DeGowin DD. *Degowin's Diagnostic Examination*. 7th ed. New York: McGraw-Hill; 2000.

Silen W. *Cope's Early Diagnosis of the Acute Abdomen*. 22nd ed. New York: Oxford University Press; 2010.

Fluids and Electrolytes

Joshua Kuethe, MD

The living organism does not really exist in the milieu exterior, but in the liquid milieu interior formed by circulating organic liquid.

—Claude Bernard

I. BASIC PHYSIOLOGY

A. BODY FLUID COMPOSITION

1. Total body water (TBW)
   a. Composed of intracellular and extracellular fluid (ECF) compartments
   b. A total of 50%–70% of total body weight
   c. Male (60%) greater than female (50%) percentage
   d. Adjusted for body habitus
      (1) In obesity, TBW is decreased by 10%–20%.
      (2) In very thin individuals, TBW is increased by 10%.
      (3) In newborns, TBW is approximately 80% but decreases to approximately 65% by 12 months of age.

2. Intracellular fluid
   a. A total of 30%–40% of total body weight
   b. Primarily found in muscle
   c. Principal cation: K^+, with smaller contributions from Mg^{2+} and Na^+; principal anions: HPO_4^- and negatively charged proteins

3. ECF
   a. ECF = interstitial fluid + intravascular fluid.
   b. Interstitial fluid is 15% of total body weight.
   c. Intravascular fluid is 5% of total body weight.
      (1) Plasma volume is 50 mL/kg of body weight.
      (2) Blood volume is 70 mL/kg of body weight.
   d. Principal cation is Na^+, and principal anions are Cl^- and HCO_3^-.

B. SERUM OSMOLALITY AND TONICITY

1. Osmolality
   a. Defined as osmoles of solute particles per kilogram of water; basically as ions per unit volume
   b. Transcompartmental movement of water occurs because certain nonpermeable molecules cannot freely migrate through the semipermeable cell membrane, thus creating a gradient.
      (1) Compounds accumulating in ECF—Na^+ and glucose
      (2) Compounds accumulating in intracellular fluid—K^+, proteins, and organic acids

23

   c. Calculated by:

$$\text{Serum osmolality (mOsm/L)} = 2\,(\text{Na}^+) + \text{glucose}/18 + \text{blood urea nitrogen}/2.8$$

2. Tonicity

   a. Tonicity is the effect of particles on cell volume; only an impermeable solute (Na^+) can alter tonicity because a freely permeable solute cannot create an oncotic gradient.

   b. The body attempts to regulate tonicity, not osmolality.

C. FLUID AND ELECTROLYTE HOMEOSTASIS

1. Baseline requirements

   a. Adult fluid requirements—35 mL/kg per day or 1500 mL/m^2 per day; titrate to maintain urine output between 0.5 and 1.0 mL/kg per hour.

   b. Adult electrolyte requirements

     (1) Na^+—100–150 mEq/day; 1–2 mEq/kg per day

     (2) K^+—50–100 mEq/day; 0.5–1 mEq/kg per day

     (3) Cl^-—90–120 mEq/day

     (4) Ca^{2+}—orally 1–3 g/day

     (5) Mg^{2+}—20 mmol/day

     (6) Phosphorus—20–30 mmol/day

   c. Pediatric hourly formula to determine fluid requirements

     (1) 0–10 kg = (4 mL × kg) per hour

     (2) 11–20 kg = 40 mL/h + (2 mL for each kg over 10 kg) per hour

     (3) More than 20 kg = 60 mL/h + (1 mL for each kg over 20 kg) per hour

<u>Example—25-kg child:</u>

$$(\text{1st 10 kg}) \times 4 = 40$$
$$+ (\text{2nd 10 kg}) \times 2 = 20$$
$$\underline{+ \text{ last 5 kg} \times 5 = 5}$$
$$25 \text{ kg total} = 65 \text{ mL/h}$$

   d. Pediatric electrolyte requirements

     (1) Na^+—3–5 mEq/kg per day

     (2) K^+—2–3 mEq/kg per day

     (3) Cl^-—5–7 mEq/kg per day

     (4) See pediatric section for more details.

   e. See specific chapters for fluid requirements/management of specific disease processes.

2. Fluid turnover and losses

   a. Gastrointestinal (GI) tract

     (1) Approximately 6000–9000 mL/day total secretion

     (2) Approximately 250 mL lost per day in stool

     (3) See Table 2.1 for specifics.

   b. Renal

     (1) Approximately 800–1500 mL/day lost

TABLE 2.1

COMPOSITION OF GASTROINTESTINAL SECRETIONS

Secretion	Volume, mL/24 h (range)	Na, mEq/L (range)	K, mEq/L (range)	Cl, mEq/L (range)	HCO₃, mEq/L (range)
Salivary gland	1500 (500–2000)	10 (2–10)	26 (20–30)	10 (8–13)	30
Stomach	1500 (100–4000)	60 (9–116)	10 (0–32)	130 (8–154)	—
Duodenum	140 (100–2000)	140	5	80	—
Ileum	3000 (100–9000)	140 (80–150)	5 (2–8)	104 (43–137)	30
Colon	—	60	30	40	—
Pancreas	— (100–800)	140 (99–185)	5 (3–7)	75 (54–95)	115
Bile	— (50–800)	145 (99–164)	5 (3–12)	100 (89–180)	35

c. Insensible losses
  (1) Approximately 400 mL/m² per day or 10 mL/kg per day for adults
  (2) Seventy-five percent via evaporate losses from skin and 25% via respiratory exchange
d. Abnormal losses
  (1) Fever—250 mL/day per degree centigrade of fever, or 15% increase in insensible losses for each degree centigrade above 37°C
  (2) Tachypnea—50% increase for each doubling of respiratory rate
  (3) GI—diarrhea, fistula, tube drainage
  (4) Third space losses—can be difficult to appreciate, often underestimated
  (5) Evaporation—ventilator, open abdomen, open wound
  (6) Operative losses—can be estimated by:

hours NPO (nothing by mouth) × baseline/maintenance intravenous fluid requirement

(preoperative deficient, if not replaced)

+ # hours of case × baseline/maintenance intravenous fluid requirement

+ operative blood loss

+ insensible losses—estimation guide:

1–3 mL/kg per hour for minor procedure

4–7 mL/kg per hour for intermediate procedure

8–12 mL/kg per hour for major procedure

II. ELECTROLYTE DISTURBANCES
A. SODIUM
1. Basic physiology
   a. Reference serum levels between 135 and 145 mEq/L
   b. Under renal regulation and is the primary solute in determining plasma osmolality

FLUIDS AND ELECTROLYTES

2

2. **Hyponatremia**
   a. Signs and symptoms—often asymptomatic until levels decline to less than 120 mEq/L or if levels acutely decline to less than 130 mEq/L
      (1) Central nervous system (CNS)—headache, fatigue, confusion, coma, seizures
      (2) GI—nausea, vomiting, diarrhea
      (3) Musculoskeletal (M/S)—weakness, muscle twitching, hyperactive deep tendon reflexes
   b. Diagnosis/causative factor
      (1) Begin by determining serum osmolality, glucose levels, and lipid levels.
      (2) Rule out isotonic hyponatremia (serum osmolality: 280–290 mOsm) due to pseudohyponatremia.
         (a) Pseudohyponatremia occurs in the presence of hypertriglyceridemia or hyperproteinemia.
      (3) Sodium reduction can be calculated by multiplying the plasma triglyceride (mg/dL) level by 0.002 *or* by multiplying the protein levels greater than 8.0 g/dL by 0.25.
      (4) Isotonic hyponatremia (serum osmolality: 280–290 mOsm) also occurs after infusions of isotonic glucose, mannitol, or glycine, or after transurethral resection of prostate (TURP).
      (5) Next, rule out hypertonic hyponatremia (serum osmolality: >290 mOsm)—occurs after hypertonic infusions of glucose, mannitol, or glycine, or after TURP. It can also occur from hyperglycemia.
         (a) For each 100 mg/dL of serum glucose greater than 100 mg/dL, serum sodium is decreased by 3 mEq/L.
      (6) Next, clinically determine the circulating volume to assist in differentiating between the forms of hypotonic hyponatremia (serum osmolality: <280 mOsm).
         (a) Hypovolemic hyponatremia can occur because of GI losses (vomiting, diarrhea, fistulas), skin losses (thermal injury), or renal losses (diuretics, diabetes insipidus, salt-wasting nephritis, peritoneal dialysis).
         (b) Isovolemic hyponatremia can occur because of water intoxication, iatrogenic causes, secretion of antidiuretic hormone, hypokalemia, drugs (sulfonylureas, carbamazepine, phenothiazines, and antidepressants), and reset thermostat.
         (c) Hypervolemic hyponatremia can occur because of congestive heart failure, nephrosis, liver failure, drugs (indomethacin, carbamazepines, vincristine, vinblastine, cyclophosphamide, and nicotine derivatives).
   c. Treatment
      (1) Correct the underlying disorder.
      (2) The following formula can be used to estimate sodium deficit:

$$Na^+ \text{ deficit (mEq/L)} = (\text{desired } Na^+ \text{ level} - \text{actual } Na^+ \text{ level}) \times TBW$$

(3) Hypovolemic hyponatremia—Replace deficit with 0.9% NaCl while monitoring frequent sodium levels to prevent too rapid of correction of subsequent hypernatremia.

(4) Water intoxication corrects readily with simple fluid restriction (<1500 mL/day).

(5) Hypervolemic hyponatremia—Most respond well to simple fluid restriction (<1500 mL/day); this may be assisted with a loop diuretic, with hourly replacements of Na^+ and K^+ while monitoring the levels.

(6) Isovolemic hyponatremia usually corrects after addressing the underlying disorder.

(7) Caution should be used in aggressively treating the symptomatic patient. Rapid infusion of hypertonic saline solutions can result in central pontine myelinolysis. Serum sodium levels should not be corrected in an excess of 0.5 mEq/L per hour to avoid this devastating complication if the patient has been symptomatic for more than 48 hours. In the asymptomatic patient, correction rates can be administered safely at 1–2 mEq/L per hour.

3. Hypernatremia

a. Always associated with a hyperosmolar state and occurs because of water loss in excess of salt loss; thus there is a free water deficit, and hypernatremia is typically delineated according to the patient's ECF volume status.

b. Signs and symptoms rarely develop if Na^+ is less than 160 mEq and osmolality is greater than 320 mOsm, unless condition develops rapidly.

(1) CNS—restlessness, irritability, delirium, mania, seizures, coma

(2) Cardiovascular (CV)—tachycardia, hypertension

c. Diagnosis/causative factor

(1) Clinically assess ECF volume

(2) Hypovolemic hypernatremia—caused by loss of hypotonic body fluid such as insensible free water loss, GI losses, diuretics, diabetes insipidus

(3) Isovolemic hypernatremia—due to the same causative factors as hypovolemic but is caused by improper correction

(4) Hypervolemic hypernatremia—most frequently iatrogenic (excessive administration of Na^+) but also seen in Conn syndrome, Cushing syndrome, steroid use, and congenital adrenal hyperplasia

d. Treatment—Rapid reversal carries a high risk for cerebral edema and uncal herniation.

(1) Address the underlying disorder.

(2) Next, determine the free water deficit:

$$H_2O \text{ deficit} = (0.6 \times \text{kg of body weight}) \times \left[(\text{serum } Na^+ \text{ (mEq/L)} / 140) - 1 \right]$$

FLUIDS AND ELECTROLYTES

2

(3) Begin by replacing half of the deficit in the first 24 hours, with the remainder in the following 2 or more days. Note that continued ongoing losses (urinary and insensible) need to be replaced concurrently.

(4) Select a hypotonic fluid such as D5W (5% dextrose in water).

B. POTASSIUM

1. Basic physiology
   a. Normal serum levels are between 3.5 and 5.1 mEq/L, and it is the major intracellular cation.
   b. Changes in K^+ have significant effects on transmembrane potential and hence cellular function.
   c. Fifty to 100 mEq of K^+ are ingested daily, with 90% excreted in urine and 10% excreted in stool.

2. Hypokalemia
   a. Signs and symptoms—generally appear only after levels are less than 2.5 mEq/L and are primarily CV
      (1) CNS—paresthesias, paralysis
      (2) CV—sensitization to digitalis and epinephrine, arrhythmias, electrocardiographic changes: low voltage, flattened T waves, ST segment depression, prolonged QT interval, and prominent U waves
      (3) GI—constipation, ileus
      (4) M/S—weakness, cramps, myalgia, rhabdomyolysis
   b. Causative factors
      (1) In surgical patient, GI (diarrhea, gastric drainage: vomiting/nasogastric tube), diuretics, and insulin administration
      (2) Redistribution to intracellular space; significant in metabolic alkalosis, insulin therapy, beta-blockers, catecholamines
      (3) Others—mucus-secreting colon tumors, magnesium deficiency, hyperaldosteronism, steroid use, anabolism, delirium tremens, hypothermia
   c. Treatment
      (1) Ensure adequate renal function before beginning replacements.
      (2) Because K^+ is primarily intracellular, small decreases in serum K^+ represent significant decreases in total body stores. This deficit can be predicted in that for every 1-mEq/L decrease from the norm, there is a 100- to 200-mEq decrease in total body stores.
      (3) Treat the alkalosis and decrease Na^+ intake.
      (4) Enteral replacement is preferred—40- to 100-mEq dosing.
         (a) Note: A banana has approximately 10 mEq K^+ per inch.
      (5) Parenteral replacement—used if patient cannot tolerate oral intake or if depletion is severe; administer no more than 10 mEq/h of KCl through a peripheral IV or no more than 20 mEq/h through a central line; this may be increased to 40 mEq/h if patient has cardiac monitoring and is in intensive care unit.

3. Hyperkalemia
  a. Signs and symptoms
    (1) CV—peaked T waves, flattened P waves, prolongation of QRS, cardiac arrest, ventricular fibrillation
    (2) M/S—weakness, paresthesias
    (3) GI—nausea, vomiting, diarrhea, intestinal colic
  b. Causative factors
    (1) Pseudohyperkalemia—can occur in hemolysis, thrombocytosis, and leukocytosis
    (2) Redistribution into extracellular space; acidosis, insulin deficiency, reperfusion syndrome, tissue necrosis—crush injuries, burns, electrocution; beta-blocker therapy, digitalis intoxication, succinylcholine
    (3) Increased total body potassium—renal insufficiency (most common in surgical patient), diabetes, spironolactone, mineralocorticoid deficiency
  c. Treatment
    (1) Mild hyperkalemia (<6.0 mEq/L and no electrocardiographic changes)
      (a) Remove exogenous sources.
      (b) Add a non–K^+-sparing diuretic (e.g., furosemide [Lasix]), and if possible, remove any medication that is capable of increasing potassium concentration.
    (2) Severe hyperkalemia (>6.0 and presence of electrocardiographic changes)
      (a) Temporizing measures (treatment for symptoms)
        (i) Calcium gluconate or calcium chloride—temporary cardiac stabilization
        (ii) Inhaled beta-agonists—causes the most rapid intracellular shift in K^+
        (iii) D50W (50 g) and 10 units intravenously of regular insulin
      (b) Therapeutic measures (decreasing total body potassium)
        (i) Kayexalate—administered orally (15 g up to 4 times daily) or rectally (30–50 g up to 4 times daily)
        (ii) Hydration and forced renal excretion with diuretics (e.g., Lasix)
        (iii) Dialysis—definitive therapy in life-threatening hyperkalemia
  Mnemonic—C Big K Di (see big K die)
  Calcium, Beta-agonists, Insulin, Glucose, Kayexalate, Dialysis, Lasix

C. CALCIUM
1. Basic physiology
  a. Normal serum levels are 8.9–10.5 mg/dL, and serum ionized levels are 4.4–5.2 mg/dL.

FLUIDS AND ELECTROLYTES

2

b. Ninety-nine percent of total body calcium is stored in bone as hydroxyapatite crystals.

c. Calcium exists in several forms in serum: 45% as free ionized Ca^{2+} (the only physiologically active form), 40% bound to proteins, and 15% bound to freely diffusible compounds.

d. Calcium metabolism is under the control of parathyroid hormone (increases Ca^{2+} bone resorption and renal reabsorption) and vitamin D (increases Ca^{2+} uptake from GI tract).

2. Hypocalcemia

a. Signs and symptoms (serum Ca^{2+} level <8.0 mg/dL or ionized Ca^{2+} level <4.0 mg/dL)

(1) CV—QT prolongation, ventricular arrhythmias

(2) M/S—cramping, paresthesias (first perioral/central, then extremities), tetany, increased deep tendon reflexes

(3) Chvostek sign—facial muscle twitching after percussion over trunk of facial nerve

(4) Trousseau sign—carpal spasm after inflating blood pressure cuff for more than 3 minutes

b. Causative factors

(1) Calcium sequestration—pancreatitis, rhabdomyolysis, packed red blood cell administration (citrate chelation)

(2) If albumin is normal, check parathyroid hormone level.

(a) Low parathyroid hormone—hypoparathyroidism, magnesium deficiency

(b) High parathyroid hormone—pancreatitis, hyperphosphatemia, renal insufficiency, fistulas, specific drugs (gentamicin, Lasix), pseudohypothyroidism, decreased vitamin D

c. Treatment

(1) Oral management—appropriate in chronic hypocalcemia

(a) Calcium carbonate

(i) Titralac—1 mL = 1 g $CaCO_3$ = 400 mg Ca^{2+}

(ii) Os-Cal—1 tablet = 1.25 g $CaCO_3$ = 500 mg Ca^{2+}

(iii) Tums—1 tablet = 0.5 g $CaCO_3$ = 200 mg Ca^{2+}

(b) Phosphate-binding antacids improve GI absorption of Ca^{2+}.

(c) Vitamin D—50,000 IU weekly for 6 weeks calciferol or other preparations; dihydrotachysterol, 1,25-dihydroxyvitamin D_3

(2) Intravenous management—appropriate in acute hypocalcemia

(a) This is not required in asymptomatic patient; 200–300 mg elemental Ca^{2+} is required to eliminate attack of tetany.

(b) One gram calcium gluconate contains 2.2 mmol Ca^{2+}.

(c) One gram $CaCl_2$ contains 6.5 mmol Ca^{2+}.

3. Hypercalcemia

a. Signs and symptoms—"stones, bones, groans, and psychic overtones"

(1) CNS—confusion, depression, psychoses, coma (psychic overtones)

    (2) GI—nausea, vomiting, anorexia, ileus, constipation, abdominal pains (groans)

    (3) Genitourinary—nephrolithiasis, polyuria (stones)

    (4) CV—hypertension, shortening of the QT interval

  b. Causative factors

    (1) Hyperparathyroidism and malignancy are the most common causes.

    (2) Other causes are milk alkali syndrome (consumption of large amounts of milk and soluble alkali—i.e., antacids), hyperthyroidism, acromegaly, pheochromocytoma, medications (thiazides, vitamin A, vitamin D), granulomatous disease, adrenal insufficiency, Paget disease of the bone, and prolonged immobilization

  c. Treatment

    (1) Mild hypercalcemia (<12 mg/dL) can be treated with restriction of calcium intake and discontinuance of offending or contributing agents.

    (2) Severe hypercalcemia requires prompt treatment.

      (a) Intravenous hydration—Most patients are dehydrated; begin with 0.9% NaCl.

      (b) Oral or intravenous phosphate inhibits bone resorption.

      (c) Diuresis with loop diuretic and aggressive intravenous hydration (>200 mL/h).

      (d) Calcitonin is useful in treating hypercalcemia associated with malignancy or primary hyperparathyroidism; usual dose is 4 units/kg subcutaneously or intramuscularly every 12–24 hours.

      (e) Pamidronate is useful in malignancy-associated hypercalcemia; usual dose is 60–90 mg.

D. MAGNESIUM

1. Basic physiology

  a. Reference serum levels are 1.7–2.3 mEq/dL.

  b. The kidney plays the greatest role in magnesium regulation.

  c. Fifty percent of total body magnesium is found in bone, 49% is found in the intracellular space, and the remaining 1% can be found in the serum. Of the serum magnesium, 60% is in the ionized form, 25% is protein bound, and 15% is complexed with nonprotein anionic species.

  d. Acute hypomagnesemia is usually accompanied by hypokalemia.

2. Hypomagnesemia

  a. Signs and symptoms

    (1) CNS—mental status changes, seizures

    (2) CV—widening of QRS complex and T wave, prolongation of PR and QT intervals, ventricular arrhythmias

    (3) M/S—weakness, fasciculations, hyperreflexia, tremors, tetany

b. Causative factors
   (1) GI losses—diarrhea, malabsorption, vomiting, biliary fistulas
   (2) Genitourinary losses—diuresis, primary hyperaldosteronism, renal tubular dysfunction
   (3) Drugs—loop diuretics, cyclosporine, amphotericin B, aminoglycosides, and cisplatin
   (4) Others—parathyroidectomy, acute myocardial infarction, and burns
c. Treatment
   (1) Mild cases (asymptomatic and >1.0 mEq/mL)—oral replacement preferred
      (a) Magnesium oxide—400-mg tablet = 20 mEq Mg^{2+}
      (b) Magnesium gluconate—500-mg tablet = 2.3 mEq Mg^{2+}
      (c) Magnesium chloride—535-mg tablet = 5.5 mEq Mg^{2+}
   (2) Severe cases (symptomatic or <1.0 mEq/mL)—intravenous replacement preferred
      (a) In the presence of arrhythmias, $1–2$ g $MgSO_4$ infused rapidly ($5–15$ minutes) followed by a continuous infusion of $1–2$ g/h.
      (b) Without symptoms, more than $4–8$ g $MgSO_4$ infused at a rate of 0.5 g/h may be required.

3. **Hypermagnesemia**
   a. Signs and symptoms
      (1) CNS—mental status changes, paralysis ($Mg^{2+} > 12$ mEq), coma
      (2) CV—atrioventricular block, prolonged QT interval, hypotension, sinus bradycardia
      (3) GI—nausea, vomiting
      (4) M/S—loss of deep tendon reflexes ($Mg^{2+} > 8$ mEq)
   b. Causative factors
      (1) Rarely occurs in the face of normal renal function
      (2) Iatrogenic (Mg^{2+} used to treat eclampsia), acute or chronic renal failure, administration of magnesium-containing antacids or laxative overuse, severe burns, crush injuries, rhabdomyolysis, severe metabolic acidosis, extracellular volume depletion
   c. Treatment
      (1) Remove offending agents.
      (2) Calcium gluconate reverses some of the life-threatening symptoms (loss of deep tendon reflexes, cardiac arrhythmias).
      (3) Intravenous hydration, correction of acid-base abnormalities, excretion with a loop diuretic, and dialysis in the patient with renal failure can be used.

E. PHOSPHORUS
1. Basic physiology
   a. Less than 1% of total body stores are found within the ECF compartment.
   b. Normal serum concentrations are between 2.5 and 4.0 mg/dL.
   c. It is under secondary control by a myriad of hormones that primarily control calcium metabolism and is primarily excreted by the kidneys.

2. Hypophosphatemia
   a. Signs and symptoms
      (1) CNS—mental status changes, weakness, flaccid paralysis
      (2) CV—cardiac arrest
      (3) M/S—bone pain
      (4) Heme—platelet and granulocyte dysfunction
   b. Causative factors
      (1) Increased renal loss—acid-base disturbances, acetazolamide, acute tubular necrosis, diabetic ketoacidosis
      (2) Decreased intestinal absorption—hypothyroidism, vitamin D deficiency, malabsorption, alcoholism, phosphate-binding antacids
      (3) Total body redistribution—refeeding syndrome, total parenteral nutrition administration
      (4) Other—after severe burns, liver resection
   c. Treatment
      (1) Mild hypophosphatemia (>1.0 mg/dL)—oral Neutra-Phos 250–500 mg every 6 hours or Phospho-Soda 5–10 mL every 8 hours (Neutra-Phos contains 250 mg phosphorus/tablet, Phospho-Soda contains 129 mg phosphorus/mL) or intravenous $NaPO_4$ or KPO_4 0.08–0.2 mmol/kg infused over 6 hours
      (2) Severe hypophosphatemia (<1.0 mg/dL)—Intravenous $NaPO_4$ or KPO_4 0.16–0.24 mmol/kg infused over 6 hours is preferred.

3. Hyperphosphatemia
   a. Signs and symptoms
      (1) M/S—tetany, soft tissue calcification
   b. Causative factors
      (1) Decreased renal excretion—renal failure
      (2) Total body redistribution—tissue trauma, acidosis
      (3) Others—antacids, vitamin D metabolites, postoperative hypoparathyroidism
   c. Treatment
      (1) Restrict intake, increase excretion with intravenous hydration and diuresis (acetazolamide), and use phosphate-binding antacids ($AlOH_2$); last, hyperphosphatemia can be corrected with hemodialysis.

III. PARENTERAL REPLACEMENT FLUID THERAPY

Table 2.2 demonstrates the composition of commonly used intravenous fluids.

A. CRYSTALLOIDS
1. Isotonic (lactated Ringer [LR] solution and 0.9% normal saline [NS] and Normosol)
   a. These are commonly used in volume resuscitation and used interchangeably, but the pH of 0.9% NS is less than LR; therefore LR is the preferred fluid in a resuscitation in which the patient is acidotic and does not have hyperkalemia, hyponatremia, hypochloremia,

---

TABLE 2.2

REPLACEMENT THERAPY—PARENTERAL FLUIDS

Solution	Na (mEq/L)	K (mEq/L)	Cl (mEq/L)	Base (mEq/L)	mOsm/L	Dextrose (g/L)	Kcal/L
D5W	—	—	—	—	278	50	170
D10W	—	—	—	—	556	100	340
D50W	—	—	—	—	2780	500	1700
0.9% NaCl	154	—	154	—	286	—	—
0.45% NaCl	77	—	77	—	143	—	—
3% NaCl	513	—	513	—	1026	—	—
D5 0.9% NaCl	154	—	154	—	564	50	170
D5 0.45% NaCl	77	—	77	—	421	50	170
D5 0.2% NaCl	39	—	39	—	350	50	170
LR	130	4	109	28	272	—	9
D5 LR	130	4	109	28	524	50	170
Normosol	140	5	98	27	295	23	170

D5W, Dextrose 5% in water; *D10W,* dextrose 10% in water; *D50W,* dextrose 50% in water; *LR,* lactated Ringer solution.

hypercalcemia, or an alkalosis. LR also is more similar to normal serum electrolyte composition, osmolality, and pH. Normosol is nearly identical to normal serum.

2. **Hypotonic (0.45% NS and D5W)**
   a. Not used in resuscitation but commonly used to correct a free water deficit
3. **Hypertonic (3% NS)**
   a. Has begun to have limited use as a volume expander in selected patient populations (some patients with head trauma); however, used primarily to correct symptomatic hyponatremia
4. **Maintenance intravenous fluid**
   a. Most commonly used is D5 0.45% NS with 20 mEq KCl added; this is simply tailored to meet the daily basal metabolic requirements of an otherwise healthy patient.

B. COLLOIDS

1. These have never been shown to be superior to crystalloids as a resuscitative fluid, only equivocal, and meta-analysis has revealed an increased mortality in patients where albumin was used as a volume expander; colloids also have not been shown to be cost-effective.
2. Albumin (100 mL of 25% and 500 mL of 5%)
   a. To be used cautiously, and not to be used in patients with an albumin level greater than 2.5 g/dL, total protein greater than 5 g/dL, or for supplementing serum albumin levels in patients with chronic disease
   b. Has benefit in limited situations (e.g., burn patients with hypoalbuminemia, resuscitation of a patient with cirrhosis)
   c. Temporarily expands the intravascular volume at least 1:1 per milliliter infused because of ability to mobilize fluid from the interstitial space into the intravascular space

3. Dextran (Dextran 40 and 70)
   a. Synthetic glucose polymer that expands the intravascular volume by 1 mL for every milliliter infused and is eliminated by the kidneys
   b. Indicated as a volume expander and thromboembolism prophylaxis
   c. Side effects include coagulopathy, laboratory test abnormalities, worsening renal function, and osmotic diuresis.
4. Hetastarch (hydroxyethyl starch, 6% solution)
   a. It is a synthetic molecule that expands the intravascular volume 1 mL for every milliliter infused and undergoes hepatic and renal elimination.
   b. It can be used as a volume expander in shock, although mortality is increased when used during sepsis.
   c. Side effects include increased amylase and an osmotic diuresis, which can be misinterpreted as achieving adequate tissue perfusion, and worsening renal function.

IV. ACID-BASE DISORDERS
A. PHYSIOLOGY
1. Normal pH is 7.35–7.45; acidemia refers to a pH less than 7.35, and alkalemia refers to a pH greater than 7.45.
2. Acid-base balance is significant because most enzymatic reactions occur optimally only at a narrow pH range.
3. Primary buffer systems
   a. Red blood cell bicarbonate-carbonate system is the most important and most rapid buffer system:

   $$HCl + NaHCO_3 \leftrightarrow NaCl + H_2CO_3 \leftrightarrow H_2O + CO_2$$

   b. Others playing a smaller role are intracellular proteins, organic phosphates, intracellular bicarbonate, and hemoglobin itself.
   c. More than half the total body alkaline buffering capacity is found within the bone.
4. Compensation systems
   a. Respiratory system eliminates volatile acids (primary = CO_2) generated during consumption of acid by the bicarbonate-carbonate system. As long as the respiratory system is not compromised, this system of acid elimination is inexhaustible.
   b. Renal system is responsible for excretion of acids and both the recovery and generation of de novo bicarbonate.

B. PRIMARY METABOLIC DISORDERS
1. Metabolic acidosis
   a. Causative factors—results primarily from the loss of alkali, accumulation of nonvolatile acids, or a decrease in the acid excretion from the kidneys
   b. Classification—is characterized as either normal (hyperchloremic) anion gap or increased anion gap acidosis; normal anion gap = 3–12:

   $$Anion\ gap = Na\ (mEq/L) - [Cl\ (mEq/L) + HCO_3\ (mEq/L)]$$

(1) Increased anion gap—ketoacidosis, alcohol intoxication, lactic acidosis, renal failure, toxin ingestion (salicylates, paraldehyde, ethylene glycol, methanol)

Mnemonic—MUDPILES:

Methanol, Uremia, Diabetic kctoacidosis, Paraldehyde, Ingestion, Lactic acidosis, Ethanol, Salicylates

(2) Normal anion gap (hyperchloremic)—renal tubular acidosis, potassium-sparing diuretics, hypoaldosteronism, diarrhea, biliary or pancreatic fluid losses, small bowel fistulas, dilutional acidosis, carbonic anhydrase inhibitors, ureteral diversions

Mnemonic—USEDCRAP:

Ureterostomy, Small bowel fistulas, Extra chloride, Diarrhea, Carbonic anhydrase inhibitors, Renal tubular acidosis, Adrenal insufficiency, Pancreatic fistulas

c. Signs and symptoms
   (1) Abdominal pain, nausea, vomiting
   (2) Decreased cardiac contractility, peripheral vasodilation, bradycardia

d. Treatment
   (1) Begin by correcting the underlying disorder.
   (2) In trauma/surgical patients, a frequent cause of metabolic acidosis is lactic acidosis from inadequate tissue perfusion, which can be corrected simply by volume resuscitation.
   (3) Without addressing the underlying disorder, the simple addition of bicarbonate will not correct the acidosis.
   (4) With mild-to-moderate acidosis, the correction of the underlying disorder will correct the acidosis, and the excessive use of bicarbonate can lead to overcorrection (alkalosis), hypernatremia, hyperosmolarity, cerebrospinal fluid acidosis, and volume overload.
   (5) For a pH less than 7.2–7.3, addition of an ampule or two of bicarbonate may be required; one ampule contains 50 mEq sodium bicarbonate.
   (6) The exact bicarbonate deficit cannot be calculated, but it can be estimated with the following formula:

$$0.4 \times wt\,(kg) \times [\text{desired bicarbonate} - \text{measured bicarbonate}\ (mEq/L)]$$

   (7) For severe acidosis, while addressing the underlying disorder, the addition of bicarbonate can be beneficial to increase the pH to greater than 7.2.

2. Metabolic alkalosis
   a. Classified as either chloride responsive or chloride unresponsive but caused by either acid loss or base gain, and aggravated by hypokalemia and volume contraction
      (1) Chloride responsive—contraction alkalosis (commonly in the surgical patient from inadequate resuscitation), diuretic use,

GI acid loss (vomiting or nasogastric tube), bicarbonate administration, villous adenoma
(2) Chloride unresponsive—severe hypokalemia, hyperaldosteronism, mineralocorticoid excess, renal failure, and chronic edema
b. Diagnosis
(1) Increased pH and bicarbonate and may be associated with compensatory hypercapnia
(2) Urine chloride levels can be measured to help to differentiate among the various causative factors. A urine chloride level less than 15 mEq/dL suggests chloride-responsive causative factors, whereas a urine chloride level greater than 15 mEq/dL indicates chloride-unresponsive causes.
c. Treatment
(1) Begin by addressing underlying causes. Volume expansion and correction of hypokalemia correct most cases. Correction with 0.9% NS facilitates improvement because of its acidity and chloride contents.
(2) In refractory cases, the use of acetazolamide (Diamox 500 mg every 6 hours) will inhibit de novo synthesis and renal reabsorption of bicarbonate.
(3) In severe cases, administer acid-containing solutions such as NH_4Cl, lysine HCl, arginine HCl, or 0.1N HCl.
(a) Calculate chloride deficit:

$$wt\ (kg) \times 0.4 \times [100 - measured\ Cl\ (mEq/L)]$$

(b) Administer over 24 hours with 0.1 N HCl.

C. PRIMARY RESPIRATORY DISORDERS
1. Respiratory acidosis
a. Causative factor—primarily from an increase in partial pressure of carbon dioxide ($PaCO_2$) secondary to inadequate ventilation.
(1) Causes of hypoventilation include respiratory center depression (a variety of causes including narcotics), chronic obstructive pulmonary disease, pulmonary disease, inadequate mechanical ventilation, and poor ventilation secondary to pain.
b. Diagnosis
(1) Decreased pH with an increased $PaCO_2$; in chronic states, will see a compensatory increase in HCO_3
c. Treatment
(1) Address underlying cause of hypoventilation.
(2) Improve minute ventilation—remove airway obstruction, pulmonary toilet, bronchodilators, avoid respiratory depressants, reverse opioid narcotics and continuous positive airway pressure/bilevel positive airway pressure
(3) Endotracheal intubation and mechanical ventilation if noninvasive measures fail; if intubated, increase minute ventilation (frequency and tidal volume).

(4) In chronic hypercapnia, particularly related to chronic obstructive pulmonary disease, hypoxemia becomes the agent driving the respiratory system; therefore the patient's hypoxemia should not be fully corrected and the hypercapnia should be slowly corrected.

2. Respiratory alkalosis
   a. Causative factor—results primarily from a decrease in $PaCO_2$ secondary to hyperventilation
      (1) Causes of hyperventilation include anxiety, pain, mechanical ventilation, CNS infections, metabolic encephalopathies, cerebrovascular accident, pulmonary embolism, hypoxia, congestive heart failure, pneumonia, cirrhosis, sepsis, closed head injury, toxins, pregnancy, and increased ventilation secondary to bronchospasm.
   b. Diagnosis
      (1) Increased pH with a decreased $PaCO_2$
   c. Treatment
      (1) Address underlying disorder.
      (2) Correct hypoxemia if present.
      (3) If acutely symptomatic and not intubated, use a rebreathing device.
      (4) In ventilated patients, decrease minute ventilation while maintaining $PaCO_2$ no less than 30 mm Hg.

D. MIXED ACID-BASE DISORDERS

1. Suspected any time pH is near-normal values with altered levels of $PaCO_2$ and HCO_3 or when compensatory changes appear to be exaggerated or insufficient

E. EVALUATION OF ACID-BASE DISORDERS (TABLE 2.3)

1. Obtain simultaneous arterial blood gases and serum electrolyte panel (use Table 2.3 to assist in reading arterial blood gases).
2. Calculate anion gap.

TABLE 2.3
ACID-BASE DISORDERS

Disorder	Primary Change	Secondary Change	Effect
Metabolic acidosis	↓ HCO_3	↓ $PaCO_2$	Last 2 digits pH = $PaCO_2$ HCO_3 + 15 = last 2 digits pH
Metabolic alkalosis	↑ HCO_3	↑ $PaCO_2$	HCO_3 + 15 = last 2 digits pH
Respiratory acidosis			
Acute	↑ $PaCO_2$	↑ HCO_3	ΔpH = 0.08 per 10 Δ in $PaCO_2$
Chronic	↑ $PaCO_2$	↑↑ HCO_3	ΔpH = 0.03 per 10 Δ in $PaCO_2$
Respiratory alkalosis			
Acute	↓ $PaCO_2$	↓ HCO_3	ΔHCO_3 = 0.2 × Δ in $PaCO_2$
Chronic	↓ $PaCO_2$	↓↓ HCO_3	ΔHCO_3 = 0.3 × Δ in $PaCO_2$

3. Calculate expected compensation from chart and locate on acid-base nomogram.
4. If compensation is not within predicted values, a mixed disorder should be expected.
5. Correlate suspected diagnosis with clinical picture.

RECOMMENDED READINGS

Nathens AB, Maier RV. Perioperative fluids and and electrolytes. In: Norton JA, Barie PS, Bollinger RR, et al., eds. *Surgery: Basic Science and Clinical Evidence*. 2nd ed. Springer; 2008:139–148.

Shires GT III. Fluid and electrolyte management of the surgical patient. In: Brunicardi FC, Andersen DK, Billiar TR, et al., eds. *Schwartz's Principles of Surgery*. 9th ed. New York: McGraw-Hill; 2010.

Nutrition

Joshua Kuethe, MD

Let thy food be thy medicine and let thy medicine be thy food.
—Hippocrates

I. NUTRITION BASICS

1. There are three sources of nutrition (normally, carbohydrates and fat provide 85% of daily energy expenditure, with protein supplying 15%).
2. Glucose yields 4 kcal/g, parenteral dextrose 3.4 kcal/g, protein 4 kcal/g, and fat 9 kcal/g (10 kcal/g for 20% intravenous [IV] fat emulsion).
3. Brain, red blood cells, white blood cells, and renal medulla are dependent on glucose in early fasting. Other tissues can use fat as an energy source.
4. One gram of nitrogen equals 6.25 g protein.
5. In healthy individuals, normal caloric needs are 25–30 kcal/kg per day, and protein needs are 0.8–1 g protein/kg per day.
6. Stressed, burned, or polytrauma patients may need as much as 55 kcal/kg per day and up to 2.5 g protein/kg per day.
7. Adequate calories in relation to nitrogen optimize protein synthesis and minimize protein catabolism. Calorie/nitrogen ratios:
   a. Most disease states—100–150:1
   b. Uremic patients—300–400:1
   c. Septic patients—100:1

II. DETERMINATION OF CALORIC NEEDS

1. Rough estimate—35 kcal/kg per day
2. Calculate basal energy expenditure (BEE) using the Harris-Benedict equation:

$$BEE \text{ (men)} = 66 + 13.7W + 5H - 6.8A$$

$$BEE \text{ (women)} = 655 + 9.6W + 1.7H - 4.7A$$

W = weight in kilogram, H = height in centimeter, and A = age
3. Calculate increase in energy needs imposed by illness or injury:
   (BEE × activity factor × injury factor) using Calvin Long:
   a. Minor operation—1.2 (20% increase)
   b. Skeletal trauma—1.35 (35% increase)
   c. Major sepsis—1.60 (60% increase)
   d. Severe thermal injury—2.10 (110% increase)

4. Calculate increase in energy needs imposed (activity factor):
   a. Confined to bed—1.2
   b. Out of bed—1.3
5. Nutrition Risk in Critically Ill (NUTRIC) score is an additional prognostic score based on six variables: age, Acute Physiology and Chronic Health Evaluation (APACHE), Sequential Organ Failure Assessment (SOFA), number of comorbidities, hospital stay until intensive care unit (ICU), and interleukin-6 (IL-6) levels.
   a. Score 6–10 indicates a high risk for malnutrition.
   b. Score 1–5 indicates a low risk for malnutrition.
   c. See Fig. 3.1.
   When all factors are considered, the two most important factors are likely recent weight loss and, in unstressed patients, serum albumin level less than 3 g/dL. Other parameters are used for corroborative purposes.

III. NUTRITIONAL ASSESSMENT

1. Assessment always starts with a thorough history and physical examination (H&P), including a Subjective Global Assessment (SGA) of Nutritional Status if patient is at risk. See Fig. 3.2 for SGA.
   a. Subjective: malnutrition defined by having two of the following criteria:
      (1) Insufficient energy intake
      (2) Unintended weight loss—mild (<5%), moderate (5–10%), or severe (>10%)
      (3) Loss of muscle mass
      (4) Loss of subcutaneous fat
      (5) Localized or generalized fluid accumulation that may mask weight loss
      (6) Diminished functional status as measured by handgrip strength (dynamometry)
   b. Physical examination findings:
      (1) Mid-arm muscle circumference, SGA fat loss, and SGA muscle wasting have been demonstrated to be better predictors of poor outcome than body mass index (BMI).
      (2) Measure height and weight, then calculate BMI (BMI = height in meters^2/weight in kilograms).
         (a) Severe malnutrition: less than 16
         (b) Moderate malnutrition: 16–17
         (c) Mild malnutrition: 17–18.5
      (3) General: loss of subcutaneous fat, any generalized fluid accumulation
      (4) Head and neck examination: hair loss, bitemporal wasting, buccal and orbital pad fat loss, conjunctival pallor, xerosis, glossitis, stomatitis, dentition, thyromegaly

3

NUTRITION

Critical Care Nutrition
www.criticalcarenutrition.com

NUTRIC Score[1]

The NUTRIC Score is designed to quantify the risk of critically ill patients developing adverse events that may be modified by aggressive nutrition therapy. The score, of 1-10, is based on 6 variables that are explained below in Table 1. The scoring system is shown in Tables 2 and 3.

Table 1: NUTRIC Score variables

Variable	Range	Points
Age	<50	0
	50 - <75	1
	≥75	2
APACHE II	<15	0
	15 - <20	1
	20-28	2
	≥28	3
SOFA	<6	0
	6 - <10	1
	≥10	2
Number of Co-morbidities	0-1	0
	≥2	1
Days from hospital to ICU admission	0 - <1	0
	≥1	1
IL-6	0 - <400	0
	≥400	1

Table 2: NUTRIC Score scoring system: if IL-6 available

Sum of points	Category	Explanation
6-10	High score	• Associated with worse clinical outcomes (mortality, ventilation). • These patients are the most likely to benefit from aggressive nutrition therapy.
0-5	Low score	• These patients have a low malnutrition risk.

Table 3: NUTRIC Score scoring system: If no IL-6 available*

Sum of points	Category	Explanation
5-9	High score	• Associated with worse clinical outcomes (mortality, ventilation). • These patients are the most likely to benefit from aggressive nutrition therapy.
0-4	Low score	• These patients have a low malnutrition risk.

*It is acceptable to not include IL-6 data when it is not routinely available; it was shown to contribute very little to the overall prediction of the NUTRIC score.[2]

[1]Heyland DK, Dhaliwal R, Jiang X, Day AG. Identifying critically ill patients who benefit the most from nutrition therapy: the development and initial validation of a novel risk assessment tool. Critical Care. 2011;15(6):R268. [2]Rahman A, Hasan RM, Agarwala R, Martin C, Day AG, Heyland DK. Identifying critically-ill patients who will benefit most from nutritional therapy: further validation of the "modified NUTRIC" nutritional risk assessment tool. Clin Nutr. 2015. [Epub ahead of print].

December 16th 2015

FIG. 3.1

Nutrition Risk in Critically Ill (NUTRIC) Score.

A. History
1. Weight change
   Overall loss in past 6 months: amount= #_____ kg, %loss= #_____
   Change in past 2 weeks: _____ increase,
                           _____ no change,
                           _____ decrease.

2. Dietary intake change (relative to normal)
   _____ no change,
   _____ change _____ duration= #_____ weeks
                   _____ type: _____ suboptimal liquid diet, _____ full liquid diet,
                           _____ hypocaloric liquids, _____ starvation.

3. Gastrointestinal symptoms (that persisted for >2 weeks)
   _____ none, _____ nausea, _____ vomiting, _____ diarrhea, _____ anorexia.

4. Functional capacity
   _____ no dysfunction (e.g., full capacity),
   _____ dysfunction _____ duration= # _____ weeks.
                         _____ type: _____ working suboptimally,
                                 _____ ambulatory,
                                 _____ bedridden.

5. Disease and its relation to nutritional requirements
   Primary diagnosis (specify) _____
   Metabolic demand (stress): _____ no stress, _____ low stress,
                   _____ moderate stress, _____ high stress.

B. Physical (for each trait specify: 0= normal, 1+= mild, 2+= moderate, 3+= severe)
   # _____ loss of subcutaneous fat (triceps, chest)
   # _____ muscle wasting (quadriceps, deltoids)
   # _____ ankle edema
   # _____ sacral edema
   # _____ ascites

C. SGA rating (select one)
   _____ A = Well nourished
   _____ B = Moderately (or suspected of being) malnourished
   _____ C = Severely malnourished

FIG. 3.2

Example of a Subjective Global Assessment Worksheet.

   (5) Cardiovascular: evidence of heart failure or high-output state
   (6) Extremities: edema, loss of muscle mass
   (7) Neurologic: evidence of peripheral neuropathy, reflexes, tetany,
       mental status, handgrip strength
   (8) Skin: ecchymoses, petechiae, pallor, pressure ulcers
2. **Objective indicators of malnutrition:** No gold standard exists, but relying heavily on short-term proteins alone is not recommended.
   a. Proteins
      (1) Albumin:
          (a) Half life $t\frac{1}{2}$: 18–20 days
          (b) Normal: greater than 3.5 g/dL
          (c) Less than 3.2 g/dL: indication of increased postoperative
              complications
          (d) Affected by hepatic and renal insufficiency as well as
              inflammatory states

    (2) Transferrin:
        (a) $t\frac{1}{2}$ 8–9 days
        (b) Provides nutritional assessment for previous 2–4 weeks
        (c) Low values only accurate in the setting of normal iron levels
        (d) Maintains validity compared with prealbumin and retinol-binding protein in renal compromise
    (3) Prealbumin:
        (a) $t\frac{1}{2}$ 2–3 days
        (b) Improvement by 2–3 mg/dL per week indicates improving nutrition status
        (c) Acute phase reactant, affected by hepatic and renal insufficiency
        (d) C-reactive protein (CRP) less than 10 improves accuracy
    (4) Retinol-binding protein:
        (a) $t\frac{1}{2}$ 12 hours
        (b) Rarely useful given short $t\frac{1}{2}$

b. Indirect calorimetry—oxygen consumption and carbon dioxide production
    (1) Determines resting energy expenditure by measuring respiratory gas exchange (i.e., O_2 consumption, CO_2 production) using the Wier equation
    (2) Gives index of fuel use: RQ = V_{CO_2}/V_{O_2}
        RQ = respiratory quotient, V_{CO_2} = CO_2 production, and V_{O_2} = O_2 consumption
        (a) RQ of 0.8–1.0 is desirable. 0.84 is ideal.
        (b) RQ of less than 0.7 suggests ketogenesis (underfeeding).
        (c) RQ of greater than 1.0 suggests lipogenesis (overfeeding).
        (d) Spuriously influenced by hyperventilation (contraindicated in clinical presentations where gas exchange is hampered or accuracy may be affected: for example, fraction of inspired oxygen (FiO_2) greater than 60, chest tubes whereby gas collection is hampered, ongoing dialysis).
    (3) RQs:
        (a) Carbohydrate = 1.0
        (b) Mixed substrate = 0.8
        (c) Lipid = 0.70

c. Nitrogen balance
    (1) To calculate 24-hour total nitrogen balance: intake − loss = (protein (g)/6.25) − (UUN + 4 g/day for estimated fecal and nonurinary nitrogen loss)
        UUN = urinary urea nitrogen collected over 24 hours
    (2) Requires accurate 24-hour urine collection and assessment of nitrogen grams given daily
    (3) Negative nitrogen balance
        (a) Protein loss or catabolism
        (b) Associated with burn injuries, starvation, or gastrointestinal (GI)/wound losses

(4) Positive nitrogen balance
   (a) Protein gain or anabolism
   (b) Associated with periods of growth

IV. PREOPERATIVE NUTRITIONAL SUPPLEMENTATION

1. Minimal benefit: low-risk ICU patients
   a. Well-nourished, mild critical illness, expected short ICU stay
2. Greater benefit: ICU patients with moderate-to-severe risk
   a. Poor nutrition status prior to admission, critically ill, longer expected ICU stay.
      (1) The malnourished patient should receive preoperative nutritional support if undergoing elective major GI surgery.
      (2) Seven days before surgery and includes enteral (preferred) or parenteral supplementation, based on caloric requirements

V. POSTOPERATIVE NUTRITIONAL SUPPLEMENTATION

1. In the malnourished patient, start supplementation as soon as possible after surgery, and continue for a minimum of 1 week.
2. A well-nourished patient should have a nutrient/energy reserve such that a 7-day nothing by mouth (NPO) status should be tolerated.
3. If oral intake is not adequate after this period (less than 60% of goal), enteric tube feedings via nasogastric or nasoenteric feeding tube or parenteral nutrition should be started.
4. If prolonged support is anticipated, a feeding gastrostomy or jejunostomy should be considered.

VI. ENTERAL NUTRITION

1. Indications
   a. Prolonged period without caloric intake
   b. Functional GI tract
   c. Inadequate oral intake
   d. Possibly avoid gut mucosal atrophy, thereby maintaining the migrating motor complex and gut-associated lymphoid tissue, and, latently, potential pathogen and toxin translocation
   e. Possibly decrease hypermetabolism in major burns and trauma

VII. SHORT-TERM SUPPLEMENTATION

1. Nasogastric
   a. Adequate gastric emptying is required.
   b. Maintain gastric residuals less than 500 mL. Note that gastric residual volume (GRV) is not a valid indicator of tolerance.

2. Postpyloric
   a. Patients with greater risk for aspiration (e.g., neurologic impairment, poor gastric motility, history of aspiration)
   b. Placement of a postpyloric feeding tube (preferably jejunal) should not delay enteral nutrition.

VIII. LONG-TERM SUPPLEMENTATION (>6 WEEKS)

1. Gastrostomy—placed operatively or percutaneously with endoscopic guidance
   a. Requires adequate gastric emptying
   b. Contraindication: evidence of reflux or impaired gag reflex
   c. Intermittent bolus feeds or continuous infusion
2. Jejunostomy—placed operatively
   a. Anticipate long-term enteral supplementation in patients for whom gastrostomy is contraindicated.
   b. This typically requires continuous infusion.
3. Gastrojejunostomy—placed operatively or percutaneously with endoscopic guidance
   a. Useful in patients with functional or mechanical gastric outlet obstruction
   b. Allows external emptying of stomach, if needed, while feeding beyond the pylorus

IX. PRODUCTS

1. Oral supplements
   a. Indications—supplementation for inadequate caloric intake
   b. Must be palatable (flavoring increases osmolarity and cost)
   c. Examples: Ensure, Ensure Plus, Boost varieties, Carnation Instant Breakfast, Great Shakes, Nutrishakes, Magic Cups
2. Tube feedings: typical advancement schedule: initiate at 25 mL/h; increase by 25 mL/h Q12 to goal as tolerated
   a. Blenderized (pureed) diet—primarily used with gastrostomy
   b. Polymeric—Isocal, Osmolite, Jevity, Fibersource HN, Replete
      (1) Complete diet intact protein; generally lactose free
      (2) Iso-osmolar, well tolerated
      (3) 1 kcal/mL
   c. High caloric density (1.5–2 kcal/mL)—Magnacal, TwoCal HN Nutren 2.0
      (1) Complete diet, intact protein; generally lactose free
      (2) Hyperosmolar—may provoke diarrhea
      (3) For patients with increased caloric need and decreased volume tolerance
   d. Monomeric—Vivonex T.E.N.: Vital, Peptamen
      (1) Amino acids or peptides as protein source

   (2) Requires minimal digestion
   (3) Improved small bowel absorption (low residue)
   (4) Some formulas are hyperosmolar.
 e. Disease-specific formulas—most are of unproven benefit.
   (1) Renal failure—Suplena, Novasource Renal, Nepro
      (a) Elemental diet, essential L-amino acids, reduced nitrogen
      (b) Hyperosmolar, 2 kcal/mL (not very palatable)
      (c) Best administered by tube (not very palatable)
   (2) Acute or chronic hepatic failure: NutriHep
      (a) Enriched with branched-chain amino acids (valine, leucine, isoleucine)
      (b) Low in aromatic and sulfur-containing amino acids
      (c) May be used as tube feeding or to supplement protein-restricted oral diet
   (3) Immunomodulatory—Impact
      (a) Enriched with immunostimulatory amino acids, lipids, and nucleic acids (see Section VI)

X. COMPLICATIONS OF ENTERAL FEEDING

1. Aspiration pneumonia
2. Feeding intolerance—evidenced by vomiting, abdominal distention or pain, cramping, diarrhea. Treat by decreasing infusion rate, changing formula, or diluting feedings.
3. Diarrhea—defined as more than five stools per day
   a. Rule out antibiotic-associated colitis.
   b. It is minimized by a continuous, appropriate administration schedule, assuming intact GI function and no pancreatic insufficiency.
   c. Rule out too-rapid advancement of hyperosmolar tube feedings.
   d. It is minimized by clean technique in formula preparation and administration (avoid bacterial overgrowth in formulation). Adhere to product expiration limit, particularly with dilute formulations.
   e. Treatment: Depending on severity, decrease administration rate or add antidiarrheal agent when infectious cause is ruled out.
      (1) Kaolin pectin (Kapectolin): safe to use even in infectious diarrhea
      (2) Diphenoxylate (Lomotil) elixir: 2.5–5 mg per gastrostomy tube every 6 hours as needed
      (3) Loperamide (Imodium) elixir: 2–4 mg every 6 hours as needed
      (4) Psyllium seed (Metamucil): 1 package in 6 oz water twice daily (bulking agent)
      (5) Nutrisource fiber: 1–2 packets daily per feeding tube
4. Metabolic: In general, the metabolic complications of hyperglycemia and refeeding syndrome are the same as for parenteral nutrition.

XI. PARENTERAL NUTRITION

1. Indications
   a. Prolonged period without caloric intake, greater than 7 days
   b. Enteral feeding is contraindicated or not tolerated.
   c. If patient exhibits protein-energy malnutrition, consider institution of parenteral nutrition as soon as possible.
   d. GI fistula—Provide adequate nutrition to compensate for GI losses. Rate of spontaneous closure is increased, but overall mortality is not affected.
   e. Short bowel syndrome—Maintain nutritional integrity/fluid and electrolyte status until remaining bowel adapts.
   f. Acute tubular necrosis—Mortality rate is decreased, with earlier recovery from renal failure. Hypercatabolism of renal failure is met by total parenteral nutrition (TPN).
2. Efficacy not completely established for the following conditions:
   a. Inflammatory bowel disease: Crohn disease limited to small bowel responds best; does not affect the course of ulcerative colitis but allows for improved postoperative course when given before ileoanal pull-through operations
   b. Anorexia nervosa
3. Role in supportive therapy—efficacy established for the following conditions:
   a. Radiation enteritis
   b. Acute GI toxicity caused by chemotherapeutic agents
   c. Hyperemesis gravidarum
4. Efficacy not yet established for the following conditions:
   a. Preoperative nutritional support for malnourished patients
   b. Cardiac cachexia
   c. Pancreatitis
   d. Respiratory insufficiency with need for prolonged ventilatory support
   e. Prolonged ileus (>5 days)
   f. Nitrogen-losing wounds

XII. BASIC COMPOSITION OF FORMULATIONS (TABLES 3.1 AND 3.2)

1. Carbohydrate—usually dextrose. Base concentrations range from 15% to 47%.
2. Amino acids are either balanced or disease specific (e.g., cardiac, hepatic).
3. Lipid emulsion
   a. They are available as 10% or 20% solutions (1 kcal/mL or 2 kcal/mL, respectively) as soybean or structured lipid (Smoflipid).
   b. Infusion of 100 g of 20% solution per week typically prevents essential fatty acid deficiency (often divided into minimum dose of twice per week).

TABLE 3.1

TOTAL PARENTERAL NUTRITION SOLUTION: COMPOSITION

Type of Solution	Amino Acids	Glucose	Lipid 20%	Calories
Standard	5% (50 g/L)	D-15 (150 g/L)	40 g	1110 kcal/L
Hepatic	4% (40 g/L)	D-25 (250 g/L)	40 g	1410 kcal/L

TABLE 3.2

ADDITIONAL COMPONENTS TO TOTAL PARENTERAL NUTRITION SOLUTION

Dose	Trace Elements (MTE-5) (Add Daily)	Type
5.0 mg	Zn	
1 mg	Cu	
10 µg	Cr	
60 mg	Se	
0.5 mg	Mn	
	Vitamins	
1 ampule every day (10 mL)	Multivitamin	
5 mg every week	Vitamin K	For patients not requiring anticoagulants
Usual	Electrolytes and insulin (limited by compatibility)	Range
20–80	Na$^+$ (mEq/L)	0–150
13–40	K$^+$ (mEq/L)	0–80
10–80	Cl (mEq/L)	0–150
4.7	Ca^{2+} (mEq/L)	0–10
15	Phos (mmol)	0–21
45–81	Acetate (mEq/L)	45–220
0–25	Regular insulin (units/bag)	0–40

Ca^{2+}, calcium ion; Cl, chlorine; Cr, chromium; Cu, copper; K^+, potassium ion; Mn, manganese; MTE-5, MultiTrace Elements 5; Na^+, sodium ion; Phos, phosphorus; Se, selenium; Zn, zinc.

   c. Check serum triglyceride level to avoid exacerbation of hypertriglyc-
      eridemia.
   d. Lipid emulsion can be substituted for carbohydrate calories in certain
      situations (decrease overall volume given, carbohydrate overfeeding,
      TPN hepatotoxicity).
   e. It is usually safe to provide 20%–60% of total calories as lipid.
4. Microcomponents
   a. Vitamins—including 5 mg vitamin K weekly
   b. Trace elements—zinc, copper, chromium, manganese, selenium (see
      Part XIX for vitamin deficiencies)
   c. Insulin and electrolytes as necessary

XIII. CENTRAL FORMULAS

1. Standard central formula: Most patients requiring parenteral nutrition can use a formula containing a final concentration of 15%–25%
   dextrose.

2. Hepatic formulation
   a. This is indicated for patients with grade 2 (impending stupor) or greater (grade 3 = stupor, grade 4 = coma) hepatic encephalopathy, or in patients with altered aminogram (quantitative serum amino acid profile) with lower branched-chain amino acids and elevated aromatic amino acids.
   b. Hepatic formulation is enriched with 35% branched-chain amino acids, alanine, arginine, and reduced amounts of aromatic and sulfur-containing amino acids.

XIV. PERIPHERAL PARENTERAL NUTRITION

1. Typically discouraged secondary to risk of phlebitis and inadequate delivery of nutrients

XV. INFUSION

1. Rate
   a. All formulations begin at 42 mL/h.
   b. Increase rate in increments of 20 mL/h every 24 hours (if blood sugar is controlled and patient does not exhibit refeeding syndrome) until goals are reached.

XVI. MONITORING

1. Vital signs every 6 hours for initial 24–48 hours
2. Fingerstick glucose determinations every 6 hours to monitor for hyperglycemia
3. Weight thrice weekly
4. Twice-weekly blood work—electrolytes, glucose, liver enzymes, calcium, phosphorus, prothrombin, complete blood count (CBC), short-turnover proteins, and CRP.

XVII. COMPLICATIONS

1. Technical
2. Catheter sepsis
3. Hyperglycemia (blood sugar >180 mg/dL)
   a. Use of fatty acids and ketones during starvation can result in transient insulin resistance when carbohydrates are introduced into the bloodstream.
   b. It may be associated with either parenteral or enteral nutrition and may lead to hyperosmolar, hyperglycemic, or nonketotic dehydration, with shock/death resulting if untreated.
   c. If blood sugar is greater than 180 mg/dL, do not increase infusion rate; administer subcutaneous regular insulin acutely (extra-TPN).

Increase insulin in TPN bag appropriately (insulin should only cover the nutrition in the parenteral nutrition itself). Rule out septic etiologies.

4. Hypoglycemia—rare complication
   a. If TPN is suddenly discontinued for any reason, IV administration of any 5% dextrose solution at the same infusion rate will prevent hypoglycemia.
   b. Rarely occurs with endogenous insulin response to high infusion rate. Treat by slowing the infusion, or in patients on cyclic TPN, lengthening the ramp down time.
   c. When discontinuing TPN, decrease current TPN bag to 42 mL/h for 1 hour before cessation of TPN (if patient has counterregulatory issues, decrease TPN over 2–3 hours before cessation).

5. Liver dysfunction
   a. Results primarily from excess carbohydrate, excess total calories, excess lipid, and, uncommonly, excess nitrogen equivalent
   b. Reversible, self-limited in adults

6. Refeeding syndrome—can occur with the onset of parenteral or enteral nutrition in patients who are chronically malnourished or who have been NPO for approximately 7 days or greater
   a. Hypophosphatemia, hypokalemia
   b. Insulin-driven phenomenon
   c. Increased adenosine triphosphate (ATP) production, glycogenesis, and protein anabolism dramatically increase potassium, magnesium, and phosphate demand
   d. Extracellular levels of phosphate can decline to less than 1 mg/dL within hours of initiating nutritional therapy.
   e. Associated with muscle weakness, increased work of breathing, paralysis, seizures, coma, cardiopulmonary decompensation, including arrhythmias, and death
   f. Hypokalemia and hypomagnesemia may also occur as a result of increased ATP production and insulin-induced intracellular shifts.
   g. Screen at-risk individuals and monitor fluid/electrolytes closely.
   h. Correct electrolytes to normalcy before instituting enteral or parenteral nutrition support.
   i. Adjunct therapy with 100 mg thiamine (enterally or parenterally) for 2–3 days may potentially blunt the refeeding effect.

XVIII. IMMUNONUTRITION

Nutritional deficits and acute stress may result in atrophy of lymphoid organs and thus impair function, leading to increased risk of infection. Immunomodulating supplementation may improve outcomes in elective surgical patients; however, there appears to be no mortality advantage.

1. Glutamine
   a. Most abundant free amino acid in the body

   b. Decreased serum levels during stress (used by kidney to form ammonia and improve acidosis)

   c. Synthesized in muscle during catabolic states

   d. Primary fuel for small intestinal enterocytes

   e. Important for maintaining healthy intestinal mucosa

   f. May protect mucosa after radiation therapy, chemotherapy, small-bowel resection

   g. Provides fuel for macrophages, T cells

   h. Contraindicated in large doses (>0.5 g/kg body weight) or in patients with hyperammonemia

2. **Arginine:** promotes T-cell proliferation, fibroblast proliferation, secretagogue for anabolic hormones

3. **Omega-3 fatty acids:** antiinflammatants

4. **Nucleotides**
   a. Provide RNA (uracil) for cell proliferation/immune function

5. **HMB** (beta-hydroxy-beta-methylbutyrate, a leucine metabolite). Promotes muscle regeneration in tandem with physical therapy

XIX. NUTRIENTS/MACROMINERALS/MICRONUTRIENTS/VITAMINS

Nutrients, minerals, and vitamins; deficiency-related symptoms; and daily requirements are listed in Table 3.3.

TABLE 3.3

NUTRIENTS/MINERALS/VITAMINS, SYMPTOMS OF DEFICIENCY, AND DAILY REQUIREMENT

Essential Fatty Acids	Deficiency	Requirements (Often Given as a Range; Based on Maximum Nongravid, Nonlactating DRI Requirement)
Linoleic and linolenic acids	Scaly, erythematous skin rash	100 g of lipid emulsion per week, usually given twice weekly
Macrominerals	**Deficiency**	**Daily Requirements**
Calcium	Acute—tetany, paresthesias, hyperreflexia, seizures, altered mental status Chronic—rickets (children), osteomalacia (adults)	1100 mg
Phosphorous	Muscle weakness, paresthesias, seizures, hemolytic anemia, impaired white blood cell function, tissue hypoxia	1055 mg
Magnesium	Hypocalcemia, tetany, ataxia, coma, psychosis, cardiac arrhythmias, hypotension	350 mg

TABLE 3.3

NUTRIENTS/MINERALS/VITAMINS, SYMPTOMS OF DEFICIENCY, AND DAILY REQUIREMENT—cont'd

Essential Fatty Acids	Deficiency	Requirements (Often Given as a Range; Based on Maximum Nongravid, Nonlactating DRI Requirement)	
Micronutrients		Enteral	Parenteral
Chromium	Glucose intolerance	35 µg	10–15 µg
Copper	Microcytic, hypochromic anemia	0.9 mg	0.3–0.5 mg
Iodine	Weakness, cold intolerance, facial swelling, pallor, hair-thinning, hoarseness, constipation	150 µg	Not well defined
Iron	Microcytic anemia	8.1 mg	Not routinely added
Manganese	Hair thinning	2.3 mg	60–100 µg
Selenium	Myositis, cardiomyopathy, collagen vascular disease	45 µg	20–60 µg
Zinc	Poor wound healing, perioral rash, hair loss, dysgeusia	11 mg	2.5–5 mg
Water-Soluble Vitamins			
Vitamin C	Bleeding gums, gingivitis, weakness of hair follicles	90 mg	200 mg
Vitamin B1 (thiamine)	Anorexia, anemia, ataxia, polyneuritis, beriberi, Wernicke encephalopathy	1.2 mg	6 mg
Vitamin B2 (riboflavin)	Photophobia, soreness/burning of lips, tongue, mouth, beefy red tongue	1.3 mg	3.6 mg
Niacin	Pellagra (glossitis, dermatitis, scaly erythematous rash, diarrhea, dementia)	14 mg	40 mg
Folate	Megaloblastic anemia	330 µg	400 µg
Pantothenic acid (B5)	Deficiency rare. Fatigue, apathy, irritability	5 mg	15 mg
Vitamin B12	Megaloblastic anemia, peripheral neuropathy	2.4 µg	5 µg
Vitamin B6	Dermatitis, glossitis, depression, confusion, convulsion	1.7 mg	4 mg
Fat-Soluble Vitamins			
Vitamin A	Xerophthalmia, immunodeficiency	900 µg	990 µg
Vitamin D	Bone resorption, osteomalacia, immune retardation	20 µg	5 µg
Vitamin E	Neuromuscular dysfunction	15 mg	10 mg
Vitamin K	Bleeding coagulopathy	120 µg	150 µg

DRI, dietary reference intake.

3

NUTRITION

RECOMMENDED READINGS

Cerra FB, Benitez MR, Blackburn GL, et al. Applied nutrition in ICU patients. A consensus statement of the American College of Chest Physicians. *Chest*. 1997;111:769–778.

Taylor BE, McClave SA, Martindale RG, et al. *Guidelines for the Provision and Assessment of Nutrition Support Therapy in the Adult Critically Ill Patient: Society of Critical Care Medicine (SCCM) and American Society for Parenteral and Enteral Nutrition (A.S.P.E.N.)*. Available at http://sccmmedia.sccm.org/documents/LearnICU/Guidelines/Nutrition-SCCM-ASPEN.pdf.

Wound Healing

Aaron Seitz, MD

Wound healing is a complex process, and every surgeon should have an understanding of the basic principles and ways to maximize healing.

I. PHASES OF WOUND HEALING

A. HEMOSTASIS (5–10 MINUTES POST INJURY)

1. Begins with endothelial injury and subsequent vasoconstriction
2. Platelet activation resulting in cytokines and growth factors released
   a. Platelet-derived growth factor (PDGF): chemotaxis
   b. Fibroblast growth factor (FGF): epithelialization
   c. Epidermal growth factor (EGF): epithelialization
   d. Vascular endothelial growth factor (VEGF): angiogenesis
   e. Transforming growth factor beta (TGF-beta): deposition of extracellular matrix
   f. Glycoproteins (fibrinogen and fibronectin), together with kinins, complement, and prostaglandins—signal the initiation of inflammation
3. Fibrin clot formation

B. INFLAMMATORY (IMMEDIATE RESPONSE: DAY 0–DAY 4 POST INJURY)

1. TGF-beta stimulates macrophage and lymphocyte chemotaxis and proliferation.
2. After hemostasis, histamine release causes vasodilation and increases vascular permeability to allow cellular migration into the wound.
3. Polymorphonuclear (PMN) leukocytes are the first to arrive (2–4 hours).
   a. Predominant cell type in early wound exudate
   b. Role of phagocytosis and protection against infection
   c. Not necessary in wound healing or collagen synthesis
   d. May actually hinder wound healing
4. Monocytes follow closely behind the PMNs and are transformed into macrophages.
   a. Vital for normal wound healing
   b. Signaling normal fibroblast production
   c. Predominant cell in wound exudate after the first 48 hours
   d. Continue débridement and conclude the inflammatory response.
   e. Secrete nitric oxide, which is bactericidal (particularly against *Staphylococcus aureus*)

C. PROLIFERATIVE (DAY 1–3 WEEKS POST INJURY)

1. Collagen deposition
   a. Fibroblasts migrate into the wound (first arrive at 24 hours post injury), stimulated mainly by PDGF.
   b. Fibroblasts synthesize and deposit collagen.
      (1) This replaces the temporary matrix.
      (2) Synthesis increases until 4 weeks after injury because of increasing numbers of fibroblasts in the wound and increased production per cell.
      (3) Increased collagen causes increased tensile strength.
2. Epithelialization
   a. Migration of cells across the wound to restore the barrier function
      (1) Increased mitotic rate
      (2) Release from the basement membrane
      (3) Creep across the open wound until they contact other epithelial cells which inhibits migration
   b. Partial-thickness wounds (some dermis intact) reepithelialize from the edges of the wound and from remaining epidermal appendages (i.e., hair follicles, sweat glands).
   c. Full-thickness wounds (no intact dermis) reepithelialize from wound margins only.
   d. Surgical incisions typically reepithelialize within 48 hours.
3. Angiogenesis
   a. Proliferation of endothelial cells to form capillaries
   b. Occurs in response to VEGF, which is secreted by macrophages and keratinocytes
   c. Nitric oxide secreted from endothelial cells—increases VEGF secretion and causes vasodilation
   d. Important to supply increased oxygen needs of healing tissue

D. MATURATION AND REMODELING (3 WEEKS–1 YEAR POST INJURY)

1. Overall collagen synthesis decreases until it reaches a point of collagen homeostasis.
2. Thin collagen fibrils (30% type III) are initially laid down parallel to the wound edge.
3. As the wound matures, tensile strength increases.
   a. At 1 week: 3%
   b. At 3 weeks 20%
   c. Final tensile strength: 80% of uninjured skin (never reaching the strength of normal skin)
   d. Type I collagen: 90%, type III: 10% (similar to uninjured skin)
4. Myofibroblasts have microfilaments similar to smooth muscle cells that contract to shrink wound and contribute to angiogenesis by decreasing metalloproteinase activity.

II. FACTORS THAT AFFECT WOUND HEALING

A. OXYGENATION

1. Fibroblasts are O_2 sensitive, require partial pressure of oxygen (PaO_2) of 30 mm Hg, and can be stimulated to proliferate and synthesize collagen if $PaO_2 > 40$ mm Hg.
2. Wound hypoxia is the most common cause of wound infection.
3. Acute anemia secondary to hemorrhage is not associated with decreased wound strength.
4. Vasoconstriction secondary to pain, temperature, hypovolemia, etc. can cause local tissue hypoxia.

B. INFECTION

1. Quantitative diagnosis of infection with 10^5 colony-forming units (cfu) per gram of tissue
2. Prolongs inflammatory phase and delays wound healing
3. Interferes with wound contraction, epithelialization, angiogenesis, and collagen deposition

C. NUTRITION

1. Malnutrition: Serum protein less than 2 g prolongs the inflammatory phase, decreases fibroplasia, and therefore delays tensile strength.
2. Deficiency of glutamine and arginine is associated with inadequate wound healing, but supplementation has not been shown to effectively reverse this process.
3. Vitamin C is an essential cofactor in collagen synthesis (no benefit to supranormal levels of vitamin C).
4. Key micronutrients include magnesium and zinc, but oral supplementation in nondeficient patients is not recommended.

D. STEROIDS

1. Steroids inhibit wound macrophages, fibroplasia, angiogenesis, and wound contraction.
2. They increase the risk for infection.
3. Vitamin A supplementation, 25,000 international units (IU) oral daily preoperatively and 4 days postoperatively, aids in promoting epithelialization and collagen synthesis.

E. SMOKING

1. Nicotine—vasoconstrictor—decreases cellular migration and oxygenation.
2. Increased partial pressure of carbon monoxide decreases O_2 carrying capacity of hemoglobin.
3. Hydrogen cyanide inhibits oxygen transport.
4. Abstinence 4 weeks before and 4 weeks after cosmetic or reconstructive surgery is recommended.

WOUND HEALING

4

F. AGE
1. Tensile strength and wound closure rates decline with increasing age.

G. FOREIGN BODIES
1. Include nonviable tissue
2. Prolong inflammation
3. Inhibit wound contraction, angiogenesis, and epithelialization

H. EDEMA
1. Inhibits perfusion and therefore inhibits healing

I. CHEMOTHERAPY
1. Historically associated with decreased wound healing, but this view is controversial
2. Little effect on healing if chemotherapy started 10–14 days after surgery

J. RADIATION
1. Acutely, radiation causes stasis and occlusion in small vessels.
2. Fibroblast injury impairs proliferation, collagen synthesis, and tensile strength; injury to fibroblasts is permanent.
3. Progressive injury: Tissues retain poor healing abilities forever.

K. DIABETES MELLITUS
1. Impairment to wound healing is multifactorial.
2. Large and small blood vessel disease results in decreased oxygen delivery.
3. Increased edema is secondary to increased venous pressure.
4. Impaired immunity results in higher rates of infection.
5. There is increased risk of poor outcomes with glucose >200 mg/dL.

L. GENERAL HEALTH
1. Obesity, coronary artery disease, chronic obstructive pulmonary disease, carcinoma, and renal or hepatic failure all impair healing potential.

III. WOUND PREPARATION

A. IRRIGATION
1. Type of solution (i.e., saline vs. soapy vs. tap water) likely does not matter.
2. There is some controversy over which method is best (i.e., low pressure vs. high pressure, pulsatile vs. non-pulsatile) but agreement on the need for copious irrigation.

B. ANTIMICROBIALS
1. Iodine-based solutions
   a. Good activity against broad spectrum of bacteria
   b. Does not impair wound healing in humans

2. Chlorhexidine
   a. Broad spectrum
   b. Recommended for preoperative preparation to decrease postoperative wound infection rates

C. DÉBRIDEMENT

1. Removal of necrotic tissue by sharp dissection back to healthy tissue is necessary for appropriate wound healing.
2. High-pressure lavage can also be used after sharp dissection is completed.
3. Use enzymatic débridement (collagenase, papain-urea) when sharp débridement is not possible.

IV. TYPES OF WOUND CLOSURE

A. PRIMARY: CLOSURE OF WOUND BY DIRECT APPROXIMATION OF WOUND EDGES

1. Braided suture provides easier handling but may increase risk of infection.
2. Triclosan-impregnated sutures are available but have not been shown to decrease rates of infection and are not recommended.
3. Tissue adhesives remove need of needle stick but should not be used for wounds under tension.
4. Intraoperatively placed dry dressings are typically left in place, after being applied under sterile conditions, for 48 hours. This allows for epithelialization to occur. Soiled dressings should be changed.
5. Most traumatic wounds can be closed primarily (after appropriate prep). Exceptions to this are infected wounds and human bites.

B. SPONTANEOUS HEALING (SECONDARY INTENTION): SPONTANEOUS WOUND CONTRACTION AND EPITHELIALIZATION

1. Negative-pressure treatment (vacuum-assisted closure)
   a. Increases wound oxygenation and granulation tissue
   b. Wound filler and negative-pressure protocols: under investigation to identify the best method
2. Hyperbaric oxygen
   a. Tissue oxygen tension is improved via hyperoxygenation.
   b. Mitosis requires at least 30 mm Hg O_2, and chronic, nonhealing wounds usually have oxygen tensions in the 5–20 mm Hg range.
   c. Hyperbaric oxygen cannot aid healing if tissue is not adequately perfused (ischemic).
3. Platelet-rich plasma
   a. High concentration of platelets in plasma results in high amounts of growth factors
   b. Used by professional athletes to speed recovery
   c. May help in chronic wound healing, but more research is necessary

WOUND HEALING

4

4. Wet-to-dry dressings
   a. Débride wound exudate and cellular debris, and prevent desiccation.
   b. Gauze is moistened with 0.9% sodium chloride.
   c. If concerned for infection/contamination, particularly with *Pseudomonas*, use Dakin solution (0.25% acetic acid). Dakin solution delays healing but decontaminates well.

C. TERTIARY HEALING
1. Delayed primary closure after allowing the wound to begin healing by secondary intention
2. May be performed any time after formation of granulation tissue, but may only be performed in clean/noninfected wound

V. MANAGEMENT OF WOUND COMPLICATIONS
A. INFECTION
1. Postsurgical wound infections usually present approximately 3 days after surgery.
2. Symptoms are erythema, induration, exudate, fever, and lymphadenopathy.
3. Most commonly caused by staphylococci or streptococci.
4. Risk increases with poor sterile technique, contaminated cases, prolonged operating room (OR) time (>5 hours), and general conditions that adversely affect wound healing (listed earlier).
5. Treatment
   a. Treat with antibiotics alone if there is only a cellulitis.
   b. Abscess requires drainage, irrigation, and débridement.

B. SEROMA
1. A seroma is sterile serous fluid collection in operative dead space.
2. It is best treated prophylactically with closed-suction drains, to be removed when output is low.
3. If a seroma forms, the fluid may be aspirated or a drain placed via ultrasound or computed tomography guidance using sterile technique. There is a small risk for infecting a sterile fluid collection when draining seroma; therefore small seromas without signs of infection are usually safe to monitor and allowed to be resorbed.

C. DEHISCENCE
1. Superficial: separation of skin and subcutaneous fat
   a. If wound is clean, may clean and close again using sterile technique. May alternatively treat as open contaminated wound and allow closure by secondary intention
2. Fascial: separation of fascia
   a. This may possibly be secondary to technical failure but can be secondary to wound infection, pulmonary disease, hemodynamic instability, age greater than 65 years, malnutrition, obesity, malignancy, ascites, steroid use, or systemic infection

b. Mortality rate is 15%–30%.
c. It may be identified by rush of serosanguineous salmon-colored fluid.
d. Small fascial separation may be monitored closely with plan to repair hernia in future.
e. If patient eviscerates, apply saline-soaked towels and repair fascia emergently in the operating room.
f. In high-risk patients with poor fascia, multiple comorbidities, or chronic steroid use, retention sutures can be placed to help to support fascial closure. These are full-thickness bites of the abdominal wall and should be left in place for approximately 3 weeks.

VI. HYPERTROPHIC SCARS AND KELOIDS

A. HYPERTROPHIC SCARS
1. Characterized by wide, raised scars that remain within the original borders of injury
2. Occur within 4 weeks of injury
3. Usually resolve over time without treatment, but corticosteroid injections may be used in certain circumstances

B. KELOIDS
1. Pathology
   a. Scar extends beyond the original borders of injury
   b. Large bundles of collagen deposited in disorganized fashion
   c. Few macrophages, but many eosinophils and mast cells
2. Epidemiology
   a. Occur within 1 year of injury
   b. Most common in African Americans—15:1 darkly pigmented skin to light skin ratio
   c. Uncommon in very young and elderly individuals
   d. High recurrence rate
3. Treatment
   a. Indication for treatment is chronic itching and skin breakdown.
   b. Silastic gel sheeting limits formation of keloids.
   c. Surgical excision with corticosteroid injections is current treatment of choice.
      (1) Excise keloid using sterile technique, and immediately inject wound with steroids.
      (2) Then treat incision site with three monthly injections after surgery.
      (3) It is shown to improve recurrence rates.
   d. Surgical excision with radiation therapy
      (1) Excise keloid, and treat with 15–20 Gy radiation within 24 hours.
      (2) Approximately five additional treatments are necessary.

4

WOUND HEALING

RECOMMENDED READINGS

Adamson R. Role of macrophages in normal wound healing: an overview. *J Wound Care.* 2009;18:349–351. http://dx.doi.org/10.12968/jowc.2009.18.8.43636.

Bucknall TE. Factors influencing wound complications: a clinical and experimental study. *Ann R Coll Surg Engl.* 1983;65:71–77.

Collins N. Glutamine and wound healing. *Adv Skin Wound Care.* 2002;15:233–234.

Coursin DB, Connery LE, Ketzler JT. Perioperative diabetic and hyperglycemic management issues. *Crit Care Med.* 2004;32:S116–S125.

Decker MR, Greenblatt DY, Havlena J, Wilke LG, Greenberg CC, Neuman HB. Impact of neoadjuvant chemotherapy on wound complications after breast surgery. *Surgery.* 2012;152:382–388. http://dx.doi.org/10.1016/j.surg.2012.05.001.

Dovi JV, He L-K, DiPietro LA. Accelerated wound closure in neutrophil-depleted mice. *J Leukoc Biol.* 2003;73:448–455.

Ehrlich HP, Krummel TM. Regulation of wound healing from a connective tissue perspective. *Wound Repair Regen.* 1996;4:203–210. http://dx.doi.org/10.1046/j.1524-475X.1996.40206.x.

Ellinger S. Can specific nutrients stimulate bowel wound healing? *Curr Opin Clin Nutr Metab Care.* 2016;19:371–376. http://dx.doi.org/10.1097/MCO.0000000000000303.

Erinjeri JP, Fong AJ, Kemeny NE, Brown KT, Getrajdman GI, Solomon SB. Timing of administration of bevacizumab chemotherapy affects wound healing after chest wall port placement. *Cancer.* 2011;117:1296–1301. http://dx.doi.org/10.1002/cncr.25573.

Fernández R, Griffiths R. Water for wound cleansing. Cochrane Database of Systematic Reviews. Wiley Online Library. *Cochrane Library.* 2012. http://dx.doi.org/10.1002/14651858.CD003861.pub3/full.

Greenhalgh DG. Wound healing and diabetes mellitus. *Clin Plast Surg.* 2003;30:37–45.

Heughan C, Grislis G, Hunt TK. The effect of anemia on wound healing. *Ann Surg.* 1974;179:163–167.

Hohn DC, MacKay RD, Halliday B, Hunt TK. Effect of O_2 tension on microbicidal function of leukocytes in wounds and in vitro. *Surg Forum.* 1976;27:18–20.

Hopf HW, Hunt TK, West JM, et al. Wound tissue oxygen tension predicts the risk of wound infection in surgical patients. *Arch Surg.* 1997;132:997–1004. http://dx.doi.org/10.1001/archsurg.1997.01430330063010.

Janis JE, Harrison B. Wound healing: part I. Basic science. *Plast Reconstr Surg.* 2014;133:199e–207e. http://dx.doi.org/10.1097/01.prs.0000437224.02985.f9.

Jonsson K, Jensen JA, Goodson WH, et al. Tissue oxygenation, anemia, and perfusion in relation to wound healing in surgical patients. *Ann Surg.* 1991;214:605–613.

Juva K, Prockop DJ, Cooper GW, Lash JW. Hydroxylation of proline and the intracellular accumulation of a polypeptide precursor of collagen. *Science.* 1966;152:92–94.

Kivisaari J, Vihersaari T, Renvall S, Niinikoski J. Energy metabolism of experimental wounds at various oxygen environments. *Ann Surg.* 1975;181:823–828.

Laato M, Lehtonen OP, Niinikoski J. Granulation tissue formation in experimental wounds inoculated with *Staphylococcus aureus*. *Acta Chir Scand.* 1985;151:313–318.

Leibovich SJ, Ross R. The role of the macrophage in wound repair. A study with hydrocortisone and antimacrophage serum. *Am J Pathol.* 1975;78:71–100.

Madden JW, Smith HC. The rate of collagen synthesis and deposition in dehisced and resutured wounds. *Surg Gynecol Obstet.* 1970;130:487–493.

Martin P, Leibovich SJ. Inflammatory cells during wound repair: the good, the bad and the ugly. *Trends Cell Biol.* 2005;15:599–607. http://dx.doi.org/10.1016/j.tcb.2005.09.002.

Mayrand D, Laforce-Lavoie A, Larochelle S, et al. Angiogenic properties of myofibroblasts isolated from normal human skin wounds. *Angiogenesis.* 2012;15:199–212. http://dx.doi.org/10.1007/s10456-012-9253-5.

Morykwas MJ, Argenta LC, Shelton-Brown EI, McGuirt W. Vacuum-assisted closure: a new method for wound control and treatment: animal studies and basic foundation. *Ann Plast Surgery*. 1997;38:553.

Noorani A, Rabey N, Walsh SR, Davies RJ. Systematic review and meta-analysis of pre-operative antisepsis with chlorhexidine versus povidone–iodine in clean-contaminated surgery. *Br J Surg*. 2010;97:1614–1620. http://dx.doi.org/10.1002/bjs.7214.

Petrisor B, Investigators F. Lavage of open fracture wounds (flow): a randomised blind-ed, multicentre pilot trial. *Orthop Proceed*. 2011;93-B:574–574.

Redler LH, Thompson SA, Hsu SH, Ahmad CS, Levine WN. Platelet-rich plasma thera-py: a systematic literature review and evidence for clinical use. *Phys Sportsmed*. 2015. http://dx.doi.org/10.3810/psm.2011.02.1861.

Ross R, Benditt EP. Wound healing and collagen formation. I. Sequential changes in components of guinea pig skin wounds observed in the electron microscope. *J Biophys Biochem Cytol*. 1961;11:677–700.

Sidle DM, Kim H. Keloids: prevention and management. *Fac Plast Surg Clin North Am*. 2011;19:505–515. http://dx.doi.org/10.1016/j.fsc.2011.06.005.

Silverstein RJ, Landsman AS. The effects of a moderate and high dose of vitamin C on wound healing in a controlled guinea pig model. *J Foot Ankle Surg*. 1999;38:333–338. http://dx.doi.org/10.1016/S1067-2516(99)80004-0.

Simpson DM, Ross R. The neutrophilic leukocyte in wound repair a study with antineutro-phil serum. *J Clin Invest*. 1972;51:2009–2023. http://dx.doi.org/10.1172/JCI107007.

Mustoe TA, Cooter RD, Gold MH, et al. International clinical recommendations on scar management. *Plast Reconstruct Surg*. 2002;110:560–571. http://dx.doi.org/10.1097/00006534-200208000-00031.

Thorn RM, Austin AJ, Greenman J, Wilkins JP. In vitro comparison of antimicrobial ac-tivity of iodine and silver dressings against biofilms. *J Wound Care*. 2009;18:343–346.

Ueno C, Hunt TK, Hopf HW. Using physiology to improve surgical wound out-comes. *Plast Reconstruct Surg*. 2006;117:59S–71S. http://dx.doi.org/10.1097/01.prs.0000225438.86758.21.

Vermeulen H, Westerbos SJ, Ubbink DT. Benefit and harm of iodine in wound care: a systematic review. *J Hospit Infect*. 2010;76:191–199. http://dx.doi.org/10.1016/j.jhin.2010.04.026.

Wukich DK, Lowery NJ, McMillen RL, Frykberg RG. Postoperative infection rates in foot and ankle surgery: a comparison of patients with and without diabetes mellitus. *J Bone Joint Surg Am*. 2010;92:287–295. http://dx.doi.org/10.2106/JBJS.I.00080.

WOUND HEALING

4

Surgical Risk Assessment

Young Kim, MD, MS

Risk comes from not knowing what you're doing.
—Warren Buffett

I. RISKS AND BENEFITS OF SURGERY

1. Whether it is a life-saving liver transplant or a cosmetic procedure, surgical intervention offers some benefit to the patient, at the risk of complications, morbidity, or even death. The surgeon must carefully weigh the relative risks and benefits of surgery before proceeding with any operation. Perioperative care requires the identification and reduction of risk factors, whether due to the patient or inherent to the operation itself.
2. Determination of risks and benefits requires careful consideration of the following factors:
   a. Disease process
      (1) Natural course if left untreated
      (2) Medical versus surgical treatment options
   b. Medical therapy
   c. Surgical therapy
      (1) Indications and contraindications
      (2) Risk factors related to surgical intervention
      (3) Technical aspect of the operation
      (4) Logistical limitations
      (5) Potential for complications
      (6) Urgency of operation
   d. Patient factors
      (1) Physiologic reserve
      (2) Risk factors related to medical comorbidities
      (3) Reducing operative risk
   e. Preoperative care
   f. Postoperative management

II. SURGICAL RISK ASSESSMENT

1. Age-related risk factors
   a. Older patients often have limited physiologic reserve or impaired function of each major organ system.
   b. "There is nothing like an operation or an injury to bring a patient up to chronological age."—W.R. Howe
2. Risk factors related to urgency of operation
   a. Risk factors

     (1) Elective procedures can be postponed until risks have been evaluated and addressed.

     (2) Urgent procedures allow a much shorter interval to address risk factors.

     (3) Emergent procedures require operation without proper evaluation and reduction of risk factors.

       (a) Emergent nature of surgery doubles risk of operative morbidity and mortality in low- and moderate-risk patients, according to one study.

  b. Reducing operative risk

     (1) Emergent procedures should not be delayed in most situations because the natural course of the disease process portends worse outcomes than the sum of the risk factors themselves.

     (2) In the case of volume-depleted patients, fluid and electrolyte replacement should occur before induction of anesthesia.

3. **Risk factors related to physical impairment**

  a. Risk factors

     (1) Impairment of organ function and severity of illness scores profoundly influence the risk for operative mortality.

  b. Evaluation of risk factors

     (1) American Society of Anesthesiologists (ASA) classification of physical status

       (a) *ASA I:* normal, healthy patient

       (b) *ASA II:* mild systemic disease

       (c) *ASA III:* severe systemic disease

       (d) *ASA IV:* severe systemic disease that is a constant threat to life

       (e) *ASA V:* moribund patient not expected to survive without operation

       (f) *ASA VI:* brain-dead organ donor

4. **Cardiovascular risk factors**

  a. Risk factors

     (1) Coronary artery disease

     (2) Congestive heart failure (CHF)

     (3) Arrhythmias

     (4) Peripheral vascular disease

     (5) Aortic stenosis

     (6) Severe hypertension

  b. Evaluation of risk factors

     (1) Goldman cardiac risk for noncardiac surgery

       (a) Risk factors (Table 5.1)

         (i) Age >70

         (ii) Recent myocardial infarction (<6 months)

         (iii) S3 gallop or jugular venous distention

         (iv) Aortic stenosis

         (v) Non-sinus rhythm *or* >5 premature atrial or ventricular complexes per minute at any time before surgery

5

SURGICAL RISK ASSESSMENT

TABLE 5.1

COMPUTING CARDIOVASCULAR RISK INDEX

Category	Factor	Score (Points)
History	Age >70 years	5
	Recent myocardial infarction (<6 months)	10
Physical examination	S3 gallop or jugular venous distention	11
	Aortic valvular stenosis	3
Electrocardiogram	Non-sinus rhythm or >5 PACs/PVCs per minute before surgery	7
Medical status	PaO$_2$ <60 mm Hg or PaCO$_2$ >50 mm Hg	3
	K <3 mEq/L or HCO$_3$ <20 mEq/L	3
	BUN >50 mg/dL or creatinine level >3 mg/dL	3
	Abnormal liver function panel	3
	Chronic liver disease	3
	Bedridden due to noncardiac cause	3
Operative factors	Intraperitoneal, intrathoracic, or aortic surgery	3
	Emergent procedure	3

BUN, Blood urea nitrogen; *PAC,* premature atrial contraction; *PVC,* premature ventricular contraction.

TABLE 5.2

GOLDMAN CLASSIFICATION OF CARDIOVASCULAR RISK

Class	Total Score	Risk of Major Complications (%)	Risk of Cardiac Death (%)
Class I	0–5	0.6	0.2
Class II	6–12	3	1
Class III	13–25	11	3
Class IV	26+	12	39

Adapted from Goldman L, Caldera DL, Nussbaum SR, et al. Multifactorial index of cardiac risk in noncardiac surgical procedures. *N Engl J Med.* 1977;297:845.

    (vi) Partial pressure of oxygen (PaO$_2$) <60 or partial pressure of carbon dioxide (PaCO$_2$) >50 mm Hg

    (vii) Hypokalemia (<3) or metabolic acidosis (<20 mEq/L)

    (viii) Impaired renal function (blood urea nitrogen [BUN] >50 or Cr >3 mg/dL)

    (ix) Abnormal liver function panel

    (x) Chronic liver disease

    (xi) Bedridden due to noncardiac causes

    (xii) Intraperitoneal, intrathoracic, or aortic surgery

    (xiii) Emergency surgical intervention

(b) Classification (Table 5.2)

    (i) Class I: 0.6% risk of major complication, 0.2% risk of cardiac death

    (ii) Class II: 3% risk of major complication, 1% risk of cardiac death

TABLE 5.3		
REVISED CARDIAC RISK INDEX		
Class	Risk Factors	Risk of Major Complication
Class I	0	0.4% (95% CI, 0.05%–1.5%)
Class II	1	0.9% (95% CI, 0.3%–2.1%)
Class III	2	6.6% (95% CI, 3.9%–10.3%)
Class IV	3+	11.0% (95% CI, 5.8%–18.4%)

CI, Confidence interval.
Adapted from Lee TH, Marcantonio ER, Mangione CM, et al. Derivation and prospective validation of a simple index for prediction of cardiac risk of major noncardiac surgery. *Circulation.* 1999;100:1043–1049.

        (iii) Class III: 11% risk of major complication, 3% risk of cardiac death
        (iv) Class IV: 12% risk of major complication, 39% risk of cardiac death
    (2) Revised Cardiac Risk Index (RCRI)
      (a) Risk factors
        (i) High-risk procedure
        (ii) History of ischemic heart disease
        (iii) History of CHF
        (iv) History of cerebrovascular disease
        (v) Preoperative treatment with insulin
        (vi) Preoperative serum creatinine >2 mg/dL
      (b) Classification (Table 5.3)
        (i) Class I: zero risk factors, 0.4% risk of major complication
        (ii) Class II: one risk factor, 0.9% risk of major complication
          (a) Consider perioperative beta-blockade.
        (iii) Class III: two risk factors, 6.6% risk of major complication
          (a) Consider perioperative beta-blockade.
        (iv) Class IV: three or more risk factors, 11.0% risk of major complication
          (a) Highly recommend perioperative beta-blockade.
          (b) If possible, defer or cancel surgery until risk factors can be assessed and reduced.
        (v) If patient risk factors are difficult to assess, consider dobutamine stress echocardiogram for further analysis.
          (a) If echocardiogram is negative, operative risk is low.
          (b) If positive, highly recommend perioperative beta-blockade.
  c. Reducing operative risk
    (1) Coronary artery disease

(a) Evaluate with electrocardiogram, exercise tolerance, dipyridamole thallium scan, multigated acquisition, or echocardiogram.

(b) Coronary angiography can be used to evaluate vessel patency.

(c) Preoperative coronary artery revascularization has been shown to decrease risk of postoperative myocardial infarction.

(2) CHF

(a) Preexisting CHF should be medically optimized (e.g., diuretics, digoxin).

(b) Preoperative assessment of pulmonary artery pressure and intraoperative transesophageal echocardiogram can be used to guide perioperative fluid management and augmentation of hemodynamic parameters (e.g., inotropes).

(3) Arrhythmias

(a) Arrhythmias should be medically optimized.

(b) Complete heart block and bradyarrhythmias may require temporary or permanent pacemaker insertion.

(c) Anticoagulation for chronic atrial fibrillation may be bridged with heparin injections during the perioperative phase.

(4) Severe hypertension

(a) Postoperative hypertension should not be relegated to surgical pain without further evaluation.

(b) Mild, nonlabile hypertension does not portend increased operative risk.

(c) Antihypertensive medications should be continued to time of surgery, except monoamine oxidase (MAO) inhibitors, which should be held 2 weeks before operation.

(d) Specific cases of severe hypertension require further workup and treatment.

(i) New-onset hypertension

(ii) Severe hypertension with diastolic blood pressure exceeding 110 mm Hg

(iii) Severe hypertension with systolic blood pressure exceeding 250 mm Hg

(iv) Unusual or unexplained causes of hypertension

5. Pulmonary risk factors

a. Risk factors

(1) Smoking (twofold risk)

(2) Chronic obstructive pulmonary disease (sixfold risk)

(3) Advanced age

(4) Industrial exposure

(5) Preexisting pulmonary disease

(6) Thoracic or upper abdominal surgery

(7) Pulmonary hypertension

(8) Obstructive sleep apnea

(9) Morbid obesity (controversial)

b. Evaluation of risk factors
   (1) Ask patient to blow out a match with unpursed lips from 20 to 25 cm away.
   (2) Ask patient to climb two flights of stairs, and then ask about shortness of breath.
   (3) Pulmonary function testing
      (a) Forced expiratory volume in 1 second (FEV_1) less than 2 L
      (b) FEV_1/forced vital capacity ratio less than 65% predicted
   (4) Arterial blood gas
      (a) $PaCO_2$ is greater than 45 mm Hg on room air
   (5) Right heart catheterization
      (a) Pulmonary artery pressure greater than 30 mm Hg
c. Reducing operative risk
   (1) Patient should discontinue smoking as long as possible before surgery.
   (2) Eight weeks of smoking cessation is required to reduce postoperative mortality.
   (3) For elective procedures, the following techniques should be taught in the office setting before surgery—chest physical therapy, incentive spirometry, deep-breathing exercises.
   (4) Chronic obstructive pulmonary disease
      (a) Initiate or continue use of bronchodilators and antibiotics.
      (b) Chest physical therapy
      (c) Perioperative systemic corticosteroids if necessary
   (5) Asthma
      (a) Initiate or continue use of bronchodilators.
      (b) Perioperative systemic corticosteroids if necessary
   (6) Pneumonia/acute pulmonary infections
      (a) Treat with pulmonary toilet and antibiotics.
      (b) Delay elective surgery until antibiotic course is complete.
   (7) Bronchiectasis
      (a) Preoperative expectorants
      (b) Pulmonary toilet, incentive spirometry
      (c) Antibiotics based on culture growth

6. Renal risk factors
   a. Risk factors
      (1) Acute renal insufficiency
         (a) BUN >50 mg/dL
         (b) Serum creatinine >3 mg/day
         (c) Note that serum BUN/creatinine abnormalities are not noted until 75%–90% of renal function has been lost.
      (2) Chronic renal failure
   b. Evaluation of risk factors
      (1) Serum BUN/creatinine levels
      (2) Daily urine output
      (3) Need for dialysis

   c. Reducing operative risk

     (1) Correct electrolyte abnormalities.

     (2) Optimize volume status.

       (a) Consider pulmonary artery pressure monitoring.

     (3) Evaluate need for continuous or intermittent hemodialysis.

       (a) Severe acidosis

       (b) Severe electrolyte derangements

       (c) Drug or metabolite intoxication

       (d) Fluid overload

       (e) Symptomatic uremia

     (4) Identify and optimize the cause of renal insufficiency.

7. Hepatic risk factors

  a. Risk factors

     (1) Cirrhosis

     (2) Acute liver failure

     (3) Chronic hepatitis

     (4) Chronic alcoholism

     (5) Portal hypertension

     (6) Esophageal varices

     (7) Uncontrolled ascites

     (8) Hepatic encephalopathy

     (9) Hepatorenal syndrome

     (10) Hepatopulmonary syndrome

  b. Evaluation of risk factors

     (1) Hepatic function panel

     (2) Esophagoscopy

     (3) Child-Pugh classification

       (a) Measures serum albumin, bilirubin, prothrombin time, hepatic encephalopathy, ascites

       (b) Class A: <5% mortality rate

       (c) Class B: 5%–10% mortality rate

       (d) Class C: 20%–50% mortality rate

     (4) Model for end-stage liver disease (MELD) score

       (a) MELD measures creatinine, international normalized ratio (INR), and bilirubin.

       (b) MELD $= 3.78 \times$ natural log [serum bilirubin (mg/dL)] $+ 11.2 \times$ natural log [INR] $+ 9.57 \times$ natural log [serum creatinine (mg/dL)] $+ 6.43$

       (c) MELD <9 has 1.9% 3-month mortality rate.

       (d) MELD 10–19 has 6.0% 3-month mortality rate.

       (e) MELD 20–29 has 19.6% 3-month mortality rate.

       (f) MELD 30–39 has 52.6% 3-month mortality rate.

       (g) MELD 40+ has 71.3% 3-month mortality rate.

  c. Reducing operative risk

     (1) Abstain from alcohol or illicit drug use.

     (2) Optimize fluid status.

    (a) Limit use of diuretics if possible.
    (b) Restrict daily free water.
    (c) Limit sodium intake to less than 2 g/day.
8. Endocrine risk factors
  a. Risk factors
    (1) Diabetes mellitus
      (a) Maintain glycemic control (glucose <180 mg/dL).
      (b) It is an independent predictor of postoperative myocardial ischemia among cardiac and noncardiac surgical patients.
      (c) Surgical stress induces secretion of hormones that increase blood glucose levels, including glucagon, epinephrine, growth hormone, and glucocorticoids.
      (d) Anesthetic agents can impair autonomic function and decrease insulin secretion.
    (2) Hyperthyroidism
    (3) Hypothyroidism
    (4) Adrenal insufficiency
  b. Evaluation of risk factors
    (1) Glycohemoglobin (Hb$_{A1C}$) levels
    (2) Thyroid function panel
    (3) Dexamethasone suppression test if there is any concern for acute adrenal insufficiency
  c. Reducing operative risk
    (1) Diabetes mellitus
      (a) For type I diabetics, schedule operations early in the day to minimize effect of fasting and ketoacidosis.
      (b) Use half the dose of long-acting insulins (e.g., Lantus) before surgery to account for nothing by mouth (NPO) time.
      (c) Avoid oral medications on day of surgery.
        (i) Metformin can cause lactic acidosis in renal failure.
        (ii) Secretagogues can cause hypoglycemia.
        (iii) Sulfonylureas are associated with increased risk of perioperative myocardial infarction.
    (2) Steroids
      (a) Indications
        (i) Preoperative dosing for adrenalectomy
        (ii) History of adrenal insufficiency
        (iii) History of adrenal or pituitary surgery
        (iv) History of radical nephrectomy for renal cell carcinoma
        (v) Steroid-dependent inflammatory bowel disease
      (b) Endogenous cortisol output
        (i) Normal adult—8–25 mg/day
        (ii) Adult undergoing major surgery—75–100 mg/day
      (c) Steroid coverage
        (i) Correct electrolytes, blood pressure, and fluid status.

5

SURGICAL RISK ASSESSMENT

(ii) If there is concern for adrenal insufficiency preoperatively, have hydrocortisone 100 mg intravenous (IV) piggyback on call to operating room.

9. **Hematologic risk factors**
   a. Risk factors for developing postoperative deep vein thrombosis (DVT) (within 30 days)
      (1) Old age (>50 years old)
      (2) History of varicose veins
      (3) History of myocardial infarction
      (4) Malignancy
      (5) Atrial fibrillation
      (6) History of ischemic stroke
      (7) Diabetes mellitus
      (8) Obesity
      (9) Prolonged immobility
      (10) Hypercoagulable diseases (e.g., factor V Leiden)
   b. Evaluation of risk factors
      (1) Wells criteria for DVT
         (a) Criteria
            (i) Lower extremity trauma, surgery, or immobilization (+1)
            (ii) Immobilization (3 days) or recent surgery (4 weeks) (+1)
            (iii) Tenderness along femoral or popliteal vein lines (+1)
            (iv) Limb swelling (+1)
            (v) Calf enlargement (>3 cm circumference, 10 cm below tibial tuberosity) (+1)
            (vi) Pitting edema (+1)
            (vii) Dilated collateral superficial veins (nonvaricose) (+1)
            (viii) Previous DVT (+1)
            (ix) Malignancy (6 months) (+1)
            (x) IV drug use (+3)
            (xi) Alternative diagnosis more likely than DVT (−2)
         (b) Total score 0–1: unlikely for DVT
         (c) Total score 2+: likely for DVT
      (2) Wells criteria for pulmonary embolism (PE)
         (a) Criteria
            (i) Clinical signs/symptoms of DVT (+3)
            (ii) PE is likely diagnosis (+3)
            (iii) Tachycardia (heart rate >100 beats/min) (+1.5)
            (iv) Immobilization (3 days) or recent surgery (4 weeks) (+1.5)
            (v) History of DVT or PE (+1.5)
            (vi) Hemoptysis (+1)
            (vii) Malignancy (6 months) (+1)
         (b) Total score 0–4: unlikely for PE
         (c) Total score 5+: likely for PE

    c. Reducing operative risk
      (1) Early ambulation
      (2) Prophylactic unfractionated or low-molecular-weight heparin
      (3) Sequential lower extremity compression devices

10. Nutritional risk factors
    a. Risk factors for severe malnutrition
      (1) Weight loss >15% over the previous 3 months
      (2) Hypoalbuminemia (<3.0 g/dL)
      (3) Anergy
      (4) Transferrin <200 mg/dL
    b. Evaluation of risk factors
      (1) Short-turnover protein panel
        (a) Prealbumin
        (b) Transferrin
        (c) Retinol-binding protein
      (2) Daily calorie counts
    c. Reducing operative risk
      (1) If malnourished, consider preoperative enteral or parenteral
         nutrition for 5–14 days to normalize short-turnover proteins.

III. PREOPERATIVE PREPARATION

1. History and physical examination (see Chapter 1)
2. Preoperative laboratory studies
    a. Complete blood count
    b. Basic metabolic panel
    c. Coagulation panel
    d. Urinalysis
    e. Type and screen
    f. Arterial blood gas if any risk of respiratory compromise or if pro-
      longed postoperative ventilator support anticipated
3. Preoperative imaging evaluation
    a. Chest radiograph (posteroanterior and lateral) unless patient is less
      than 35 years or has a previously normal X-ray within the past 6
      months
    b. Electrocardiogram if older than 35 years or has cardiac risk
      factors
4. Skin preparation
    a. Remove hair on the day of surgery with an electric clipper.
    b. Shaving the night before surgery is associated with compensatory
      bacterial proliferation and increased risk of wound infection.
    c. Provide preoperative scrub or shower of the operative site with a
      germicidal soap (e.g., Hibiclens).
5. Preoperative antibiotics
    a. Administer antibiotics 30 minutes before skin incision to optimize
      blood level of the medication.

TABLE 5.4

ANTIBIOTIC PROPHYLAXIS OF BACTERIAL ENDOCARDITIS

Antibiotic Agent	Adult Dosing	Pediatric Dosing
Amoxicillin (PO)	3 g 1 h before and 1.5 g 6 h after procedure	50 mg/kg 1 h before and 25 mg/kg 6 h after procedure
Erythromycin (PO)—if allergic to penicillins	1 g 2 h before and 500 mg 6 h after procedure	20 mg/kg 2 h before and 10 mg/kg 6 h after procedure
Ampicillin (IV/IM)	2 g 30 min before procedure	50 mg/kg 30 min before procedure
Gentamicin (IV/IM)	1.5 mg/kg 30 min before procedure	2 mg/kg 30 min before procedure
Vancomycin (IV)—if allergic to penicillins	1 g 1 h before procedure	20 mg/kg 1 h before procedure

Prevention for dental, upper respiratory, genitourinary, and gastrointestinal procedures. Add gentamicin to IV vancomycin for gastrointestinal and genitourinary procedures.

PO, Oral; *IM,* intramuscular; *IV,* intravenous.

  b. Indications for prophylactic antibiotics
    (1) Clean procedures
      (a) Most cardiac, thoracic, vascular, neurosurgical, orthopedic, and ophthalmic procedures—cefazolin 1–2 g IV or vancomycin 1 g IV
    (2) Clean-contaminated procedures
      (a) Gastrointestinal, genitourinary, gynecologic, respiratory tract, and head/neck procedures—cefazolin 1–2 g IV
      (b) Colorectal procedures—oral neomycin and erythromycin, and cefoxitin or cefotetan 1–2 g IV
    (3) Contaminated or dirty procedures
      (a) Cefoxitin or cefotetan 1–2 g IV with or without gentamicin 1.5 mg/kg IV every 8 hours, or clindamycin 600 mg IV every 6 hours and gentamicin 1.5 mg/kg IV every 8 hours
  c. There are special considerations for patients with prosthetic heart valves or prior valvular heart disease, with respect to endocarditis prophylaxis.
  d. Redose antibiotic if operation lasts longer than 4 hours or twice the half-life of the antimicrobial agent.
  e. Prophylactic antibiotics should not exceed 24-hour duration.
  6. Bacterial endocarditis prophylaxis
    a. Indications for endocarditis prophylaxis include the following:
      (1) Prosthetic heart valves
      (2) Congenital valve disease
      (3) Rheumatic valve disease
      (4) History of endocarditis
      (5) Idiopathic hypertrophic subaortic stenosis
      (6) Mitral valve prolapse with murmur (Barlow syndrome)
    b. Antibiotic recommendations (Table 5.4)
      (1) Oral regimens are more convenient and safer for the patient.

      (2) Parenteral medications are more likely to be effective and recommended for patients with higher risk of bacterial endocarditis.

      (3) A single dose of parenteral antimicrobials is adequate for most dental and diagnostic procedures of short duration.

7. **Respiratory care**
   a. Teach incentive spirometry and deep breathing exercises before surgery.
   b. Use bronchodilators for moderate-to-severe chronic obstructive pulmonary disease.

8. **Bowel preparation**
   a. Nonbowel operation
      (1) Recommend period of fasting (usually at midnight or 8 hours before procedure) and, if indicated, nasogastric decompression of the stomach before induction of anesthesia.
      (2) This reduces risk of complications due to aspiration.
   b. Bowel operation
      (1) Goals of bowel preparation
         (a) Remove all solid and most liquid contents from the bowel.
         (b) Reduce bacterial population of the bowel in anticipation of complications that may result from wound contamination.
      (2) Bowel preparation may be helpful if the gastrointestinal lumen is intentionally or accidentally entered (e.g., enterotomy).
      (3) Various gastric diseases cause bacterial overgrowth within the stomach, and oral antibiotic preparation (e.g., neomycin) should be considered.
         (a) Prolonged H_2-blocker usage
         (b) Achlorhydria
         (c) Gastric carcinoma
         (d) Obstructive peptic ulcer disease
      (4) Standard bowel preparation
         (a) Clear liquid diet 48 hours before the procedure
         (b) On the day of surgery
             (i) 10:00 a.m.—45 mL Fleet Phospho-Soda, 8 oz water
             (ii) 11:00 a.m.—8 oz water
             (iii) 12:00 p.m.—8 oz water
             (iv) 1:00 p.m.—8 oz water, neomycin 500 mg, metronidazole 750 mg
             (v) 2:00 p.m.—8 oz water
             (vi) 3:00 p.m.—neomycin 500 mg, metronidazole 750 mg
             (vii) 5:00 p.m.—four bisacodyl 5-mg tablets
             (viii) 7:00 p.m.—one bisacodyl 10-mg rectal suppository
             (ix) 10:00 p.m.—neomycin 500 mg, metronidazole 750 mg
         (c) If the stool contains remnant solid material, then administer one bottle of oral magnesium citrate

9. **Access and monitoring**
   a. IV access
      (1) At least one 18-gauge IV catheter is required to initiate anesthesia.
      (2) Consider central venous access if peripheral access is limited.

b. Intraarterial catheters can be used to frequently monitor blood pressure, blood glucose, and arterial blood gases.
c. Pulmonary artery catheters may help with monitoring of overall fluid status and other hemodynamic parameters.

10. **Other considerations**
   a. IV maintenance fluids while NPO
   b. Mechanical and chemical thromboembolic prophylaxis
   c. Maintenance medications may be given on the morning of surgery.
      (1) Antihypertensives (e.g., beta-blockers)
      (2) Cardiac medications
      (3) Anticonvulsants
   d. Perioperative glucose management
      (1) Use half the dose of long-lasting insulins.
      (2) Hold oral diabetic medications.
      (3) Maintain an ideal glucose level of less than 180 mg/dL.
   e. Subacute bacterial endocarditis prophylaxis
   f. Perioperative steroid management
   g. Preoperative discussion regarding stoma creation and, if possible, consultation to a wound care nurse specializing in stoma management

IV. POSTOPERATIVE CARE

1. **Pulmonary management**
   a. Postoperative pulmonary complications cause significant perioperative morbidity and mortality, with consequent prolonging of hospital and intensive care unit (ICU) stay.
   b. Complications
      (1) Atelectasis
      (2) Aspiration events
      (3) Pneumonia
      (4) Prolonged mechanical ventilation
      (5) Respiratory failure
      (6) Worsening of underlying lung disease
   c. Risk factors
      (1) Increased incidence of complications with proximity of incision to diaphragm
      (2) Duration of operation longer than 3–4 hours
      (3) Type of anesthesia and use of neuromuscular blockade
   d. Reducing postoperative risk
      (1) Early ambulation
      (2) Aggressive pulmonary toilet
         (a) Incentive spirometry
         (b) Deep breathing
         (c) Chest physical therapy
      (3) Adequate analgesia

(a) Epidural analgesia in upper abdominal incisions decreases the incidence of pulmonary complications.
(b) Advantages of epidural narcotics
  (i) Longer duration of action
  (ii) Minimal side effects (e.g., sedation, respiratory depression)
(c) Local anesthetics may be added to epidural narcotics for a multimodal approach to pain control.
(d) Patient-controlled analgesia (PCA) can also be used to minimize postoperative narcotic use.

2. **Hematologic management**
  a. Complications
    (1) DVT
    (2) PE
    (3) Inadequate hemostasis (e.g., hemoperitoneum)
    (4) Ischemic stroke
  b. Reducing postoperative risk
    (1) Early ambulation
    (2) Sequential compression devices
    (3) Heparin chemoprophylaxis
      (a) Absolute contraindications—active bleeding, severe bleeding diathesis, severe thrombocytopenia (<20,000/µL), neurosurgery, recent ocular surgery (within 10 days), intracranial hemorrhage (e.g., subdural hematoma) within 48 hours
      (b) Relative contraindications—mild-to-moderate bleeding diathesis, moderate thrombocytopenia (20,000–100,000/µL), brain metastasis, recent major trauma, major abdominal surgery within past 2 days, gastrointestinal or genitourinary bleeding, infective endocarditis, malignant hypertension

3. **Renal management**
  a. Complications
    (1) Oliguria or anuria
    (2) Electrolyte abnormalities
    (3) Acid-base imbalances
    (4) Symptomatic or severe uremia
  b. Reducing postoperative risk
    (1) Hyperkalemia with electrocardiogram changes
      (a) IV calcium
      (b) Dextrose (half ampule of 50 dextrose [D50]) followed by insulin (10 units)
      (c) Kayexalate (5 g) oral or per rectum
      (d) Hemodialysis if refractory

4. **Endocrine management**
  a. Complications
    (1) Hyperglycemia
    (2) Hypoglycemia
    (3) Acute adrenal insufficiency

  b. Reducing postoperative risk
   (1) American Diabetes Association recommendations for target inpatient blood glucose concentrations
      (a) General surgical patient—random less than 180 mg/dL, fasting 90–126 mg/dL
         (i) Better glycemic control equates to lower infection rates
      (b) Cardiac surgical patient—less than 150 mg/dL
         (i) Better glycemic control reduces mortality and sternal wound infections
      (c) Critically ill patient—80–110 mg/dL
   (2) Steroid coverage for adrenal insufficiency
      (a) Hydrocortisone phosphate or hemisuccinate—100 mg IV piggyback preoperatively, then every 6 hours for the first 24 hours
      (b) If response is adequate, then reduce dosage to 50 mg every 6 hours for the next 24 hours, then taper to maintenance dosage over 3–5 days
         (i) Resume home-dose steroids when able to take oral medications
      (c) If fever, hypotension, or other complications occur, maintain or increase hydrocortisone dosage to 200–400 mg for 24 hours.
      (d) If there is evidence of potassium wasting, consider switching to methylprednisolone (Solu-Medrol).
      (e) Note that high-dose steroid regimens can impair wound healing, increase catabolism, induce electrolyte imbalances, and increase infectious complications.
5. Management of postoperative fever
  a. All pyrogens converge on the release of interleukin-1, a proinflammatory cytokine, which affects thermoregulatory neurons in the anterior hypothalamus
  b. Common causes of fever (the five Ws)
   (1) *W*ind—atelectasis, pneumonia
   (2) *W*ater—urinary tract infection
   (3) *W*ound infection
   (4) *W*alking—thrombophlebitis
   (5) *W*onder drugs—drug-induced fever
  c. Timing of fever
   (1) Less than 24 hours—classically relegated to atelectasis due to inability to clear pulmonary secretions, but more likely be due to effect of systemic inflammatory cytokine release after major surgery
   (2) 24–48 hours—respiratory complications, catheter-related infection
   (3) 48–72 hours—bloodstream infection, thrombophlebitis, wound infection, urinary tract infection, pneumonitis, intraabdominal abscess, postoperative pancreatitis, drug allergy, *Candida* sepsis if receiving total parenteral nutrition, other causes

6. **Management of wound complications**
   a. Wound infection
      (1) Etiology
          (a) Most commonly due to skin flora *(Staphylococcus, Streptococcus)*
          (b) Less commonly secondary to *Enterococcus*, *Pseudomonas, Proteus,* or *Klebsiella*
      (2) Incidence
          (a) Clean, atraumatic, uninfected wound—3.3%–4.0%
          (b) Clean wounds without emergent operation, drained wounds, stab wounds—7.4%
          (c) Controlled entrance into bronchus, gastrointestinal tract, or oropharyngeal cavity—10.8%
          (d) Perforated viscus—28.3%
      (3) Risk factors
          (a) Advanced age
          (b) Steroids
          (c) Obesity
          (d) Duration of operation
          (e) Malnutrition
      (4) Prevention
          (a) Proper skin preparation
          (b) Bowel preparation if indicated
          (c) Prophylactic antibiotics
          (d) Meticulous technique with minimal tissue handling
          (e) Temperature control
          (f) Appropriate drainage
          (g) Irrigation with antibiotic solutions is controversial
      (5) Management
          (a) Depends on degree of infection
          (b) Ranges from opening the incision to radical débridement
          (c) Antibiotics for gram-positive cocci (cefazolin or cephalexin) indicated if there is surrounding cellulitis and edema
   b. Wound hematoma
      (1) Etiology
          (a) Inadequate hemostasis
      (2) Risk factors
          (a) Anticoagulation
          (b) Fibrinolysis
          (c) Polycythemia vera
          (d) Myeloproliferative disorders
          (e) Hypocoagulable disorders
      (3) Management
          (a) If discovered early or hemodynamically unstable—return to operating room for hematoma evacuation and hemostasis
          (b) If discovered late—warm compresses and expectant management

 c. Fascial dehiscence
  (1) Etiology
   (a) Usually due to technical error
   (b) Incidence of 0.5%–3.0%
  (2) Risk factors
   (a) Malnutrition
   (b) Hypoproteinemia
   (c) Morbid obesity
   (d) Steroid use
   (e) Malignancy
   (f) Uremia
   (g) Diabetes mellitus
   (h) Increased abdominal pressure
  (3) Management
   (a) Fluid resuscitation
   (b) Application of sterile dressing
   (c) Return to operating room for débridement and repair

RECOMMENDED READINGS

Fleisher L, et al. ACC/AHA 2006 guideline update on perioperative cardiovascular evaluation for noncardiac surgery: focused update on perioperative beta-blocker therapy. *J Am Coll Cardiol*. 2006;47:2343–2355.

Goldman L, Caldera DL, Nussbaum SR, et al. Multifactorial index of cardiac risk in noncardiac surgical procedures. *N Engl J Med*. 1977;297:845.

Lee TH, Marcantonio ER, Mangione CM, et al. Derivation and prospective validation of a simple index for prediction of cardiac risk of major noncardiac surgery. *Circulation*. 1999;100:1043–1049.

Van den Berghe G, Wilmer A, Hermans G, et al. Intensive insulin therapy in the medical ICU. *N Engl J Med*. 2006;354:449–461.

Wells PS, Owen C, Doucette S, Fergusson D, Tran H. Does this patient have deep vein thrombosis? *JAMA*. 2006;295:199–207.

Suture Types, Needle Types, and Instruments

Drew D. Jung, MD

Give us the tools, and we will finish the job.

—Winston Churchill

Despite sufficient knowledge of anatomy, pathophysiology, and disease processes, a surgeon will be lost in the operating room without a comprehensive knowledge of the surgical tools at his or her disposal. Learning the nomenclature and specific utility of all the various tools in the operating room can be a daunting task for a surgeon in training. The focus of this chapter is to outline the most common tools encountered. It is by no means an exhaustive list, and thus it is imperative to stay up to date as new suture material, needles, and instruments are developed.

I. SUTURE MATERIAL

A. THE OPTIMAL SUTURE

1. **Easy to handle**
   a. Properties inherent to the suture material. Some suture is more rigid than others. Some suture has high degree of memory—it retains its coiled shape from packaging. Manipulation should require minimal concentration and should have a high degree of ease when securing knots.
2. **High tensile strength**
   a. Tensile strength is defined as the maximal stress the suture material can withstand before breaking.
   b. Suture with high tensile strength can secure tough tissue or tissue prone to high shear and mechanical forces.
3. **Minimal tissue reaction**
   a. Suture results in local tissue inflammation due to presence of a foreign body. Ideal suture has minimal local tissue inflammation.
4. **Antimicrobial properties**
   a. Suture can harbor microbes within the individual strands. Ideally, suture material should limit the number of microbes it introduces to the body or can be coated with antimicrobial substances.
5. **High plasticity and elasticity**
   a. Plasticity is defined as the ability to be easily shaped or molded.
   b. Elasticity is defined as the ability of a material to resume its normal shape after being stretched or compressed.
   c. These qualities allow suture to adapt to anchoring tissue as it expands and contracts.
6. **Low cost**

B. SUTURE CHARACTERISTICS

1. Absorbable versus nonabsorbable (Tables 6.1 and 6.2)
   a. Absorbable sutures will be broken down and dissolve over time. This will result in loss of tensile strength as the suture is absorbed.

TABLE 6.1

COMMON ABSORBABLE SUTURES

Suture	Material	Filament	Tissue Reaction	Tensile Strength	Complete Absorption (Days)
Catgut	Cow or sheep intestinal submucosa	Twisted	Moderate	Poor	80
Chromic catgut	Same as above plus tanned with chromic salts to delay absorption	Twisted	Moderate	Poor	>120
Polyglycolic acid	Polymer of glycolic acid	Braided or monofilament	Low	Good	90–120
Polyglactic acid	Copolymer of glycolide and L-lactide	Braided	Low	Good	60–90
Polydioxanone	Polymer of paradioxanone	Monofilament	Low	Greatest	180
Polytrimethylene carbonate	Copolymer of glycolide and trimethylene carbonate	Monofilament	Low	Good	180–210

Data from Tajirian AL. A review of sutures and other skin closure materials. *J Cosmet Laser Ther.* 2010;12:296–302.

TABLE 6.2

COMMON NONABSORBABLE SUTURES

Suture	Material	Filament	Tissue Reaction	Tensile Strength	Handling
Surgical silk	Silk	Braided or twisted	High	Low	Good
Nylon	Polymers of nylon	Monofilament or braided (rare)	Low	High	Poor
Polypropylene	Polymers of propylene	Monofilament	Least	Good	Poor
Braided polyester	Braided polyethylene terephthalate	Braided	Low	High	Good
Polybutester	Copolymer of polyglycol terephthalate and polybutylene terephthalate	Monofilament	Low	High	Good (high elasticity)

Data from Tajirian AL. A review of sutures and other skin closure materials. *J Cosmet Laser Ther.* 2010;12:296–302.

Absorbable sutures are further subdivided by the length of time it takes for the suture to be dissolved, which can range from days to weeks.
b. Nonabsorbable suture is not naturally broken down and retains much of its tensile strength over time.

2. **Synthetic versus natural**
   a. Either can be absorbable or nonabsorbable.
   b. Synthetic material that is nonabsorbable is inert. Absorbable material has a predictable pattern of absorption. They usually are monofilament—thus are easy to handle.
   c. Natural material has very good handling but is associated with tissue reaction

3. **Monofilament versus polyfilament**
   a. Monofilament has a smooth surface, causes less tissue trauma, does not harbor bacteria, and does not draw water up via capillary action. It is more prone to stretching.
   b. Polyfilament (braided) suture is stronger, more pliable, has good handling, and results in stronger knots. However, it can harbor bacteria, causes tissue trauma, and draws water up via capillary action.

4. **Size**
   a. Range is from 10-0 to 7.
   b. The smallest is 10-0; 7 is the largest.
   c. Smaller suture size may require magnification assistance (loupes, microscope).
   d. The larger the suture is, the greater the tensile strength is.
   e. Each type of suture comes in various sizes. The specific vendor can be contacted to figure out the various sizes available for purchase.
   f. General uses for suture size
      (1) Size: 10-0 to 8-0
         (a) Diameter: 0.02–0.04 mm
         (b) Common in ophthalmic surgery, microsurgery, small nerve and vascular injury (usually in the hand)
      (2) Size: 7-0 to 6-0
         (a) Diameter: 0.05–0.07 mm
         (b) Repairing small vessels and nerves, vascular grafts
      (3) Size: 5-0 to 4-0
         (a) Diameter: 0.1–0.15 mm
         (b) Larger vessels (abdominal aorta), skin closure
      (4) Size: 3-0 to 2-0
         (a) Diameter: 0.2–0.3 mm
         (b) Skin closure, bowel repair/anastomosis, vessel ligation
      (5) Size: 0 to 1
         (a) Diameter: 0.35–0.4 mm
         (b) Closing fascia, joint capsules, deep layers of back
      (6) Size: 2 to 5
         (a) Diameter: 0.5–0.7 mm
         (b) Tendon repair, orthopedic surgery

SUTURE TYPES, NEEDLE TYPES, AND INSTRUMENTS

6

    (7) Size: 6 to 7

        (a) Diameter: 0.8–0.9 mm

        (b) Available only in surgical steel; closure of sternotomy

5. **Plasticity**

  a. Ability of suture to retain new form/length after stretching

6. **Elasticity**

  a. Ability of suture to retain original form/length after stretching

C. ABSORBABLE SUTURE

1. **Loses majority of tensile strength within 60 days**
2. **Broken down enzymatically or hydrolytically**

  a. When undergoing absorption, suture first loses tensile strength and then loses mass (i.e., a suture will persist long after its functional use has been eliminated). An absorbable suture will usually persist (unless manually removed) anywhere from 60 to 210 days, depending on the material.

3. **Natural absorbable suture**

  a. Plain catgut

    (1) Made from purified collagen from bovine intestines

    (2) Polyfilament

    (3) Tensile strength lasts 7–10 days

    (4) Stored in a solution of alcohol and water to maintain moisture, handling, and tensile strength

  b. Chromic catgut

    (1) Made from purified collagen from bovine intestines

    (2) Polyfilament

    (3) Coated with chromic acid salts

    (4) Due to coating, absorption of suture is prolonged compared with plain catgut. Tensile strength lasts 21–28 days.

    (5) Does not need to be stored in alcohol solution; allows improved handling and smoothness when tying

  c. Fast catgut

    (1) Made from purified collagen from bovine intestines

    (2) Polyfilament

    (3) Heat treated to hasten suture degradation

    (4) Tensile strength lasts for 3–5 days.

    (5) Intended for skin closure only

4. **Synthetic absorbable suture**

  a. In general, synthetic absorbable sutures hold tensile strength longer than natural absorbable sutures due to decreased inflammatory response and decreased tissue reaction.

  b. Polyglactic acid (Vicryl, Ethicon, Cincinnati, OH)

    (1) Biodegradable copolymer synthesized from glycolic acid and lactide

    (2) Single strands of the copolymer are braided to form a single suture. Braiding allows for excellent handling, high knot security, and high initial tensile strength. A downside to the braided

suture is that the space between the individual strands draw in extracellular fluid and can harbor bacteria, which may lead to increased wound infection.

(3) Tensile strength is 75% at 14 days and 25% at 28 days.

(4) Also available is irradiated polyglycolic acid (Vicryl Rapide, Ethicon).

    (a) Increases suture degradation

    (b) Tensile strength 50% at 5 days

c. Polyglycolic acid (Dexon, Covidien, Dublin, Ireland)

    (1) Biodegradable polymer synthesized from glycolic acid

    (2) Braided suture

    (3) Tensile strength 89% at 7 days, 63% at 14 days, 17% at 21 days

    (4) Low tissue reactivity, good tensile strength, excellent knot security, excellent handling

d. Poliglecaprone (Monocryl, Ethicon)

    (1) Biodegradable copolymer synthesized from glycolic acid and epsilon-caprolactone

    (2) Monofilament

    (3) Tensile strength 60% at 7 days, 30% at 14 days

    (4) Low tissue reactivity, good tensile strength, good knot security, handling of smaller sizes of suture may be difficult due to high degree of memory

    (5) Generally used for epidermal approximation for skin closure

e. Polydioxanone (PDS; Ethicon)

    (1) Biodegradable polymer synthesized from poly(p-dioxanone)

    (2) Monofilament

    (3) Tensile strength 80% by 14 days, 70% by 28 days, 60% by 42 days

    (4) Low tissue reactivity, excellent tensile strength, moderate knot security, good handling but does have high degree of memory

    (5) Best used in tissue that requires prolonged approximation (abdominal fascia)

f. Polytrimethylene carbonate (Maxon, Covidien)

    (1) Biodegradable copolymer synthesized from glycolic acid and trimethylene carbonate

    (2) Monofilament

    (3) Tensile strength 75% at 14 days, 50% at 28 days, 25% at 42 days

    (4) Similar to PDS but with much easier handling due to minimal memory

D. NONABSORBABLE SUTURE

1. Not affected by hydrolysis or proteolysis
2. Tensile strength intact for much longer than absorbable sutures
3. Generally used for skin closures, tendon and nerve repair, vascular ligation and repair

SUTURE TYPES, NEEDLE TYPES, AND INSTRUMENTS

6

4. **Natural nonabsorbable suture**
   a. Surgical silk (Permahand, Ethicon; Sofsilk, Covidien)
      (1) Composed of fibroin, an organic protein derived from domesti-cated *Bombyx mori* (silkworm)
      (2) Braided
      (3) Dyed black for easier visibility
      (4) Coated with either wax or silicone
         (a) Minimizes water absorption and tissue friction
      (5) Tensile strength is gradually lost over time as more water is absorbed and is completely lost by 1 year.
      (6) Extremely easy to handle, good knot security
5. **Synthetic nonabsorbable suture**
   a. Nylon (Ethilon, Ethicon; Dermalon, Covidien)
      (1) First synthetic suture, composed of nylon 6
      (2) Monofilament
      (3) Tensile strength lost at rate of 15%–20% annually
      (4) High tensile strength, low tissue reactivity, excellent knot secu-rity, high elasticity, difficult to handle due to high memory
         (a) May be soaked in alcohol to reduce memory
   b. Polypropylene (Prolene, Ethicon; Surgilene, Covidien)
      (1) Made from catalytic polymerization of propylene
      (2) Monofilament
      (3) Higher tensile strength compared with nylon; does not lose strength over time
      (4) Low tissue reactivity, low knot security, high plasticity
   c. Surgical steel
      (1) Synthetic alloy consisting of chromium, nickel, molybdenum
      (2) Monofilament
      (3) Good tensile strength and corrosion resistance
      (4) Used in orthopedics and cardiac surgery (closure of sternotomy); very difficult to handle comparatively

E. SUMMARY

1. Suture material is chosen based on type of tissue being approximated. In general, nonabsorbable suture is used on tissues for which high ten-sile strength is needed (tendons/ligaments) or externally on the skin and removed at a later date. Absorbable suture is chosen based on how long tensile strength is required (i.e., how quickly the tissue will heal and no longer require approximation by suture).
2. Suture choices for common general surgery indications
   a. Skin closure
      (1) A 3-0 absorbable suture (e.g., Vicryl) is used to approximate the subcutaneous tissue and Scarpa fascia.
      (2) Epidermis is approximated either with a running absorbable mono-filament (e.g., 4-0 Monocryl) or with an interrupted nonabsorbable monofilament (e.g., Nylon, usually a larger size 1, 0, 1-0, 2-0).

b. Abdominal wall fascia is generally closed with looped 0 PDS (a large synthetic absorbable suture).

c. Bowel anastomosis is performed using 3-0 Prolene to approximate the mucosal and submucosal layers and 3-0 silks to oversew the anastomotic suture line with serosa.

d. Vascular anastomosis is performed using 6-0 or 7-0 Prolene (nonabsorbable synthetic monofilament). This prevents trauma to the blood vessel when running the suture through the tissue. In addition, the lack of capillary action prevents the suture from swelling and contracting, which would result in tissue trauma and anastomotic leaks. Material with high tensile strength and elasticity is needed to protect the anastomosis from pulsatile pressure.

II. NEEDLES

1. Classified by needle point, shape, thickness, and suture attachment
2. Each type of suture can come on various needles (Fig. 6.1).
3. Needle point
   a. Cutting
      (1) Three cutting edges
      (2) Allows easy passage through dense, tough tissue
      (3) Repetitive use will dull the needle point.
      (4) Avoid grasping the tip of a cutting needle to prevent unintended blunting.
   b. Tapered
      (1) Round body
         (a) Spreads tissue without cutting
         (b) Used on less dense/fibrous tissue
         (c) Commonly used for anastomoses
      (2) Cutting
         (a) Combines round body tapered needle with advantages of cutting
         (b) Cutting tip allows easy penetration of denser tissue.
         (c) Tapered body prevents further cutting as needle is pulled through tissue.
         (d) Commonly used for sclerotic vessels or tendon repair
   c. Blunt
      (1) Tapered body with rounded tip
      (2) Prevents damage to friable tissue
      (3) Commonly used on liver and kidney
4. Needle shape
   a. Straight needle
      (1) Designed to be used by hand without the aid of a needle driver or forceps
      (2) Used when tissue is easily accessible (i.e., skin)

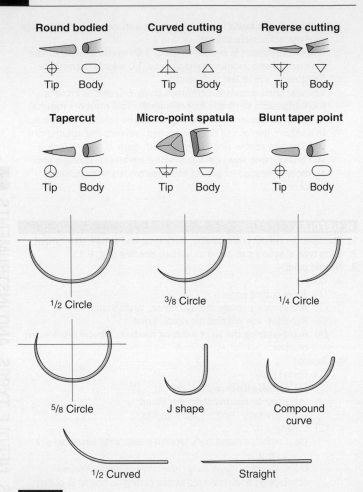

Round bodied

Tip   Body

Curved cutting

Tip   Body

Reverse cutting

Tip   Body

Tapercut

Tip   Body

Micro-point spatula

Tip   Body

Blunt taper point

Tip   Body

1/2 Circle

3/8 Circle

1/4 Circle

5/8 Circle

J shape

Compound curve

1/2 Curved

Straight

FIG. 6.1

Various shapes of needles. (Adapted from www.stayguardwoundcare.com.)

  b. Curved needle
    (1) Requires assistance of a needle driver
    (2) Comes in various arcs
      (a) 1/4, 3/8, 1/2, 5/8 of a circle
    (3) The greater the curvature, the deeper the needle penetration
5. Needle body
  a. Heavy

(1) Resistant to bending

(2) Best for going through tough tissue (i.e., abdominal fascia)

b. General

(1) Withstands bending with routine use

c. Vascular

(1) The size of the needle body is similar to the size of the suture. This ensures that the hole made by the needle piercing the vessel is completely filled by the suture to prevent bleeding.

6. **Attachment**

a. Eyed needle

(1) Requires suture to be threaded by a member of the surgical team

b. Swaged needle

(1) Suture is inserted into the base of the needle.

(2) Available in control-release (commonly called a "pop-off" needle). The needle can be easily removed from the suture to facilitate hand tying.

7. **Commonly used needles**

a. RB1—small, tapered point, ½ circle, commonly used for vascular anastomoses

b. CT1—larger, thick, tapered point, ½ circle, most common general closure needle

c. SH—tapered point, ½ circle, larger than RB1, most commonly used for bowel anastomoses

d. CTX—similar to CT1, but larger and thicker

III. INSTRUMENTS

1. **Needle holder—designed to grasp needle and assist with suturing**

2. **Scissors**

a. Heavy scissors (Mayo)

(1) Mainly used for cutting suture but can be used for some general abdominal dissection and débridement of necrotic soft tissue

b. Fine scissors (Metzenbaum, Potts, Iris)

(1) Smaller tips allow for improved precision.

(2) They are used for assistance with general dissection.

(3) Metzenbaum scissors are used for dividing tissue and dissection in subcutaneous and intraabdominal tissue. Potts and Iris scissors are much more fine tipped than Metzenbaum scissors and are generally used for very precise dissection (in the hand, around nerves/tendons).

3. **Dissecting forceps (Adson, Bonney, DeBakey, rat tooth)**

a. Designed to grasp tissue to aid with dissection, suturing

b. Must be handled gently because excessive force can damage tissue

c. Toothed versus blunt

6

SUTURE TYPES, NEEDLE TYPES, AND INSTRUMENTS

(1) Toothed graspers used on tougher tissue; allow improved handling of tissue
(2) Blunt graspers used with delicate tissue and the presence of teeth can lead to inadvertent damage.

4. Tissue forceps
   a. Designed to grasp tissue and aid with manipulation and retraction
   b. Most forceps are designed for use on specific tissue, and inappropriate use can result in damage to tissue.
   c. Allis forceps—toothed forceps with broad grasping area, general forceps used to retract, elevate, manipulate soft tissue
   d. Kocher forceps—strong, toothed forceps used for grasping fascia
   e. Babcock—blunt grasper designed for bowel manipulation
   f. Ringed forceps—commonly used to grasp surgical gauze/sponges to assist with dissection or cleaning surgical field

5. Hemostats (mosquito, Kelly, burlisher, right angle)
   a. Used to clamp tissues/vessels to control hemorrhage or assist with ligation
   b. Can also be used to assist with general tissue dissection

6. Retractors
   a. Used for retraction of tissue to improve exposure
   b. Available in various shapes and sizes
   c. Handheld retractors
   d. Self-retaining retractors
      (1) They have a locking mechanism that eliminates the need for manual retraction. This will free up hands of the surgeon and assistant.
      (2) A set of retractors that requires assembly before use. In general, a post is attached to the operating table rail. A circular metal ring is attached to the post and suspended in the air over the operating field. Multiple retractors are secured to the metal ring and used to retract the abdominal wall.

7. Suction (Yankauer, Frasier, Pool)
   a. Used to remove fluid and blood from surgical field

8. Scalpels
   a. Used for skin incisions and occasionally sharp dissection
   b. #10 blade—broad base, used for large incisions
   c. #11 blade—V-shaped, used for stab incisions (incision and drainage, trocar placement)
   d. #15 blade—essentially a smaller version of a #10, used for smaller incisions, precise débridement and dissection, plastic/cosmetic procedures)

RECOMMENDED READINGS

Patel KA. Sutures, ligatures and staples. *Surgery (Oxford)*. 2008;26:48–53.
Tajirian AL. A review of sutures and other skin closure materials. *J Cosmet Laser Ther*. 2010;12:296–302.

Anesthesia

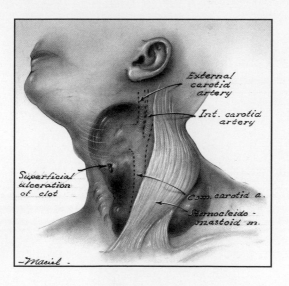

External carotid artery

Int. carotid artery

Superficial ulceration of clot

Com. carotid a.

Sternocleido-mastoid m.

-Maciel-

PART II

Anesthesia

Local Anesthesia

Fernando Ovalle Jr., MD

The safest sedation is no sedation.

—Anonymous

Local anesthesia is not only a common adjunct to higher levels of sedation but may also be an effective stand-alone method of anesthesia in many situations. When used appropriately, local anesthesia can simplify the treatment of many surgical ailments without the dangers and costs of general anesthesia. The surgeon should have an understanding of the risks, benefits, and appropriate applications. Understanding anatomy and the limits of regional anesthesia is important for appropriate clinical use.

I. INJECTABLE AGENTS

A. MECHANISM OF ACTION

1. Block conduction in nerves by impairing propagation of action potential (sodium channel mediated)
   a. Only uncharged forms enter peripheral nerves; thus local anesthetics perform better in alkaline environments.
   b. Infected and inflamed fields can be treated more effectively by alkalinizing the solution with bicarbonate (HCO_3) (see later for preparation).
   c. After the agent reaches the cytoplasm, the ionized form is able to block sodium channels.
2. Differential blockade of nerve fibers
   a. Myelinated and smaller nerves are most affected.
   b. Clinical sequence of sensations anesthetized based on order of nerve fibers blocked is autonomic/vasodilation > pain > temperature > pressure > motor function.

B. CLASSES

1. Amides
   a. Metabolism is hepatic.
   b. Elimination half-life is 2–3 hours.
   c. True allergy is rare.
   d. These include a second letter *i* in their name (i.e., lidocaine).
   e. Examples are lidocaine, bupivacaine, prilocaine, and ropivacaine.
2. Esters
   a. Metabolism is by pseudocholinesterases, which create a short plasma half-life.
   b. These do not contain a second letter *i* in their name.
   c. Examples are procaine, chloroprocaine, cocaine, and tetracaine.
3. Commonly available local anesthetics
   a. Table 7.1

TABLE 7.1

PROPERTIES OF COMMONLY AVAILABLE LOCAL ANESTHETICS

Name	Class	Onset (min)	Duration (h) (Without/With Epinephrine)	Max Dose (mg/kg) (Without/With Epinephrine)
Procaine (Novocaine)	Ester	2–5	0.25–1	7
Chloroprocaine (Nesacaine)	Ester	<1	0.5	11
Lidocaine (Xylocaine)	Amide	2–5	1–2/2–4	4.5/7
Bupivacaine (Marcaine)	Amide	5–15	3–4/4–8	2.5/3
Liposomal bupivacaine (Exparel)	Amide (slow release)	5–15	Up to 72 h	266 mg total (amount in 20-mL vial)
Ropivacaine (Naropin)	Amide	10–15	2–6	2.5

4. Commonly used solutions
   a. Lidocaine (quick onset, shorter duration) and bupivacaine (slightly longer onset, longer duration) are the most common local anesthetics used.
   b. Quickly calculating maximum dosage
      (1) Convert concentration of local from percentage to mg/cc by multiplying by 10.
         (a) Example: 1% lidocaine = 1 g/100 cc = 10 mg/1 cc (or 0.1 cc/mg)
   c. Multiply patient's weight (kg) by listed dose maximum (mg/kg), and then divide by local anesthetic concentration (mg/cc).
      (1) Example: Using 1% lidocaine with epinephrine (7 mg/kg max dose) on a 70-kg patient: [(70 kg × 7 mg/kg)] / [10 mg/cc] = 49 cc until toxic
   d. Standard solutions:
      (1) For the majority of adult emergency room procedures, a solution of 1% lidocaine with epinephrine works quickly, lasts for a long enough period of time to comfortably perform a procedure, and can be given in enough quantity to avoid problems with toxicity.
      (2) In multitrauma patients or in children, in whom the amount of needed local anesthetic increases and/or the weight of the patient decreases, the need for less concentrated formulations of lidocaine (such as 0.5% and 0.25%) becomes more important to avoid toxicity.
      (3) For combination short- and long-term pain control, prepare a syringe with a 1:1 mixture of 1% lidocaine and 0.5% bupivacaine (may also include bicarbonate as previously discussed to reduce pain of injection).

C. TOXICITY

1. Central nervous system toxicity
   a. Prodromal symptoms: light-headedness, dizziness, metallic taste in mouth, circumoral numbness, and tinnitus
   b. Severe toxicity: seizures, loss of consciousness
2. Cardiovascular toxicity
   a. Symptoms: tachyarrhythmia or bradyarrhythmia, ventricular fibrillation, hypotension
3. Prevention
   a. Avoid excessive doses (calculate maximum dose based on patient's weight).
   b. Avoid intravascular injection (aspirate before injecting to confirm needle tip is not intravascular).
4. Management
   a. Give no more local anesthetic.
   b. Supportive management with airway protection, supplemental oxygen, benzodiazepines for seizure treatment, intravenous (IV) fluid administration for cardiovascular support, arrhythmia treatment according to advanced cardiac life support (ACLS) guidelines
   c. Lipid emulsion therapy
      (1) IV infusion of a 20% lipid emulsion (e.g., Intralipid 20%) has become an accepted part of treatment for systemic toxicity from local anesthetics and particularly for cardiac arrest that is unresponsive to standard therapy.
      (2) American Society of Regional Anesthesia and Pain Medicine (ASRA) guidelines recommend considering the use of lipid emulsion therapy at the first signs of systemic toxicity from local anesthetics, after airway management.
         (a) Give bolus of 1.5 mL/kg over 1 minute.
         (b) Convert to an infusion at a rate of 0.25 mL/kg per minute for 20–60 minutes, or until hemodynamic stability is restored.

D. USE OF EPINEPHRINE

1. Utility
   a. Used in conjunction with local anesthetic to provide hemostasis
   b. Delays absorption of the local anesthetic into the systemic circulation
   c. Allows for a greater concentration of local anesthetic to be used before reaching toxic levels (see Table 7.1)
2. Safety
   a. Subcutaneous injection of epinephrine in combination with local anesthetics to distal areas (such as fingers and toes) has been shown to be safe without evidence of necrosis over multiple studies.
   b. Current recommendations include low-dose use of epinephrine, typically injected at a concentration of 1:100,000–400,000.
   c. Avoid circumferential injection if possible.

7

LOCAL ANESTHESIA

3. Optimal timing between injection and incision
   a. The time until maximal cutaneous vasoconstriction after injection of lidocaine with epinephrine is historically reported as 7–10 minutes.
   b. If optimal visualization is desired, waiting longer to make an incision after injection with epinephrine must be considered and weighed against delaying the start of the procedure.

II. TECHNIQUES

A. BEFORE INJECTING LOCAL ANESTHETIC IN TRAUMATIC INJURIES, BE SURE TO PERFORM AND DOCUMENT A DETAILED SENSORY EXAMINATION, WHICH MAY BE SUBSEQUENTLY MASKED BY YOUR BLOCK

B. OPTIMAL TIMING BETWEEN INJECTION AND INCISION

1. The time until maximal cutaneous vasoconstriction after injection of lidocaine with epinephrine is historically reported as 7–10 minutes.
2. If optimal visualization is desired, waiting longer to make an incision after injection with epinephrine must be considered and weighed against delaying the start of the procedure.

C. GENERAL TECHNIQUES TO DECREASE PAIN

1. Use smaller gauge needles (25 G or smaller).
2. If there is an open wound/laceration, inject through open skin edges.
3. If injecting through intact skin,
   a. Orient needle perpendicular to skin and inject 0.5–1 cc immediately below the dermis.
   b. When area is deemed anesthetized, redirect the needle more parallel to the skin, progressing and injecting slowly along the path of planned infiltration to ensure the anesthetic remains ahead of the needle at all times.
4. Add bicarbonate (8.4% solution) to alkalinize the solution and reduce the burning pain associated with the lower pH of the anesthetic.
   a. In a 10-cc syringe, add 1 cc of bicarbonate to 9 cc of local anesthetic.

D. FIELD BLOCKS

1. A field block involves blocking nerves circumferentially around the periphery of a wound. It is useful for wounds without a specific nerve or nerves that can be blocked directly.

E. NERVE BLOCKS FOR THE FACE

1. Supratrochlear and supraorbital nerve block (V1)
   a. The supraorbital and supratrochlear nerves and extensions of the frontal branch of the first division of the trigeminal after it exits the supraorbital fissure. Together, they supply sensory innervation to the anterior scalp.

b. The supraorbital foramen can be located at the superior orbital rim above the pupil in midline gaze. Palpate the foramen while retracting the brow laterally.

c. Enter the lateral aspect of the middle third of the brow, and aim for the foramen.

d. Inject 2 mL at this point. Keep your other hand at the orbital rim to protect the orbit. Advance the needle, continuing a wheal until the nasal bone is contacted; 2–5 mL of desired local agent should be used.

2. Infraorbital nerve block (V2)

a. The infraorbital nerve is an extension of the second division of the trigeminal. It provides sensation to the lower eyelid, upper lip, the tip and lateral aspect of the nose, and part of the nasal septum.

b. The infraorbital foramen can be located just approximately 1 cm below the orbital rim, in line with the midpoint of the pupil in midline gaze.

c. An intraoral route is generally preferred; inject a wheal into the gingivobuccal sulcus just above the maxillary first premolar. While palpating the foramen externally, advance the needle to contact maxilla adjacent to the foramen. Keep a finger firmly on the orbital rim to protect the orbit.

d. Inject 1–2 mL while your external digit feels the wheal expand.

3. Inferior alveolar nerve block (V3)

a. There are multiple approaches to anesthetize the inferior alveolar nerve through intraoral injections. The preferred approach to access the nerve high in its course is percutaneous. This is preferable in trauma to the mouth and mandible because the patient may not tolerate intraoral injection.

b. Just below the zygoma, the sigmoid notch of the mandible can be palpated 2.5 cm anterior to the tragus. Ask the patient to open and close his or her mouth; the condyle will bump against your finger.

c. Administer a subcutaneous wheal at the midpoint of the sigmoid notch.

d. With a long fine-gauge needle, such as a 25-G spinal needle, enter straight through the anterior portion of the sigmoid notch, and advance until it hits the pterygoid plate. Note the needle position, and retract the needle almost out of the skin. Advance the needle to the same depth, aiming 1 cm posterior to the previous point of pterygoid contact. Aspirate and inject 3–4 mL.

e. The anesthetized area includes most of the cheek from the preauricular area to the mandibular border, the mandible to midline.

f. Alternatively, the intraoral approach can be performed. With the patient's mouth maximally opened, identify the maxillary second molar. The syringe should angle such that it crosses the contralateral oral commissure. Advance the needle approximately 2.5 cm until the condyle is encountered, and aspirate. Withdraw 1 mm and advance superiorly. Aspirate again and, if negative, inject 2–3 mL of local.

7

LOCAL ANESTHESIA

4. **Mental nerve block (terminal V3)**
   a. The mental foramen varies in position from 1 cm distal to 1 cm mesial to the second mandibular bicuspid, most commonly found between the apices of the first and second mandibular premolars.
   b. Effective blocks are achieved by engaging the nerve within 1 cm of the foramen. An intraoral approach is preferred. Apply lateral traction on the lower lip near the canine. The nerve is sometimes visible or palpable through the mucosa while on traction.
   c. Injection of 2 mL submucosal in this area provides anesthesia to the ipsilateral lower lip.
   d. To completely anesthetize the chin, block the distal branches of the mental nerve and the mylohyoid branches by inserting the needle anterior to the canine and passing the inferior border of the mandible. Inject 2 mL using a fanning technique. These regions are all covered by an inferior alveolar nerve (V3) block.

5. **Dorsal nasal block**
   a. The dorsal nasal nerve, a branch of the anterior ethmoidal, emerges at the inferior border of the nasal bone approximately 6 mm from midline. Bilateral injection at these points (or a wheal across the cranial dorsum of the nose) anesthetizes the nasal tip and cartilaginous dorsum.

6. **Zygomaticotemporal and zygomaticofacial block**
   a. The zygomaticotemporal and zygomaticofacial nerves exit foramens on the concave lateral orbital rim. They are addressed by palpating the zygomaticofrontal suture and inserting a needle 0.5 cm inferior to the suture and 1 cm posterior to the superolateral orbital rim.
   b. Aiming 1 cm below to the lateral canthus, the zygoma is encountered; 2–3 mL of local anesthesia is injected while withdrawing the needle.
   c. Area of anesthesia includes the temporal scalp abutting the area of supraorbital innervation and the zygomatic arch. The zygomaticofacial block includes a wedge of the lateral malar check area overlying the zygoma.

7. **Great auricular nerve block**
   a. To identify the greater auricular nerve, have the patient turn his or her head against your hand placed on the ipsilateral forehead.
   b. At the midpoint of the sternocleidomastoid (SCM), 6.5 cm from the inferior aspect of the external auditory canal, the nerve can be reliably located.
   c. Inject 2 mL of local anesthesia just over the muscle at this point. Anesthesia is provided to the lower third of the ear, postauricular skin, and a variable area of the tragus down toward the mandibular angle. The ear should be addressed as a field block because there are multiple nerve contributions. Injecting a large wheal anterior and posterior connecting with each other will anesthetize the entire ear.

F. NERVE BLOCKS FOR THE UPPER EXTREMITY

1. When performing nerve blocks, ask patients to describe any electrical/shooting pains, which may indicate the needle tip is positioned inside the nerve. If this occurs, reposition the needle before injecting.

2. Digital block
   a. Provides anesthesia for fingers from base to tip by blocking the digital nerves bilaterally.
   b. Start by injecting a wheal to either side of the base of the proximal phalanx of the finger to be anesthetized.
   c. Insert the needle adjacent to the phalanx, and advance until you observe the needle tent the volar skin.
   d. Inject a 2-mL wheal and slowly remove the needle, delivering another milliliter.
   e. Next, without exiting the skin, create a wheal across the dorsum of the finger, and repeat the procedure through anesthetized skin to bathe the contralateral digital nerve.

3. Wrist block (provides complete hand anesthesia)
   a. It targets the median and ulnar nerves and the dorsal sensory branch of the radial nerve.
   b. Depending on the area of injury or procedure, only parts of the wrist block may be necessary. The individual distributions of and approaches to the median, ulnar, and radial nerves are outlined below.

4. Median nerve block
   a. The median nerve sits just below and radial to the palmaris longus under the flexor retinaculum, and its sensory branches innervate the radial three and a half digits, as well corresponding area on the palm.
   b. Injection landmarks include the palmaris longus if present and the flexor carpi radialis at the wrist crease.
   c. Ulnar to the palmaris longus at the level of the distal wrist crease, inject a subcutaneous wheal to anesthetize the skin; then advance the needle through the fascia. A "click" may or may not be noted.
   d. Advance at a 45- to 60-degree angle, aiming at the base of the fourth finger to contact the bone of the distal carpal row.
   e. Withdraw the needle approximately 2 mm, aspirate, and inject 2–4 mL local anesthesia with gentle pressure. If the local does not flow freely, reposition the needle.
   f. Injecting in a fanning manner by performing initial injection, then repeating, aiming toward the third digit, may improve success.

5. Ulnar nerve block
   a. The ulnar nerve sits between the flexor carpi ulnaris and the ulnar artery, and its sensory branches innervate the ulnar one and a half digits and corresponding area on the palm.
   b. The flexor carpi ulnaris tendon can be easily identified by having the patient forcefully flex and ulnarly deviate the wrist.
   c. The preferred approach is to enter the ulnar (medially) aspect of the wrist just dorsal (deep/underneath) to the flexor carpi ulnaris after administering a skin wheal.

7

LOCAL ANESTHESIA

   d. Insert the needle 5–10 mm aiming radially, aspirate, and inject 3–5 mL of local anesthesia. An additional 2 mL is useful subcutaneously to block cutaneous branches to the hypothenar area.

6. **Radial nerve block**
   a. The dorsal sensory branches of the radial nerve are multiple and less predictable than the other nerves described. They innervate most of the dorsum of the hand and wrist.
   b. To anesthetize the radial nerve–innervated portion of the hand, use a subcutaneous field block from the radial styloid to the radial dorsum of the wrist; approximately 5 mL is required.

III. TOPICAL AGENTS

A. **TOPICAL ANESTHESIA CAN AVOID THE PAIN AND ANXIETY OF NEEDLE INJECTION AND IS ESPECIALLY USEFUL IN THE PEDIATRIC POPULATION. IT CAN ALSO BE USED AS AN ADJUNCT TO DECREASE SUPERFICIAL SKIN PAIN BEFORE PERFORMING MORE TARGETED NERVE BLOCK WITH AN INJECTABLE LOCAL ANESTHETIC AGENT.**

B. **SYSTEMIC BLOOD LEVELS OF THESE COMPOUNDED TOPICAL ANESTHETICS DEPEND ON THE ABSORPTION, PATIENT SIZE, RATE OF ELIMINATION, AND TYPE OF SURFACE (I.E., MUCOSAL VERSUS EXTRAMUCOSAL AND INTACT VERSUS BROKEN SKIN). TOPICAL AGENTS GENERALLY HAVE A MUCH LONGER TIME OF ONSET THAN INJECTABLES.**

C. **COMMONLY USED PRODUCTS (10)**

1. **TAC (tetracaine 0.5%, adrenaline 1:2000, cocaine 11.8%)**
   a. Effective on face and scalp in approximately 30 minutes
   b. Effectiveness comparable to lidocaine injection
   c. Concern with cocaine absorption on mucosal surfaces has limited use

2. **LET (lidocaine 4%, epinephrine 1:2000, tetracaine 0.5%)**
   a. More cost effective and improved safety over TAC
   b. Effective in 20–30 minutes when applied to open lacerations
   c. Not recommended for use on lacerations greater than 6 cm or complicated wounds

3. **EMLA (eutectic mixture of local anesthetics) consists of 2.5% lidocaine, 2.5% prilocaine, a thickener, an emulsifier, and distilled water adjusted to a pH level of 9.4**
   a. Approved for use on intact skin/nonmucosal surfaces and must be covered by an occlusive dressing to absorb optimally
   b. Provides anesthesia in 45–90 minutes

RECOMMENDED READINGS

Chowdhry S, Seidenstricker L, Cooney DS, et al. Do not use epinephrine in digital blocks: myth or truth? Part II. A retrospective review of 1111 cases. *Plast Reconstr Surg.* 2010;126:2031–2034.

Firoz B, Davis N, Goldberg LH. Local anesthesia using buffered 0.5% lidocaine with 1:200,000 epinephrine for tumors of the digits treated with Mohs micrographic surgery. *J Am Acad Dermatol.* 2009;61:639–643.

Kaweski S. Topical anesthetic creams. *Plast Reconstr Surg.* 2008;121:2161–2165.

Lalonde D, Bell M, Benoit P, et al. A multicenter prospective study of 3,110 consecutive cases of elective epinephrine use in the fingers and hand: the Dalhousie Project clinical phase. *J Hand Surg Am.* 2005;30:1061–1067.

Larrabee Jr WF, Lanier BJ, Miekle D. Effect of epinephrine on local cutaneous blood flow. *Head Neck.* 1987;9:287–289.

McKee DE, Lalonde DH, Thoma A, et al. Optimal time delay between epinephrine injection and incision to minimize bleeding. *Plast Reconstr Surg.* 2013;131:811–814.

Mustoe TA, Buck DW, Lalonde DH. The safe management of anesthesia, sedation, and pain in plastic surgery. *Plast Reconstr Surg.* 2010;126:165e–176e.

Neal JM, Mulroy MF, Weinberg GL. American Society of Regional Anesthesia and Pain Medicine checklist for managing local anesthetic systemic toxicity: 2012 version. *Reg Anesth Pain Med.* 2012;37:16–18.

7

LOCAL ANESTHESIA

Conscious Sedation

Bobby L. Johnson, MD

Some of you say that religion makes people happy. So does laughing gas.

—Clarence Darrow

The ability to understand and administer conscious sedation to perform invasive procedures is a necessity for the practicing surgeon. It is no longer solely the role of the anesthesiologist to provide sedation and analgesia for patients undergoing less complex but still painful or stimulating procedures. A surgeon must be familiar with the pharmacology, physiology, and techniques necessary to safely deliver sedation.

I. INTRODUCTION

A. DEFINITION

1. Sedation is "a minimally depressed level of consciousness that retains the patient's ability to independently and continuously maintain an airway and respond appropriately to physical stimulation and verbal commands" (American Dental Association Council on Education).
2. Sedation comprises a continuum from minimal sedation to general anesthesia (American Society of Anesthesiologists Guidelines) (Table 8.1).

B. APPLICATIONS (SELECTED)

1. Intensive care unit (ICU)/emergency department procedures
2. Central venous line insertions
3. Chest tube insertions
4. Endoscopic procedures
5. Hernia reductions
6. Patients with extensive burns

II. PREPROCEDURAL EVALUATION

A. HISTORY

1. General history and review of systems, including tobacco, alcohol, and drug use history
2. Previous anesthetics and any adverse outcomes
3. Airway abnormalities (e.g., obstructive sleep apnea, severe snoring, stridor, and previous tracheostomy)
4. Chromosomal abnormalities and/or syndromes (e.g., Down syndrome)
5. Gastroesophageal reflux disease/hiatal hernia
6. Obesity
7. Adequate intravenous (IV) access in situ
8. Last meal (food and drink) (see Section II.C)

8

TABLE 8.1				
SEDATION GUIDELINES				
	Minimal Sedation (Anxiolysis)	Moderate Sedation/Analgesia (Conscious Sedation)	Deep Sedation/ Analgesia	General Anesthesia
Responsiveness	Normal response to verbal stimulation	Purposeful[a] response to verbal or tactile stimulation	Purposeful[a] response after repeated or painful stimulation	Unarousable, even with painful stimulus
Airway	Unaffected	No intervention required	Intervention may be required	Intervention often required
Spontaneous ventilation	Unaffected	Adequate	May be inadequate	Frequently inadequate
Cardiovascular function	Unaffected	Usually maintained	Usually maintained	May be impaired

[a]Because sedation is a continuum, it is not always possible to predict how an individual patient will respond. Hence practitioners intending to produce a given level of sedation should be able to rescue patients whose level of sedation becomes deeper than initially intended.

Data from document developed by the American Society of Anesthesiologists (ASA); approved by the ASA House of Delegates, October 13, 1999.

B. AIRWAY EXAMINATION

1. General assessment of patient (e.g., body habitus, presence of cervical collar)
2. Mallampati examination (Fig. 8.1)
3. Mouth opening (adults should have 3- to 4-cm distance between upper and lower incisors)
4. Thyromental distance (distance from thyroid cartilage to mandible; should be at least 5 cm in adults)
5. Neck extension
6. Assessment for any cervical spine abnormalities or disorders associated with atlantooccipital instability
7. Lack of extension or significantly reduced extension may indicate difficulty with direct laryngoscopy
8. Any craniofacial/bony abnormalities
   a. Receding mandible
   b. High, arched palate
   c. Syndromes (e.g., Pierre Robin, Treacher Collins)
9. Dentition
10. Facial hair (presence of a beard or other significant facial hair may signal difficult mask ventilation)

C. AMERICAN SOCIETY OF ANESTHESIOLOGISTS FASTING GUIDELINES (TABLE 8.2)

1. Need to follow for all elective procedures
2. May be modified in emergency situations at discretion of practitioner

8

CONSCIOUS SEDATION

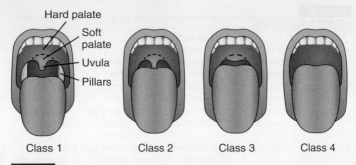

FIG. 8.1

Mallampati classification: class I—faucial pillars, soft palate, and uvula are visible; class II—faucial pillars and soft palate are visible, and uvula view is obstructed by base of tongue; class III—only soft and hard palates are visible; and class IV—only hard palate is visible.

TABLE 8.2

SUMMARY OF FASTING RECOMMENDATIONS TO REDUCE THE RISK FOR PULMONARY ASPIRATION[a]

Ingested Material	Minimum Fasting Period (h)[b]
Clear liquids[c]	2
Breast milk	4
Infant formula	6
Nonhuman milk[d]	6
Light meal[e]	6

[a]These recommendations apply to healthy patients who are undergoing elective procedures. They are not intended for women in labor. Following the guidelines does not guarantee complete gastric emptying.

[b]The fasting periods noted apply to all ages.

[c]Examples of clear liquids include water, fruit juices without pulp, carbonated beverages, clear tea, and black coffee.

[d]Because nonhuman milk is similar to solids in gastric emptying time, the amount ingested must be considered when determining an appropriate fasting period.

[e]A light meal typically consists of toast and clear liquids. Meals that include fried or fatty foods or meat may prolong gastric emptying time. Both the amount and types of foods ingested must be considered when determining an appropriate fasting period.

III. MONITORING

A. BEST ACHIEVED BY SOMEONE OTHER THAN PERSON PERFORMING PROCEDURE

B. PREPROCEDURE
1. Vital signs
2. SpO$_2$
3. Places supplemental oxygen

C. CLINICAL ASSESSMENT
1. Most important monitor
2. Needs to be ongoing

3. Vital signs once every 5 (q5) minutes
4. Level of consciousness q5 minutes

D. CONTINUOUS PULSE OXIMETRY

E. CONTINUOUS ELECTROCARDIOGRAM
1. For evaluation of abnormal cardiac rhythms
2. Can monitor for bradycardia or tachycardia

F. BLOOD PRESSURE
1. Intermittent sphygmomanometry
2. Or monitoring via arterial line

G. CAPNOGRAPHY (USUALLY WITH DEEP SEDATION OR GENERAL ANESTHESIA ONLY; NOT AVAILABLE IN ALL PATIENT CARE AREAS)

H. APPROPRIATE ALARMS ON MONITOR

IV. AVAILABILITY OF EMERGENCY MEDICAL EQUIPMENT AND PERSONNEL

A. IMMEDIATE ACCESS TO SUCTION, BAG-MASK VENTILATION, INTUBATION MATERIALS, DEFIBRILLATOR, AND EMERGENCY (ADVANCED CARDIAC LIFE SUPPORT) MEDICATIONS

B. ANESTHESIA OR OTHER TRAINED AIRWAY STAFF IN CLOSE PROXIMITY

V. TRAINING IN AIRWAY MANAGEMENT

A. ABILITY TO PROVIDE ESCALATING LEVELS OF AIRWAY SUPPORT

B. EXPERIENCE IN CONTROLLED SETTING WITH SKILLED EXPERTS

C. KNOWLEDGE OF AIRWAY ADJUNCTS AND THEIR APPROPRIATE USE

VI. MEDICATIONS

A. GENERAL PRINCIPLES
1. Establish goals/end points of sedation.
2. Drugs should be given in small, incremental doses and titrated to end points of analgesia/sedation.
3. Allow time for onset before repeating.
4. Benzodiazepines and opiates have synergistic effects.
5. For non-IV routes (e.g., oral/rectal/intramuscular [IM]), allow adequate time for absorption (repeat doses not recommended due to unpredictable absorption).

8

CONSCIOUS SEDATION

B. NARCOTICS

1. Narcotics are used for both analgesia and sedation.
2. All produce dose-dependent respiratory depression, with increased risk in those at extremes of age.
3. Other common side effects include but are not limited to orthostatic hypotension, pruritus, nausea and vomiting, constipation, and urinary retention.
4. Doses provided are for adults; see pediatric literature for pediatric dosing:
   a. Morphine sulfate
      (1) Prototypic narcotic
      (2) Initial dose: 2–5 mg IV
      (3) Onset of effect: 5–10 minutes (peak 20–30 minutes)
      (4) Duration of effect: 3–4 hours
      (5) Can cause significant pruritus
   b. Fentanyl (Sublimaze)
      (1) A hundred times more potent than morphine
      (2) Initial dose: 25–50 μg IV
      (3) Onset in 1–3 minutes
      (4) Duration of effect: 30–60 minutes
      (5) Chest wall rigidity at large doses
      (6) Quick on, quick off
   c. Hydromorphone (Dilaudid)
      (1) Approximately 5 times more potent than morphine
      (2) Initial dose: 0.2–0.4 mg IV
      (3) Onset in approximately 15 minutes; peaks at 1 hour
      (4) Lacks histamine release associated with morphine
   d. Meperidine (Demerol)
      (1) One-tenth as potent as morphine
      (2) Initial dose: 12.5–50 mg IV
      (3) Onset time: approximately 5 minutes
      (4) Duration of effect: 2–3 hours (peak 10–20 minutes)
      (5) Helpful with postoperative shivering

C. BENZODIAZEPINES

1. Enhance affinity of receptors for γ-aminobutyric acid (GABA)
2. Produce sedation and anterograde amnesia
3. Anxiolytic and behavioral disinhibitor
4. Side effects: respiratory depression and disorientation
5. CAUTION: may potentiate sedative effects of narcotics; may have paradoxical or exaggerated effects in patients at extremes of age
6. Doses provided are for adults; see pediatric literature for pediatric dosing.
   a. Midazolam (Versed)
      (1) Initial dose of 0.5–2 mg IV
      (2) Onset within 30–60 seconds
      (3) Peak effect at 3–5 minutes
      (4) Duration of sedation (varies): 15–80 minutes
      (5) Elimination half-life is 2–4 hours

      (6) Metabolized by cytochrome P-450 system, excreted by kidney
      (7) Caution for respiratory depression and hypotension
  b. Diazepam (Valium)
      (1) Dose: 2–5 mg IV
      (2) Slower onset (1–3 minutes)
      (3) Duration of effect: 0.5–2 hours
      (4) Several active metabolites prolong effects
      (5) Elimination half-life is 15–21 hours
  c. Lorazepam (Ativan)
      (1) Dose: 0.5–1 mg IV
      (2) Slow onset (5–15 minutes)

D. OTHER COMMON NONBARBITURATE MEDICATIONS

1. **Ketamine**
   a. Primarily an *N*-methyl-D-aspartate (NMDA) antagonist
   b. Dissociative sedative/anesthetic
   c. Initial dose of 0.5–1 mg/kg IV
   d. Onset in 1–3 minutes
   e. Duration of sedation: 10–20 minutes
   f. Little effect on cardiac and respiratory function
   g. Can produce hallucinations
2. **Dexmedetomidine (Precedex)**
   a. Alpha2-adrenergic agonist
   b. Initial dose: 1 µg/kg IV over 10 minutes
   c. Onset of action: 4–6 minutes
   d. Duration of action: 10–20 minutes
   e. Very little respiratory depression and patients often still able to follow commands
   f. Some analgesic properties, but patients will likely need adjuncts for adequate pain control
3. **Propofol (Diprivan)**
   a. Primarily a $GABA_A$ potentiator and sodium channel blocker
   b. Potent IV sedative
   c. No analgesic properties
   d. Use not recommended for light-to-moderate sedation
   e. Causes profound, rapid decline in level of consciousness, producing a state of general anesthesia if not carefully titrated
   f. To administer, practitioners must be able to rescue patient from any level of sedation, including general anesthesia.

VII. REVERSAL MEDICATIONS

A. NALOXONE (NARCAN)

1. Opioid antagonist
2. Dose: 40–100 µg IV (adult dose)
3. Side effects: pulmonary edema, tachycardia, hypertension, arrhythmias, nausea/vomiting, pain

8

CONSCIOUS SEDATION

4. CAUTION: Short duration of action (30–45 minutes) makes redosing often necessary.

B. FLUMAZENIL (ROMAZICON)
1. Benzodiazepine competitive antagonist
2. Initial dose: 0.01 mg/kg IV (maximum, 0.2 mg)
3. Subsequent doses of 0.005–0.01 mg/kg per dose to maximum cumulative dose of 1 mg administered at 60-second intervals
4. Side effects: acute anxiety, hypertension, tachycardia
5. Caution: Duration of action is 30–60 minutes, necessitating redosing.

VIII. RECOVERY AND DISCHARGE
A. GENERAL PRINCIPLES
1. Patients must remain in areas where monitoring is feasible.
2. Patients should be monitored closely at intervals determined by the practitioner until discharge criteria are met.
3. Personnel capable of recognizing and managing complications must be present at all times.

B. DISCHARGE GUIDELINES
1. Vital signs are stable and within acceptable limits for individual patient.
2. Patient is alert and oriented or at baseline mental status.
3. Sufficient time has elapsed since last medication or reversal agent dosage to allow for recovery.
4. Outpatients must have appropriate guardian to escort home and remain with patient for at least 24 hours.
5. Outpatients must receive written instructions for care at home, diet, restrictions, etc.

RECOMMENDED READINGS
Hansen TG. Sedative medications outside the operating room and the pharmacology of sedatives. *Curr Opin Anesthesiol*. 2015;28:446–452.

Hession P, Joshi G. Sedation: not quite that simple. *Anesthesiol Clin*. 2010;28(2):281–294.

Mallampati RS, Gatt SP, Gugino LD, et al. A clinical sign to predict difficult tracheal intubation: a prospective study. *Can Anaesth Soc J*. 1985;32:429–434.

Practice guidelines for preoperative fasting and the use of pharmacologic agents to reduce the risk of pulmonary aspiration: application to healthy patients undergoing elective procedures: a report by The American Society of Anesthesiologists Task Force on Preoperative Fasting. *Anesthesiology*. 1999;90:896–905.

General Anesthesia

Lauren M. Baumann, MD

Although an anesthesiologist plays a critical role in the perioperative management of patients, it is important that the surgeon be familiar with the general principles of anesthesia and their potential impact on the surgical patient. Surgical care of the patient begins in the preoperative period and extends through the postoperative recovery; therefore understanding by the surgeon of anesthetic techniques and recognition and management of complications is essential. Communication between the surgeon and the anesthesiologist is paramount to good perioperative outcomes.

9

I. PREOPERATIVE ASSESSMENT AND PREPARATION

A. SURGICAL INTERVENTION OR PROCEDURE BEING PERFORMED
1. Careful attention must be paid to verification of site.

B. HISTORY AND CHART REVIEW
1. Anesthesia history
   a. Past procedures requiring general or regional anesthesia: difficult airway, success of specific techniques, complications?
   b. Personal or family history of malignant hyperthermia
   c. History of postoperative nausea and vomiting (PONV)
   d. History of difficult intubation
2. Current medications
   a. Special attention paid to anticoagulants, beta-blockers, antihypertensives, diuretics, oral hypoglycemics, and antidepressants, especially monoamine oxidase inhibitors
3. Drug allergies (including latex)
4. Review of systems
   a. Particular attention should be paid to pulmonary and cardiovascular history, including an assessment of functional status with documentation of level of activity.
5. Consults
   a. Previous evaluation by medicine, cardiology, or anesthesia department
6. Fasting status
   a. "Nothing by mouth (NPO) status" (see Chapter 16 for American Society of Anesthesiologists Guidelines)

C. PHYSICAL EXAMINATION
1. Vital signs, including height and weight
2. Airway examination
   a. Size of tongue versus pharynx (Mallampati classes I–IV; see Chapter 16)
   b. Cervical spine mobility
   c. Anterior mandibular space—distance from the notch of the thyroid cartilage to the tip of the mentum (thyromental distance) while the head is

maximally extended; less than 6 cm (receding mandible, short muscular neck) increases the risk for difficulty encountered during intubation.
   d. Dentition—noting loose, chipped, cracked teeth and dentures or dental appliances
3. Neurologic examination—noting preexisting deficits, asymmetry
4. Cardiovascular examination—noting murmurs, S3 gallop, jugular venous distention
5. Respiratory examination
6. Examination of regional anesthesia site (if applicable)
   a. Locating surface anatomy and noting abnormalities including signs of localized infection

D. LABORATORY DATA
1. Complete blood cell count if history of anemia or ongoing bleeding
2. Electrolytes (Na^+, K^+), blood urea nitrogen, and creatinine for patients with a history of renal disease or currently taking diuretics
3. Prothrombin time, international normalized ratio, and partial thromboplastin time if patient is taking anticoagulants or has history of coagulopathy

E. RADIOLOGY, CARDIOLOGY, OTHER PREOPERATIVE TESTING
1. Review relevant imaging (plain radiographs, computed tomography, magnetic resonance imaging, ultrasound)
2. Echocardiogram, exercise or chemical stress test, electrocardiogram (EKG), cardiac catheterization results
3. Pulmonary function tests (particularly if single lung ventilation is needed)

F. ASSESSMENT
1. Make a detailed problem list including pertinent anesthetic, surgical, and medical issues.
2. Assign American Society of Anesthesiologists Physical Classification Status using Emergency designation if appropriate (Table 9.1).

G. ANESTHETIC PLAN
1. Determine appropriate anesthetic technique (see Section II).
2. Determine whether invasive monitoring (arterial line, central venous line, pulmonary artery catheter, transesophageal echocardiography, etc.) is necessary.
3. Decide on method for postoperative pain control (intravenous [IV] narcotics, epidural, or nerve block).
4. Make preliminary decision on patient's postoperative destination (postanesthetic care unit or intensive care unit [ICU]).
5. Determine whether special equipment is necessary (double-lumen endotracheal tube [ETT], fiberoptic bronchoscope, etc.).
6. Explain associated risks and benefits to patient/guardian, and document conversation in the chart.

TABLE 9.1

AMERICAN SOCIETY OF ANESTHESIOLOGISTS (ASA) CLASSIFICATION SYSTEM[a]

ASA I	A normal healthy patient
ASA II	A patient with mild systemic disease
ASA III	A patient with severe systemic disease
ASA IV	A patient with severe systemic disease that is a constant threat to life
ASA V	A moribund patient who is not expected to survive without the operation
ASA VI	A declared brain-dead patient whose organs are being removed for donor purposes

[a]The addition of "E" denotes emergency surgery, when delay in treatment would lead to a significant increase in the threat to life or body part.

H. INDICATIONS FOR DELAYING OR POSTPONING ELECTIVE SURGERY

1. Uncontrolled medical disease (cardiac, respiratory, hepatic, renal, endocrine)
2. Upper respiratory infection
3. Patient noncompliance with fasting guidelines

I. PREOPERATIVE PREPARATION

1. IV access (at least 18 or 20 gauge); may need more than one
2. Placement of invasive lines, epidurals, etc.
3. Administration of preoperative medications (see Section III)

J. PREOPERATIVE MEDICATION GOALS

1. Anxiety relief, sedation, analgesia, and amnesia
2. Control of oral and bronchial secretions
3. Increased gastric pH and decreased gastric secretions; antiemetic effects
4. Preparation for airway manipulations (aerosolized lidocaine, viscous lidocaine)

II. INTRAOPERATIVE MANAGEMENT

A. EQUIPMENT

The equipment listed in this section should be present whenever an anesthetic is administered. This list is not comprehensive, and additional equipment may be necessary depending on the patient and clinical situation.

1. Standard monitors
   a. Noninvasive blood pressure
   b. Pulse oximetry
   c. EKG—leads II and V5
   d. Capnography
   e. Oxygen analyzer
   f. Temperature
2. Anesthesia machine
   a. Suction
   b. Spare oxygen tank

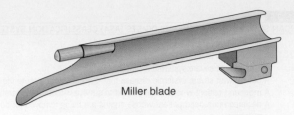

Miller blade

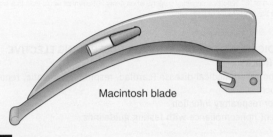

Macintosh blade

FIG. 9.1
Laryngoscope blades.

3. Airway
   a. Laryngoscope handles (short and long)
   b. Laryngoscope blades (Miller 2 and 3; Macintosh 3 and 4; Fig. 9.1)
   c. Oral airways—multiple sizes
   d. Endotracheal tubes—multiple sizes
   e. Stylets
   f. Nasal airways
   g. Oxygen delivery devices (nasal cannulas and face masks)
   h. Ambu bag
   i. Stethoscope

B. TECHNIQUES OF ANESTHESIA
1. General anesthesia
   a. Inhalational versus IV induction
   b. Airway—nasotracheal, orotracheal, laryngeal mask airway, mask
   c. Maintenance—inhalational versus IV
   d. Analgesia
   e. Neuromuscular blockers
      (1) Intraoperative monitoring with train-of-four, may use ulnar or orbicularis orbis muscle
2. Regional anesthesia
   a. Spinal
      (1) Injection of local anesthetic into subarachnoid space
      (2) Level of anesthesia—controlled by specific gravity of injected mixture, contour of the spinal canal, and patient position

    (3) Complications—diminished sympathetic tone, vasodilation, hypotension, decreased cardiac output, spinal headache, hypoventilation (thoracic level), total spinal (block above C3), urinary retention

    (4) Contraindications—coagulopathy, infection at insertion site, neurologic dysfunction, hypovolemia, patient refusal

b. Epidural

    (1) Injection of local anesthetic into potential space bordered by dura mater and spinal canal periosteum (level of placement depends on surgical site and dermatomal coverage needed)

    (2) Complications—**hypotension**, infection (superficial or epidural space), epidural hematoma, local anesthetic toxicity (larger volume needed in epidural space), intravascular injection of local anesthetics (epidural space has extensive venous plexus)

    (3) Contraindications—coagulopathy, infection at insertion site, neurologic dysfunction, and hypovolemia

c. Combined spinal/epidural
Combined spinal/epidural anesthesia takes advantage of the beneficial aspects of both, that is, a rapid, reliable block with spinal anesthesia and the ability to supplement the block and provide postoperative pain relief with an epidural.

d. Caudal—injection of local anesthetic at S5 through sacrococcygeal ligament

e. Peripheral nerve blocks; local/field blocks with or without sedation

3. Monitored anesthesia care

  a. Sedation and analgesia

  b. Continuous monitoring

4. Bier block (IV regional anesthesia)

  a. This is excellent for forearm, hand, or foot procedures.

  b. One hour is usually the limit.

  c. Double-pneumatic tourniquet is applied above elbow (or calf).

  d. Initially inflate above venous pressure to distend vein; then venipuncture with 22-gauge IV line.

  e. Release tourniquet, exsanguinate extremity with elevation and wrap with elastic bandage, and inflate distal tourniquet and then proximal tourniquet.

  f. Inject catheter with 0.5% lidocaine injection.

  g. With onset of tourniquet pain (at 45 minutes), inflate distal tourniquet and release proximal tourniquet for slow release of lidocaine into systemic circulation.

C. INTRAOPERATIVE COMPLICATIONS

Anesthesiologists are trained to recognize and prevent hemodynamic, respiratory, airway, and other difficulties that could potentially lead to intraoperative catastrophes.

1. Hemodynamic

  a. Hypotension/hypertension (bleeding, hypovolemia, etc.)

    (1) May consider arterial catheter or other invasive monitor

9

GENERAL ANESTHESIA

       (2) Important to maintain hemodynamic stability to maintain adequate perfusion, particularly in areas of anastomosis

  b. Arrhythmias (tachycardia, bradycardia, other cardiac arrhythmias)

       (1) Need constant EKG monitoring; look for any signs of ischemia

2. **Respiratory**

  a. Hypoxia

       (1) Constant monitoring of functional oxygen saturation (SpO_2), airway pressures, and minute volumes

  b. Hypercarbia

       (1) Difference between end-tidal CO_2 ($ETCO_2$) and partial pressure of carbon dioxide ($PaCO_2$) is 2–5 mm Hg.

       (2) Representative of dead space on ventilator. If $ETCO_2$ increases, consider complication such as pulmonary air embolism, thromboembolism, or decreased cardiac output.

  c. Bronchospasm

3. **Airway**

  a. Difficult airway and airway trauma from intubation

  b. Pulmonary aspiration of gastric contents

  c. Laryngospasm

4. **Temperature**

  a. Temperature stability and normothermia (36°C) are critical.

       (1) Hypothermia may lead to increased morbidity, including coagulopathy and increased surgical site infection.

  b. The monitoring of temperature may be esophageal, cutaneous, rectal, etc.

  c. Most effective warming techniques are forced-air (Bair Hugger) and circulating water warmers.

5. **Malignant hyperthermia**

Malignant hyperthermia is characterized by a hypermetabolic state and has a genetic predisposition. It is presumed that a defect in the calcium release channel sustains greater concentrations of calcium in the myoplasm, causing persistent skeletal muscle contraction after administration of succinylcholine or volatile anesthetics, or both. Definitive diagnosis is by muscle biopsy.

  a. Prophylaxis—Avoid malignant hyperthermia-triggering drugs (volatile gases, succinylcholine) in patients with suspected family history.

  b. Clinical signs

       (1) Masseter rigidity after succinylcholine administration

       (2) Unexplained tachycardia and tachypnea

       (3) Arrhythmias

       (4) Cyanosis

       (5) Metabolic or respiratory acidosis or both **(increased $ETCO_2$ is an early sign)**

       (6) Fever—late sign (may reach 107°F)

  c. Treatment

       (1) Terminate volatile inhaled agents and succinylcholine; administer nontriggering IV anesthetics (opiates, ketamine, barbiturates, or nondepolarizing blockade).

(2) Notify surgeon and request termination of the surgical procedure when possible.

(3) Rapidly administer Dantrolene—start with 2.5 mg/kg up to total 10 mg/kg.

(4) Hyperventilate with 100% O_2 at 10 L/min to flush inhaled anesthetics.

(5) Consider $NaHCO_3$, guided by arterial pH, if base deficit is greater than 8.

(6) Treat hyperkalemia with $NaHCO_3$, regular insulin (10 units), and 50% dextrose (50 mL).

(7) Initiate active cooling—cooled saline, cold gastric lavage, or surface cooling.

d. Postoperative monitoring

(1) Transfer patient to ICU, with careful monitoring of temperature, $ETCO_2$, minute ventilation, heart rate (HR), blood gas, K^+, and creatine kinase (CK).

(2) Late complications include consumptive coagulopathy, acute renal failure, hypothermia, skeletal muscle swelling, and neurologic sequelae.

III. PHARMACEUTICALS

A. IV ANESTHESIA

IV anesthetics may be used as induction agents, supplemental anesthetic agents, or sole anesthetic agents. For most patients, choice of anesthetic agent is relatively simple. However, there are certain scenarios that may suggest or prohibit the use of a specific agent. See Table 9.2 for a list of commonly used IV anesthetic agents and their special considerations.

B. NEUROMUSCULAR BLOCKING DRUGS

Patients must be adequately anesthetized before administration of neuromuscular blocking drugs because they are without analgesic or anesthetic effects. In addition, their airway must be secure with adequate ventilator assistance. The choice of neuromuscular blocking agent depends on the desired speed of onset, duration of effect, route of elimination, and potential side effects. Clinically, the degree of neuromuscular blockade is monitored by visually monitoring a twitch response after electrical stimulation of a peripheral motor nerve (ulnar or facial nerve branch).

1. **Depolarizing agents mimic the action of acetylcholine, producing depolarization of the postjunctional membrane.**
2. **Nondepolarizing agents compete with acetylcholine for postjunctional receptors and prevent changes in membrane ion permeability. They are classified clinically as long, intermediate, and short acting (Table 9.3).**

C. REVERSAL OF NEUROMUSCULAR BLOCKADE

Nondepolarizing agents can be antagonized by anticholinesterase drugs. Atropine or glycopyrrolate should be added to block muscarinic side effects (e.g., salivation, bronchospasm, bradycardia).

TABLE 9.2

INTRAVENOUS ANESTHESIA

Agent	Details and Pharma-cology	Dose (mg/kg)	Side Effects	Warning!—Use With Caution
Thiopental	Acts on γ-aminobutyric acid receptor; immediate onset. May have slow emergence with high doses.	2–5	Hypotension; peripheral vasodilation; tachycardia	Hypovolemia, coronary artery disease
Etomidate	Acts on γ-aminobutyric acid receptor; rapid onset for induction; good cardiovascular stability.	0.1–0.3	Burns on injection; myoclonus; adrenocortical suppression (with continuous infusion)	Hypovolemia
Ketamine	Acts on N-methyl-D-aspartate, opioid and other receptors. Provides dissociative anesthesia; good bronchodilator with preserved airway reflexes. Does not provide visceral analgesia.	1–2	Hypertension (HTN); tachycardia; apnea; emergence hallucinations (pretreat with benzodiazepines)	Coronary artery disease, severe hypovolemia
Propofol	Acts on γ-aminobutyric acid receptor; has immediate onset and rapid emergence; pharmacokinetics unchanged by hepatic or renal failure.	1–2	Burns on injection; hypotension; respiratory depression and/or apnea	Hypovolemia, coronary artery disease
Midazolam	Enhances effect on γ-aminobutyric acid receptor; sedation with anterograde amnesia; good anxiolytic; anticonvulsant; onset 30–60 s	0.15–0.3	Sedation and respiratory depression; may enhance effects of narcotics	Hypovolemia

Detailed pharmacology and other information on benzodiazepines and narcotics can be found in Chapter 16.

1. **Edrophonium:** Always use with atropine because onset and duration are similar.
2. **Neostigmine:** Always use with glycopyrrolate.
3. **Pyridostigmine**

D. INHALATIONAL ANESTHESIA

Minimum alveolar concentration is the minimum concentration of anesthesia that prevents movement in 50% of patients in response to a noxious stimulus (skin incision). Speed of onset depends on alveolar partial pressure (Pa) of

TABLE 9.3

NEUROMUSCULAR BLOCKING AGENTS

Agent	Duration	Comments/Side Effects	Metabolism
Depolarizing Agents			
Succinylcholine	Short	Rapid onset. May cause hyperkalemia (burns, spinal injury, trauma), dysrhythmia, bradycardia, malignant hypertension (see Section II.C).	Metabolized by pseudocholinesterase, renal excretion
Nondepolarizing Agents			
Pancuronium	Long	Interacts with halothane; may cause ventricular irritability, tachycardia, HTN. Rarely used.	Biliary and renal excretion
Atracurium	Short	Laudanosine (metabolite) buildup may cause seizures. Rarely used.	Ester hydrolysis and Hoffman elimination—OK for use in hepatic or renal failure
Vecuronium	Intermediate	Fewer cardiovascular effects	Biliary and renal excretion
Rocuronium	Intermediate	Rapid onset	Biliary and renal excretion
Cisatracurium	Intermediate	No adverse hemodynamic effects	Hoffman elimination—degradation is pH and temperature dependent

the anesthetic, blood solubility, cardiac output, and alveolar-to-venous partial pressure difference.

1. Nitrous oxide
   a. Nonflammable and odorless (good patient acceptability); rapid recovery with low potency; decreases minimum alveolar concentration of volatile agents
   b. Complications—diffusion hypoxia (provide O_2 after surgery to prevent hypoxia), expansion of air-filled cavities (e.g., bowel [dangerous in bowel obstruction]), and pneumothorax
2. Sevoflurane
   a. Rapid induction and emergence, inhalational induction
   b. Complications—decreases systemic vascular resistance and arterial blood pressure and interacts with CO_2 absorbers (soda lime, barium lime) to produce compound A, which is potentially toxic to the kidneys
3. Isoflurane
   a. Complications—pungent, not suitable for inhalational induction; decreased systemic vascular resistance and arterial blood pressure; increased heart rate
4. Desflurane
   a. New inhalation agent with rapid induction and rapid recovery (similar to that of N_2O)

9

GENERAL ANESTHESIA

   b. Hemodynamic effects similar to isoflurane
   c. Complications—sympathetic activation with rapid increases in concentration

E. LOCAL ANESTHETICS

1. Uses
   a. Analgesia/anesthesia without risks of general anesthesia
   b. Used in spinal, epidural, regional, and local anesthesia
2. Dosage considerations
   a. Limit total anesthetic dosage to prevent seizures and arrhythmias or cardiac arrest.
   b. Add vasoconstrictor to slow vascular absorption.
   c. Avoid inadvertent vascular injection by preinjection aspiration.
   d. Impending toxicity may be indicated by muscle twitching, restlessness, or sleepiness.
3. Treatment of toxicity and precautions
   a. Trendelenburg position, O_2, IV diazepam (5–10 mg), thiopental (50–100 mg)
   b. Never inject solutions containing epinephrine into digits, ear, tip of nose, or penis because they may cause local ischemic necrosis.
4. Commonly used local anesthetics
   a. Lidocaine—dosage maximum: 7 mg/kg with epinephrine, 4.5 mg/kg without epinephrine
   b. Mepivacaine—dosage maximum: 7 mg/kg with epinephrine, 4.5 mg/kg without epinephrine
   c. Bupivacaine—dosage maximum: 2.5 mg/kg
   d. Ropivacaine—dosage maximum: 3 mg/kg
5. Systemic toxicity effects—numbness of the tongue, visual disturbances, unconsciousness, seizures, central nervous system depression, coma, and respiratory arrest

IV. POSTOPERATIVE MANAGEMENT

A. PAIN MANAGEMENT

1. Nonsteroidal antiinflammatory drugs (contraindicated in renal disease and failure and patients with history of peptic ulcer disease)
   a. Ketorolac
   b. Ibuprofen
2. Narcotic analgesics
   a. Oral narcotics
      (1) Oxycodone ± acetaminophen
      (2) Hydrocodone ± acetaminophen
   b. IV narcotics
      (1) Intermittent boluses (nurse administered)
      (2) Patient-controlled analgesia
      It allows the patient to self-administer narcotics (morphine, hydromorphone) with a programmable infusion pump and attempts to

provide optimal pain relief and safety by avoiding peak and trough levels out of the therapeutic range caused by delays in administration, improper dosage, and pharmacokinetic and pharmacodynamic variability. Pumps are programmed to deliver intermittent boluses on demand, a continuous infusion, or a continuous background infusion with intermittent bolus doses. The dose, dose interval, and infusion rate are determined by the physician. Potential complications are respiratory depression, tolerance, nausea, vomiting, and pruritus.

3. Intrathecal analgesia
   a. This provides short-term analgesia (24 hours).
   b. Morphine is the drug of choice; dosage is 0.5 mg or less.
   c. It is limited to single-dose administration by risk for spinal headache and nerve damage from multiple punctures.
   d. Side effects are respiratory depression, nausea, and vomiting.

4. Epidural analgesia
   Epidural analgesia attempts to provide pain relief without high systemic levels and side effects of analgesics. Narcotics, local anesthetics, or both can be used.
   a. Advantages
      (1) Prevents muscle spasm and splinting, avoiding pulmonary complications
      (2) Allows earlier ambulation
      (3) Possible earlier return of gastrointestinal function after surgery
      (4) Excellent for patients with chest trauma, including rib fractures, pulmonary contusion, and flail chest
   b. Adverse side effects
      (1) Local anesthetics—**hypotension**, motor block, systemic toxicity, urinary retention
      (2) Narcotics—**respiratory depression**, pruritus, nausea, vomiting, urinary retention
   c. Dosing
      (1) Intermittent dosing causes peak systemic levels above those required for analgesia, causing more side effects.
      (2) Continuous infusion prevents peaks and troughs of intermittent dosing.
      (3) Combining infusions of local anesthetics and narcotics reduces the total dose of each, reducing the chance of adverse side effects.
   d. Postoperative management
      (1) Careful monitoring of blood pressure, urine output, and respiratory rate
      (2) Judicious fluid resuscitation for hypotension; patient at high risk of pulmonary edema, particularly after thoracic surgery
      (3) May need to decrease rate of epidural or split narcotic and local anesthetic if patient has persistent hypotension despite adequate intravascular volume

B. RESPIRATORY MONITORING

1. Hypoxia

   a. This may be related to sedation, pain, and splinting or atelectasis.

   b. Monitor SpO_2 continuously. Supplemental oxygen and/or more invasive respiratory support may be needed.

   c. Treat underlying etiology.

   d. If unable to safely wean O_2 to less than 4–6 L nasal cannula, consider transfer to ICU or step-down rather than floor status.

2. Obstruction

   a. Obstruction is the most common cause of hypoxia postoperatively.

   b. It is commonly caused by the tongue or oropharyngeal soft tissues from residual anesthesia and muscle relaxants. Position patient appropriately with head tilt and jaw thrust.

   c. Continuous positive airway pressure (CPAP), bag-mask ventilation, or sedation with reintubation may be needed for laryngospasm.

   d. For vomit, blood, or other debris in airway, perform suctioning.

C. HEMODYNAMIC INSTABILITY

1. Hypotension

   a. Most commonly due to hypovolemia, left ventricular dysfunction, or arrhythmia. Also consider drug reactions, adrenal insufficiency, and transfusion reaction.

   b. Manage with IV fluid administration, ionotropic agents, Trendelenburg positioning, and supplemental O_2.

2. Hypertension

   a. Secondary to pain, anxiety, or poorly managed essential hypertension

D. POSTOPERATIVE NAUSEA AND VOMITING

PONV is a major concern for patients and is a major problem in the postanesthesia recovery unit. Multimodal therapy is best for a patient with a history of PONV.

1. Risk factors

   a. Female sex

   b. Nonsmoker

   c. Intraoperative opioid administration

   d. History of PONV

   e. Type of surgery (laparoscopic, strabismus surgery, inner or middle ear)

2. Treatment [common side effect]

   a. Serotonin (5-HT$_3$) receptor antagonists

      (1) Ondansetron [headache]

      (2) Dolasetron

   b. Metoclopramide

   c. Dexamethasone [hyperglycemia]

   d. Droperidol [extrapyramidal effects]

   e. Promethazine [sedation, dry mouth]

   f. Scopolamine patch [pupillary constriction if patient touches eyes; may be unilateral]

RECOMMENDED READINGS

American Society of Anesthesiologists online. Available at: www.asahq.org.

American Society of Anesthesiologists: Standards guidelines and statements. Standards for basic anesthetic monitoring. Committee of Origin: Standards and Practice Parameters (Approved by the ASA House of Delegates on October 21, 1986, and last amended on October 20, 2010 with an effective date of July 1, 2011). (http://www.asahq.org/~/media/sites/asahq/files/public/resources/standards-guidelines/standards-for-basic-anesthetic-monitoring.pdf).

Lee TH, et al. Derivation and prospective validation of a simple index for prediction of cardiac risk of major noncardiac surgery. *Circulation*. 1999;100:1043–1049.

Morgan E, Mikhail M, Murray M. *Clinical Anesthesiology*. 5th ed. New York: McGraw-Hill; 2013.

Wolters U, et al. ASA classification and perioperative variables as predictors of postoperative outcome. *Brit J Anaesth*. 1996;77:217–222.

GENERAL ANESTHESIA

9

PART III

Surgical Critical Care

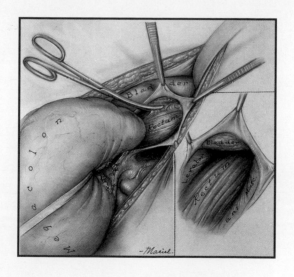

Surgical Critical Care

Surgical Infection

Aaron Seitz, MD

Within one linear centimeter of your lower colon, there lives and works more bacteria than all humans who have ever been born. Yet many people continue to assert that it is we who are in charge of the world.

—Neil deGrasse Tyson

Surgical infection has been around as long as surgical procedures have been performed. Advances in our understanding of infections began to expand exponentially in the 19th century from discoveries by physicians and scientists, such as Ignaz Semmelweis, who discovered that puerperal fever rates in obstetric patients could be reduced by hand washing, Joseph Lister, with his principles of antisepsis and use of carbolic acid to prevent infection, Charles McBurney, who pioneered "source control" with development of the appendectomy, or William Altemeier and his *Manual of Control of Infection in Surgical Patients.*

I. BACKGROUND AND SCOPE OF PROBLEM

1. In 1991 the *New England Journal of Medicine* published "The Nature of Adverse Events in Hospitalized Patients," which reported a 3.7% rate of disabling injuries caused by medical treatment (wound infections made up 14%).
2. In 1999 the Institute of Medicine published, "To Err Is Human: Building a Safer Health System."
   a. Cited studies that claimed number of deaths in the United States from medical errors may be higher than deaths from automobile accidents. This accelerated the development of health care quality improvement initiatives.
   b. Subsequently, the Healthcare Research and Quality Act of 1999 was passed and the Agency for Healthcare Research and Quality was branded. Progress was made in reducing morbidity due to medication errors but was slow in reducing infections.
3. In 2005 the National Nosocomial Infections Surveillance was renamed National Healthcare Safety Network (NHSN).
   a. It serves as the most widely used health care–associated infection (HAI) tracking system.
   b. Centers for Medicaid and Medicare Services (CMS) imposes financial penalties on hospitals that do not participate in NHSN reporting.

4. In 2007 research was published estimating the number of HAIs and resulting deaths in US hospitals.
   a. Rate of 4.5 infections per 100 hospital admissions was reported.
   b. Of deaths from patients with HAIs, 63% were attributed to the infection.
5. In 2008 the US Department of Health and Human Services established the Federal Steering Committee for the Prevention of HAI with the ultimate goal of eliminating HAIs.
6. In 2009 they released the National Action Plan to Prevent HAIs: Road Map to Elimination with 5-year target goals, which included:
   a. 50% reduction in central line–associated bloodstream infections (CLABSIs)—successful,
   b. 30% reduction in *Clostridium difficile* hospitalizations—unsuccessful,
   c. 25% reduction in catheter-associated urinary tract infections (CAUTIs)—unsuccessful,
   d. 25% reduction in surgical site infections (SSIs)—unsuccessful,
   e. 95% adherence to Surgical Care Improvement Project (SCIP) measures—successful and subsequently retired.
7. Cost analysis published in 2012 estimated costs per case for the following:
   a. CLABSIs—$45,814
   b. Ventilator-associated pneumonia (VAP)—$40,144
   c. SSIs—$20,785
   d. *C. difficile* infections—$11,285
   e. CAUTIs—$896
8. In 2012 the final rule implementing a hospital inpatient value-based purchasing program went into effect that rewards hospitals for performance in quality measures instead of rewarding the act of reporting on them.
9. Road Map to Eliminate HAI: 2013 Action Plan Conference was held with proposed 2020 targets, which included:
   a. 50% reduction in CLABSIs from 2015 baseline,
   b. 25% reduction of CAUTIs from 2015 baseline,
   c. 30% reduction in facility-onset *C. difficile* from 2015 baseline,
   d. 30% reduction in SSI admission and readmission from 2015 baseline.
10. In 2014 updated multistate prevalence statistics from surveys taken from 2009 to 2011 to assess for HAIs were reported in the *New England Journal of Medicine.*
    a. Four percent of patients were diagnosed with at least one HAI.
       (1) Pneumonia accounted for 22%.
       (2) SSIs accounted for 22%.
       (3) Gastrointestinal infections (primarily *C. difficile*) accounted for 17%.
       (4) Device-related infections accounted for 25%.

11. In 2016 the Centers for Disease Control and Prevention (CDC) released the National and State Healthcare Associated Infections Progress Report. It reported the following statistics for acute care hospitals:
   a. Fifty percent reduction in CLABSIs compared with the national baseline
   b. No reduction in CAUTIs compared with the national baseline
   c. Seventeen percent reduction in SSIs compared with the national baseline
   d. Eight percent reduction in *C. difficile* infections compared with the national baseline

II. MOST COMMON INFECTIONS AFFECTING SURGICAL PATIENTS

A. CENTRAL LINE–ASSOCIATED BLOODSTREAM INFECTION

1. Definition: CLABSI is a laboratory-confirmed bloodstream infection in which a central line was in place for greater than 2 calendar days on day of diagnosis. It also includes bloodstream infections in which the line was removed the day before diagnosis if the line was previously in place for greater than 2 calendar days.

2. Epidemiology and pathogenesis
   a. Four percent of short-term, noncuffed central venous catheters lead to bloodstream infections, compared with 0.1% of peripheral intravenous (IV) lines, 0.8% of arterial lines, and 2.4% of peripherally inserted central catheters (PICCs).
   b. Intensive care unit (ICU) length of stay is increased approximately 10 days secondary to nosocomial bloodstream infection.
   c. Top five causative agents include
      (1) *Staphylococcus aureus*
      (2) Coagulase-negative staphylococcus
      (3) *Candida* spp.
   d. Most CLABSIs from short-term central venous catheters are extraluminally acquired and result from skin flora

3. Prevention of CLABSI
   a. Healthcare Infection Control Practices Advisory Committee (HICPAC) (part of the CDC) published guidelines in 2011. Highlights as they pertain to surgical residents are as follows:
      (1) Perform hand hygiene before procedure.
      (2) Use maximal sterile barrier precautions (sterile gloves, cap, gown, mask, drapes, etc.) for placement of central venous catheters.
      (3) Wear new sterile gloves when handling new catheter in guidewire exchange.
      (4) Prep skin with greater than 0.5% chlorhexidine for central venous catheter placement.
      (5) Subclavian placement is recommended instead of internal jugular or femoral venous placement for nontunneled central venous catheter insertion to minimize infectious risk.

10

SURGICAL INFECTION

       (a) Risk of infection is 4.5% with subclavian placement versus 20% associated with femoral venous placement or 8.6% with internal jugular placement.

       (b) Infectious risk must be weighed against risk of pneumothorax or perforation of great vessels ($<1\%$ but often fatal).

       (c) Subclavian placement should be avoided in patients on hemodialysis or with advanced kidney disease.

    (6) Ultrasound guidance used by trained personnel is recommended in placement of internal jugular catheters.

    (7) Chlorhexidine-impregnated dressing sponge may be indicated for your facility.

    (8) Promptly remove catheter that is no longer essential.

    (9) Replace catheters placed without aseptic technique (emergent) within 48 hours.

    (10) Routine central catheter replacement is not recommended.

    (11) Replacement of central venous catheter for infectious cause should not be performed over a guidewire.

4. Treatment

  a. Catheter removal and appropriate IV antimicrobial therapy

  b. Not recommended—routine tip culture and subsequent treatment for a positive result

B. SURGICAL SITE INFECTIONS

1. Definitions and diagnosis

  a. Timing: SSI is infection associated with the surgical site that occurs within 30 days of operation or within 1 year if surgical implant was used.

  b. CDC changed diagnosis of surgical wound infection to SSI and published the following categories for diagnosis and study:

    (1) Superficial incisional SSI: involving the skin or subcutaneous tissues with purulent drainage and/or organisms isolated and/or signs and symptoms of pain, erythema, hyperthermia, or swelling. Does not include stitch abscess or infected burn wound

    (2) Deep incisional SSI: involving the fascial or muscle layers

    (3) Organ/space SSI: diagnosis of abscess by physical examination, radiology, or reoperation and/or purulent drainage and/or organisms cultured from organ or body space

  c. Classification of surgical wounds

    (1) Class I or clean: uninfected operative wound in which no inflammation is encountered or mucosal tract violated

    (2) Class II or clean-contaminated: mucosal (respiratory, genitourinary, alimentary) tract entered without unusual contamination

    (3) Class III or contaminated: open, fresh, or accidental wounds, gross spillage from gastrointestinal tract, inflammation encountered

    (4) Class IV or dirty: old traumatic wounds and those involving clinical infection or perforated viscus

2. Epidemiology and pathogenesis
   a. SSIs account for approximately 20% of HAIs.
   b. SSI prevention is associated with 4% absolute risk reduction in mortality.
   c. Rates are decreasing as a result of a national effort to reduce incidence (see earlier), but SSI remains most common and most costly HAI.
   d. Pathogen prevalence is dependent upon procedure type, but some generalizations can be made.
      (1) *S. aureus* and coagulase-negative *Staphylococcus* are most prevalent for most operations.
      (2) Gram-negative rods are most prevalent for abdominal operations.
      (3) Enterococci are associated with $\frac{1}{3}$ of transplant operations.

3. Prevention
   a. Principles are based on the HICPAC guidelines published in 1999 and then updated in 2008. A 2014 update was published independently. Highlights as they pertain to surgical residents are as follows:
      (1) Encourage tobacco cessation at least 30 days before operation.
      (2) Reduce hemoglobin A1c levels in diabetic patients to less than 7% before surgery, if possible.
      (3) Do not delay surgery for administration of total parenteral nutrition because this may actually increase infection risk.
      (4) Administer oral antimicrobials in addition to subsequent preoperative parenteral prophylaxis to reduce risk of SSI in colorectal patients. Note that oral antimicrobials have been shown to be effective only when used in conjunction with mechanical bowel prep.
      (5) Use appropriate antimicrobial prophylaxis.
         (a) Antibiotics may not be indicated for procedures expecting class I surgical wounds and no use of surgical implants.
         (b) Administer antibiotics within 1 hour of incision or 2 hours if vancomycin or quinolone is used. Antibiotics administered less than 30 minutes before incision may provide a 1% absolute risk reduction when compared with administration 31–60 minutes prior.
         (c) Choice of prophylactic antibiotics administered consistent with the following recommendations:
            (i) Weight-based dosing adjustments for obese patients
            (ii) Redosing of antibiotic for prolonged surgical procedures (>2 half-lives or excessive blood loss)
            (iii) Prophylactic antibiotics discontinued within 24 hours of surgery or 48 hours for cardiac surgery
            (iv) In clean and clean-contaminated procedures, no additional prophylactic antibiotic administered after skin closure
      (6) Remove hair appropriately (only as needed, using electric clippers, performed just before surgery).

(7) Use alcohol-containing preoperative skin cleansing agents.

(8) Use a surgery safety checklist similar or identical to the World Health Organization 19-point checklist (3% absolute risk reduction in SSI).

(9) Use plastic wound protectors for gastrointestinal and biliary surgery (45% relative risk reduction).

(10) Asepsis and good surgical technique are as follows:
   (a) Wear appropriate surgical attire.
   (b) Handle tissue gently, maintain effective hemostasis, minimize devitalized tissue and foreign bodies, and eradicate dead space at the surgical site.

(11) Use intraoperative wound irrigation with iodine or antibiotic-based solutions.

(12) Maintain normothermia intraoperatively and in the immediate preoperative and postoperative period.

(13) Leave incision to heal by secondary intention or delayed primary closure if class III or IV wound.

(14) If drainage is necessary, use a closed suction drain via incision separate from surgical incision, with removal as soon as possible.

(15) Control postoperative morning glucose for cardiac surgery patients.

(16) Protect incision postoperatively for 48 hours, with use of sterile technique if dressing must be replaced before this time.

b. Unresolved and controversial issues
   (1) Methicillin-resistant *S. aureus* (MRSA) decolonization protocols with mupirocin may be indicated in cardiac and orthopedic surgery populations to decrease rates of SSI and may be reasonable for high-risk patients but should not be used routinely, due to the risk of resistance development and propagation.
   (2) Showering with antiseptic at least 1 day before operation may not reduce the rate of SSI.
   (3) Maintaining oxygenation with supplemental and supranormal oxygen postoperatively and intraoperatively, respectively, may not reduce SSI rate, although a meta-analysis in 2009 reported a 3% absolute risk reduction for SSI with use of supplemental oxygen.
   (4) HICPAC 2013 draft guidelines update for prevention of SSI:
      (a) Antimicrobial (triclosan-coated) sutures: Do not use for prevention of SSI.
      (b) Topical antimicrobials before or immediately after wound closure: Do not use for prevention of SSI.
      (c) Topical antimicrobial (cyanoacrylate) sealants: Do not use for prevention of SSI.
      (d) Topical antimicrobial dressings: Further research is needed.

4. Treatment
   a. Updated guidelines were published by the Infectious Disease Society of America (ISDA) in 2014. (The following highlights pertain to surgical residents.)
      (1) Fever greater than 38°C in first 4 days
         (a) If systemic signs of infection and visible drainage or marked inflammation of wound are present, then send Gram stain to rule out streptococci and clostridia.
         (b) If positive, proceed to urgent or emergent wound debridement and treatment with vancomycin, broad-spectrum penicillin, and clindamycin.
      (2) Fever greater than 38°C after first 4 days with erythema and/or induration
         (a) Open the incision.
         (b) If fever resolves, leukocytosis is less than 12,000, and erythema is less than 5 cm from incision, then no antibiotics are indicated because there is no difference in clinical outcome, although there is a greater rate of wound sterilization with administration of systemic antibiotics.
         (c) If fever, leukocytosis, or cellulitis persists, begin appropriate systemic antibiotics and dressing changes.

C. CATHETER-ASSOCIATED URINARY TRACT INFECTIONS
1. Definitions and diagnosis
   a. CAUTI (adults and children >1 year old): must have indwelling urinary catheter in place for greater than 2 days or removed for less than one day before diagnosis
      (1) Symptomatic urinary tract infection (SUTI) must meet the following:
         (a) At least one of the following:
            (i) Fever greater than 38°C
            (ii) Suprapubic tenderness with no other causes
            (iii) Costovertebral angle pain or tenderness with no other causes
         (b) AND urine culture with no more than two species, one of which has colony counts of greater than 10^5 colony-forming units (CFU)/mL
      (2) Asymptomatic bacteremic urinary tract infection (ABUTI)
         (a) Urine culture with no more than two species, one of which has colony counts of greater than 10^5 CFU/mL
         (b) Blood culture with at least one matching bacterium
      (3) Does not include bacteria found on urinalysis or in culture without aforementioned symptoms (i.e., asymptomatic bacteriuria [ASB])
      (4) Pyuria is not diagnostic of and should not be used as an indication for antimicrobial treatment, but the absence of pyuria in a symptomatic patient excludes CAUTI.

(5) Malodorous or cloudy urine has not been associated with CAUTI and is not an indication for urine culture or treatment with antimicrobials.

(6) Urinalysis positive for nitrite provides 92% specificity for clinically relevant infection but provides poor sensitivity (29%). Thus urinalysis is a poor screening test to rule out CAUTI.

2. Epidemiology and pathogenesis
   a. Historically, health care–associated urinary tract infection was most common HAI (32%).
   b. CAUTI was most recently reported as fourth most common HAI (13%).
   c. Fifteen percent of nosocomial bacteremia is attributable to the urinary tract and is associated with a 10% mortality.
   d. Top three causative agents include:
      (1) *Escherichia coli* (21%)
      (2) *Candida* (21%)
      (3) *Enterococcus* (15%)

3. Prevention
   a. CAUTI–HICPAC published guidelines in 2009. The following are highlights as they pertain to surgical residents:
      (1) Maintain awareness to implement prompt removal. When studied, providers were unaware of patient catheterization in 28% of surveys.
      (2) Use urinary catheters in surgical patients only as necessary, not routinely. Accepted indications include but are not limited to:
         (a) Obstruction of urinary tract distal to bladder
         (b) Postoperatively from bladder or prostate surgery
         (c) Close monitoring of volume status in critically ill patients (i.e., patients with hypoxemia, hypotension, congestive heart failure, need for inotropic support, repeat diuretic use, etc.)
         (d) Need for monitoring in uncooperative patient
         (e) Continuous bladder irrigations for urinary tract hemorrhage
         (f) Postoperative care after spinal anesthesia
         (g) Palliative care for terminally ill
      (3) Avoid use of urinary catheters for treatment of incontinence unless it is for protection of decubitus wound.
      (4) For operative patients with an indwelling catheter, remove within 24 hours unless continued use is appropriately indicated. Duration of catheterization is directly correlated with CAUTI incidence.
      (5) Consider alternative methods of urinary drainage, including external catheterization and intermittent catheterization.
      (6) Use aseptic technique (hand hygiene, sterile gloves, drape, sponges, antiseptic solution for periurethral cleaning) for insertion.
      (7) After aseptic insertion, maintain closed drainage. If leakage occurs, replace catheter and drainage system.

4. Treatment
   a. Remove catheter, or replace catheter if catheter is still required.
   b. Seven days of antimicrobial therapy are recommended if prompt resolution of symptoms occurs, 10–14 days for those with delayed response.
   c. Five-day regimen of levofloxacin may be considered in patients who are not critically ill.
   d. Three-day regimen may be considered for women younger than 65 years without upper urinary tract symptoms in whom the catheter has been removed.
   e. No treatment is indicated for ASB, with two exceptions:
      (1) Pregnant patients
      (2) Patients who underwent traumatic genitourinary procedures resulting in mucosal bleeding

D. **CLOSTRIDIUM DIFFICILE** INFECTION
1. Definitions and diagnosis
   a. Diagnostic criteria
      (1) Clinically significant diarrhea (sustained change in bowel movement consistency and/or frequency and/or abdominal cramping without other etiology)
      (2) OR toxic megacolon without other etiology
      (3) AND stool positive for *C. difficile* toxin or *C. difficile* organisms OR pseudomembranous colitis identified by endoscopy, surgery, or histopathology
   b. Disease severity (important for treatment decision)
      (1) Mild to moderate: aforementioned diagnostic criteria without meeting severe or complicated criteria
      (2) Severe: serum albumin less than 3 g/dL plus ONE of white blood cell (WBC) greater than 15×10^3 cells/μL or abdominal tenderness
      (3) Severe and complicated: any one of the following:
         (a) ICU admission
         (b) Hypotension
         (c) Fever greater than 38.5°C
         (d) Ileus or distension
         (e) Altered mental status
         (f) Leukocytosis greater than 35×10^3 cells/μL or leukopenia less than 2×10^3 cells/μL
         (g) Lactate greater than 2.2 mM
         (h) End-organ failure
      (4) Recurrent *C. difficile* infection
2. Epidemiology and pathogenesis
   a. *C. difficile* is most common pathogen causing HAI.
   b. Mean length of hospital stay is increased up to 5.5 days.

   c. Attributable mortality associated with *C. difficile* infection is 5%–10%.

   d. Antibiotics classified as high risk because of their propensity for subsequent *C. difficile* infection:

     (1) Second-generation cephalosporins

     (2) Third-generation cephalosporins

     (3) Fluoroquinolones

     (4) Clindamycin

3. Prevention

   a. Initial guidelines were published by the ISDA in 2008 and updated in 2014. The following are highlights as they pertain to surgical residents.

     (1) Antimicrobial stewardship and usage restrictions

     (2) Wear full barrier precautions (gown and gloves) when interacting with *C. difficile*–infected patients.

     (3) Hand hygiene before and after interacting with *C. difficile*–infected patients. Handwashing with soap and water is not a recommended prevention strategy to reduce the rate of *C. difficile* infections in nonoutbreak facilities because there have not been any studies showing decreased rates of *C. difficile* after implementing soap and water handwashing policies.

     (4) In contrast, alcohol-based handwash has been shown to decrease rates of MRSA and vancomycin-resistant enterococcus (VRE).

     (5) Use dedicated patient-care equipment (i.e., stethoscope).

     (6) Do not perform test of cure for appropriately treated patients because clinically cured patients can have toxigenic *C. difficile* in their stool for several weeks.

     (7) Continue contact precautions for 48 hours after diarrhea resolves.

     (8) Probiotic prophylaxis is controversial but may be a low-risk strategy to prevent *C. difficile* infection (3.5% absolute risk reduction) for patients with no relative contraindications to probiotic use.

4. Treatment

   a. Pharmacologic

     (1) Mild to moderate: Treat with metronidazole 500 mg orally (PO) three times a day (TID) for 10 days. If there is no response in 5–7 days, switch to vancomycin.

     (2) Severe: Treat with vancomycin 125 mg PO four times a day (QID) for 10 days.

     (3) Severe and complicated: Treat with vancomycin 500 mg PO QID, metronidazole 500 mg IV every 8 hours (Q8H), and vancomycin 500 mg in 500-mL enema QID.

     (4) Recurrent: Repeat metronidazole or vancomycin, with fecal transplant considered after three recurrences.

b. Surgical
  (1) Decision to intervene surgically should be considered if one of the following is present:
    (a) Hypotension requiring vasoactive medication use
    (b) End-organ dysfunction
    (c) Leukocytosis greater than 50×10^3 cells/µL
    (d) Lactate greater than 5 mM
    (e) Complicated disease with failure to improve after 5 days
  (2) Operative intervention
    (a) Subtotal colectomy with end ileostomy is effective.
    (b) Minimally invasive loop ileostomy with on-table colonic lavage with polyethylene glycol 3350/electrolyte, followed by postoperative antegrade vancomycin flushes, has also been shown to be effective.

E. VENTILATOR-ASSOCIATED PNEUMONIA
1. Definitions and diagnosis
  a. ISDA published management guidelines in 2016. The following are highlights pertinent to surgical residents.
    (1) Diagnostic criteria
      (a) Lung infiltrate on chest radiograph
      (b) New-onset fever and/or purulent sputum and/or leukocytosis and/or new hypoxemia
      (c) Greater than 48 hours after intubation
    (2) Protocol recommendations
      (a) Obtain respiratory secretion samples on all patients—noninvasive methods are preferred (i.e., endotracheal aspiration), but invasive methods (i.e., bronchoscopy) are also acceptable.
      (b) Obtain blood cultures for any patient suspected of VAP because it may alter antibiotic management.
2. Epidemiology and pathogenesis
  a. VAP is one of the most common HAIs, causing significant morbidity and mortality in critically ill patients. It affects 10%–25% of mechanically ventilated patients and carries up to a 13% attributable mortality.
  b. VAP adds 5–7 days to ICU length of stay and increases length of hospitalization by 10–12 days.
  c. Most common pathogens are as follows:
    (1) Early onset
      (a) *Streptococcus pneumoniae*
      (b) *Haemophilus influenzae*
      (c) Methicillin-sensitive *S. aureus*
      (d) Gram-negative bacilli
    (2) Late onset
      (a) MRSA
      (b) *Pseudomonas aeruginosa*
      (c) *Acinetobacter baumannii*

SURGICAL INFECTION

10

3. Prevention
    a. Semirecumbent positioning
    b. Daily sedation wake-wean trials
    c. Small bowel tube feeding
    d. Prophylactic probiotics
    e. Early tracheostomy
4. Treatment (based on ISDA 2016 guidelines)
    a. Empiric antibiotic coverage should be broad spectrum to include *S. aureus*, *P. aeruginosa*, and gram-negative bacilli.
        (1) Include only MRSA coverage if greater than 10%–20% *S. aureus* isolates from unit are methicillin resistant.
        (2) Double cover *P. aeruginosa* only if ONE of the following is present:
            (a) Prior IV antibiotic use within 90 days
            (b) Septic shock at time of VAP
            (c) Adult respiratory distress syndrome (ARDS) before VAP diagnosis
            (d) Greater than 5 days of hospitalization
            (e) Requiring acute renal replacement therapy
    b. Deescalate broad-spectrum empiric antibiotic therapy to isolated bacteria and susceptibility.
    c. Length of therapy is 7 days.
    d. Discontinue antibiotics if invasive sampling resulted in growth below the defined threshold for VAP diagnosis (i.e., 10^4 CFU/mL).

F. PURULENT SKIN AND SOFT TISSUE INFECTIONS
1. Diagnosis
    a. Physical examination: painful, tender, fluctuant red nodules
    b. Imaging: may be diagnosed by computed tomography (CT) scan or magnetic resonance imaging (MRI)
    c. Severity stratification
        (1) Mild: no signs of systemic infection
        (2) Moderate: signs of systemic infection (i.e., fever >38°C, tachypnea >24 breaths/min, tachycardia >90 beats/min, leukocytosis >12×10^3 cells/μL or <400 cells/μL)
        (3) Severe: associated with sepsis
2. Epidemiology and pathogenesis
    a. Can be polymicrobial, but usually *S. aureus*
    b. MRSA becoming more common
3. Treatment
    a. Mild: incision and drainage with probing of cavity to break up loculations
    b. Moderate: incision and drainage, Gram stain/culture, and sensitivity of drainage with treatment with oral antibiotics
    c. Severe: incision and drainage, Gram stain/culture, and sensitivity of drainage with treatment with IV antibiotics

G. NECROTIZING SOFT TISSUE INFECTION

1. Definitions and diagnosis
   a. Preferred diagnostic terminology: necrotizing soft tissue infection, which includes infection of skin, subcutaneous tissues, fascia, and/or muscle. Many previously defined terms often still used colloquially. They are presented here for historical perspective.
      (1) Gas gangrene: clostridial anaerobic myonecrosis
      (2) Necrotizing fasciitis: extensive necrosis of the superficial fascia (not deep fascia as commonly assumed) regardless of bacterial etiology with widespread undermining of surrounding tissue
      (3) Fournier gangrene: described in 1883 as fulminant gangrene of the penis and scrotum defined by sudden onset, rapid progression, and the absence of a definite cause
         (a) This term is frequently used to describe necrotizing soft tissue infection of the perineum, regardless of gender of the patient.
      (4) Flesh-eating bacteria: term sensationalized by the media, initially used as a dramatic description of Fournier gangrene
   b. Diagnosis can be achieved by multiple methods.
      (1) Most important element in diagnosis is high index of suspicion. High-risk patients include uncontrolled diabetics, the morbidly obese, and IV drug users.
      (2) Laboratory
         (a) Admission leukocytosis less than 15.4×10^3 cells/μL AND serum Na$^+$ greater than 135 mM provide 99% negative predictive value for necrotizing infection.
         (b) Wong et al. published a laboratory-based scoring tool that provides 92% positive predictive value and 96% negative predictive value.
         (c) Gram stain from wound may help to identify clostridial infections. However, use of laboratory testing should not delay surgical treatment.
      (3) Imaging (x-ray, CT scan, ultrasound, MRI) can support diagnosis but should not delay treatment if preimaging probability is high.
      (4) Clinical examination
         (a) High fever, tachycardia almost universally present
         (b) May have crepitus, tenderness out of proportion to examination, blisters, and/or ecchymosis
         (c) If associated with surgical incision: "dishwater" purulent drainage
         (d) Finger test: used after making a small incision. Positive if subcutaneous tissues easily dissected from deep fascia.

2. Epidemiology and pathogenesis
   a. US incidence of 500–1500 cases per year
   b. Most common etiologic agents:
      (1) Clostridial: *C. perfringens*, *C. novyi*, *C. septicum* (70% associated with malignancy)
      (2) Nonclostridial: usually polymicrobial, but group A *Streptococcus* may be found as sole etiologic agent

3. Treatment
   a. Early, complete, and aggressive surgical debridement of necrotic tissue with second look within 24–48 hours of initial operation
   b. Broad-spectrum antibiotics to cover gram-positive, gram-negative, and anaerobic organisms, plus clindamycin to inhibit toxin production
   c. Aggressive physiologic support in ICU
   d. Hyperbaric oxygen use and IV immunoglobulin for group A streptococcal infections are controversial.

H. INTRAABDOMINAL INFECTIONS

1. Primary microbial peritonitis
   a. More common among patients with ascites
   b. Diagnosis—paracentesis with presence of bacteria on Gram stain and greater than 100 WBC/mL
   c. Treatment with 14–21 days of antibiotics specific to pathogen
2. Secondary microbial peritonitis
   a. Associated with hollow viscus perforation (i.e., appendicitis, diverticulitis, perforation, etc.)
   b. Treatment with source control, debridement of necrotic organ, and IV antibiotics
3. Intraabdominal abscess
   a. Common after secondary microbial peritonitis
   b. Treatment with drainage ± antibiotics. Percutaneous drainage preferred if possible, but open drainage may be necessary with multiple abscesses or inability to perform percutaneous image-guided procedure. Antibiotics used in patients with systemic signs of infection.
4. Hepatic/splenic abscesses
   a. 80% pyogenic, 20% parasitic or fungal
   b. Most commonly caused by manipulation of biliary tract
   c. Treatment
      (1) Small (<1-cm abscess): samples for Gram stain/culture and sensitivity and 4–6 weeks of antibiotics
      (2) Large: percutaneous drainage ± antibiotics
      (3) Recurrent: repeat drainage but may need unroofing and marsupialization (hepatic) or splenectomy (splenic)
5. Secondary pancreatic infections (infected pancreatic necrosis or pancreatic abscess)
   a. Occur in 10%–15% of patients with severe pancreatitis with necrosis. Of note, prophylactic antibiotics for sterile pancreatic necrosis are discouraged.
   b. Gold standard of treatment is open necrosectomy with repeat debridements; however, this caries a significant morbidity (30%) and mortality (5%) rate. Minimally invasive approaches (i.e., endoscopic, laparoscopic, etc.) have also been studied with good results but are institutionally and regionally dependent upon local expertise.

III. SEPSIS

1. **Definitions**
   a. Sepsis is a life-threatening organ dysfunction caused by dysregulated host response to infection.
   b. Historically sepsis was a spectrum of disease states ranging from fulminant infection with hemodynamic instability, to mild forms of inflammatory response. Previously the definition of sepsis was based on evidence of or suspected infection associated with two or more of the following systemic inflammatory response syndrome (SIRS) criteria:
      (1) Body temperature greater than 38°C or less than 36°C
      (2) Heart rate greater than 90 beats/min
      (3) Hyperventilation with respiratory rate greater than 20 breaths/min or arterial partial pressure of carbon dioxide ($PaCO_2$) less than 32 mm Hg
      (4) WBC count greater than 12×10^3 cells/µL or less than 4×10^3 cells/µL
   c. Task force convened in 2014 by the European Society of Intensive Care Medicine and the Society of Critical Care Medicine to evaluate utility of previous definitions and to create new ones as needed.
      (1) SIRS criteria were discarded as diagnostic criteria, as well as subset definition of "severe sepsis."
      (2) Task force emphasized use of the new Sequential Organ Failure Assessment (SOFA) score for evaluating sepsis. Each of the following categories (see next) is given a score of 0–4 points, based on organ dysfunction. SOFA score ≥2 associated with 10% mortality risk.
         (a) Respiratory—PaO_2 to FiO_2 ratio
         (b) Coagulation—platelet count
         (c) Liver—serum bilirubin
         (d) Cardiovascular—blood pressure
         (e) Central nervous system—Glasgow Coma Score (GCS)
         (f) Renal—serum creatinine or urine output
      (3) New "quick SOFA" (qSOFA) scoring system, although less robust SOFA score, can be assessed quickly and repeatedly and may be useful for bedside assessment. Each category (see next) is given a score of 0 or 1 based on the clinical examination of the patient. qSOFA ≥2 in non-ICU patients are associated with poor outcomes.
         (a) Respiratory rate greater than 22/min
         (b) Altered mentation
         (c) Systolic blood pressure less than 100 mm Hg

2. **Diagnosis**
   a. Patient with suspected infection: Evaluate with qSOFA.
   b. qSOFA ≥2: Consider increasing monitoring or level of care, and order additional lab tests to calculate SOFA.
   c. SOFA ≥2: Diagnose sepsis.
   d. Despite adequate fluid resuscitation, vasoactive medication required to maintain mean arterial pressure (MAP) greater than 65 and serum

> lactate greater than 2 mM: Diagnose septic shock (associated with > 40% in hospital mortality).

3. **Epidemiology:**
   a. Primary cause of death from infection
   b. Increasing incidence
   c. Accounts for 5% of US hospital costs
4. **Pathogenesis: systems affected**
   a. Cardiovascular
      (1) Decreased peripheral vascular resistance and increased capillary leak caused by systemic proinflammatory cytokines
      (2) Decreased preload caused by peripheral venodilation
      (3) Increased cardiac index driven primarily by tachycardia
   b. Respiratory
      (1) Acute lung injury—neutrophil-moderated injury secondary to pneumonia or other infectious processes
      (2) Acute respiratory distress syndrome caused by capillary leak and cytokine activation
   c. Immune
      (1) Proinflammatory cytokines
         (a) Tumor necrosis factor-α—released by macrophages and T cells
         (b) Interleukin-1β (IL-1β)—both local and systemic stimulation
         (c) IL-2—activates other lymphocyte subpopulations
         (d) IL-6—end-organ dysfunction
      (2) Antiinflammatory cytokines: IL-10
      (3) Complement system activation
      (4) Neutrophil (polymorphonuclear neutrophils) activation
   d. Endocrine
      (1) Hypothalamic–pituitary axis activation
         (a) Adrenal: increased cortisol release, increased epinephrine release
         (b) Increased antidiuretic hormone and vasopressin release
      (2) Renin-angiotensin-aldosterone system activation
      (3) Hyperglycemia
         (a) Increased glucagon and catecholamine secretion, which leads to decreased serum insulin in early sepsis
         (b) Peripheral insulin resistance in late sepsis
   e. Hematologic
      (1) Leukocytosis/leukopenia
      (2) Activation/upregulation of the coagulation cascade → disseminated intravascular coagulopathy
      (3) Thrombocytopenia
      (4) Neurologic—mental status changes (e.g., delirium)
5. **Treatment**
   a. Guidelines published in "Surviving Sepsis Campaign: International Guidelines for Management of Severe Sepsis and Septic

Shock: 2012." The following are highlights pertinent to surgical residents.

(1) "Early goal-directed therapy" with resuscitation of the septic patient during the first 6 hours
   (a) Volume repletion should be at least 30 mL/kg crystalloid challenge, to be repeated if hemodynamics continue to improve.
   (b) Albumin may be considered if substantial amounts of crystalloid are being used.
   (c) Avoid hetastarch.
   (d) Goals should include the following: central venous pressure (CVP) 8–12 mm Hg, MAP greater than 65 mm Hg, UOP greater than 0.5 mL/kg per hour, venous oxygen saturation (S_VO_2) 65%, normalized lactate
   (e) If goals are achieved, there is 16% absolute risk reduction in 28-day mortality.
(2) Blood cultures before antibiotics
(3) Broad-spectrum antibiotic therapy within 1 hour of recognition of sepsis
(4) Imaging studies to confirm source of infection
(5) Source control within 12 hours of diagnosis
(6) Norepinephrine as first-choice vasoactive medication to maintain MAP greater than 65 mm Hg
   (a) Epinephrine is second agent.
   (b) Vasopressin (0.03 units/min) can be used as second agent or to decrease dose of norepinephrine.
   (c) Avoid dopamine except in extreme circumstances.
   (d) Dobutamine may be indicated after appropriate fluid resuscitation in the presence of elevated cardiac filling pressures. It may also be used to augment oxygen delivery if S_VO_2 is less than 65% after appropriate fluid resuscitation.
(7) IV corticosteroids only in presence of shock unresponsive to vasopressor therapy
   (a) Do not use adrenocorticotropic hormone (ACTH) stimulation test to identify candidates, because accurate testing methods have not been identified.
   (b) Use continuous flow IV hydrocortisone 200 mg/day and taper when vasopressor therapy is concluded.
   (c) Clinical response to steroids in true adrenal insufficiency is rapid (within 1–2 hours). In the absence of response, steroids should be discontinued.
(8) Hemoglobin goal 7–9 g/dL in absence of tissue hypoperfusion, ischemic coronary artery disease, or active hemorrhage. A goal of 10 g/dL may be attempted if S_VO_2 less than 65% after appropriate crystalloid resuscitation.

10

SURGICAL INFECTION

(9) Protocolled approach to blood glucose when two consecutive blood glucose levels greater than 180 mg/dL with a target of less than 180 mg/dL

(10) Deep vein thrombosis prophylaxis

(11) Stress ulcer prophylaxis in patients with bleeding risk

(12) Reassessment of antimicrobial therapy daily for deescalation

(13) Oral/enteral feeding within first 48 hours, or IV glucose if unable to use gastrointestinal (GI) tract

RECOMMENDED READINGS

Bratzler DW, Dellinger EP, Olsen KM, et al. Clinical practice guidelines for antimicrobial prophylaxis in surgery. *Am J Health-Syst Pharm.* 2013;70(3):195–283.

Nelson RL, Gladman E, Barbateskovic M. Antimicrobial prophylaxis for colorectal surgery. *Cochrane Database Syst Rev.* 2014; 9(5):CD001181.

Rivers E, Nguyen B, Havstad S, et al. Early goal-directed therapy in the treatment of severe sepsis and septic shock. *N Engl J Med.* 2001;345(19):1368–1377.

Singer M, Deutschman CS, Seymour CW, et al. The third international consensus definitions for sepsis and septic shock (Sepsis-3). *J Am Med Assoc.* 2016;315(8):801–810.

Hemorrhage and Coagulation

Peter L. Jernigan, MD

For the life of the flesh is in the blood.

—Leviticus 17:11

I. GENERAL TOPICS

A. NORMAL BLOOD VOLUME AND COMPOSITION

1. Total blood volume (TBV) = 70 mL/kg total body weight (80 mL/kg for newborns)
2. Total volume red blood cells (RBCs) = TBV × hematocrit
   a. Approximately 26 mL/kg for male patients, 24 mL/kg for female patients
   b. Can be measured using chromium-tagged erythrocytes, but this is not often performed clinically
3. Total plasma volume = TBV × (1 − hematocrit)

B. CLASSES OF HEMORRHAGIC SHOCK (TABLE 11.1)

1. Class I and II classically are managed with crystalloid.
2. Class III and IV typically require blood products.

C. TYPING, SCREENING, AND CROSSMATCHING

1. Typing—serologic compatibility established for donor and recipient A, B, O, and Rh antigen groups
2. Screening—tests recipient blood for presence of common antibodies (indirect Coombs test)

TABLE 11.1
CLASSES OF HEMORRHAGIC SHOCK

	I	II	III	IV
Blood loss (mL)	<750	750–1500	1500–2000	>2000
Blood loss (% blood volume)	<15	15–30	30–40	>40
Pulse rate/min	<100	100–120	120–140	>140
Blood pressure	Normal	Normal	Decreased	Decreased
Pulse pressure	Normal	Decreased	Decreased	Decreased
Respiratory rate/min	14–20	20–30	30–40	>35
Urine/output (mL/h)	>30	20–30	5–15	Negligible
Mental status	Normal	Mildly anxious	Anxious, confused	Confused, lethargic

11

143

3. Crossmatching—tests for compatibility of recipient blood with a specific blood product to be infused. Test mixes donor's RBCs and recipient's serum, drawn less than 72 hours before test takes place.

D. GENERAL BLOOD PRODUCT ADMINISTRATION GUIDELINES

1. Allow 30 minutes for frozen products to thaw or for cold products to be warmed. Products should be warmed to 33°C–35°C before or during infusion.
2. Ensure the patient has appropriate intravenous or intraosseous access.
3. Before administration of blood product, the patient's name, medical record number, blood product ordered, blood type, and product's expiration date should be checked, ideally by two people together.
4. Use a standard blood filter to remove clots or large aggregates of cells.
5. Check vital signs at minimum before beginning infusion, 15 minutes into infusion, and after completion of transfusion of each unit.

II. LABORATORY TESTS AND REFERENCE VALUES

A. COMPLETE BLOOD COUNT

1. Hemoglobin (13.5–18.0 g/dL in males, 12.0–16.0 g/dL in females); hematocrit (40%–54% in males, 38%–47% in females)
2. Platelets: from 150,000 to 400,000/mm^3; 50,000/mm^3 is required for normal hemostasis.

B. PROTHROMBIN TIME

1. Evaluates production of vitamin K–dependent factors (II, VII, IX, X); indicates function of extrinsic pathway
2. Increased when functional volume of one or more factors is less than 50% (reference range, 12–14 seconds)

C. INTERNATIONAL NORMALIZED RATIO

1. Developed because of laboratory variations in prothrombin time (PT) results caused by variations in thromboplastin (PT test reagent) activity; used to modulate warfarin therapy (reference, 1.0)

D. ACTIVATED PARTIAL THROMBOPLASTIN TIME

1. Evaluates function of intrinsic pathway
2. Increased when functional volume of one or more factors is less than 50% (reference range, 40–60 seconds, varies by laboratory)

E. ACTIVATED CLOTTING TIME

1. Similar to activated partial thromboplastin time (aPTT) but designed to measure clotting time after administration of heparin. It correlates linearly with concentration of heparin in blood. Normal range 70–180 seconds, and therapeutic range varies with indication.

F. BLEEDING TIME
1. Evaluates platelet function and blood vessel integrity (reference range, 2.5–5.5 minutes)
2. Assessed with small cut on patient's skin

G. PLATELET FUNCTION TESTS
1. Multiple available technologies, including several point-of-care tests
2. Alternative to bleeding time for diagnosis of congenital and acquired platelet disorders

H. THROMBIN TIME
1. Measures polymerization of fibrinogen

I. FIBRINOGEN
1. Normal fibrinogen levels are 200–400 mg/dL, functional level is greater than 150 mg/dL. Affects PT and aPTT when less than 50 mg/dL

J. VISCOELASTIC TESTS
1. Point-of-care functional assessment of clot formation, strength, and lysis. Two available technologies: thromboelastography (TEG) and rotational thromboelastometry (ROTEM)
   a. Similar technology and comparable results (Fig. 11.1)
   b. TEG more prevalent in North America; ROTEM more prevalent in Europe

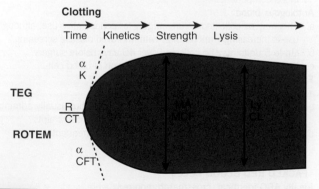

FIG. 11.1
Schematic thromboelastography (TEG) (upper half)/rotational thromboelastometry (ROTEM) (lower half) tracing indicating the commonly reported variables reaction time (R)/clotting time (CT), clot formation time (K/CFT), alpha angle (α), maximum amplitude (MA)/maximum clot firmness (MCF), and lysis (Ly)/clot lysis (CL). (From Johansson PI, Stissing T, Bochsen L, Ostrowski SR. Thromboelastography and thromboelastometry in assessing coagulopathy in trauma. *Scand J Trauma Resusc Emerg Med.* 2009;17:45, fig. 1.)

2. Useful to distinguish between medical and surgical bleeding and to guide ongoing blood product resuscitation

III. SPECIFIC BLOOD PRODUCTS

A. WHOLE BLOOD
1. Must be ABO identical, crossmatch required
2. Banked whole blood usually stored in 500-mL units
3. Stored at 4°C in citrate/phosphate/dextrose preservative for up to 21 days
4. Contains all blood components
   a. This is a poor source of platelets, which lose function after stored for 24 hours in whole blood.
   b. Clotting factors are stable in whole blood for up to 12 days, except factors V and VIII.
   c. Storage lesion: Intracellular 2,3-diphosphoglycerate (DPG) and adenosine triphosphate are reduced during storage; hemoglobin dissociation curve shifts to the left (more affinity for oxygen); pH decreases; and lactate, ammonia, and potassium increase.
5. Indications
   a. Used during mass casualty or military operations. May be supplied by fresh donations
   b. Burn surgery—used perioperatively when large losses of blood, platelets, and bleeding factors are expected
   c. Decreases donor exposure but generally less widely available than blood components
6. Autologous blood
   a. This may be collected before surgery for perioperative use, although use is increasingly uncommon with improved disease screening.
   b. Up to 5 units may be collected over 40 days before surgery.
   c. Erythropoietin is given to hasten generation of blood cells.
7. Fresh whole blood
   a. Administered within 48 hours of donation
   b. May be more effective than component therapy but usually administered untested for infectious disease due to time constraints
   c. "Walking blood bank"—group of donors tested frequently when transfusions are likely (military operations)

B. PACKED RED BLOOD CELLS
1. Ideally ABO identical, crossmatch required
   a. For emergency transfusions, type-specific and O-negative RBCs are equally safe for transfusion.
   b. After 4 units of O-negative blood, risk for hemolysis significantly increases.
2. One unit of packed red blood cells (pRBCs) has volume of 250–350 mL.
3. Stored at 4°C. Shelf life depends on storage solution (21 days for citrate/phosphate/dextrose solutions, 42 days for additive solutions).

4. Contains concentrated RBCs, hematocrit 60%–65%
   a. Effects on intracellular adenosine triphosphate and DPG are lessened but not eliminated.
   b. Leukocyte-reduced pRBCs are standard in most Western countries, although variable in the United States.
5. Transfusion of 1 unit pRBCs should increase hemoglobin level by 1 g/dL or hematocrit value 3%–4% in adults. In children, transfusion of 10 mL/kg pRBCs should increase hemoglobin level by 2 g/dL.
6. Indications
   a. Evidence of hemorrhagic shock
   b. Acute hemorrhage with hemodynamic instability or evidence of inadequate oxygen delivery (low venous oxygen saturation [S_vO_2], base deficit, lactic acidosis)
   c. In the critical care setting, transfusion should be based on evidence of impaired oxygen delivery (DO_2) to tissues, rather than on hemoglobin or hematocrit measures.
   d. A "restrictive" transfusion strategy (transfuse for hemoglobin <7 g/dL) is generally favored in patients with hemodynamically stable anemia and has been demonstrated to be safe even in critically ill patients.
   e. In the setting of acute myocardial ischemia a "liberal" transfusion strategy may be beneficial (transfuse for hemoglobin <8 g/dL).
   f. pRBCs should not be transfused for treatment of chronic anemia or anemia of pregnancy. Chronic anemia may be treated with iron or erythropoietin, and transfusion is rarely required because patients have adjusted to low hemoglobin level.
   g. Prophylactic preoperative pRBC transfusion based on expected intraoperative blood loss is not indicated.
   h. The decision to transfuse should always be based on overall clinical assessment and not just hemoglobin or hematocrit.
7. Cell Salvage (Cell Saver)
   a. Blood collected intraoperatively from cavities uncontaminated by malignant cells or infectious agents, centrifuged, and washed to contain only RBCs. Must be used within 4 hours of collection

C. FRESH FROZEN PLASMA
1. ABO compatibility required, Rh type unimportant, no crossmatch required
2. Aliquoted into 250-mL units from whole blood
3. Frozen to −18°C within 8–24 hours of collection, may be stored for 24 hours at 1°C–6°C
4. Contains 200 units of all coagulation factors (1 unit/mL), estimated 40% recovered function after transfusion
   a. Factors V and VIII less stable than vitamin K–dependent factors, begin depreciating after thawing
5. Estimated 10% increase in all functional factors with 4 units fresh frozen plasma (FFP)

11

HEMORRHAGE AND COAGULATION

6. Indications
   a. Correction of significant coagulopathy in a patient who is actively bleeding or undergoing an invasive procedure (PT >3 seconds beyond normal range, international normalized ratio [INR] >1.5)
   b. Treatment or prevention of dilutional coagulopathy with massive transfusion
   c. Emergent reversal of warfarin
   d. Treatment of coagulopathies from liver failure or disseminated intravascular coagulation
   e. Treatment of congenital coagulation factor deficiencies if no specific component therapies available

D. PLATELETS

1. ABO compatibility preferred, Rh type unimportant, no crossmatch required
   a. Patients who undergo frequent transfusions can develop antibodies to transfused platelets or other proteins, significantly decreasing effectiveness of transfusion.
   b. When refractoriness develops, human leukocyte antigen–matched platelets often are used.
2. Package consists of 6 units (each approximately 50 mL) pooled from individual donors (six times increased risk for transmission of infectious disease) or an apheresis unit from a single donor.
3. Store at 20°C–24°C, and use within 5 days of donation.
4. Each packet contains stable clotting factors (except factors V and VIII) from 1 to 2 units of FFP.
5. Each six-pack increases platelet count by 5000–10,000/mm^3.
6. Indications
   a. Clinical bleeding occurs with functional platelet counts less than 50,000/mm^3 (i.e., transfusion of normal platelets may be necessary to overcome congenital or acquired disorders causing abnormal platelet function).
   b. Correct functional platelet count to 50,000/mm^3 in preparation for surgical procedure or to 30,000/mm^3 in preparation for lumbar puncture or central line placement.
   c. There is no role for prophylactic transfusion for any platelet count without clinical bleeding.
   d. Platelet function is measured clinically by bleeding time; bleeding time longer than two times upper limit of normal with clinical bleeding is indication for platelet transfusion.

E. CRYOPRECIPITATE

1. ABO compatibility preferred but not required, Rh type unimportant, no crossmatch required.
2. Typically transfused as pooled "unit" consisting of 15- to 20-mL units from six individual donors
3. Made from precipitate of thawed FFP; must be transfused within 4 hours

4. Each individual unit contains 80–150 units factor VIII/von Willebrand factor (vWF), 250–350 mg fibrinogen (pooled "unit" contains 5–6 times these amounts).
    a. Fibrinogen in 1 unit FFP equals amount in 2 units cryoprecipitate.
5. One pooled unit increases fibrinogen by approximately 50 mg/dL.
6. Indications
    a. Correction of clinical coagulopathy with fibrinogen concentration less than 80 mg/dL
    b. Expect fibrinogen deficiency after massive transfusion of other blood products.
    c. May be given for hemophilia A, von Willebrand disease if no specific component therapies available

IV. MASSIVE TRANSFUSION AND DAMAGE CONTROL RESUSCITATION

A. **DEFINITION OF MASSIVE TRANSFUSION VARIES, BUT MOST COMMONLY USED IS 10 OR MORE UNITS OF BLOOD PRODUCTS IN THE FIRST 24 HOURS**
B. **PREDICTORS OF NEED FOR MASSIVE TRANSFUSION**
1. Numerous scoring systems exist for prediction. Many require laboratory results and complex calculations.
2. Assessment of blood consumption (ABC) score is a nonlaboratory score validated in civilian trauma.
    a. Systolic blood pressure less than 90 mm Hg, heart rate greater than 120 beats/min, penetrating injury mechanism, and positive focused abdominal sonography for trauma (FAST) examination
    b. Two or more criteria are predictive of requiring massive transfusion.
3. Potential predictors from other studies: base deficit ≥6, temperature <35.5°C, INR >1.5, hemoglobin <11 g/dL
C. **PRESENCE AND IMPLEMENTATION OF STANDARDIZED PROTOCOLS IMPROVE SURVIVAL IN PATIENTS REQUIRING MASSIVE TRANSFUSION.**
D. **DAMAGE CONTROL RESUSCITATION IS A STRATEGY TO LIMIT ONGOING BLEEDING BY ADDRESSING HYPOTHERMIA, ACIDOSIS, AND COAGULOPATHY.**
1. Infusion of crystalloid is limited to prevent dilutional coagulopathy.
2. The patient and all fluids are warmed.
3. Blood products are transfused in a balanced ratio (1:1:1 plasma to platelets to pRBCs).
4. Any ongoing hemorrhage must be controlled surgically.

V. TRANSFUSION REACTIONS

A. **IMMUNE MEDIATED**
1. Acute hemolytic reaction occurs when recipient plasma contains antibodies to donor RBCs because of ABO incompatibility (pRBCs, whole blood).
    a. Incidence is 1:250,000–1:1,000,000 transfusions.

11

HEMORRHAGE AND COAGULATION

b. Characterized by immediate fever, chills, dyspnea, back pain, bleeding, and shock initially, with renal failure occurring later in course. Anesthetized patients may experience only hypotension or bleeding.

c. Treat with volume expansion, diuresis, and urine alkalinization after immediately stopping transfusion. Reaction can occur after transfusion of only 10 mL; severity increases with amount transfused.

d. Hemoglobinemia (pink plasma) and hemoglobinuria will occur within minutes. Decreased haptoglobin indicates hemolysis. Direct agglutination test (Coombs test) will be positive as long as residual incompatible RBCs persist in circulation.

e. Delayed hemolytic reaction can occur 2–10 days after transfusion when recipient's antibody titer recovers; reaction is characterized by mild anemia and hyperbilirubinemia.

2. Febrile nonhemolytic reaction occurs when recipient plasma contains antibodies to leukocytes in donor unit (pRBCs, whole blood).

a. Incidence is 1:100 transfusions.

b. It is characterized by a 1°C increase in body temperature 1–6 hours after start of infusion.

c. Stop transfusion until hemolytic reaction is ruled out by absence of hemoglobinemia or hemoglobinuria; rule out other causes of fever.

d. There is decreased occurrence when leukocyte-reduced pRBCs are used.

3. Allergic reaction to donor components (any transfusion)

a. It is characterized by itching, urticaria, wheezing, and angioedema.

b. Treat with antihistamines, acetaminophen, and continue transfusion. Premedicate for future transfusions and use washed, leukocyte-reduced products.

c. Patients with history of immunoglobulin A (IgA) deficiency without history of transfusion may have an anaphylactic reaction.

4. Alloimmunization to RBCs, leukocytes, platelets, or other protein components (human leukocyte antigen class I antigens) can occur after multiple transfusions (especially with human leukocyte antigen–unmatched products).

a. No immediate complications but sensitizes patient and increases risk for adverse event during future transfusions

b. Can prevent by using all ABO-matched products and washed/leukocyte-reduced pRBCs

5. Transfusion-related acute lung injury occurs when donor antibodies attack recipient leukocytes, leading to immune complex deposition in pulmonary capillary beds (any transfusion).

a. 1:5000 transfusions

b. Presents as pulmonary edema, acute respiratory distress syndrome–like syndrome, secondary to rapid increase in pulmonary capillary permeability, usually within 2–6 hours of infusion

c. Treat supportively; may require intubation and mechanical ventilation for 2–4 days while insult resolves
d. More commonly occurs with transfusion of plasma, especially from multiparous female donors
6. **Graft-versus-host disease occurs in immunocompromised patients when donor leukocytes attack recipient tissues (pRBCs, whole blood).**
   a. It is characterized by multiorgan system failure; mortality rate is greater than 90%.
   b. Stop transfusion; supportive treatment. Use of leukocyte-reduced, irradiated blood reduces occurrence.

B. **NONIMMUNOLOGIC REACTIONS**
1. **Transmission of infectious disease is the same for whole blood, pRBCs, and FFP (US data).**
   a. Human immunodeficiency virus transmission: 1:2,000,000 transfusions
   b. Hepatitis B transmission: 1:270,000 transfusions
   c. Hepatitis C transmission: 1:230,000 transfusions
   d. Case reports of cytomegalovirus, Epstein-Barr virus, and West Nile virus transmission
2. **Bacterial contamination occurs rarely, most often in platelets because they are stored at higher temperature (1:12,000 transfusions).**
3. **Multiple retrospective studies suggest link between transfusion and rates of nosocomial infection, pneumonia, length of stay, and mortality.**
   a. One theory suggests that recipient leukocytes become tolerant because of infusion of donor leukocytes with similar but nonidentical human leukocyte antigen patterns.
   b. Another theory suggests that donor leukocytes or components released during transfusion downregulate recipient leukocyte response.
4. **Hemosiderosis occurs with repeated pRBC transfusion.**
   a. Each unit of pRBCs contains 250 mg iron.
   b. Treatment with deferoxamine chelates iron to promote its excretion.
5. **Potassium abnormalities are caused by alterations in normal action of the sodium-potassium pump in pRBCs.**
   a. Initial hyperkalemia during transfusion because pRBC pumps are inactive during storage, leading to increased potassium in supernatant of unit
   b. Often followed by hypokalemia because pumps in transfused RBCs become active and drive extracellular potassium into cells
6. **Hypocalcemia is caused by citrate preservative in all blood products complexing with ionized calcium for excretion. Usually transient, self-limited effect, unless multiple transfusions are being performed**

VI. SURGICAL COAGULOPATHY—GENERAL CONSIDERATIONS
A. **COAGULATION CASCADE (FIG. 11.2)**
B. **MEDICAL HISTORY TO DETERMINE RISK FOR BLEEDING**
1. Family history of coagulopathy/bleeding diathesis
2. Personal history

11

HEMORRHAGE AND COAGULATION

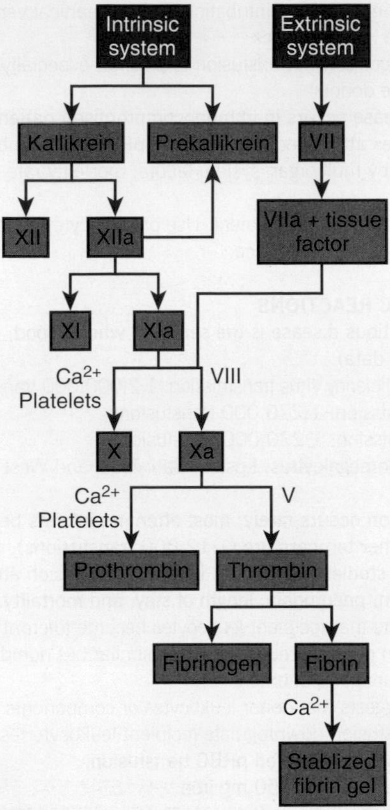

FIG. 11.2
Coagulation cascade.

a. Postoperative or postprocedural bleeding/hemarthrosis/intramuscular bleeds (indicates coagulation factor disorder) and/or easy bruising/mucosal bleeding (indicates platelet disorder)
b. History of cirrhosis or liver failure
c. Medications
   (1) Nonsteroidal antiinflammatory drugs
   (2) Antiplatelet agent: aspirin, clopidogrel (Plavix)
   (3) Warfarin
   (4) Novel oral anticoagulants, direct thrombin or factor Xa inhibitors: dabigatran (Pradaxa), rivaroxaban (Xarelto), apixaban (Eliquis), edoxaban (Savaysa)

VII. CONGENITAL BLEEDING DISORDERS

A. HEMOPHILIA A

1. X-linked deficiency of factor VIII, intrinsic pathway dysfunction with increase of aPTT
2. For surgery, requires 75%–100% factor VIII activity for 7–10 days perioperatively
3. One factor VIII unit contains 1% factor VIII activity.
4. Dose of factor VIII concentrate (must be dosed every 12 hours): [desired factor VIII activity (%) − current factor VIII activity (%)] × [total plasma volume (mL)/100] = number of units to be infused
5. Can also treat with desmopressin 0.3 μg/kg intravenous daily (induces release of vWF from endothelial cells, increasing levels of factor VIII)
6. Can treat with cryoprecipitate if other therapies are not available

B. HEMOPHILIA B (CHRISTMAS DISEASE)

1. X-linked deficiency of factor IX, intrinsic pathway dysfunction with increase of aPTT
2. For surgery, requires 75%–100% factor IX activity for 7–10 days perioperatively
3. A total of 1.5 factor IX units contain 1% factor IX activity, then use aforementioned formula; must be dosed every 18 hours

C. VON WILLEBRAND DISEASE

1. Autosomal dominant deficiency in functional vWF, which is a subendothelial protein with two functions: (1) binder of platelets to endothelium, and (2) carrier for factor VIII
2. Multiple types
   a. Type 1 (60%–80% of patients): quantitative deficiency of vWF, usually mild symptoms
   b. Type 2 (15%–30% of patients): qualitative deficiency of vWF, mild-to-moderate symptoms
   c. Type 3 (5%–10% of patients): quantitative deficiency of vWF, severe symptoms including spontaneous bleeding
   d. Acquired von Willebrand disease: secondary to autoimmune disease, heart disease, cancer, or medications
3. Treat with 0.3 μg/kg desmopressin intravenous daily; will see effect in 30–90 minutes; must wait 24 hours between doses to allow levels to recover.
4. Some factor VIII concentrate solutions also contain vWF.
5. May be treated with cryoprecipitate in severe refractory cases

D. THROMBASTHENIA (GLANZMANN DISEASE), BERNARD-SOULIER SYNDROME

1. There is absence of platelet surface proteins necessary for binding and aggregation.
2. Treat with platelet transfusion.

11

HEMORRHAGE AND COAGULATION

VIII. ACQUIRED BLEEDING DISORDERS

A. VITAMIN K DEFICIENCY

1. This is caused by warfarin use, poor nutrition, reduction of normal intestinal flora, total parenteral nutrition, and biliary obstruction.
2. Treat with vitamin K, 10 mg intravenous or subcutaneous once (correction in 6–8 hours). May also give vitamin K, 10 mg orally, with correction in 24 hours.
3. Treat with FFP infusion for immediate correction (duration 8–12 hours).

B. HYPOTHERMIA

1. Activity of all coagulation factors and platelets is severely impaired at temperatures less than 35.5°C.

C. LIVER FAILURE

1. Caused by decreased synthesis of vitamin K–dependent clotting factors and factor V (including fibrinogen with advanced disease). Correct with FFP (will not correct with vitamin K alone).

D. END-STAGE RENAL DISEASE

1. Causes platelet dysfunction secondary to uremia. Treat with desmopressin, dialysis, or chronic, low-dose estrogen therapy.

E. DISSEMINATED INTRAVASCULAR COAGULATION

1. Caused by concurrent coagulation and clot lysis in small vessels (consumptive coagulopathy)
2. Can occur with sepsis, trauma, obstetric complications, malignancy, burns, anaphylaxis, infection
3. Laboratory—increased PT, aPTT, bleeding time; decreased platelets, fibrinogen; increased fibrin degradation products (D dimer)
4. Coagulation cascade activated in small vessels, leading to fibrin deposition. Results in consumptive coagulopathy, consumptive thrombocytopenia, hemolytic anemia, local tissue ischemia, followed by hemorrhage
5. Treat underlying cause. Transfusions to correct specific deficits; do not transfuse platelets until less than 50,000 mm^3.

F. ACQUIRED THROMBOCYTOPENIA

1. Decreased production because of folate/B12 deficiency, leukemia, radiation, chemotherapy, acute ethanol intoxication, and viral infection
2. Shortened survival because of immune thrombocytopenia, thrombotic thrombocytopenic purpura, disseminated intravascular coagulation, and hemolytic uremic syndrome. Treat with steroids, intravenous immunoglobulin, or plasmapheresis with guidance by a hematologist.
3. Transfuse platelets for clinical bleeding or procedure.

G. HEPARIN-INDUCED THROMBOCYTOPENIA—SPECIAL CASE OF DRUG-INDUCED IMMUNE THROMBOCYTOPENIA

1. Caused by formation of antibodies to heparin-platelet factor 4 (PF4) complexes, which bind to platelets, causing clumping (consumptive thrombocytopenia, venous thrombosis 70%, arterial thrombosis 15%)
2. Occurs less frequently with use of low-molecular-weight heparin (LMWH)
3. 4T scoring system for diagnosis: 1–3 = low probability, 4–5 = intermediate probability, 6–8 = high probability
   a. Thrombocytopenia: two points—greater than 50% drop in platelet count and nadir ≥20; one point—30%-50% platelet drop and nadir 10–19
   b. Timing: two points—clear onset 5–10 days after heparin or ≤1 day with previous heparin exposure in last 30 days; one point—onset day 5–10 but less clear trend, onset after day 10, or ≤1 day with previous heparin exposure 30–100 days prior
   c. Thrombosis: two points—new confirmed thrombosis, skin necrosis, or acute systemic response after heparin bolus; one point—progressive or recurrent thrombosis, non-necrotizing skin lesions, or suspected thrombosis
   d. Other causes of thrombocytopenia: two points—none; one point—possible
4. Definitive diagnosis by positive serotonin release assay and PF4/polyanion enzyme immunoassay for antibodies OR positive heparin-induced platelet activation test
5. Treat with immediate cessation of heparin and initiation of alternate method of anticoagulation to prevent further thrombosis (argatroban or lepirudin). Be cautious of heparin-bonded catheters or other sources of heparin.

H. HYPERFIBRINOLYSIS

1. Hyperfibrinolysis may be congenital or acquired (severe trauma, sepsis, liver failure, cardiopulmonary bypass, major surgery) and lead to severe bleeding.
2. Fibrinogen degradation products interfere with fibrin polymerization and platelet aggregation.
3. D dimer, fibrin split products, and plasmin/alpha2-antiplasmin complexes are all nonspecific markers.
4. Hyperfibrinolysis can be diagnosed with viscoelastic tests (TEG/ROTEM).
5. Treatment with lysine analogs (ε-aminocaproic acid and tranexamic acid [TXA]) may decrease need for transfusion.

IX. MEDICATIONS

A. ANTIPLATELET AGENTS

1. Aspirin
   a. It inhibits platelet aggregation and degranulation by irreversibly preventing production of thromboxane A_2 by cyclooxygenase.
   b. Hold for 5–7 days before procedure.

2. Nonsteroidal antiinflammatory drugs
   a. They inhibit platelet aggregation and degranulation by reversibly preventing production of thromboxane A_2 by cyclooxygenase.
   b. Hold for 2 days before procedure.
3. Clopidogrel (Plavix)
   a. It inhibits platelet aggregation by irreversibly inhibiting platelet binding of adenosine diphosphate (ADP) and ADP-mediated activation of glycoprotein IIb/IIIa complex.
   b. Hold for 5–7 days before procedure.
4. Transfuse platelets for immediate correction of medication effects.

B. HEPARINS
1. Unfractionated heparin
   a. Enhances inhibitory effects of antithrombin III on thrombin and factor Xa
   b. Administered as continuous intravenous infusion to keep aPTT between 1.5 and 2.5 times upper limit of normal
   c. May be administered subcutaneously for DVT prophylaxis
   d. Surgical procedures may take place with aPTT less than 1.3 times upper limit of normal.
2. LMWH
   a. LMWH enhances inhibitory effects of antithrombin III on factor Xa; more stable therapeutic anticoagulation than unfractionated heparin, and thus routine monitoring is not required.
   b. Increased effects are seen in renal failure.
   c. Monitor anti–factor Xa activity (not aPTT) to determine therapeutic effect.
3. Hold therapeutic doses of heparin and LMWH 8–12 hours before procedures.
4. For immediate correction, administer 1 mg protamine intravenously for every 100 units of heparin most recently administered. Half dose for each hour since heparin administration (less effective in counteracting LMWH).

C. WARFARIN
1. It inhibits vitamin K cycle (production of factors II, VII, IX, and X).
2. Administer orally, and adjust dose for target INR.
3. Hold warfarin 5–7 days before procedure. Check INR to ensure less than 1.5.
4. For urgent procedure, administer 10 mg vitamin K orally once (effects in 24 hours).
5. For emergency, administer 10 mg vitamin K intravenously or subcutaneously once (effect in 6–8 hours) and FFP (immediate effect).

D. DIRECT THROMBIN INHIBITORS
1. Administered as continuous intravenous infusion (except dabigatran, see later)

2. No known reversal agents. FFP, recombinant factor VIIa, and pro-thrombin complex concentrates have been used for emergent reversal with varying success.
3. Bivalirudin
   a. Titrated for aPTT ratio (patient's measured aPTT/laboratory median reference aPTT value) of 1.5–2.5
   b. Short half-life (10–90 minutes)
   c. Renally excreted, so increased effects seen with renal insufficiency
4. Argatroban
   a. Administered as intravenous infusion and monitored by aPTT
   b. Increased effects seen in hepatic failure
   c. Discontinue infusion 2–4 hours before procedure (aPTTs usually return to reference levels within this time frame).
   d. Can artificially elevate INR. Must be considered when transitioning to warfarin

E. FACTOR Xa INHIBITORS (FONDAPARINUX)
1. Fondaparinux administered as subcutaneous injection (oral formulations described later)
2. Does not typically affect PT or PTT
3. Renal metabolism. Half-life 17–21 hours in normal renal function

F. NEW ORAL ANTICOAGULANTS
1. Direct thrombin inhibitors (dabigatran) and direct factor Xa inhibitors (rivaroxaban, apixaban, edoxaban)
2. US Food and Drug Administration (FDA)-approved for anticoagulation in atrial fibrillation
3. No lab monitoring required and lower risk of hemorrhagic stroke versus warfarin
4. Half-life of each drug is different. Generally stop 24–48 hours before procedure.
5. Reversal agents now available
   a. Idarucizumab: monoclonal antibody that preferentially binds and inhibits dabigatran
   b. Andexanet alfa: factor Xa decoy protein that reverses factor Xa inhibitors

G. ANTIFIBRINOLYTICS
1. ε-Aminocaproic acid and TXA block plasmin binding to fibrin and prevent breakdown of clot.
2. Indications
   a. Prophylaxis against postoperative bleeding (cardiac, liver, orthopedic, or other operations with high risk for postoperative bleeding)
   b. Ongoing bleeding with evidence of fibrinolysis on TEG or ROTEM
   c. TXA for major traumatic injury with hemorrhagic shock or suspected fibrinolysis (hypothermia, acidosis, coagulopathy, thrombocytopenia); should be given within 3 hours of injury

11

HEMORRHAGE AND COAGULATION

RECOMMENDED READINGS

CRASH-2 Trial Collaborators, Shakur H, Roberts I, et al. Effects of tranexamic acid on death, vascular occlusive events, and blood transfusion in trauma patients with significant haemorrhage (CRASH-2): a randomized, placebo-controlled trial. *Lancet*. 2010;376:23–32.

Hébert PC, Wells G, Blajchman MA, et al. A Multicenter, randomized, controlled clinical trial of transfusion requirements in critical care. *N Engl J Med*. 1999;340:409–417.

Holcomb JB, Tilley BC, Baraniuk S, et al. Transfusion of plasma, platelets, and red blood cells in a 1:1:1 vs a 1:1:2 ratio and mortality in patients with severe trauma: the PROPPR randomized clinical trial. *JAMA*. 2015;313:471–482.

Napolitano LM, Kurek S, Luchette FA, et al. Clinical practice guideline: red blood cell transfusion in adult trauma and critical care. *Crit Care Med*. 2009;37:3124–3157.

Practice guidelines for perioperative blood management: an updated report by the American Society of Anesthesiologists Task Force on Perioperative Blood Management. *Anesthesiology*. 2015;122:241–275.

Shock

Amanda M. Pugh, MD

> *The person, although severely injured, congratulates himself upon having made an excellent escape, and flatters himself that he is not only in no danger, but that he will soon be well; in fact, to look at him one would hardly suppose, at first sight, that there was anything serious the matter with him; the countenance appears well, the breathing is good, the pulse is but little affected, except that it is too soft and frequent, and the mind, calm and collected, possesses its wonted vigor, the patient asking and answering questions very much as in health. But a more careful examination soon serves to show that deep mischief is lurking in the system; that the machinery of life has been rudely unhinged, and the whole system profoundly shocked; in a word, that the nervous fluid has been exhausted, and that there is not enough power in the constitution to reproduce and maintain it.*

> —Samuel Gross, *A System of Surgery*

12

Shock is often wrongly thought of as hypotension. Rather, it is defined as a state of inadequate delivery of oxygen and nutrients necessary for normal tissue and cellular functioning, leading to cellular hypoxia and death.

I. PATHOPHYSIOLOGY

The body's physiologic response depends on the etiology of shock (hemorrhagic/hypovolemic, cardiac failure, sepsis, or neurogenic injury). Regardless of etiology, the initial response is a result of inadequate oxygen delivery in relation to local oxygen demand causing a conversion from aerobic to anaerobic metabolism. This results in the production and accumulation of lactic acid and the development of metabolic acidosis. If this state persists, cellular adenosine triphosphate is depleted, sodium and potassium leave the cell, and the cell membrane loses its potential. With continued energy depletion, cellular death occurs. Cellular death leads to an inflammatory response that perpetuates shock. The body has regulatory mechanisms that initially compensate for the changes, but with persistent hypoperfusion, the body will enter a decompensation phase, and eventually the irreversible stages of shock.

II. HEMODYNAMIC CONSIDERATIONS

Physiologic response is based on maintaining cerebral and coronary perfusion, so appropriate management of a patient in shock is a basic and essential skill required by all surgeons. This requires an understanding of basic hemodynamics and the changes that occur to intravascular volume with modification of preload, afterload, and myocardial contractility in the various forms of shock.

A. IMPORTANT RELATIONSHIPS

1. MAP = CO × SVR, where MAP = mean arterial pressure, CO = cardiac output, and SVR = systemic vascular resistance.
2. CO = HR × SV, where CO = cardiac output, HR = heart rate, and SV = stroke volume.
3. Stroke volume is determined by preload, myocardial contractility, and afterload.
4. The Frank-Starling curve relates left ventricular end-diastolic volume (LVEDV; preload) to stroke volume. Up to a certain level (the "flat" portion of the curve), increased preload leads to increased stroke volume, with subsequently increased cardiac output. With the exception of septic shock, all other forms of shock have a low cardiac output.

B. PRELOAD

1. Preload is a measure of the filling of the ventricle and, theoretically, is an indication of the LVEDV.
2. As an alternative, the central venous pressure (CVP) can be used as an indirect measurement of central blood volume except when there is right ventricular dysfunction. For this reason, in many older patients with cardiac disease or pulmonary dysfunction, CVP is an inaccurate assessment of left-sided filling volume.
3. Pulmonary artery (Swan-Ganz) catheters measure pulmonary capillary wedge pressure, an estimation of left ventricular end-diastolic pressure, which in turn should reflect LVEDV. These assumptions may be inaccurate in patients with mitral valve disease, aortic insufficiency, pulmonary venous pathology, and altered left ventricular compliance. Optimal pulmonary capillary wedge pressure is 8–15 mm Hg, but this varies with the individual.

C. AFTERLOAD

1. Afterload is defined as the resistance against which the heart muscle must contract or pump.
2. The main determination of afterload is arterial pressure, which influences the ejection fraction. The ejection fraction can be maintained after an increase in afterload by an increase in preload. However, this compensation is lost in shock.
3. Afterload can be estimated by calculating the SVR.

$$SVR = [(MAP - CVP) \times 80]/CO$$

where MAP = mean arterial pressure, CVP = central venous pressure, and CO = cardiac output.

III. ORGAN RESPONSE TO SHOCK

A. NEUROENDOCRINE RESPONSE

1. It is an involuntary response originating from the hypothalamus, autonomic nervous system, and endocrine glands to maintain coronary and cerebral perfusion.
2. Initiated by hypoxia, hypotension, and hypovolemia as detected by baroreceptors and chemoreceptors. Baroreceptors sense pressure changes in the atria, aortic arch, and carotid bodies resulting in disinhibition of the autonomic nervous system and sympathetic activation.
3. Activation of the sympathetic response releases epinephrine and norepinephrine.
4. Catecholamines stimulate beta1-adrenergic receptors increasing cardiac output by increasing heart rate and cardiac contractility, and alpha1-adrenergic receptors causing an increase in blood pressure through vasoconstriction.
5. Catecholamines also alter insulin and glucose metabolism, ultimately increasing the availability of glucose for metabolism.
6. Activation of the hypothalamic-pituitary-adrenal axis causes an increase in adrenocorticotropic hormone (ACTH), which in turn stimulates the release of cortisol and aldosterone from the adrenal cortex establishing a catabolic state.
7. Increased levels of cortisol cause increases in gluconeogenesis and lipolysis while decreasing peripheral use of glucose and amino acids.
8. The pancreas produces less insulin, whereas glucagon production is increased. This causes an increase in hepatic gluconeogenesis.
9. This simultaneous and combined response results in stress-related hyperglycemia and refraction to insulin.
10. The renin-angiotensin system is also stimulated, causing an increase in aldosterone, which in turn increases sodium and water. The final result is low-volume, concentrated urine.
11. Vasopressin is released by the posterior pituitary gland, causing a direct increase in water resorption in the distal renal tubules.

B. MICROVASCULAR DYSFUNCTION

1. Vasoconstriction occurs selectively to decrease perfusion to dermal, renal, muscle, and splanchnic vascular beds to keep adequate perfusion to central organs, such as the brain and heart.
2. Capillary endothelial layer is usually compromised in shock states.
   a. Circulating inflammatory mediators, by-products of infection, lipopolysaccharide, thrombin, tumor necrosis factor-α, interleukin-1, nitric oxide, and endothelin-1 all cause capillary leak.
   b. Exact mechanism is still not clear, and the only current treatment is early resuscitation of volume status, rapid elimination of infectious and necrotic tissue, and vasopressors for inotropic support if cardiovascular function is compromised.

12

SHOCK

C. INFLAMMATORY RESPONSE

1. Shock triggers a massive systemic inflammatory response syndrome (SIRS).
   a. Activated leukocytes, platelets, endothelial cells, and macrophages are main players.
      (1) These cells generate amplifying inflammatory mediators with widespread physiologic consequences.
2. Coagulation and complement cascades are triggered.
3. Capillary leak causes fluid extravasation into noninjured tissues remote from the primary site of injury.
4. Creates a hyperdynamic inflammatory response that can lead to SIRS, acute respiratory distress syndrome (ARDS), and multiorgan system failure.

D. PULMONARY

1. The lungs are the most sensitive organ to injury and usually the first organ system to fail, leading to the development of ARDS.
2. ARDS is initiated and perpetuated by the aforementioned inflammatory changes.
3. Ultimately leads to a decrease in pulmonary compliance, surfactant abnormalities, and alveolar collapse.
   a. Functional residual capacity decreases and pulmonary insufficiency develops.
   b. Increase in pulmonary vascular resistance leads to an increase in cardiac workload and more strain on the cardiopulmonary system.

E. RENAL

1. Hypotension during the early phases of injury causes renal vasoconstriction.
   a. An increase in the afferent arteriole resistance causes a decrease in glomerular filtration rate with an increase in aldosterone and vasopressin.
   b. Persistent oliguria can lead to acute tubular necrosis (ATN) and multiorgan system failure.

IV. MULTIORGAN DYSFUNCTION SYNDROME

A. DEFINITION

Multiorgan dysfunction is a syndrome of progressive but potentially reversible insufficiency involving two or more organ systems that arises after resuscitation from an acute disruption of normal homeostasis.

B. CAUSES

1. Can result from prolonged or inadequately controlled shock
2. Is the most common cause of mortality in a surgical intensive care unit

C. PREVENTIVE MEASURES

1. Hemodynamic support—maintenance of adequate tissue oxygenation and substrate delivery
2. Nutritional support—provision of adequate nutrition and reversal of catabolism
3. Prevention of infection—maintenance of optimal antimicrobial defenses and prompt antimicrobial therapy at first sign of infection

V. SHOCK STATES

Blalock (1934) divided shock states into four basic categories, based on causative factor: (1) hypovolemic, (2) septic, (3) neurogenic, and (4) cardiogenic shock. With some additional subcategories, these divisions are still useful. The basic hemodynamic profiles of each type of shock are outlined in Table 12.1 and are described in greater detail in this section.

A. HYPOVOLEMIC SHOCK

1. Subdivided into hemorrhagic, traumatic, and nonhemorrhagic (e.g., burn shock)

   Signs and symptoms depend on degree of volume depletion, speed of volume depletion, duration of shock, and the body's compensatory reactions. Severity of shock and clinical presentation can be stratified according to the amount of fluid lost. Although the classifications presented in Table 12.2 are generally applied to hemorrhagic shock, they are useful in assessing the severity of shock.

   Note: *Young patients, who have particularly effective compensatory responses, may be able to maintain a normal blood pressure and heart rate up to the point of cardiovascular collapse and arrest. Older patients on beta-blockers also may not have reflex tachycardia. It is important to recognize early signs of shock in these patients.*

   a. Hemorrhagic shock
      Clinical signs of shock (hypotension, tachycardia, weak pulses, and/or cool, clammy skin) occur after at least 25% blood loss. See Table 12.2.

TABLE 12.1
HEMODYNAMIC PROFILES IN SHOCK

Type of Shock	HR	CVP	PCWP	CO	SVR
Hypovolemic	↑↓	↓	↓	↓	↑
Septic	—	—	—	—	—
Hyperdynamic	↑	↓	↓	↑	↓
Hypodynamic	↑↓	↑↓	↑↓	↓	↑
Neurogenic	↑	↓	↓	↓	↓
Cardiogenic	↑↓	↑	↑	↓	↑

CO, Cardiac output; *CVP*, central venous pressure; *HR*, heart rate; *PCWP*, pulmonary capillary wedge pressure; *SVR*, systemic vascular resistance.

TABLE 12.2

CLASSES OF HYPOVOLEMIC SHOCK

Class	Amount of Blood Loss (mL)	Blood Loss (%)	Heart Rate (beats/min)	Blood Pressure Pres-sure	Blood Pressure	Pulse	Respiratory Rate (breaths/min)	Urinary Out-put (mL/h)	Mental Status
I	<750	<15	<100	Normal	Normal	Normal to ↑	14–20	>30	Slightly anxious
II	750–1500	15–30	>100	Normal	Normal	↓	20–30	20–30	Mildly anxious
III	1500–2000	30–40	>120	↓	↓	↓	30–40	5–15	Anxious, confused
IV	>2000	>40	>140	↓			>35	Negligible	Confused, lethargic

(1) Treatment
  (a) Remember ABCs—first establish airway to ensure adequate oxygenation and ventilation.
  (b) Control external hemorrhage, if present.
  (c) Intravenous access and administration of crystalloid, preferably lactated Ringer solution. Lactate buffers hydrogen ions from ischemic tissues that are washed out with reperfusion. Serum lactate and base deficit are indicators of decreased tissue perfusion and acidosis, which can be used to guide resuscitation. Patients with hypovolemia may demonstrate increased afterload caused by compensatory peripheral vasoconstriction to maintain adequate blood flow to vital organs. Reducing afterload in this setting is inappropriate until steps to correct volume status have been completed.
  (d) Blood products transfusion. Recent data support the use of a 1:1:1 transfusion protocol (1 unit packed red blood cells [PRBCs], 1 unit plasma, 6-pack platelets). It is important to remember that the initial hemoglobin may not represent true blood loss. Early initiation of a massive transfusion protocol may assist in obtaining and administering blood product rapidly.
  (e) Operative control of hemorrhage if necessary. For traumatic hemorrhage always consider the places that will hold volumes of blood large enough to cause hypotension → thoracic cavity, peritoneum, retroperitoneum, thigh, and external.
  (f) Avoid hypothermia and acidosis, which disrupt the coagulation pathway.
  (g) Always rule out gastrointestinal tract as etiology of nontraumatic hemorrhage.
b. Traumatic shock
  (1) Due to ischemic changes from hypovolemia and devitalized tissue from mechanism of injury, there is a proinflammatory response similar to that seen in septic shock.
c. Nonhemorrhagic hypovolemic shock
  (1) It is similar to hemorrhagic shock, except that blood transfusion is usually not necessary.
  (2) Examples include third-space losses in bowel obstruction, gastrointestinal losses from diarrhea, emesis, biliary drainage, pancreatic fistula, and burns.
  (3) After the initial resuscitation effort with normal saline or lactated Ringer's solution (LR) is completed, replacement fluids should be crystalloid with appropriate electrolyte composition of fluid lost. Usually D5 ½ normal saline + 20 mEq KCl/L is used for gastrointestinal losses proximal to ligament of Treitz and LR for losses distal.

B. SEPTIC SHOCK
1. It implies hemodynamic instability caused by host inflammatory response to infection.

12

SHOCK

Classification of severity of septic shock includes:
   a. Sepsis—systemic signs of shock with diagnosis of infectious source
   b. Severe sepsis—sepsis with organ dysfunction
   c. Septic shock—severe sepsis with persistent hypotension requiring vasopressor support despite fluid resuscitation
2. Local response to infection includes rubor, calor, dolor, and tumor. Systemic responses in this setting include vasodilation, altered mental status, fever, capillary leak, and organ dysfunction.
3. Host mediators implicated in pathogenesis of septic shock include multiple cytokines (e.g., tumor necrosis factor-α and interleukin-1), reactive oxygen radicals, vasoactive peptides, the complement cascade, and platelet-activating factor.
4. It may result from infection with gram-positive or gram-negative bacteria, fungi, virus, or protozoa that initiates inflammatory, metabolic, endocrinologic, and immunologic pathways.
5. Response (see Table 12.1) may be hyperdynamic (compensated) or hypodynamic (uncompensated).
6. Decreased afterload is also present in septic shock due to inappropriate vasodilation that causes relative hypovolemia. In these instances, vasopressors are often used to improve vascular tone to help to maintain adequate perfusion.
7. Gram-positive—massive fluid losses secondary to dissemination of potent exotoxin, often without bacteremia
   a. Causative organisms include *Clostridium, Staphylococcus,* and *Streptococcus.*
   b. Characterized by hypotension with normal urine output and unaltered mental status. Acidosis is infrequent.
   c. The prognosis is generally good with treatment.
   d. Treatment includes intravenous fluids to correct volume deficit, appropriate antibiotics, and surgical drainage or debridement, if necessary.
8. Gram-negative—initiated by endotoxins in cell walls of gram-negative bacteria
   a. Causative organisms include gastrointestinal flora, including coliforms and anaerobic bacilli, such as *Klebsiella, Enterobacteriaceae, Serratia,* and *Bacteroides.*
   b. Common sources in order of decreasing frequency—urinary tract, pulmonary, alimentary tract, burns, and soft tissue infections. Always be suspicious for catheter-related sepsis.
   c. Endotoxin, or lipopolysaccharide, in the outer membrane of gram-negative bacteria can elicit marked host inflammatory response even in the absence of viable bacteria.
9. **Fungal—causative organisms are commonly *Candida* spp.**
   a. Seen in neutropenic, immunosuppressed, polytrauma, or burn patients
   b. Risk factors include parenteral nutrition, invasive monitors, and broad-spectrum antibiotics.

        c. When *Candida* organisms reach the intravascular compartment, widespread dissemination can occur.
            (1) Fungi lodge in the microcirculation, forming microabscesses.
            (2) Characterized by high fevers and rigors
            (3) Blood cultures negative in 50% of patients
        d. Treat with an antifungal agent (e.g., amphotericin B).
    10. Human immunodeficiency virus infection should always be of consideration when dealing with trauma patients who are in septic shock with an unknown source.
    11. Treatment
        a. Early identification of the infectious etiology and initiation of appropriate antibiotic treatment with fluid resuscitation are important. Guidelines include:
            (1) Within 3 hours: Obtain blood cultures, start empiric antibiotics, obtain baseline lactate, and give a bolus of at least 30 mL/kg crystalloid.
            (2) Within 6 hours: Add vasopressors if persistent hypotension or lactic acidosis continues, trend lactate, and measure CVP for endpoint resuscitation goals.
        b. Foley catheter to monitor urine output
        c. Invasive hemodynamic monitoring—arterial line and central venous line
        d. Vasopressors as needed. First line therapy consisting of norepinephrine followed by the addition of vasopressin
        e. In patients who remain hypotensive after adequate fluid resuscitation and remain on high-dose vasopressor therapy, treatment with intravenous corticosteroids (hydrocortisone 200–300 mg/day) for 7 days in three to four divided doses or by continuous infusion should be considered if adrenal insufficiency is suspected.
        f. Support of individual organ systems

C. NEUROGENIC SHOCK
1. Usually results from spinal cord injury, regional anesthetic agent, or autonomic blockade. Diagnosis is based on history and neurologic examination.
2. Hemodynamics
    a. Loss of vasomotor control
    b. Expansion of venous capacitance bed with peripheral pooling of blood
    c. Inadequate ventricular filling
3. Manifestations
    a. Warm, well-perfused skin
    b. Low blood pressure
    c. Low or normal urine output
    d. Bradycardia may be present if adrenergic nerves to heart are blocked, above T4, preventing the normal reflex tachycardia response to decreased pressures.

12

SHOCK

4. Treatment
   a. Correct ventricular filling pressure with intravenous fluids.
   b. Use vasoconstrictors to restore venous tone (vasopressin, phenylephrine [Neo-Synephrine], dopamine, etc.) and potentially heart rate.

Note: *Vasculature to those parts of the body with an intact autonomic nervous system may constrict excessively, resulting in ischemia to vital organs or necrosis of fingers.*

   c. Use Trendelenburg position if necessary.
   d. Maintain body temperature.

D. CARDIOGENIC SHOCK

Cardiogenic shock can be thought of as pump failure, and the etiology can either be myocardial dysfunction from primary (e.g., myocardial infarction) or from secondary (e.g., compressive) causative factors. Hemodynamically a systolic blood pressure less than 90 mm Hg, cardiac index less than 2.2 L/min per m^2, and PWP greater than 15 mm Hg are usually clinically seen.

1. **Primary myocardial dysfunction**
   a. It includes myocardial infarction, dysrhythmias, valvular dysfunction, and myocardial failure.
   b. Compromised myocardial contractility is the chief pathology in primary cardiogenic shock. Treatment is directed toward increasing myocardial function with various inotropic agents.
   c. Treatment
      (1) Identify and correct hemodynamically significant arrhythmias.
      (2) Optimize filling pressures.
      (3) If SVR is increased, initiate afterload reduction with nitroglycerin or nitroprusside. By reducing afterload, cardiac output can be optimized for a given preload and contractility. This is especially useful in cardiogenic shock when myocardial function is reduced. A reduction in afterload can greatly improve cardiac output.
      (4) If SVR is low or normal, initiate inotropic support with dopamine or dobutamine. Amrinone and milrinone are phosphodiesterase inhibitors used in resistant cardiogenic shock.
      (5) In practice, afterload reduction and inotropic support are often performed concurrently due to the secondary effects of inotropic support. Inotropes will cause an increase in afterload and tachycardia, which increases myocardial O$_2$ consumption and can further exacerbate ischemia.
      (6) If inotropic support fails, consider intraaortic balloon pump or ventricular assist device, which decreases afterload and increases diastolic cardiac perfusion without increasing myocardial O$_2$ demand.
      (7) In the setting of acute myocardial infarction, consider interventional cardiac catheterization, percutaneous catheter-based interventions, thrombolytic therapy, or surgical treatment. Surgical intervention with coronary artery bypass grafting is indicated

in patients who do not respond to treatment with percutaneous coronary intervention.

2. Secondary myocardial dysfunction, also known as obstructive shock
   a. It includes tension pneumothorax, cardiac tamponade, vena cava obstruction, and pulmonary embolus.
   b. Treatment of the underlying problem should alleviate shock.
   c. In the setting of trauma, distended neck veins should suggest secondary myocardial dysfunction (cardiac compression) and should be acted on immediately. Absence of distended neck veins does not rule out cardiac compression in a patient with hypovolemia. Distention may become evident only after adequate fluid resuscitation.
      (1) Common causes
          (a) Tension pneumothorax—shift of trachea to uninvolved side, decreased breath sounds, distended neck veins. This is not a radiographic diagnosis. These findings should prompt immediate intervention.
          (b) Cardiac tamponade—hypotension, muffled heart sounds, distended neck veins (Beck triad); low voltage on electrocardiogram and enlarged cardiac silhouette on chest radiograph (classic "water bottle" shape)
      (2) Associated findings may include pulsus paradoxus (decline in systolic blood pressure >10 mm Hg with inspiration).
      (3) Treatment is by fluid administration and correction of underlying mechanism.
          (a) Tension pneumothorax: Decompress with 14-gauge angiocatheter in second intercostal space, midclavicular line; definitive treatment is by chest tube placement in fifth intercostal space, anterior axillary line.
          (b) Acute cardiac tamponade: If hemodynamically stable, perform pericardiocentesis or pericardial window. If the patient is hemodynamically unstable, consider prompt operative thoracotomy or sternotomy.

E. HYPOADRENAL SHOCK/ADRENAL INSUFFICIENCY
1. Adrenal cortical hormones provide natural resistance to shock during times of stress and injury.
2. A reduction in blood volume and chemistry of these hormones can mimic hypovolemic shock.
   a. Leads to decreased capillary tone and permeability
3. It can be verified by checking cortisol levels lesser than 15 mg/dL.
   a. It can also be measured after an ACTH stimulation test.
      (1) Any measurement less than 5 mg/dL or less than 9-mg/dL increase would constitute deficiency.
   b. The diagnosis is difficult due to the relative lack of classic addisonian symptoms, and a high degree of suspicion is needed.
4. Correct by administering physiologic doses of steroids.

12

SHOCK

VI. VASOACTIVE AGENTS

1. **Inotropic agents and vasopressors**

   Note: *These agents should not be used as a substitute for adequate volume resuscitation.*

   a. Dopamine—effects are dose dependent.
      (1) For 3–5 µg/kg per minute (renal dose), renal artery vasodilation may enhance splanchnic perfusion and promote diuresis.
      (2) For 5–10 µg/kg per minute, there is stimulation of cardiac alpha-receptors, with increased contractility and cardiac output. Increased heart rate is seen with increasing dosage.
      (3) Doses greater than 10 µg/kg per minute increase alpha-adrenergic effects, with increased MAP and SVR caused by peripheral vasoconstriction.
   b. Dobutamine—synthetic dopamine analog with beta1 and beta2 effects; also acts as a mild vasodilator in addition to its inotropic effects; usual dosage is 5–15 µg/kg per minute.
   c. Amrinone—phosphodiesterase inhibitor that increases cyclic adenosine monophosphate. It has inotropic effects and also reduces afterload.
   d. Norepinephrine (Levophed)—exerts both alpha and beta effects. Beta effects predominate at lower doses, with increased heart rate and contractility; dose-dependent increases in alpha effect are seen, with vasoconstriction at increasing dosages.
   e. Epinephrine—at lower dosages (0.01 µg/kg per minute), there are beta1-mediated increases in heart rate and contractility. Vasoconstriction occurs with increasing dosages. There are concerns about increased myocardial oxygen demands with use.
   f. Phenylephrine (Neo-Synephrine) has alpha1 effect (vasoconstriction).
   g. Vasopressin—direct vasoconstrictor without inotropic or chronotropic effects may result in decreased cardiac output and splanchnic flow. Typical doses range from 0.01 to –0.04 unit/min.

2. **Vasodilators**

   a. Nitroglycerin—Primary effect is venodilation via direct action on vascular smooth muscle; increases venous capacitance.
   b. Nitroprusside acts directly on both arterial and venous smooth muscle.

RECOMMENDED READING

Zuckerbraun BS, Peitzman AB, Billiar TR, et al. Shock. In: Brunicardi F, Andersen DK, Billiar TR, et al., eds. *Schwartz's Principles of Surgery.* 10th ed. New York: McGraw-Hill; 2014.

Cardiopulmonary Monitoring

Paul T. Kim, MD

In the event of a cardiac arrest, the first procedure is to take your own pulse.

—Samuel Shem

The goal of cardiopulmonary monitoring is to assess the adequacy of the cardiac and pulmonary systems in meeting the metabolic needs of the patient. Although these goals may appear simple, this monitoring can become amazingly complicated in practice. The most important idea to grasp is that no single measurement can exist in isolation; all data must be considered with other data and the presentation of the patient. The ideal monitor is noninvasive, reliable, and conveys physiologic information in "real time." Often, in critically ill patients, noninvasive monitoring is either unreliable or inaccurate and invasive monitoring is required.

I. CARDIAC MONITORING
A. CARDIAC RHYTHMS
1. Continuous electrocardiogram (EKG)—allows for rapid recognition and analysis of heart rate, rhythm and various amplitudes and intervals
2. EKG abnormalities (Figs. 13.1–13.7)
   a. ST segment changes
      (1) ST segment depression is seen in subendocardial myocardial infarction (MI) and myocardial ischemia.
      (2) ST segment elevation is seen in transmural MI.
   b. T wave changes
      (1) Peaked T waves are seen with hyperkalemia.
      (2) Inverted T waves can be seen in many cardiac and noncardiac conditions, such as MI, myocarditis, and myocardial contusion.
      (3) Biphasic T waves can be seen in hypokalemia or ischemia.

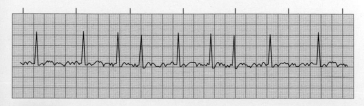

FIG. 13.1
Atrial fibrillation.

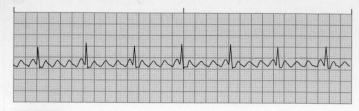

FIG. 13.2
Atrial flutter.

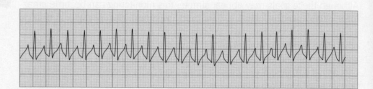

FIG. 13.3
Supraventricular tachycardia.

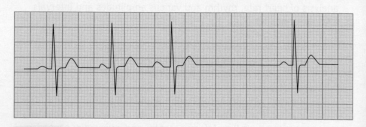

FIG. 13.4
Mobitz I second-degree heart block.

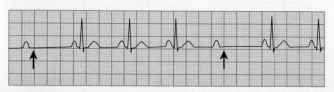

FIG. 13.5
Mobitz II second-degree heart block.

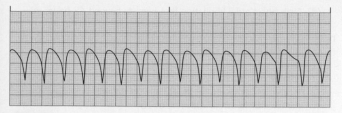

FIG. 13.6
Ventricular tachycardia.

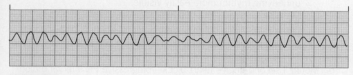

FIG. 13.7
Ventricular fibrillation.

   c. QTc interval
      (1) Prolonged QTc interval (>440 ms) is associated with in-
          creased risk of ventricular arrhythmias, such as torsades de
          pointes.
      (2) Prolonged QTc can be caused by various electrolyte disturbances
          and by drugs, such as antipsychotics (haloperidol, quetiapine),
          antidepressants (amitriptyline, nortriptyline, bupropion), anti-
          histamines (loratadine, diphenhydramine), and antiarrhythmics
          (amiodarone).
3. Common cardiac arrhythmias
   a. Atrial fibrillation: irregularly irregular ventricular rate with the absence
      of discernible P waves
      (1) Hemodynamically unstable patients require immediate synchro-
          nized direct current cardioversion.
      (2) In stable patients, rhythm control can often be achieved pharma-
          cologically with beta-blockers, calcium channel blockers, digoxin,
          or antiarrhythmics, such as amiodarone.
      (3) If rhythm control is unattainable, rate control is the next goal.
          Although current American Heart Association guidelines suggest
          similar outcomes for rate and rhythm control for patients with
          new onset atrial fibrillation, surgical patients frequently have an
          inciting event (operation, acute volume overload) and potential
          contraindications for anticoagulation that may make rate control
          more desirable.

    (4) New-onset atrial fibrillation that persists beyond 48 hours may require anticoagulation to prevent sequelae of embolization.

b. Atrial flutter: narrow complex tachycardia caused by reentry circuit in right atrium, typical rate of 130–170 (approximately 150 most common)

    (1) Treatment is similar to atrial fibrillation.

    (2) Have high suspicion for atrial flutter in patients with narrow complex tachycardia with rate of 150.

c. Supraventricular tachycardia (SVT): narrow complex sinus tachycardia, typical rate of 170–280 (higher than in atrial flutter)

    (1) Adenosine can help to differentiate SVT from atrial flutter and sinus tachycardia as the slowing of the ventricular rate makes the underlying rhythm more easily visible.

    (2) Mainstay of treatment is identification and treatment of the underlying cause, but rate-control agents such as beta-blockers, calcium channel blockers, or amiodarone can also be used if the SVT is symptomatic.

d. Mobitz I second-degree heart block—progressive PR interval prolongation before a nonconducted P wave

    (1) It may be asymptomatic or symptomatic, but hemodynamically stable patients should be closely monitored with transcutaneous pacing pads in place.

    (2) Hemodynamically unstable patients should be promptly treated with atropine and temporary transcutaneous cardiac pacing started.

    (3) Patients may eventually require permanent pacemaker placement if heart block does not resolve.

e. Mobitz II second-degree heart block—PR interval unchanged before a nonconducted P wave

    (1) Treatment is similar to Mobitz I heart block.

    (2) However, Mobitz II has a higher likelihood of progressing into third-degree heart block, and therefore more aggressive treatment is indicated.

f. Ventricular tachycardia: wide QRS complex (>120 ms) tachycardia with atrioventricular dissociation

    (1) Stable patients can be chemically cardioverted with antiarrhythmics, such as lidocaine or amiodarone.

    (2) Hemodynamically unstable patients require immediate synchronized direct current cardioversion.

    (3) All wide complex tachycardias should be treated as ventricular tachycardia until proven otherwise.

g. Ventricular fibrillation: irregular ventricular rhythm with no distinction between QRS complex, ST segment, and T waves

    (1) When recognized, immediate treatment is asynchronous defibrillation, then follow advanced cardiac life support (ACLS) protocol if rhythm is sustained after defibrillation.

B. BLOOD PRESSURE MONITORING

1. Sphygmomanometer—Indirect measurement of arterial blood pressure based on the assumption that pressures in the cuff are equal to pressures in the encompassed artery. The accuracy depends on the correct choice of cuff size and may be unreliable in patients with atherosclerotic disease.

2. Arterial catheter
   a. Advantages—This allows for continuous direct measurement of arterial blood pressure and arterial access for blood sampling.
   b. Limitations/complications—Air bubbles in the catheter-transducer system or clotting in the catheter can lead to decreased resonant frequency and erroneous measurements. Measurement also can be positional. Possible complications include thrombosis and distal ischemia, hematoma, stricture, arteriovenous fistula, or infection.
   c. Arterial pressure measurements can vary based on the location of the artery (i.e., aorta vs. radial), but mean arterial pressure (MAP) should be the same regardless of the distance of the artery from the heart and may be more clinically relevant than systolic or diastolic blood pressure.

C. HEMODYNAMIC MONITORING BASIC PRINCIPLES

1. Most often, hemodynamic monitoring is used to evaluate patients with potential inadequate oxygen delivery, whether that be caused by volume status, cardiac function, or high demands. Oxygen delivery is calculated by the following formula:

$$DO_2 = CaO_2 \times CO \times 10$$

where CaO_2 = arterial content of oxygen and CO = cardiac output. Although most values contributing to arterial oxygen content are known or easily determined, the factors that affect cardiac output are more complex, and this is where additional monitoring devices have the most utility. The ideal method of hemodynamic monitoring would be noninvasive, accurate, and continuous and give information about multiple components of oxygen delivery. Although many methods of evaluating the hemodynamic status of a patient have been developed, we have yet to find an ideal mode that meets all of these requirements. Overall, the information we seek from hemodynamic monitoring devices usually can fall into three basic categories:
   a. Intravascular volume status
   b. Cardiac function
   c. Adequacy of oxygen delivery

2. Basic clinical examination of the patient: Assessment of pulse, blood pressure, and urine output can offer a rapid assessment of the adequacy of perfusion.
   a. Intravascular volume status
      (1) Neck vein distension
      (2) Passive leg raise—predictor of fluid responsiveness but requires measuring either cardiac output, stroke volume, or pulse pressure

13

CARDIOPULMONARY MONITORING

    (a) Patient is placed in a semirecumbent position.

    (b) The legs are passively raised to 45 degrees, and stroke volume, cardiac output, or pulse pressure are monitored for change.

    (c) Maximal effect occurs at 30–90 seconds, and a 10% increase in stroke volume, cardiac output, or pulse pressure suggests that the patient would be responsive to fluids.

    (d) Utility is limited in severely hypovolemic patients and those with positional restrictions.

  b. Cardiac function—difficult to ascertain on simple physical examination. Tachycardia may represent a compensatory response to hypovolemia but may also be a result of cardiac failure.

  c. Adequacy of perfusion—adequate urine output can indicate sufficient renal perfusion, which is often sacrificed under situations in which brain and cardiac perfusion must be preserved. This can be unreliable in patients with intrinsic renal disease or those receiving diuretics.

3. In critically ill patients, clinical examination provides limited information, and additional monitoring devices are frequently required. We will discuss representative examples from the current methods of hemodynamic monitoring later, but new devices are constantly being developed, and existing devices are continually being updated. However, in general, these devices still provide data answering the three aforementioned questions. As a guide, these parameters are as follows:

  a. Parameters that assess preload (volume status): central venous pressure (CVP, estimation of right atrial filling pressure), pulmonary artery wedge pressure (PAWP, estimation of left atrial filling pressure), stroke volume (SV), right and left ventricular end-diastolic volume (RVEDV and LVEDV, respectively), stroke volume variation (SVV), pulse pressure variation (PPV), global end-diastolic volume (GEDV), intrathoracic blood volume (ITBV)

  b. Parameters that assess afterload: systemic vascular resistance (SVR), pulmonary vascular resistance (PVR)

  c. Parameters that assess contractility: cardiac output (CO), cardiac index (CI), right and left ventricular ejection fractions

  d. Parameters that assess oxygenation: hemoglobin, partial pressure of arterial oxygen and CO_2 (Pao_2, $Paco_2$), mixed venous oxygen saturation (Svo_2), central venous oxygen saturation ($Scvo_2$)

D. SPECIFIC DEVICES FOR CARDIAC MONITORING

1. Echocardiogram
  a. Transthoracic echocardiogram (TTE)
    (1) Measurements
      (a) Volume status can be assessed by looking at cardiac chamber sizes and the diameter of the inferior vena cava (IVC).

(i) Collapsed cardiac chambers and/or small (<1.2 cm) or collapsed IVC indicate low volume status.

(ii) However, IVC diameter <1.2 cm has a sensitivity of only 25% for hypovolemia.

(b) Cardiac function: Global function as well as regional wall motion abnormalities can be measured. Echocardiogram can also differentiate right heart from left heart function in cases where there is a discrepancy.

(2) Advantages

(a) Can be performed quickly at bedside

(b) Noninvasive

(3) Limitations/complications

(a) Patient's body habitus can limit the views of a bedside echocardiogram.

(b) Accuracy is highly dependent on operator skill and experience.

b. Transesophageal echocardiogram (TEE)

(1) Measurements—Similar to TTE, TEE can provide information about intravascular volume status and cardiac function. TEE also provides superior visualization of the heart, especially the posterior heart structures including valves as the transducer is in much closer proximity to the heart.

(2) Advantages—TEE provides real-time measurement of CO, SV, ventricular systolic function, volume assessment, and anatomic abnormalities, although measurements are valid only at that particular point in time.

(3) Limitations/complications

(a) Accuracy is highly dependent on operator skill and experience.

(b) Complications include dental, hypopharyngeal or esophageal injuries, malpositioning of endotracheal tube, or upper gastrointestinal (GI) bleeding.

(c) It should not be used in patients with known esophageal stricture, esophageal varices, or recent esophageal surgery.

2. **Venous catheter–based monitoring**

a. Central venous catheter

(1) Measurements

(a) Volume status: Trends in CVP may be useful in monitoring resuscitation, but single measurements may be inaccurate and of limited utility in the critically ill patient.

(b) Cardiac function: It does not give any information about cardiac function.

(c) Oxygen delivery: Although many papers, including the guidelines for sepsis, use central venous saturation as a measurement of adequacy of oxygen delivery, this value only reflects saturation in either the superior or IVC, depending on the location of the catheter (see mixed venous saturation later).

13

CARDIOPULMONARY MONITORING

(2) Advantages
  (a) Allows for continuous measurement of CVP and evaluation of trended data
  (b) Provides central venous access for certain solutions and medications, as well as central venous blood sampling
(3) Limitations/complications
  (a) Invasive procedure with potential for pneumothorax, hemothorax, and/or arterial puncture
  (b) Risks of infection
b. Pulmonary artery catheter (PAC)
  (1) Description—PAC contains multiple lumens/ports, thermistor and thermal filament for CO monitoring, and balloon for PAWP or pulmonary artery occlusion (PAO) pressure measurement. Proximal infusion port and right atrial lumen can be used for infusing fluids and drugs, as well as measuring right atrial pressures. Pulmonary artery (PA) lumen allows for measurement of PA pressures.
    (a) The catheter is inserted into a large vein (internal jugular, subclavian, or femoral vein) and advanced through the right atrium, the right ventricle, and into the PA.
    (b) It is the gold standard for cardiac output monitoring. It uses thermodilution technique as mentioned later.
  (2) Measurements
    (a) Volume status:
      (i) CVP
      (ii) PAWP or PAO—measured at the very end of the catheter, distal to the balloon. Although measurement of PAO is not directly related to left atrial (LA) pressures, the catheter functions on the assumption that the pulmonary vascular system is a low-pressure system, and therefore LA pressures are effectively transmitted to PAO measurements.
      (iii) RVEDV, SV—calculated values that give information regarding volume status
    (b) Cardiac function: CO and CI are measured by thermodilution in which the change in temperature of blood passing by the thermistor is used to calculate flow and cardiac output. Historically, this was performed by injection of cold saline at a proximal port. Modern-day PACs have a built-in thermal filament that heats surrounding blood in the right ventricle, and temperature change is detected by the thermistor located at the tip of the catheter. These types of catheters can often provide continuous, rather than static, CO monitoring.
    (c) Oxygen delivery:
      (i) Svo_2—The Swan-Ganz catheter is the only hemodynamic monitoring device that can measure a true mixed venous saturation, as this is defined by the saturation in

the PA. Unlike venous saturations obtained from central venous catheters, the oxygen content in the PA reflects the return from both the SVC and IVC.

(ii) Svo_2 provides an index of tissue perfusion and oxygenation. Increasing Svo_2 correlates positively with cardiac output and tissue perfusion and negatively with systemic shunt states (e.g., sepsis and hepatic failure).

(iii) Although Svo_2 cannot reflect changes in regional perfusion, a decreasing Svo_2 is a generally ominous sign. Knowledge of the Svo_2 will also allow calculation of arteriovenous oxygen content and physiologic shunt (Qsp/Qt), both of which can assist in managing respiratory failure.

(3) Advantages
   (a) Able to monitor advanced hemodynamic parameters to determine cardiac and pulmonary function, as well as overall fluid status.
   (b) Specialized catheters allow atrial, ventricular, or atrioventricular sequential cardiac pacing.
   (c) Continuous evaluation of variables

(4) Limitations/complications
   (a) Other parameters (i.e., peripheral resistance) are calculated from the measured values noted previously. Therefore their best utility is to assess trends.
   (b) PAWP is an estimation of left-heart filling pressure based on pulmonary vasculature being a low-pressure system. Thus cardiac and pulmonary disease states, such as valvular diseases or pulmonary hypertension, may lead to inaccurate measurements.
   (c) Respiratory failure requiring high levels of positive end-expiratory pressure increases intrathoracic measurements (including all measurements and calculations obtained from PA catheter) to an unknown and unpredictable degree.
   (d) For patients with low cardiac output, right-sided cardiomegaly, or unusual anatomy, or who are accessed from the left internal jugular vein, it may be difficult to achieve proper placement of the catheter.
   (e) In addition to the risks of central venous catheter insertion, PA catheters can cause cardiac dysrhythmias, as well as PA rupture.

3. Arterial pulse contour analysis–based monitoring
   a. FloTrac/Vigileo
      (1) Description—analyzes arterial line waveform using a specific proprietary algorithm that converts the pressure signal into a flow measurement based on assumptions about arterial compliance. This then allows for calculations of cardiac output.

(a) It does not require external calibration that refers to methods such as thermodilution or drug-dilution techniques that are performed to calibrate cardiac output monitoring devices for accurate measurements.

(2) Measurements

   (a) Volume status:

      (i) SVV and PPV are naturally occurring phenomena in which the arterial pulse pressure and stroke volume fall during inspiration and rise during expiration due to changes in intrathoracic pressure.

      (ii) SVV and PPV are indicators of relative preload responsiveness. If there is 13%–15% variation during inspiration, the patient is likely hypovolemic and will respond to volume. Conversely, if there is <10% variation, the patient is unlikely to be volume responsive.

      (iii) SV

   (b) Cardiac function: CO, CI—Unlike devices that use thermodilution, instruments based on arterial waveform analysis do not measure but instead calculate CO using proprietary algorithms that vary from company to company.

(3) Advantages

   (a) Much less invasive compared with PA catheter because it requires only an arterial line.

   (b) Provides continuous CO, SV, SVR, SVV, and PPV (Table 13.1 for normal values)

   (c) Does not require external calibration

(4) Limitations/complications

   (a) It requires good arterial waveform for accurate analysis.

   (b) Inaccurate in patients with hemodynamic instability or rapid vascular motor tone changes. In hemodynamically unstable patients, calibrated devices may be more useful.

   (c) Because there is no external calibration, the data may be less accurate than monitors with calibration.

TABLE 13.1

REFERENCE VALUES FOR VARIOUS HEMODYNAMIC PARAMETERS

Central venous pressure (CVP)	0–8 mm Hg
Pulmonary artery pressure (PAP)	15–30/6–12 mm Hg
Pulmonary artery wedge pressure (PAWP)	6–12 mm Hg
Cardiac output (CO)	4.0–8.0 L/min
Cardiac index (CI)	2.5–4 L/min/m^2
Mixed venous oxygen saturation (Svo$_2$)	70–80%
Stroke volume variations (SVV)	≤10%
Pulse pressure variations (PPV)	≤10%
Global end-diastolic volume index (GEDVI)	680–800 mL/m^2
Intrathoracic blood volume index (ITBVI)	850–1000 mL/m^2

b. Pulse contour cardiac output (PiCCO)
   (1) Description—hybrid-type device that provides continuous cardiac monitoring through arterial waveform analysis like FloTrac/Vigileo but is externally calibrated through transpulmonary thermodilution technique
       (a) Thermodilution technique—Cold saline is injected through the central line, and change in temperature is measured downstream via an arterial line to calculate cardiac output.
       (b) That measurement is then used to calibrate the cardiac output measurements calculated from arterial contour analysis.
   (2) Measurements
       (a) Volume status: SVV, PPV, GEDV, ITBV
           (i) SVV and PPV are similar to parameters measured by other arterial waveform analysis devices.
           (ii) GEDV is an estimate of end-diastolic volume in all four cardiac chambers and ITBV consists of GEDV plus pulmonary blood volume. These two measures are calculated via thermodilution technique noted previously and represent preload volume.
           (iii) Low GEDV or ITBV indicates hypovolemia.
           (iv) SV
       (b) Cardiac function: CO, CI
       (c) Oxygen delivery: $Scvo_2$—not as accurate as Svo_2 as it only contains SVC blood sample (see PAC section earlier).
   (3) Advantages
       (a) It provides continuous CO, SV, SVV, SVR, PPV, GEDV, and ITBV (see Table 13.1 for normal values).
       (b) External calibration may make calculated CO more accurate.
   (4) Limitations/complications
       (a) Unreliable in patients with poor arterial signal, rapid changes in vascular tones, arrhythmia, severe peripheral vascular disease, aortic valve pathology, and mechanical circulatory assist devices
       (b) Requires arterial line and central venous catheter
c. Lithium dilution cardiac output (LiDCO)
   (1) Description—provides continuous cardiac monitoring through arterial waveform analysis, which is externally calibrated via lithium dilution technique
       (a) Lithium is injected peripherally, and blood samples are drawn to plot a lithium concentration time curve to obtain the cardiac output.
       (b) As with PiCCO, this measurement is used to calibrate the cardiac output values calculated from arterial contour analysis.
   (2) Measurements
       (a) Volume status: SVV, PPV, ITBV, SV
       (b) Cardiac function: CO, CI
       (c) Oxygen delivery: $Scvo_2$

13

CARDIOPULMONARY MONITORING

(3) Advantages
  (a) Requires only arterial line and a peripheral venous line
  (b) Provides continuous CO, SV, SVV, SVR, PPV, and ITBV (see Table 13.1 for normal values)
(4) Limitations/complications
  (a) It is inaccurate in patients with poor arterial signal, aortic regurgitation, arrhythmia, and severe peripheral vasoconstriction.
  (b) Calibration can be affected by nondepolarizing muscle relaxant and lithium therapy.
  (c) It is contraindicated in patients less than 40 kg or in first trimester of pregnancy.

4. **Bioreactance**
  a. Nicom, Cheetah
    (1) Description—measures the phase changes in an alternating electrical current crossing the patient's torso, which has been shown to correlate with pulsatile changes in aortic fluid volume. Four electrodes are placed on the patient's chest, and a 75-kHz electrical signal is generated on one side and detected across the chest by the other electrode. The delay in transmission is then measured by the device—the higher the cardiac stroke volume, the more significant the phase shifts become. Because the signal is only affected by pulsatile flow, the delay can be used to calculate how much blood is coming out of the LV into the aorta, or stroke volume.
    (2) Measurements
      (a) Volume status: SV
      (b) Cardiac function: CO, CI
      (c) Oxygen delivery: none
    (3) Advantages: noninvasive continuous monitoring of cardiac output, stroke volume
    (4) Limitations/complications
      (a) It depends highly on positioning of the electrodes.
      (b) Limitations include electrical interference (i.e., electrocautery), fluid in thorax (pleural effusions, pulmonary edema, pericardial tamponade), changes in peripheral vascular resistance, obesity, arrhythmias, and motion artifacts.
      (c) Validation studies suggest poor correlation compared with PA catheter.

II. PULMONARY MONITORING
A. PULSE OXIMETRY
1. Noninvasive method to measure capillary hemoglobin saturation using a light absorption of red (600–750 nm) and infrared (850–1000 nm) light absorption characteristics of oxygenated and deoxygenated hemoglobin. A light emitter and detector are placed on a translucent site with good blood

flow (e.g., fingernail bed, earlobe, nasal ala), and the ratio of red/infrared signal detection is then converted to an arterial oxygenation saturation (Spo_2) value based on calibration curves from healthy individuals.

2. Limitations:
   a. Hypotension or hypothermia resulting from poor peripheral perfusion can lead to inadequate signal.
   b. Motion artifact can interfere with signal detection due to unstable waveform.
   c. Carbon monoxide poisoning or smokers can have artificially high readings.
   d. Nail polish and artificial fingernails can interfere with oximetry readings.

B. **APNEA MONITORING—DETECTS CHEST WALL MOTION BY SENSING A CHANGE IN THE ELECTRICAL IMPEDANCE ACROSS THE CHEST WALL; ALARMS ARE USUALLY SET TO DETECT BRADYPNEA OR APNEA**

C. **CAPNOGRAPHY**
1. End-tidal carbon dioxide in exhaled air is directly measured.
2. Continuous measurement of end-tidal carbon dioxide is an indicator of adequate tidal volume and clearance of metabolic by-products.
3. After being calibrated to an arterial blood gas, end-tidal CO_2 monitoring is useful to determine trends in CO_2 production and clearance.

D. **ARTERIAL OR VENOUS BLOOD GAS**
1. It allows determination of oxygen delivery and consumption and clearance of metabolic waste products.
2. It reflects oxygenation, ventilation, and acid-base status.
3. A complete discussion of blood gas interpretation can be found in Chapter 14.

III. IMPORTANT FORMULAS

A. **CARDIAC OUTPUT**

$$CO = HR \times SV$$

HR = heart rate; SV = stroke volume
Reference range = 4–8 L/min

B. **ARTERIAL CONTENT OF OXYGEN**

$$CaO_2 = (1.39 \times Hg \times Spo_2) + (Pao_2 \times 0.0031)$$

Hg = hemoglobin level; Spo_2 = arterial oxygen saturation; Pao_2 = arterial partial pressure of oxygen
Reference value = 18 mL/dL

13

CARDIOPULMONARY MONITORING

C. OXYGEN DELIVERY

$$DO_2 = CaO_2 \times CO \times 10$$

CaO_2 = arterial content of oxygen; CO = cardiac output
Reference value = 1000 mL/min

D. OXYGEN CONSUMPTION

$$VO_2 = (CO \times CaO_2) - (CO \times CvO_2)$$

CaO_2 = arterial content of oxygen; CvO_2 = venous content of oxygen; CO =
cardiac output
Reference value = 125 mL/min/m²

RECOMMENDED READINGS

Holcroft JW, Anderson JT. Cardiopulmonary monitoring. In: Souba WW, Fink MP, Jurkovich GJ, et al., eds. *ACS Surgery: Principles and Practice*. New York: WebMD; 2007.

Marino PL, ed. *The ICU Book*. 4th ed. New York: Lippincott Williams & Wilkins; 2013.

Monnet X, Marik P, Teboul JL. Passive leg raising for predicting fluid responsiveness: a systematic review and meta-analysis. *Intensive Care Med*. 2016;42:1935–1947.

Monnet X, Teboul JL. Passive leg raising: five rules, not a drop of fluid! *Crit Care*. 2015; 19:18.

Sasai T, Tokioka H, Fukushima T, et al. Reliability of central venous pressure to assess left ventricular preload for fluid resuscitation in patients with septic shock. *J Intensive Care*. 2014;2:58.

Schlöglhofer T, Gilly H, Schima H. Semi-invasive measurement of cardiac output based on pulse contour: a review and analysis. *Can J Anaesth*. 2014;61:452–479.

Thiele RH, Bartels K, Gan TJ. Cardiac output monitoring: a contemporary assessment and review. *Crit Care Med*. 2015;43:177–185.

Vincent JL, Rhodes A, Perel A, et al. Clinical review: update on hemodynamic monitoring—a consensus of 16. *Crit Care*. 2011;15:229.

Mechanical Ventilation

Paul T. Kim, MD

Development in most fields of medicine appears to occur according to sound scientific principles. However, exceptions can be found, and the development of mechanical ventilatory support is one of them.

—J. Rasanen

The goal of mechanical ventilation is to facilitate gas exchange for tissue oxygen delivery, provide ventilation for removal of carbon dioxide, unload the work of the respiratory muscles, and minimize the detrimental effects of both endotracheal intubation and mechanical ventilation. The procedures and indications for endotracheal intubation, tracheostomy placement, and cricothyroidotomy are addressed later in this handbook.

I. DETERMINING NEED FOR MECHANICAL VENTILATION

A. AIRWAY INSTABILITY
1. From operative procedure, head injury, intoxication, among other causes, usually only requiring temporary support

B. RESPIRATORY FAILURE
1. From acute respiratory distress syndrome, chronic obstructive pulmonary disease, pulmonary edema, among other causes, usually requiring prolonged support

C. GUIDELINES
1. The first indication is consideration of intubation.
2. Intubation is NOT a sign of weakness.
3. Ventilation is not "addictive."
4. Remember, mechanical ventilation is a support measure, not a cure for cardiopulmonary disease. Inappropriate use can lead to ventilator-induced lung injury and increased mortality.

II. VENTILATION VERSUS OXYGENATION

A. VENTILATION
1. The purpose of ventilation is to eliminate CO_2, a function of minute ventilation (selected on the ventilator with respiratory rate and tidal volume [V_T]). Minute ventilation (V_E) has two components, alveolar ventilation (⅔ of V_T) and dead space ventilation (⅓ of V_T); normal V_E is 6 L/min, driven at brainstem by $Paco_2$ and pH. In lung disease, physiologic dead space can be much higher and a dead space to tidal

volume ratio (V_D/V_T) greater than 0.6 is predictive of mortality in acute respiratory distress syndrome (ARDS).

B. OXYGENATION

1. Oxygenation is a function of ventilation and perfusion (V/Q) matching, evaluated by calculating alveolar-arterial (A-a) gradient ($Pao_2 - Pao_2$), where Fio_2 is the fraction of inspired oxygen:

$$[Pao_2 = Fio_2 \times (\text{barometric pressure} - P_{H_2O}) - Pao_2/RQ]$$

Reference range is 8–12 mm Hg
Estimate: P/F ratio (Pao_2/Fio_2), which at sea level is $100/0.21 = 500$.

III. NONINVASIVE POSITIVE PRESSURE VENTILATION

A. POSITIVE PRESSURE VENTILATION

1. Provided via face mask with either continuous positive airway pressure (CPAP) or positive pressure ventilation (continuous mandatory ventilation [CMV], pressure support ventilation [PSV], proportional assist ventilation [PAV])

B. INITIAL SETTINGS

1. Usually 5 cm H_2O positive end-expiratory pressure (PEEP) and 5–10 cm H_2O pressure support

C. ADVANTAGES

1. Most studies have described advantages of noninvasive positive pressure ventilation in patients with immediately reversible causes of respiratory insufficiency (exacerbations of chronic obstructive pulmonary disease or cardiogenic pulmonary edema).

D. RESERVED

1. For those patients who have a presumed temporary respiratory insufficiency from a rapidly reversible cause (narcotic overdose, multiple rib fractures, exacerbations of congestive heart failure, or chronic obstructive pulmonary disease). Improvement in symptoms in the first 2 hours demonstrates success. If there is no improvement in the first 2 hours, intubation should be performed.

IV. CONVENTIONAL MECHANICAL VENTILATION

Several parameters may be manipulated to limit the functions of the ventilator; however, the most common and default arrangement is time trigger (mandatory ventilation) or flow trigger (spontaneous ventilation), volume cycled, and pressure limited for each breath.

A. MODES OF VENTILATION

1. Assist control: This ensures delivery of a minimum (mandatory) V_E but also allows additional patient-triggered (spontaneous) breaths; each

breath, regardless of the trigger (time or patient initiated), is completely supported to desired volume or pressure. Major limitation is that agitated patients may become hyperventilated (with respiratory alkalosis or development of auto-PEEP) if the respiratory rate is rapid.

2. Intermittent mandatory ventilation: Only a selected number of breaths are fully supported to desired volume or pressure; additional breaths are reliant on patient effort with delivered pressure support. Often used as a bridge to spontaneous respirations, but experience has demonstrated this to be a suboptimal approach to liberation from the ventilator.

3. Pressure control ventilation: Either physician or patient determines respiratory rate; once triggered (time or flow), the ventilator will deliver a preselected pressure, which will result in a variable volume depending on the pulmonary compliance. Pressure control ventilation is useful for poorly compliant lungs to decrease the risk for barotrauma, although it may lead to increased $Paco_2$ (permissive hypercapnia).

4. Pressure support ventilation: The simplest form of pressure-limited ventilation, it is used to augment spontaneous breathing, not to provide full ventilatory support. The patient determines both respiratory rate and inspiratory time at a physician-selected pressure support. Exhalation occurs passively. This mode most closely resembles spontaneous unassisted breathing and should be the mode of choice in the patient with a spontaneous respiratory drive.

5. In patients who are breathing rapidly during assist/control ventilation and show evidence of respiratory alkalosis or auto-PEEP, a change to intermittent mandatory ventilation should prove beneficial; however, in patients with respiratory muscle weakness or cardiac dysfunction, assist/control should be favored.

B. VENTILATOR STRATEGIES

1. Oxygenation
   a. Fio_2: This parameter is usually adjusted initially when a patient has difficulty oxygenating (decreased Spo_2 [arterial saturation as measured during pulse oximetry] or Pao_2). Although Fio_2 less than 60% is well tolerated, prolonged periods at greater than 60% can result in nitrogen washout, adsorption atelectasis, increased pulmonary shunt, and pulmonary fibrosis. Elevated Fio_2 should be avoided and the Fio_2 required to maintain normoxia targeted.
   b. PEEP: Used to prevent alveolar collapse during expiration and preserve functional residual capacity. PEEP of 5 cm H_2O reduces work of breathing, improves oxygenation in intubated patients, and helps to prevent leakage of fluid around the endotracheal (ET) tube cuff. Increasing PEEP may be helpful for recruitment of alveoli and to optimize the V/Q interface (if more alveoli are open and oxygenated, then more oxygen can diffuse into the blood). An important caveat is that increasing PEEP can have detrimental hemodynamic effects

(see later). Best PEEP is best determined using stepwise increases in PEEP and assessing the effects on oxygen delivery (DO_2) and respiratory mechanics (compliance), not simply aiming for increased arterial oxygenation.

2. Ventilation
   a. An initial ventilator setting of respiratory rate of 12–15 breaths/min and V_T of 5–8 mL/kg should ensure adequate clearance of CO_2.
   b. If $Paco_2$ level remains increased, increasing the respiratory rate to 20–24 breaths/min will likely correct the hypercapnia while preserving a reasonable pulmonary airway pressure. If this maneuver does not correct the hypercapnia, consider excessive production of CO_2 as a complicating factor (obtain metabolic cart to assess for overfeeding; see later).
   c. When all maneuvers fail and CO_2 level continues to increase, remember there is little physiologic detriment if the pH remains greater than 7.20.

C. LIBERATION FROM MECHANICAL VENTILATION

1. Nurse- or respiratory therapist–driven protocols with daily spontaneous breathing trials (SBTs) have shown the best results in early liberation from mechanical ventilation.
2. Weaning strategies: When the clinical scenario improves (patient is awake, able to take spontaneous breaths, and arterial oxygenation is acceptable [Pao_2 >80 mm Hg on Fio_2 ≤40%] with minimal ventilatory support), then the process of liberation begins.
3. SBTs: This is best determined daily over 30 minutes with the patient breathing through the ventilator circuit with minimal PEEP only; the patient will determine respiratory rate, V_T, and minute ventilation. If arterial blood gas shows acceptable values (Pao_2 >80 mm Hg and with acceptable pH), then the patient is ready for extubation.
4. Rapid shallow breathing index: Another parameter used is the rapid shallow breathing index. If frequency/V_T is <105, then a high likelihood exists that the patient is ready for extubation (e.g., respiratory rate of 20 and V_T of 0.500 L = rapid shallow breathing index of 40). If the patient passes the SBT, then seriously consider extubation.
5. Failure of SBT is demonstrated by tachypnea, increased work of breathing, dysrhythmias, or hemodynamic instability.

D. FAILURE TO LIBERATE FROM MECHANICAL VENTILATION

If the patient does not pass the SBT, it is important to determine why the patient did not pass.

1. Mental status: Patients should be awake and alert for best success of liberation.
2. Airway protection: Patients should be able to protect the airway by coughing, swallowing secretions, and calling for help.

3. Secretion control: Excessive secretions may further compromise a tenuous airway.
4. Respiratory muscle fatigue: This usually requires 24 hours of rest on ventilator with respiratory rate of 20–25 breaths/min to completely off-load the work of breathing.
5. Electrolyte abnormalities: Phosphorus and magnesium in particular can contribute to continued ventilator dependence.
6. It is usually best medicine to wait 24 hours before attempting another SBT after a failed SBT.

V. EFFECTS ON CARDIAC PERFORMANCE

A. ENDOTRACHEAL INTUBATION AND MECHANICAL VENTILATION PLACE IMPORTANT PHYSIOLOGIC DEMANDS ON PATIENTS

B. THE SHIFT FROM NEGATIVE PRESSURE TO POSITIVE PRESSURE VENTILATION CAN COMPROMISE PRELOAD BY

1. Decreasing the pressure gradient for venous inflow into the thorax
2. Reducing ventricular distensibility, thus decreasing ventricular filling during diastole
3. Compressing the pulmonary veins, thus increasing right heart afterload, possibly to the extent that it dilates the right heart, shifts the ventricular septum, and thus decreases left ventricular chamber size (known as ventricular interdependence)

C. POSITIVE PRESSURE VENTILATION

1. Can decrease afterload by augmenting the pressure gradient between the left ventricle and the extrathoracic outflow tract (decreases left ventricular transmural pressure)

D. THE EFFECTS OF POSITIVE PRESSURE VENTILATION ON CARDIAC PERFORMANCE

1. Tends to reduce ventricular filling during diastole but enhance ventricular emptying during systole. These effects can be countered in most hypovolemic patients with fluid administration. However, patients with cardiac failure will not respond to fluid administration.

VI. NEED FOR TRACHEOSTOMY

In patients who repeatedly do not pass the SBT, consideration should be given to tracheostomy to decrease the complications associated with long-term endotracheal intubation (tracheal stenosis, ventilator-associated pneumonia, prolonged intensive care unit stay, etc.). Another group of patients to be considered for tracheostomy is patients with a high likelihood of requiring prolonged mechanical ventilatory support. It is our policy to perform early (<7 days) bedside percutaneous tracheostomy as often as possible in these patients.

14

MECHANICAL VENTILATION

VII. VENTILATOR CAUTIONS

A. DEFINITION OF ACUTE RESPIRATORY DISTRESS SYNDROME

1. Acute onset: within 1 week of a known clinical insult or new or worsening respiratory symptoms
2. Bilateral chest infiltrates on chest radiograph
3. Respiratory failure not fully explained by cardiac failure or fluid overload
4. Mild: P/F ratio ≤300 mm Hg but >200 mm Hg with PEEP or CPAP ≥5 cm H_2O
5. Moderate: P/F ratio ≤200 mm Hg but >100 mm Hg with PEEP ≥5 cm H_2O
6. Severe: P/F ratio ≤100 mm Hg ≥5 cm H_2O

B. ACUTE LUNG INJURY/ACUTE RESPIRATORY DISTRESS SYNDROME TREATED WITH PROTECTIVE LUNG STRATEGY

1. Limit lung volumes to 6 mL/kg (predicted body weight).
2. Limit pulmonary plateau pressure to 30 cm H_2O.
3. Use PEEP to limit Fio_2 to 0.60.
4. Transient levels of increased PEEP can be used to recruit additional alveoli (recruitment maneuver).

C. VENTILATOR-ASSOCIATED PNEUMONIA

1. Evidence of pneumonia after 3–5 days of mechanical ventilation
   a. Fever
   b. Increased white blood cell count
   c. Purulent sputum production
   d. New infiltrate on chest radiograph
2. The previous criteria combined with bronchoscopically obtained specimen with greater than 100,000 colonies/mL
3. Protocol-driven therapy: initial broad-spectrum antimicrobials and deescalation of therapy when culture results dictate a specific organism and sensitivities

VIII. PEARLS

A. STANDARD INITIAL VENTILATOR SETTINGS

Assist/control rate: 12
V_T: 6 mL/kg (predicted body weight)
Pressure support: 10 cm H_2O—pressure support is inactive in the assist control (AC) mode
PEEP: 5 cm H_2O
Fio_2: 0.60

Obtain arterial blood gas in 30–60 minutes, and make appropriate changes.

Normal inspiratory/expiratory ratio is 1:3, with 15 breaths/min; this is 1 second of inspiration and 3 seconds of expiration. Pao_2 greater than 60 mm Hg usually equates to Spo_2 greater than 90%.

RECOMMENDED READINGS

Marino PL, ed. *The ICU Book*. 2nd ed. New York: Lippincott Williams & Wilkins; 1988.
Sena MJ, Nathens AB. Mechanical ventilation. In: Souba WW, Fink MP, Jurkovich GJ, et al., eds. *ACS Surgery: Principles and Practice*. New York: WebMD; 2005.

PART IV

Trauma Surgery

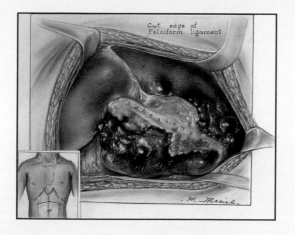

PART IV

Trauma Surgery

Primary and Secondary Survey

Meghan C. Daly, MD

Push it. Examine all things intensely and relentlessly.
—Annie Dillard

I. EPIDEMIOLOGY

A. MORTALITY
Trauma is the third leading cause of death in the United States for all ages and the leading cause of deaths in persons younger than 45 years.
1. A total of 50% of deaths occur within minutes after injury.
2. A total of 30% of deaths occur within 24 hours of injury.
3. The remainder of deaths occur days to weeks after injury.

B. MECHANISMS OF INJURY
1. **Motor vehicle crash or collision (MVC)**
   a. It is the leading cause of death.
   b. Adolescents and young adults are at greatest risk for fatal MVCs.
   c. Alcohol intoxication is a major factor in fatal MVCs in adolescents and young adults.
2. **Firearms**
   a. Approximately 33,000 deaths occur secondary to firearms annually.
3. **Falls**
   a. Falls are the leading cause of nonfatal injury in children younger than 14 years.
   b. A total of 27% of adults older than 65 years will fall each year.
4. **Industrial accidents and burns are also significant.**

II. MANAGEMENT OF THE TRAUMA PATIENT

A. PRIMARY SURVEY
Initial evaluation of the trauma patient
1. Brief history—mechanism of injury, time of injury, vital signs in the field, and medical history
2. ABCDEs
   a. **A**irway: If the patient is alert and answers the questions with a clear voice, the airway is intact. If the patient's airway is not secure, rapid sequence endotracheal intubation or a definitive surgical airway should be established. Repeated assessment of airway patency is crucial. Special considerations include:
      (1) Mental status: Glasgow Coma Scale (GCS) (Table 15.1) score of less than 8 usually requires intubation for airway protection. Agitation or combativeness may be signs of hypoxia or profound shock.

TABLE 15.1	
GLASGOW COMA SCALE	
Eye Opening	
Opens spontaneously	4
Opens to command	3
Opens to pain	2
No response	1
Verbal	
Oriented	5
Confused	4
Inappropriate words	3
Incomprehensible sounds	2
No response	1
Motor	
Follows commands	6
Localizes pain	5
Withdraws from pain	4
Flexion with pain (decorticate)	3
Extension with pain (decerebrate)	2
No response	1

(2) Facial trauma: Upper airway landmarks can be distorted by soft tissue damage or blood.

(3) Protect cervical spine.

(4) A surgical airway (i.e., cricothyroidotomy) is established when edema of the glottis, fracture of the larynx, or severe oropharyngeal hemorrhage obstructs the airway or an endotracheal tube (ET) cannot be placed through the vocal cords. Surgical cricothyroidotomy is performed by making a skin incision that extends through the cricothyroid membrane, dilating, and inserting a small ET or tracheostomy tube.

b. **B**reathing: Assess oxygen saturation via pulse oximetry. Anemia, hypotension, and hypothermia can affect the reliability of the pulse oximeter. Palpation, percussion, auscultation, and inspection of chest cavity should be performed. Injuries that severely impair ventilation include: tension pneumothorax, flail chest with pulmonary contusion, massive hemothorax, and open pneumothorax.

c. **C**irculation and hemorrhage control: Shock is defined as inadequate tissue perfusion to support metabolic demands. The trauma patient can present with hypovolemic, cardiogenic, or neurogenic shock, or a combination of all three. Two large-bore (16–18 gauge) peripheral intravenous lines should be established.

(1) Vital signs: Tachycardia can be the first sign of hypovolemic shock. Blood pressure can be misleading because in hypovolemic shock, hypotension is not seen until 30%–40% of the blood volume is lost. Absence of tachycardia may be present in patients taking beta-blockers or digoxin, those in spinal shock, or in older adults.

TABLE 15.2

CLASSIFICATION OF HEMORRHAGE

Parameter	I	II	III	IV
Blood loss (mL)	<750	750–1500	1500–2000	>2000
Blood loss (%)	<15	15–30	30–40	>40
Pulse rate	<100	>100	>120	>140
Blood pressure	Normal	Normal	Decreased	Deceased
Respiratory rate	14–20	20–30	30–40	>35
Urine output (mL/h)	>30	20–30	5–15	Negligible
Central nervous system symptoms	Normal	Anxious	Confused	Lethargic
Fluid	Crystalloid	Crystalloid	Blood	Blood

15

PRIMARY AND SECONDARY SURVEY

  (2) Physical examination: Level of consciousness, skin color, capillary refill, and pulses must be assessed.
  (3) Hypovolemic shock: This is caused by loss of blood volume (Table 15.2 for classes of shock). Major areas of internal hemorrhage include: chest, abdomen, retroperitoneum, pelvis, and long bones. Source of bleeding can be identified via physical examination and imaging (chest x-ray, pelvic x-ray, or focused assessment sonography in trauma [FAST]). One to 2 L of isotonic fluids are given initially unless the patient has predictors for requiring a massive transfusion. Predictors for massive transfusion include a penetrating mechanism of injury, a systolic blood pressure (SBP) <90 mm Hg, heart rate >120, and a positive FAST examination. If a massive transfusion is anticipated, resuscitation should be done with a balanced 1:1:1 (packed red blood cells [PRBC]:fresh frozen plasma [FFP]:platelets) transfusion strategy to mimic whole blood.
  (4) Cardiogenic shock: This is caused by blunt or penetrating cardiac injury; it can also be caused by tension pneumothorax, which is treated with needle decompression and subsequent chest tube placement. Patients in cardiogenic shock may have cardiac tamponade, which is associated with *Beck triad:* hypotension, muffled heart sounds, and distended neck veins. Cardiac tamponade can be initially managed with pericardiocentesis.
  (5) Neurogenic shock: This is caused by injuries to the spinal cord that result in loss of sympathetic tone, vasodilatation, and inability to mount a tachycardic response. Neurogenic shock is treated with fluid resuscitation and vasopressors.
 d. **D**isability: After the airway, breathing, and circulation are assessed, the mental status and neurologic function are evaluated. The GCS is a standardized method of classifying level of consciousness.
 e. **E**xposure: All clothing should be completely removed to perform a thorough assessment. Warm blankets and warmed fluid should be used to decrease hypothermia.

B. FURTHER EVALUATION AND TRANSFER

1. Transfer of trauma patients: Some trauma facilities do not have the resources to deal with certain injuries. The patient should be stabilized and transferred by air or ground depending on the distance and injury severity.
2. Additional studies/diagnostics
   a. Foley catheter to monitor urine output. Contraindicated if blood is present at urethral meatus, scrotal or penile hematoma, or high-riding prostate on rectal examination. If any contraindications, perform retrograde urethrogram to determine whether urethral injury is present. If no extravasation, a Foley catheter may be safely inserted.
   b. Nasogastric tubes can be helpful for decompression. Massive gastric distension can contribute to nausea, vomiting, aspiration, tachycardia, and hypotension. Intubated patients should receive a nasogastric tube. Orogastric tubes are preferred over nasogastric tubes in patients with midface trauma.
   c. Radiographic studies: In patients who are critically ill, it is important to obtain only studies that will affect management. A portable chest and pelvic radiograph can provide valuable information in the unstable patient. Patients being transported for studies or procedures must have an established airway, be hemodynamically stable, and be on a cardiopulmonary monitor.
   d. Laboratory evaluation: Draw a standard trauma laboratory panel while establishing intravenous access. Recommend: type and screen, complete blood cell count, electrolyte panel, and coagulation tests. Lactic acid and base deficit are helpful to monitor the degree of shock. Thromboelastography (TEG) may guide resuscitation and blood product use.

C. SECONDARY SURVEY

Survey consists of a complete history and physical examination. It does not begin until the primary survey is complete, resuscitative efforts are underway, and normalization of vital functions has been demonstrated. Often the secondary survey is delayed until a definitive operation has been performed.

1. History includes complete questioning of the patient, prehospital personnel, and family. The important aspects of history are in the pneumonic AMPLE:
   a. **A**—Allergies
   b. **M**—Medications
   c. **P**—Past illness and pregnancy
   d. **L**—Last meal
   e. **E**—Events and environment related to the injury
2. Specific considerations
   a. Firearms: It can be beneficial to know type of weapon, number of shots heard, and distance of victim from gun.

   b. MVCs: Important questions include position of victim in car, whether the patient was ejected from the vehicle, extrication time, direction of impact, speed of vehicle, loss of consciousness, restraint use (seatbelts, air bags), and outcome of others passengers in the car.

   c. Fall: Important questions include height of fall, landing surface, position body landed on, and loss of consciousness.

3. Physical examination: complete and thorough physical examination. Sequence is as follows: head, maxillofacial structures, cervical spine and neck, chest, abdomen, perineum/rectum/vagina, musculoskeletal system, and neurologic system. Missed injuries can be minimized by maintaining a high index of suspicion and continually monitoring the patient's status.

III. PEDIATRIC TRAUMA

Children have different mechanisms of injury, hemodynamic responses to stress, communication barriers, relatively small total blood volume, increased metabolic requirements for growth, and problems with thermoregulation.

A. MECHANISMS OF INJURY
1. MVCs are the leading cause of mortality in this age group.

B. PRIMARY SURVEY

The ABCDEs are followed; however, there are some specific considerations:

1. Airway: Children have a shorter neck, short trachea, large tongue, and floppy epiglottis. The proper size ET should be placed.
   a. An oversized ET can cause future tracheal stenosis.
   b. An undersized ET tube will not allow for adequate ventilation.
   c. ET size is determined by diameter of child's fifth digit or calculated as follows: (age in years + 16)/4.
   d. Cuff pressures less than 30 mm Hg are considered safe.

2. Breathing: Children are primarily diaphragmatic breathers, and any interference with diaphragm excursion will interfere with breathing.
   a. Children swallow air when crying, which can cause gastric distension and decrease left hemidiaphragm movement. Gastric decompression should be accomplished early.
   b. Tension pneumothorax can progress quickly to respiratory failure.

3. Circulation: Tachycardia is usually the first sign of hypovolemia. Table 15.3 details the normal vital signs of children. Other signs of hypovolemic shock include changes in mentation, decreased capillary refill, skin pallor, and hypothermia.

4. Intravenous access: Antecubital lines should be the first attempted location but can be challenging in children. Other sites include:
   a. Femoral line
   b. Saphenous vein cut-down at the ankle
   c. Intraosseous infusion in tibia or sternum.

15

PRIMARY AND SECONDARY SURVEY

TABLE 15.3

VITAL PARAMETERS BY AGE

Age Group	Respiratory Rate	Heart Rate (Beats/Min)	Systolic Blood Pressure (mm Hg)
Newborn	30–50	120–160	50–70
1–12 months	20–30	80–140	70–100
13–36 months	20–30	80–130	80–110
3–5 years	20–30	80–120	80–110
6–12 years	20–30	70–110	80–120
13+ years	12–20	55–105	110–120

IV. TRAUMA AND PREGNANCY

Trauma is the leading cause of death during pregnancy. It is important for the trauma surgeon to be aware of the unique set of physiologic variables of gravid women.

A. EPIDEMIOLOGY

1. MVCs, falls, and assaults are the leading causes of trauma.
2. MVCs, falls, and firearms are the leading causes of fetal death.

B. ANATOMIC AND PHYSIOLOGIC CHANGES DURING PREGNANCY
(Table 15.4.)

C. MATERNAL EVALUATION

The mother is always the priority in care and treatment because the most common cause of fetal demise is maternal death.

1. **Primary survey**
   a. ABC: Securing the airway and providing adequate oxygenation is important to decrease maternal catecholamines, which can cause vasoconstriction and maternal/placental insufficiency.
   b. Supine hypotensive syndrome
      (1) Caused by aortocaval compression by the uterus.
      (2) Place mother in left lateral decubitus position while keeping the spine neutral.
   c. Signs of shock can be delayed because of physiologic hypervolemia.

D. FETAL ASSESSMENT

1. **Heart rate: Reference range is 120–160 beats/min.**
   a. Doppler instrument detects heart rate by 12 weeks of gestation.
   b. Initial response to stress is tachycardia followed by bradycardia in severe distress.
   c. Cardiotechnographic monitors assess fetal heart rate and uterine contractions.
2. Fetal exposure to radiation: all necessary radiographic tests should be done if they will benefit the mother.

TABLE 15.4

ANATOMIC AND PHYSIOLOGIC CHANGES DURING PREGNANCY

System	Change	Implication
Cardiovascular	↓ Peripheral vascular resistance, ↓ venous return, ↓ blood pressure (10–15 mm Hg)	Supine hypotensive syndrome (10–15 mm Hg)
Blood volume	Plasma and blood volume, white blood cell count to 20,000/L	Physiologic hypervolemia
Coagulation	Hypercoagulable, clotting factors, ↓ fibrinolysis	Venous thromboembolism
Respiratory	Diaphragm excursion, tidal volume, minute ventilation, ↓ Pco_2	Chronic compensated respiratory alkalosis
Gastrointestinal	↓ Motility, ↓ gastroesophageal sphincter competency	Risk for aspiration
Renal	Glomerular filtration rate, creatinine, ↓ blood urea nitrogen	Hydronephrosis and hydroureter
Endocrine	Parathyroid hormone, calcitonin	Calcium absorption

Pco_2, Partial pressure of carbon dioxide.

a. Less than 3 weeks: Death of embryo can result.
b. Three to 16 weeks: Radiation can affect organogenesis.
c. More than 16 weeks: Neurologic deficits are most common.
d. X-ray exposure: Cumulative radiation dosage should be limited to 5–10 rads during pregnancy.
e. When possible, shield the uterus with a lead apron when taking radiographs.

V. PENETRATING NECK TRAUMA

Penetrating neck trauma is usually caused by firearms or stabbings. The neck has been divided into three anatomic zones. After the ABCDEs are evaluated, neck trauma should be managed based on the anatomic zone. Refractory shock warrants immediate exploration. Injuries to zone II often require operative exploration, although nonoperative management after computed tomography (CT) imaging is becoming increasingly used. Injuries in zones I and III can be difficult to expose. Preoperative imaging in these zones can be helpful to guide operative management.

A. ZONE I
1. Horizontal between clavicles and cricoid cartilage

B. ZONE II
1. Cricoid cartilage to angle of mandible

C. ZONE III
1. Angle of mandible to base of skull

D. NECK EXPLORATION
1. Make longitudinal incision along the anterior border of the sternocleidomastoid.
2. Retract the sternocleidomastoid laterally.
3. Dissect cervical fascia, and identify and examine the internal jugular vein.
   a. Most commonly injured vascular structure in the neck is the internal jugular vein.
4. Ligate the facial vein along the anterior border of the neck.
5. Identify and open carotid sheath.
6. Examine the carotid artery for injuries.
   a. Identify the vagus nerve.
   b. Gain proximal and distal control of the carotid artery if injured.
   c. Carotid artery injuries should be repaired. Carotid ligation, if necessary, is generally tolerated (indicated when patient is in extremis or has complete neurologic deficit before surgical intervention).

RECOMMENDED READINGS

Gupta M, Schriger DL, Hiatt JR, et al. Selective use of computed tomography compared with routine whole body imaging in patients with blunt trauma. *Ann Emerg Med*. 2011;58:407–416.

Kotwal RS, Howard JT, Orman JA, et al. The effect of a golden hour policy on the morbidity and mortality of combat casualties. *JAMA Surg*. 2016;151:15.

MacKenzie EJ, Rivara FP, Jurkovich GJ, et al. A national evaluation of the effect of trauma-center care on mortality. *N Engl J Med*. 2006;354:366–678.

Trunkey D. Initial treatment of patients with extensive trauma. *N Engl J Med*. 1991;324:1259–1263.

Abdominal Trauma

Amanda M. Pugh, MD

I. PATHOPHYSIOLOGY

1. Significant blunt force, deceleration, and penetrating wounds should be considered to have intraperitoneal injuries until ruled out by further diagnostic evaluation.
2. The abdominal cavity can hold a significant amount of blood without obvious signs, so a high level of suspicion is warranted based on type of trauma.
3. Trauma mortality has a trimodal distribution.
   a. First peak: This occurs seconds to minutes after trauma due to overwhelming injury involving the brain, spinal cord, heart, airway, and great vessels (aortic transection).
   b. Second peak: the "golden hour" after trauma, during which intervention has greatest impact. Deaths in this period result from intracranial hemorrhage, hemothorax, tension pneumothorax, ruptured spleen, severe liver lacerations, femur fractures, and other multiorgan injuries.
   c. Third peak: This occurs several days to weeks after trauma due to sepsis and multiorgan failure.
4. Blunt trauma
   a. Mechanism of injury
      (1) Direct blow—crushing injuries that can rupture organs
      (2) Deceleration—tearing injuries, such as liver or spleen at attaching ligaments
   b. Key questions—speed of vehicle, angle of impact, fate of other passengers, use of seat belt, airbag deployment, extraction time, and height of fall
   c. During evaluation always look for a seat belt sign, which if present should increase suspicion of intraabdominal blunt trauma injuries.
5. Penetrating trauma
   a. Mechanism of injury
      (1) Stab wounds—if located between nipples and perineum should be evaluated for intraperitoneal injury
      (2) Gunshot wounds—injury based on velocity, trajectory, and fragmentation
         (a) Low velocity—injuries depend on the bullet tract
         (b) High velocity—impart more kinetic injury to abdominal organs and have increased damage around the bullet track ($KE = \frac{1}{2}\,mv^2$, where KE represents kinetic energy, m represents mass of the moving particle, and v^2 represents volume of the particle squared)
         (c) Shotgun—injury based on type of shot and distance from the gun

16

b. Explosives—usually involves penetrating and blunt injuries due to force of blast
c. Key questions—timing of injury, caliber/size of weapon used, distance from gun barrel, number of wounds

II. DIAGNOSIS

1. Diagnosis is based on the standard Advanced Trauma Life Support (ATLS) primary approach that includes a structured primary and secondary survey (refer to Chapter 15).
2. Location of injury, mechanism of injury, and hemodynamic stability should be considered during the assessment and evaluation of the patient.
3. Indications for laparotomy
   a. Hemodynamic instability or peritoneal irritation
   b. Blunt trauma
      (1) Hypotension that is suspected to be secondary to intraabdominal injury (do not waste time in the emergency department with more than a radiograph and type and crossmatch if hypotension persists)
      (2) Positive focused assessment sonography in trauma (FAST) with hypotension
      (3) Diaphragmatic rupture or free air
      (4) Computed tomographic (CT) scan showing extravasation from liver or spleen injury, renal pedicle injury, pancreatic hematoma, mesenteric hematoma, or large amount of free fluid in pelvis not explained by solid organ injury (suggestive of small bowel injury)
   c. Penetrating trauma *(in addition to previously described indications)*
   d. Gunshot wound (GSW) penetrating "the box" bordered by nipple line superiorly, perineum and gluteal folds inferiorly, and flank (posterior axillary line) laterally
   e. Stab wounds that penetrate the anterior abdominal wall fascia. Violation of the fascia can be verified with:
      (1) Local wound exploration (although the false negative rate is nearly 30%)
      (2) FAST, although if negative it does not exclude injury
      (3) Diagnostic peritoneal lavage (DPL), which can be useful to identify injuries when patients have small amounts of free fluid without obvious injury
      (4) Diagnostic laparoscopy
4. Secondary survey adjuncts—operative decision making
   a. Plain film radiographs—urgent chest, abdominal, and pelvic (anteroposterior view)
      (1) Evaluate for associated thoracic injury (diaphragm injury, hemothorax/pneumothorax).
      (2) Place paper clip markers at penetrating injuries; assess missile trajectory.

    (3) Evaluate for free intraabdominal air.

    (4) Evaluate for pelvic fracture.

b. FAST—ultrasound probe placed over four interfaces to look for free fluid: pericardium, hepatorenal fossa, splenorenal fossa, and pelvis/pouch of Douglas

    (1) This study is used to evaluate for hemoperitoneum in patients who have hemodynamic changes but no obvious indication for laparotomy.

    (2) Advantages over DPL are rapid (2–3 minutes to complete), relative localization of injury, noninvasive, inexpensive, and inclusion of pericardium evaluation

    (3) Skilled users can appreciate hemothorax, pneumothorax, and inferior vena cava (IVC) fullness.

    (4) Limitations are sensitivity anywhere from 44% to 91% in ruling out solid organ injury, does not examine retroperitoneum, and is less sensitive than DPL for small amounts of intraperitoneal blood. The minimum amount of fluid required for a positive examination is at least 200–400 mL.

    (5) Regardless of FAST findings, hemodynamically stable patients with abdominal pain or unreliable examination will get CT scan to look for missed solid organ or retroperitoneal injury.

c. DPL

    (1) DPL is another study to evaluate for hemoperitoneum, although FAST has replaced it for the most part.

    (2) Indications include evaluation for small bowel injury when fluid seen on CT is not explained by solid organ injury bleeding, when CT is not available, and for stab wounds with uncertain depth. Any evidence of gross blood, bile, or gastrointestinal (GI) contents indicates a laparotomy.

    (3) Contraindications include prior abdominal operations, coagulopathy, and obesity. The stomach and bladder should be decompressed first to avoid injury.

    (4) An infraumbilical technique is usually performed; however, a supraumbilical technique should be used when a patient has pelvic fractures or pregnancy.

    (5) Peritoneal lavage fluid should be sent for analysis if no gross contamination is present. Results are positive if there is >100,000 red blood cells (RBCs), >500 white blood cells (WBCs), or a positive Gram stain.

d. Abdomen/pelvis CT scan with intravenous (IV) contrast

    (1) This is only for hemodynamically stabilized patients who have no prior indication for laparotomy.

    (2) It is useful because many injuries can be missed with DPL and FAST (including solid organ hematomas, diaphragmatic, pancreatic, and retroperitoneal injuries) and because many injuries can be managed without surgery (observation or embolization).

16

ABDOMINAL TRAUMA

(3) Oral contrast is not typically given—no definite improvement in detecting small bowel injury, increases delay in obtaining CT scan, and aspiration risk.

(4) Early pancreas and small bowel injuries are the most commonly missed diagnoses on CT scanning.

III. TREATMENT

1. Continue with initial resuscitation measures. When diagnostic steps are complete, triage nonoperative patients (discharge, floor, intensive care unit [ICU]). When indications for laparotomy are met, proceed as outlined in the following sections.

2. Basic operative maneuvers
   a. Request special equipment as needed (Cell Saver, vascular tray, rigid sigmoidoscope, etc.).
   b. Administer broad-spectrum IV antibiotics before incision for prophylaxis.
   c. Wide prep—sternal notch to anterior thighs (access to the chest if needed and access to proximal greater saphenous vein for graft if needed)
   d. Midline laparotomy—Goals are to control hemorrhage, control contamination, and then definitive repair of injury. Rapidly inspect all four quadrants, and pack if bleeding. Apply pressure to bleeding areas or ligate bleeding vessels. Use clamps or single sutures to control contamination.
      (1) Clot often represents the site of injury.
      (2) Right upper quadrant (RUQ)—Palpate liver and visualize diaphragm and kidney (usually dividing the falciform ligament for better visualization and avoidance of traction).
      (3) Left upper quadrant—Palpate/visualize spleen and visualize diaphragm.
      (4) Lower quadrants—Look for obvious bladder or bowel injury.
      (5) Eviscerate and run small bowel from ligament of Treitz to ileocecal valve, examining both sides and the mesentery.
      (6) Run colon from cecum to peritoneal reflection.
      (7) Inspect the retroperitoneum for hematomas.
   e. Special considerations
      (1) Kocher maneuver—mobilization of first and second portion of duodenum by dissection through lateral attachments. Indications include bile staining or bruising of second portion of duodenum or concern for pancreas injury on CT scan.
      (2) Cattell-Braasch maneuver (right medial visceral rotation)—continuation of Kocher maneuver by taking down lateral attachments of ascending colon along right paracolic gutter and reflecting colon medial with dissection anterior to Gerota fascia. It is indicated for exposure of right colon injuries and aortic/IVC injuries below the superior mesenteric artery.

    (3) Mobilize spleen if there is concern about left upper quadrant bleeding or injury and/or distal pancreas injury.

    (4) Mattox maneuver (left medial visceral rotation): Take down splenorenal ligament and left peritoneal reflection along white line of Toldt, extending down to distal sigmoid colon. It is indicated for exposure of entire aorta, including origin of celiac axis, superior mesenteric artery, left iliac, and left renal arteries.

  f. Abdominal closure options

    (1) Primary fascial closure

    (2) There are many temporary closure options in setting of large-volume resuscitation or planned take back for second look.

    (3) Vicryl mesh closure is used if fascia cannot be reapproximated after the aforementioned temporary closures; it provides absorbable covering of omentum and bowel that will eventually granulate and can be skin grafted.

3. Damage control laparotomy

  a. Standard of care for the patient who presents in extremis and/or develops the triad of death during the operation (acidosis, coagulopathy, hypothermia)

  b. Stage 1: operative control of hemorrhage and contamination

    (1) Solid organ injury tamponade (packing)

    (2) Repair/ligation of accessible blood vessels

    (3) Perforated bowel occlusion/resection

    (4) External tube drainage (bile/pancreatic ducts and ureters)

    (5) Rapid temporary closure of abdominal cavity

  c. Stage 2: ongoing resuscitation in the ICU setting

  d. Stage 3: reexploration and definitive treatment

  e. Stage 4: definitive abdominal wall closure

16

ABDOMINAL TRAUMA

IV. ORGAN-SPECIFIC INJURY MANAGEMENT (TABLE 16.1 LISTS INJURY STAGING THAT OFTEN GUIDES THERAPY)

1. Diaphragm

  a. Penetrating injuries to the diaphragm vary in size and location.

  b. Blunt injuries are usually large linear tears, and 75% occur on the left because of the blocking effect of the liver on the right and usually involve the central tendon. On x-ray film, look for blurring of the diaphragm, nasogastric tube coursing up into the chest, or hemothorax. Ultrasound can also be helpful to detect bowel in the chest.

  c. An abdominal approach is usually used to evaluate for other intraperitoneal injuries. They usually can be repaired with a running primary closure using a *permanent suture.*

  d. Grade V injury may require AlloDerm patch or Marlex (polypropylene) mesh to span defect. The diaphragm can also be reattached more cephalad in the thoracic cavity.

TABLE 16.1

ORGAN INJURY GRADING SCALE

Organ	I	II	III	IV	V
			Grade		
Diaphragm	Contusion	L <2 cm	L = 2–10 cm	L >10 cm or tissue loss <25 cm²	Tissue loss <25 cm²
Liver	H <10% surface area, L <1 cm depth	H 10%–50% surface area, L = 1–3 cm depth, <10 cm length	H >50% surface area, expanding or ruptured, L >3 cm depth	H with active bleeding, L involving 25%–75% parenchyma	L >75% of lobe or >3 segments in single lobe, vena caval, or central hepatic vein injury (Note: grade VI = hepatic avulsion)
Spleen	H <10% surface area, L <1 cm depth	H 10%–50% surface area or <5 cm diameter, L = 1–3 cm depth not involving trabecular vessels	H >50% surface area or >5 cm diameter, expanding or ruptured, L >3 cm depth or involving trabecular vessels	H with active bleeding, L involving segmental/hilar vessels devascularizing >25% of spleen	Completely devascularized or shattered spleen
Stomach	H <3 cm, partial-thickness L	H >3 cm, L >3 cm	L >3 cm	L involving vessels on greater or lesser curvature	Extensive rupture (>50%), devascularization

16

ABDOMINAL TRAUMA

Pancreas	Small H/L without duct injury	Large H/L without injury or tissue loss	Distal transection or L with duct injury	Proximal transection/parenchymal L involving ampulla	Massive head disruption
Duodenum	H in one segment, partial-thickness L without perforation	H in multiple segments, small L <50% circumference	Large L (50%–75% circumference D2, 50%–100% circumference other segments)	Very large L of D2 (75%–100% circumference), rupture of ampulla or distal CBD	Massive duodeno-pancreatic injury or devascularization of duodenum
Jejunum/Ileum	H without devascularization, partial-thickness L without transection	Small L <50% circumference	Large L (>50% circumference without transection)	Transection	Segmental tissue loss, devascularization
Colon	Contusion, H, partial-thickness L	Small L (<50% circumference)	Large L (>50% circumference)	Transection	Transection with devascularized segment, tissue loss
Rectum	Contusion, H, partial-thickness L	Small L (<50% circumference)	Large L (>50% circumference)	Full-thickness L with perineal extension	Devascularized segment
Kidney	Contusion, hematoma	Nonexpanding perirenal H, L <1 cm, no urine extravasation	L >1 cm but without collecting system rupture or urine extravasation	L through renal cortex to collecting system, injury to main renal artery	Shattered, devascularized

CBD, Common bile duct; H, hematoma; L, laceration.

2. **Stomach**
   a. Suspect injury when CT scanning shows unexplained intraperitoneal fluid, pneumoperitoneum, stomach wall thickening or stranding, or extravasation of oral contrast. Intraoperatively, visualize anterior gastric surface from the gastroesophageal junction to the pylorus. If injury seen or suspected, open gastrocolic ligament to enter lesser sac and visualize posterior surface. A posterior injury is the most common injury missed.
   b. Grade I: Unroof and evacuate hematoma because this may be hiding a deeper injury. Perform seromuscular closure with interrupted sutures.
   c. Grade II–III: Repair primarily in a two-layer fashion.
   d. Grade IV–V: Perform partial gastrectomy and gastroduodenostomy or gastrojejunostomy to reestablish enteric drainage.

3. **Liver**
   a. The large size of the liver makes it more likely to be injured during blunt trauma than other organs. It is also commonly injured in penetrating injuries to the RUQ.
   b. Many low-grade liver lacerations or hematomas diagnosed with CT without active extravasation of contrast can be managed nonoperatively in the stable patient. They require close monitoring, serial (every 4–6 hours) hematocrits until stable, and a high index of suspicion for postinjury complications, including infected hematoma and biloma.
      (1) Adjuncts that are helpful in nonoperative management are angioembolization and endoscopic retrograde cholangiopancreatography (ERCP). Indications for angiography include hemodynamic changes requiring 4 units packed RBC (pRBC) in 6 hours or 6 units in 24 hours.
   c. Hypotension and ongoing transfusion requirements are indications for operative exploration and repair. If injury is discovered intraoperatively, attempt to control bleeding with packing first, then proceed based on grade of the injury.
   d. Basic maneuvers for profuse bleeding from RUQ:
      (1) First line therapy is to pack the liver (above and below). Many liver injuries will not need direct repair but will tamponade and clot because of the low-pressure system.
      (2) If packing and pressure do not control hemorrhage, the Pringle maneuver can help to differentiate the source of the injury. This is done by clamping the hepatoduodenal ligament, which includes the portal vein, hepatic arteries, and common bile duct (CBD). Limit duration of continuous clamping, but you can clamp up to an hour without irreversible injury.
      (3) The Pringle maneuver will usually control bleeding from the hepatic artery and/or the portal vein. If this fails, an injury to the hepatic veins or retrohepatic IVC should be considered.

e. Grade I–II injuries—Admit patient to the surgical intensive care unit (SICU) and monitor closely unless hemodynamically unstable, which mandates a laparotomy. If operative management is required, use of electrocautery, topical clotting agents (Surgicel or FloSeal), and packing with omentum can help to stop bleeding. Drains are usually not required, and abdomen can be closed after other injuries are treated.

f. Grade III–V injuries when Pringle maneuver controls bleeding (usually hepatic arteries or portal vein)—Treat topical bleeding as in grade I or II (see previous), ligate parenchymal bleeding vessels with silk sutures, and reapproximate liver parenchyma with chromic sutures.

   (1) If packs are left in, remove during take-back laparotomy in 1–2 days.

   (2) Injuries that involve the hepatic artery or portal vein:

      (a) Ligation from celiac axis to common hepatic artery is applicable due to collateral blood flow. However, the proper hepatic artery requires repair.

      (b) Selective ligation of right/left hepatic artery or portal vein is tolerated. A cholecystectomy is required if right hepatic artery is ligated.

g. Grade III–V injuries when Pringle maneuver does not control bleeding—Significant ongoing bleeding indicates injury to hepatic vein or vena cava. Get better exposure by taking down additional attaching coronary and triangular ligaments, extend laparotomy to median sternotomy to gain exposure above and below diaphragm, stop bleeding with one of the methods below, then definitively repair the bleeding vessels either at that time or during take-back laparotomy after patient is stabilized.

   (1) Hemostasis adjuncts for venous bleeding

      (a) Place additional packing, especially if the right lobe is injured. The goal is to use the anterior chest wall, the diaphragm, and the retroperitoneum to circumferentially compress the liver parenchyma for an extended period. Due to location of the left lobe of the liver, packing is less useful. If packing controls hemorrhage, the patient should be stabilized in the SICU and a hepatic vein stent should be considered for definitive repair.

      (b) If bleeding continues after packing, direct repair may be required. Hepatic vascular isolation can be accomplished by suprahepatic/infrahepatic clamping of vena cava, temporary shunting, or venovenous bypass.

h. Definitive repair

   (1) Hepatic parenchymal sutures—Chromic sutures are used on the liver. Shallow lacerations can be approximated using a running suture. Horizontal mattress sutures are used for deeper lacerations (with or without pledgets). If it works, this is far less invasive than other methods.

16

ABDOMINAL TRAUMA

(a) Criticized as a source of hepatic necrosis (ischemia)
(b) Can be used to close entrance and exit wounds of penetrating injuries, but this risks future infected intrahepatic hematoma
(2) Hepatotomy with selective ligation of bleeding vessels
(a) Can be extended to anatomic liver resection if needed, such as large left lobe injuries not amenable to successful packing compression or when large segment of liver is deemed nonviable. Anatomic hepatic resection is associated with high mortality rate (50%) in the setting of trauma.
(3) Hepatic artery ligation or angioembolization for deep arterial bleeding
(4) Nonviable hepatic tissue should be debrided bluntly after patient is stable and can tolerate the unavoidable blood loss.

i. Postoperative management—Overall mortality rate of patients with hepatic injuries is nearly 10%. Mortality rate is greater as grade of injury increases and is greater in blunt trauma. Infection rates are greater in penetrating injuries.
(1) Delayed hemorrhage (usually occurs within 48 hours)— Etiology is usually a missed vascular injury and requires returning to the operating room or angiography for attempted embolization if patient is coagulopathic.
(2) Perihepatic infection—fever or increased WBC count 3–4 days after injury. First need to rule out common things, such as pneumonia, infected line, urinary tract infection, then get CT scan with oral and IV contrast, and do CT-guided percutaneous drainage as needed.
(3) Biliary leak—Suspect with increasing bilirubin level and persistent or worsening RUQ pain. Usually resolves with time and nothing by mouth (NPO). If no resolution, do endoscopic retrograde cholangiopancreatography with stent placement to ensure that enteric route is least resistant path of bile drainage.
(a) Biloma—Sterile ones will be resorbed (discovered incidentally on CT); however, infected ones should be treated like abscesses (percutaneous drainage).
(b) Biliary ascites—suggests major bile duct injury. Explore, wash out, and attempt definitive repair over T tube if necessary.
(c) Biliary fistula—Perform ERCP with sphincterotomy.
(4) Hepatic artery pseudoaneurysm—result of untreated arterial injury and has a potential to rupture. RUQ pain, upper GI bleed, and jaundice suggest rupture into a bile duct causing hemobilia. Portal hypertension is observed with rupture into the portal vein. Hepatic arteriography is required for embolization of pseudoaneurysm.

4. **Spleen**
   a. Concern for the rare but often fatal overwhelming postsplenectomy infection from encapsulated bacteria (*Streptococcus pneumoniae, Haemophilus influenzae, Neisseria meningitides*) has led to an increase in nonoperative management of splenic injuries, especially in pediatric trauma. Injury is easily graded on CT scan with IV contrast. If discovered operatively, decide between splenic repair (splenorrhaphy) or splenectomy.
   b. Splenectomy—Dissection is often done bluntly with fingers in the unstable patient with brisk bleeding from the left upper quadrant.
      (1) Indications: hilar injuries, greater than grade II injury with coagulopathy, and severe damage to parenchyma
   c. Splenic artery embolization—selective versus complete. The area embolized will infarct and may result in chronic pain.
   d. Postoperative management
      (1) Vaccines to cover encapsulated bacteria should be given within 2 weeks of injury or immediately before patient is discharged.
      (2) Infection is an important postoperative complication to recognize. It is normal to have an increase in platelets and WBCs directly after surgery. However, by postoperative day (POD) 5, if platelet to WBC ratio <20 or WBC >15, then an infectious work-up should be considered.
5. **Pancreas and duodenum**
   a. The key determinants of outcome include delay in diagnosis and the integrity of the pancreatic duct. Have a high index of suspicion based on mechanism (steering wheel, handlebar, or GSW to epigastrium). CT is only 70%–80% sensitive and specific. Look for subtle findings including fluid between splenic vein and the pancreatic body, fluid in the lesser sac, thickened left anterior renal fascia, or retroperitoneal blood or air. Amylase levels are unreliable for diagnosis within first 3 hours. Explore all patients operatively if pancreas injury suspected.
   b. Duodenal hematoma—Main issue is bowel obstruction. Most resolve with conservative management (NPO and nasogastric tube decompression) within 2 weeks. Use of total parenteral nutrition should be considered if obstructed longer than 5 days. Exploration is required if remains obstructed longer than 3 weeks. If diagnosed with laparotomy, evacuate.
   c. Duodenal perforation or laceration
      (1) Grades I–II—Small injuries can be repaired primarily with a running suture. Consider pyloric exclusion if there is associated pancreas injury.
      (2) Grade III—Perform primary suture repair when possible, but treatment of larger injuries is based on location of injury.
         (a) First portion of duodenum can be mobilized and repaired with an end-to-end anastomosis.

16

ABDOMINAL TRAUMA

    (b) Second portion of duodenum: Small injuries may be patched, otherwise a Roux-en-Y duodenojejunostomy with the duodenum oversewn is required because of the lack of mobilization near the pancreas.

    (c) Third and fourth portions of duodenum: Resect portion with the injury, and perform a duodenojejunostomy.

  (3) Grades IV–V—trauma Whipple

d. Pancreas injury

  (1) Management depends on location of damage and if there is a ductal injury.

  (2) Contusions are managed nonoperatively.

  (3) Grades I and II—Goal is hemostasis and adequate drainage. If no duct injury is seen, place Jackson-Pratt (JP) drains and get out. Remove JP drains when drain amylase is less than serum amylase. Pancreatic fistula is defined by drain output persisting more than 3 days and amylase content ≥3 times serum amylase (see management of pancreatic fistula later).

  (4) Grade III—distal pancreatectomy

    (a) Place feeding jejunostomy for injuries with grade ≥III; begin elemental tube feeds early.

    (b) Ductal transection can be diagnosed by exploration or ERCP/ magnetic resonance cholangiopancreatography (MRCP).

  (5) Grade IV—If duct injury is indeterminate on local exploration, consider intraoperative pancreatic ductography either via needle into gallbladder or duodenotomy and ampulla cannulation.

    (a) Stable patient—Oversew salvageable portion of proximal pancreas stump, Roux-en-Y choledochojejunostomy.

    (b) Unstable patient—Get hemostasis, drain widely, get out. Postoperative endoscopic retrograde cholangiopancreatography to define injury and possibly place duct stent.

    (c) Consider pyloric exclusion—Perform diversion with a gastrojejunostomy in complex duodenal and pancreatic injuries.

  (6) Grade V—trauma Whipple; high morbidity and mortality rates. Strongly consider two-stage operation with first stage for resection and second operation after stabilization for reconstruction.

  (7) Postoperative management—Complication rates for injuries to this organ are high (20%–40%).

    (a) Fistula—diagnosed with persistent drain output greater than 30 mL/day and drain to serum amylase ratio >3 after POD 5. Low-output fistulas (<200 mL/day) usually resolve with conservative management. High-output fistulas (>700 mL/ day) need endoscopic retrograde cholangiopancreatography to guide operative treatment or stenting. Octreotide decreases volume of output but not time for closure.

(b) Pancreatitis/secondary hemorrhage—It is rare and may require reoperation or embolization.

(c) Abscess—Consider percutaneous drainage versus surgical debridement.

(d) Pseudocyst—results when duct injuries are missed or treated with external drains only. ERCP can be used to evaluate for a ductal injury. If persistent or painful, fenestrate into GI tract (cystogastrostomy or cystojejunostomy).

6. Small bowel (jejunum and ileum)
   a. Suspect when CT shows significant intraperitoneal fluid without liver or splenic injury, or Chance fracture (thoracic or lumbar fracture dislocation).
   b. Fix simple (grades I–II) injuries—use single-layer Lembert sutures for serosal tears/hematomas and two-layer closure for injuries up to 50% of circumference if the closure will not significantly narrow the bowel lumen.
   c. Resect complex injuries (grades III–V).
      (1) Usually stapled, functional side-to-side anastomosis for the sake of time
      (2) May need to create ostomy if delayed diagnosis, unstable patient
      (3) Preservation of ileocecal valve if possible if significant length of bowel is being resected
         (a) Less than 200-cm jejunum and ileum at risk for short bowel syndrome

7. Colon
   a. Partial thickness (grade I)—Perform seromuscular closure with silk sutures.
   b. Full thickness nondestructive (grades II–III)—Repair by primary closure.
   c. Destructive injury in stable patient (grades IV–V)—Resect destroyed segment, and do primary anastomosis (usually side-to-side stapled).
   d. Destructive injury in unstable patient (transfusion of more than six units pRBCs, delayed diagnosis with fecal peritonitis, in shock)—Resect with end colostomy (Hartmann procedure) or resection with anastomosis and proximal diversion.
   e. Postoperative management
      (a) Consider delayed primary closure of abdominal wound in the setting of gross stool spillage. The ideal time for delayed closure of these wounds is PODs 3–5. Secondary skin closure is also an option to avoid the risk for wound infection and subsequent hernia risk.
      (b) Colostomy takedown—usually wait until at least 3 months after injury.

16

ABDOMINAL TRAUMA

8. **Rectum**
   a. Most common mechanisms of injury include penetration with foreign object and GSW to the pelvis/buttocks or perineum. Digital rectal examination is mandatory, looking for gross blood and palpating for rectal wall defect or hematoma. This should be followed by rigid sigmoidoscopy (easier done in the operating room than the emergency department) if injury is suspected.
   b. Rectal injuries to anterior or lateral side walls of upper two thirds of rectum should be treated just as colon injuries.
   c. Rectal injuries to extraperitoneal surfaces (lower third and entire posterior rectum)
      (1) Due to the pelvis, access to extraperitoneal injuries is limited.
      (2) If accessible, it should be repaired primarily.
      (3) If unable to access, then diversion is necessary with either a loop ileostomy or sigmoid loop colostomy.
      (4) Presacral drainage should be considered with extensive injuries, but is not mandatory; if not performed percutaneous drainage may be needed in a delayed fashion.
   d. Colon and rectal complications
      (1) Intraabdominal/pelvic abscess—treated with percutaneous drainage
      (2) Fistula—most resolve with conservative management
9. **Kidney, ureters, bladder (see chapter on urology)**
   a. Urology service is usually called for injuries to the genitourinary system.
   b. Diagnosis: Suspect injury in the setting of hematuria; CT is the gold standard.
10. **Retroperitoneal hematomas and major vessel injuries**
    a. Zone I (midline along aorta)—Management for blunt and penetrating is the same.
       (1) Superior to the transverse mesocolon
          (a) Small aorta injuries—Repair with 4-0 Prolene or polytetrafluoroethylene graft.
          (b) Proximal left gastric, splenic, and common hepatic artery injuries can be ligated.
          (c) Superior mesenteric artery injuries—Reimplant in distal aorta away from likely injured pancreas.
          (d) Proximal renal artery injuries—Repair/reimplant if less than 4 hours from injury; otherwise ligate.
          (e) Superior mesenteric vein—Repair with 5-0 Prolene if possible; leave abdomen open if superior mesenteric vein ligated.
       (2) Inferior to transverse mesocolon—aorta injury
          (a) Repair primarily or with graft, cover with a viable omental pedicle to prevent aortoenteric fistula.
       (3) Inferior to mesocolon: IVC injury—Suspect when bleeding from base of the mesentery of hepatic flexure or ascending colon or asymmetric hematoma (R > L).

(a) Repair primarily with 4-0 Prolene or bovine pericardial patch.

(b) Infrarenal IVC can be ligated in destructive injuries, but watch for leg compartment syndrome.

b. Zone II (laterally including the kidneys)

(1) Blunt injury: The only reason to open a hematoma in this setting is if it is ruptured, pulsatile, or rapidly expanding, even if CT shows an injured kidney. Repair as in penetrating injury (next).

(2) Penetrating injury: Obtain proximal control of renal vessel with vessel loop first, then open hematoma and repair according to renal injury section (see previous description).

c. Zone III (pelvis)

(1) Blunt injury: Open hematoma only if ruptured, pulsatile, or rapidly expanding, or if there is loss of ipsilateral iliac or femoral pulse. Repair as in penetrating injury (next).

(2) Penetrating injury: Expose bifurcation of aorta and IVC. Control proximal iliac distal external iliac vessels with vessel loops, clamp internal iliac vessels, open hematoma, and attempt to repair.

(a) Ligation is simplest, quickest maneuver in setting of exsanguination, but it is associated with 50% amputation rate. This can be reduced by femorofemoral crossover graft within 6 hours.

(b) Stable patients: Options based on extent of destruction include lateral arteriorrhaphy, bovine pericardium patch angioplasty, complete transection, and primary end-to-end anastomosis versus polytetrafluoroethylene graft.

(c) Unstable patient: Consider temporary intraluminal shunt, then definitive repair within 6 hours.

V. SPECIAL CIRCUMSTANCES

1. Abdominal compartment syndrome

a. Adverse physiologic consequences of increased intraabdominal pressure (>25 mm Hg)

b. Risk factors: packing remaining in the abdomen after initial laparotomy, bowel edema caused by massive crystalloid resuscitation and/or reperfusion injury, ongoing intraabdominal bleeding, and primary fascial closure

c. Diagnosis

(1) Hypotension—impaired venous return, impaired cardiac compliance, reduced cardiac output

(2) Hypoxia and increased airway pressures—Lung compression from elevated diaphragms decreases ventilation.

(3) Oliguria—Renal vein and parenchymal compression impairs renal function.

16

ABDOMINAL TRAUMA

    (4) Monitor abdominal examination and intraabdominal pressures (transduced bladder pressure).

  d. Treatment

    (1) Open the abdomen—at bedside if patient crashing or in the operating room urgently.

2. **Pregnancy**

  a. These patients are hypervolemic at baseline, which thus can mask more significant blood loss before showing signs of shock. Their pelvic veins are enlarged, making them at greater risk in the setting of pelvic fractures. The fetus cannot survive without the mother— treat her first.

  b. Initial assessment/diagnosis—Place patient on left side or just elevate right hip as soon as safely possible from spinal standpoint to avoid caval compression by gravid uterus.

    (1) Volume status—liberal crystalloid and blood resuscitation for the sake of the fetus

    (2) Assess fundal height, uterine tenderness, vaginal bleeding, and amniotic fluid in vagina.

    (3) Look for fetal heartbeat and fetal movement during FAST examination.

    (4) Use radiography as indicated in nonpregnant patients; if DPL done, use open technique above the uterus.

  c. Operative treatment

    (1) Uterine rupture—Explore (with potential for emergency C-section) unstable patients or if imaging shows extended fetal extremities, abnormal fetal position, or free intraperitoneal air.

    (2) Perimortem C-section—For more than 24 weeks' gestation, ideally perform starting 4 minutes after mother's cardiac arrest while cardiopulmonary resuscitation continues during and after C-section. Do not perform in unstable patient because of anticipated cardiac arrest.

  d. Management

    (1) Consult obstetrician on all pregnant trauma patients, although he or she may not monitor nonviable (<20 week) pregnancies.

    (2) If more than 20 weeks' gestation, cardiotocographic monitoring for minimum of 6 hours, longer if anything concerning such as contractions, nonreassuring heartbeat, or if mother is seriously injured. Watch for signs of placental abruption and disseminated intravascular coagulopathy.

    (3) Kleihauer-Betke test is a blood test that measures fetal hemoglobin in mother's blood.

      (a) Used to dose Rh immunoglobulin to inhibit formation of Rh antibodies in the Rh-negative mother

RECOMMENDED READINGS

American College of Surgeons. *ATLS Advanced Trauma Life Support Program for Doctors.* 9th ed. Chicago: American College of Surgeons.

Burlew CN, Burlew MEE, Cothren C, Moore EE. Trauma. In: Brunicardi F, Andersen DK, Billiar TR, et al., eds. *Schwartz's Principles of Surgery.* 10th ed. New York: McGraw-Hill; 2014.

16

ABDOMINAL TRAUMA

Thoracic Trauma

Nick Charles Levinsky Jr., MD

No new method and no new discovery can overcome the natural difficulties that attend a wound of the heart.

—James Paget, 1896

I. EPIDEMIOLOGY OF THORACIC TRAUMA

A. THORACIC TRAUMA

Thoracic trauma ranks third in incidence behind head and extremity trauma, with motor vehicle crashes being the most common mechanism in the United States. These injuries are directly responsible for 15%–25% of trauma deaths and contribute to 25%–50% of the remaining trauma-related deaths. Blunt trauma makes up the majority of thoracic trauma (~60%–70%), with few patients presenting with isolated chest trauma. The proportion of blunt versus penetrating trauma varies with location, with an increased proportion of penetrating trauma in more urban areas.

B. AFRICAN-AMERICAN MALES

African-American males have a 1 in 20 chance of being shot or stabbed before the age of 30 in urban America.

C. MOTORCYCLE ACCIDENTS

A total of 75% of fatally injured riders had some type of thoracic injury.

II. PHYSICAL EXAMINATION OF THE CHEST

A. CHEST AUSCULTATION

1. Absent or diminished breath sounds may indicate pneumothorax or hemothorax and may be unilateral or bilateral. A small pneumothorax may only demonstrate absent breath sounds at the apex, and presence of breath sounds does not eliminate the possibility of a pneumothorax.

B. POINT TENDERNESS

1. Clinical evidence of rib fractures
2. May not see rib fractures on plain chest radiograph

C. FLAIL CHEST

1. Paradoxical chest wall movement of the flail segment

D. SUBCUTANEOUS EMPHYSEMA

1. Pulmonary laceration is most common cause (such as from a fractured rib).
2. Concurrent pneumothorax should be expected.
3. Consider less common causes such as esophageal or tracheobronchial injury.

E. DULLNESS VERSUS RESONANCE ON PERCUSSION
1. Hemothorax versus pneumothorax
2. May be difficult to ascertain in a crowded and noisy trauma bay

F. SEAT BELT SIGNS
1. Seen across the chest, but pathology could be elsewhere

III. ADJUNCTS TO THE PHYSICAL EXAMINATION
A. CHEST RADIOGRAPHS
1. A negative chest x-ray (CXR) does not rule out occult pathology, and a pneumothorax can be present even if not seen (especially if x-ray is in supine position).
2. Widened mediastinum: "Textbook definition" is 8 cm or greater.
   a. This raises concern for aortic injury.
   b. More often than not, this is related to other findings—pericardial fat pad, thymus, patient positioning/habitus—but this finding warrants further evaluation.
3. Rib fractures may be radiographically occult.
4. Pneumothorax: Look for a "lung line."
   a. Tension pneumothorax should be a clinical diagnosis.
5. Hemothorax: The costophrenic angle will be obscured by >300 mL of blood.
6. Pneumomediastinum is most commonly due to pulmonary injury with pneumothorax.
   a. This raises concern for possible esophageal or airway injury.
7. Sternal fracture may require lateral film to be identified.
8. Diaphragm injury
   a. May demonstrate hollow viscus above the diaphragm (gastric bubble, bowel gas pattern)
   b. May visualize nasogastric (NG) tube above the diaphragm
   c. Left diaphragm may appear elevated above the right.

B. COMPUTED TOMOGRAPHY SCAN OF THE CHEST WITH INTRAVENOUS CONTRAST
1. Should have a relatively low threshold to obtain CT scan of the chest in the hemodynamically stable patient with significant chest wall trauma.
2. Contrast study will identify vascular injury, such as dissection, transection, or pseudoaneurysm.
3. Occult pneumothorax may be identified on computed tomography (CT).
4. The initial chest radiograph can be inadequate secondary to being an anteroposterior film while the patient is lying supine.
5. Pulmonary contusion can also be identified.

IV. PATHOPHYSIOLOGY OF THORACIC TRAUMA
1. Consequences are secondary to the result of effects on respiratory and hemodynamic functions.

17

THORACIC TRAUMA

2. Death is secondary to impairment of oxygen delivery, transport, or both.
   a. Pulmonary gas exchange
   b. Cardiac output
   c. Hemoglobin concentration
   d. Oxygen-hemoglobin affinity
3. Majority of interventions during resuscitation are:
   a. Airway protection: necessary to ventilate, oxygenate, and prevent aspiration
   b. Ventilatory and oxygenation support: to prevent hypoxemic arrest
   c. Decompression of tension pneumothorax: to prevent obstructive shock and subsequent cardiac arrest
   d. Control of hemorrhage: to prevent worsening hemorrhagic shock, acidosis, and eventual arrest

V. BLUNT CHEST TRAUMA

1. Rib fractures:
   a. They are extremely painful and lead to splinting and decreased tidal volumes.
   b. They may result in atelectasis, poor pulmonary toileting followed by pneumonia, and subsequent respiratory failure.
   c. Treat with multimodality pain control and aggressive pulmonary volume expansion.
      (1) Consider thoracic epidural placement or intercostal nerve block
      (2) Treat with scheduled acetaminophen, patient-controlled narcotic analgesia, intravenous (IV) and oral (PO) narcotics as necessary (PRN), and topical lidocaine patches.
      (3) Use hourly incentive spirometry and other pulmonary volume expansion maneuvers.
   d. Sharp rib fragments may injure lung or intercostal vascular bundles, resulting in pneumothorax or hemothorax.
   e. These fractures often occur with concurrent pulmonary contusion (due to impact) leading to decreased oxygenation.
2. Flail chest: at least two fractures per rib in two or more consecutive ribs, resulting in "free-floating" segment of chest wall
   a. Mortality is as high as 40% in patients with associated pulmonary contusions.
   b. This may show paradoxical chest wall movement on respiration (flail segment moves opposite direction of the rest of the chest wall during respiration).
   c. Treat similarly to rib fractures.
   d. Surgical fixation is controversial but may be useful in the following situations:
      (1) Failure to wean from the ventilator
      (2) Patients undergoing elective thoracotomy for other reasons
      (3) Long-term nonunion and associated symptoms

    e. Surgical fixation has been associated with decreased ventilator days, pneumonia and sepsis, need for tracheostomy, and possibly mortality.

3. **Sternal fracture: usually no specific treatment required unless displaced**
   a. May require lateral chest films or CT scan to identify
   b. High risk of underlying cardiac contusion or other injuries

4. **Pulmonary contusions: extremely common after rib fractures (prevalent in 25%–35% of blunt chest traumas)**
   a. These contusions lead to ventilation/perfusion mismatch due to alveolar damage and subsequent alveolar inflammation, edema, and hemorrhage.
   b. They are identifiable on chest radiograph or CT as patchy consolidations or ground-glass opacities not restricted by anatomic boundaries of the pulmonary lobes.
   c. Initial treatment is supportive with pulmonary volume expansion maneuvers (incentive spirometry, etc.) and supplemental oxygen; in addition, minimize crystalloid resuscitation as able.
   d. Patient may demonstrate worsening respiratory function 24–72 hours after initial injury as contusion evolves, necessitating intubation and ventilator support for subsequent respiratory failure.

5. **Cardiac contusions: may present with arrhythmias in the trauma bay or shortly thereafter**
   a. Obtain electrocardiogram (EKG): usually present with persistent tachycardia, minor ST or T wave abnormalities, or premature atrial contractions (PACs)/premature ventricular contractions (PVCs), but more severe injuries may demonstrate heart block, severe ischemic changes, new bundle branch blocks, depressed ejection fraction (right ventricle more commonly), or ventricular arrhythmias. Cardiac contusion was present in 29%–56% of patients when diagnosed via EKG.
   b. Trend troponins: Troponin appears to be more sensitive and specific than creatine kinase MB (CK-MB) and may reach peak levels sooner in trauma than in myocardial infarction. Cardiac contusion was present in 15%–24% of patients when diagnosis was based on troponin elevation.
   c. Telemetry monitoring for 24–48 hours if abnormal admission EKG or troponin elevation: Up to 95% of ventricular arrhythmias and cardiac failures occurred within the first 48 hours after injury. Eastern Association for the Surgery of Trauma (EAST) guidelines dictate no need for telemetry if the patient has a normal EKG on presentation.
   d. Echocardiogram may be helpful to evaluate cardiac function if patient is unstable.
   e. Patient may present with concurrent rib fractures or sternal fracture; however, sternal fracture has been shown to be a poor predictor of cardiac contusion and is not an indication for cardiac monitoring.

6. **Aortic injury: can occur secondary to blunt or penetrating injury**
   a. The majority of aortic transections occur just distal to the take-off of the left subclavian artery due to deceleration injury.

b. The vast majority (80%) of people with blunt aortic injuries exsanguinate at the scene. Only 20% survive to the hospital, with 10% surviving the first 24 hours in-hospital.
c. It may be seen as widened mediastinum on radiograph; contrast CT of the chest is imaging study of choice. Imaging findings include:
   (1) Tracheal deviation
   (2) Left mainstem bronchial depression
   (3) Left apical capping (a curved density at the lung apex on CXR indicative of hematoma)
   (4) Widened mediastinum
   (5) Mediastinal hematoma with contrast extravasation
   (6) False aortic lumen
d. Patient must have aggressive blood pressure and heart rate control with an agent such as esmolol to maintain systolic blood pressure less than 100–120 mm Hg and heart rate approximately 60 beats/min (nicardipine as second agent, followed by nitroglycerin/nitroprusside for additional control). This is challenging in a patient with multisystem injuries, and optimal heart rate control may not be achievable.
e. Traditional management involved emergent posterolateral thoracotomy and replacement of the injured segment of aorta with a prosthetic graft. Thoracic endovascular aortic repair (TEVAR) is increasingly becoming the gold standard. Stent deployment across an aortic injury is safe and effective. TEVAR has demonstrated decreased rates of mortality and paraplegia, with comparable (to improved) risk of stroke when compared with open repair. Benefits of TEVAR also include:
   (1) It does not require systemic anticoagulation.
   (2) The need for single lung ventilation is avoided.
   (3) Positioning of the patient is also less of an issue in patients with multiple injuries.
   (4) However, there is risk of stent endoleaks, and therefore long-term following is often required.
f. Urgent repair within 24 hours after stabilization of other life-threatening injuries, rather than emergent repair, preceded by appropriate preoperative blood pressure control has been shown to improve outcomes, likely due to improved resuscitation before surgery.

7. **Diaphragm injuries**
   a. These occur in approximately 2%–4% of all abdominal injuries.
   b. These likely occur with equal frequency between blunt and penetrating injuries, although historical reports would favor blunt injuries over penetrating trauma.
   c. A high index of suspicion is required to diagnose these injuries.
   d. Dyspnea, orthopnea, and chest pain can have referred pain to scapula.
   e. Gastric distention with ipsilateral lung collapse occurs in extreme situations.

f. Diagnosis can be difficult; however, several studies may be used.
   (1) Chest radiograph—May see gastric bubble or loops of bowel in the chest, often mistaken for a pneumothorax. Placement of NG tube can help to diagnose because it may show NG placement above the diaphragm.
   (2) CT scan
   (3) Fluoroscopy—mobility of left hemidiaphragm (most commonly injured)
   (4) Bowel sounds in the chest on auscultation
   (5) Cardiac displacement

g. Repair
   (1) Early diagnosis—repair via laparotomy with horizontal mattress sutures; recommend nonabsorbable monofilament, but almost any permanent suture will suffice. This also requires placement of a chest tube to drain pleura.
   (2) If other injuries have been ruled out, diagnostic laparoscopy with repair is an option. This is best with occult injury in a stable patient, such as in a patient with a stab wound to the left chest undergoing diagnostic laparoscopy.
   (3) Late diagnosis (>1 week)—repair via thoracotomy or thoracoscopic surgery. Adhesions to the lung must be taken down.

VI. PENETRATING CHEST TRAUMA

1. This results in localized anatomic disruption to blood vessels and tissues.
   a. Injuries within "the box"—heart and great vessel involvement is likely.

Pearl: *"The box" is anatomically medial to the nipples and between the costal margin and clavicles.*

2. Track of projectile may be difficult to predict despite entry and exit wounds—possibility for ricochet, multiple projectiles, and inability to recreate scene (often entrance and exit wounds are not known).
3. High-velocity projectiles (>1000 feet/s) produce profound tissue damage due to dissipation of kinetic energy and the creation of a "temporary cavity" as projectile decelerates through tissues.
4. Hemorrhage
   a. Arterial bleeding may stop by arterial retraction and vasoconstriction.
   b. Venous bleeding may arrest by tamponade as IV pressure decreases.
   c. Identified and treated most often with tube thoracostomy. Indications for emergent thoracotomy include:
      (1) Initial chest tube output exceeding 1500 mL of blood

17

THORACIC TRAUMA

    (2) Bloody drainage exceeding 200–250 mL/h for 3 consecutive hours

    (3) Shock without other etiology

5. **Pericardial tamponade may occur secondary to myocardial laceration or injury to the coronary vessels.**

  a. Results in decreased right atrioventricular filling, which leads to decreased cardiac output

  b. Systemic hypotension, tachycardia, distended neck veins, and muffled heart tones—all pathognomonic

  c. Early stage: filling pressures maintained by aggressive fluid resuscitation maintaining blood pressure and overcoming the effect of the tamponade

  d. Late stage: precipitous and profound hypotension because patient is no longer able to compensate

6. **Pneumothorax: Lung collapses secondary to parenchymal injury from penetrating trauma or blunt trauma (sharp fragments from rib fractures).**

  a. If parenchymal defect is smaller than glottis, the pneumothorax is usually small and ventilation is preserved. However, if the defect is larger than the glottis, the air will pass preferentially through the injury site, leading to a large pneumothorax ("sucking chest wound").

  b. Small pneumothoraces less than 1 cm may be managed conservatively if there is no respiratory compromise.

  c. Larger or symptomatic pneumothoraces should be treated with tube thoracostomy (chest tube placement).

  d. Tension pneumothorax is a clinical diagnosis and an *immediate threat to life.*

    (1) Diagnose by tracheal deviation, distended neck veins, diminished lung sounds, and hemodynamic instability.

    (2) Perform immediate needle decompression as a temporizing measure prior to emergent chest tube placement.

    (3) Needle thoracostomy: Perform when a tension pneumothorax is suspected:

      (a) Locate the second intercostal space in the mid-clavicular line on side of the tension pneumothorax.

      (b) Insert a 14-G IV cannula until air is aspirated or a gush of air is noted.

      (c) Remove the needle, leaving the cannula in place to relieve the tension.

      (d) Then proceed to definitive chest tube placement.

      (e) The fourth intercostal space at the anterior axillary line may need to be used in larger patients to access the pleural space.

      (f) The procedure is associated with a 33%–73% failure rate, as well as complications such as intrathoracic hemorrhage.

  e. Occult pneumothorax is diagnosed on chest CT, but not evident on chest radiograph. No treatment is necessary if small and asymptomatic.

7. Air embolism (estimated incidence rate of 4%–14%) is caused by direct communication between blood vessels and airways or lung parenchyma.
   a. Air embolizing to the cerebral arteries, coronaries, or heart chambers may be catastrophic.
   b. Air embolism may lead to sudden circulatory collapse after tracheal intubation and initiation of positive pressure ventilation.
   c. Unexplained neurologic deficits or seizures may indicate a cerebral air embolism.
   d. If associated with unilateral lung injury, treat with immediate thoracotomy and placement of clamp around the hilum to prevent further passage of air into the systemic circulation.
   e. Selective ventilation of the uninjured lung may also be lifesaving.
8. A total of 90% of great vessel injuries are due to penetrating trauma, with increased risk with penetrating trauma to "the box."
   a. Depending on nature of injury and hemorrhage, these may be repaired primarily; endovascular repairs are becoming more common.
   b. Treat aortic injury as detailed previously.
9. Cardiac injury may result in rapid accumulation of blood within the pericardium and pericardial tamponade with as little as 50 mL of blood.
   a. Beck's triad is hypotension, distended neck veins, and muffled heart sounds.
      (1) This may also be diagnosed with ultrasound on focused assessment with sonography for trauma (FAST) examination.
      (2) If hemodynamically unstable, patient requires emergent pericardiocentesis followed by definitive treatment.
      (3) If patient becomes pulseless, perform resuscitative thoracotomy to evacuate pericardium.
   b. Survivable injuries may be repaired primarily. Hemorrhage control is achieved via clamping, finger occlusion, skin stapling of ventricular wall, or Foley bulb occlusion of defect.
   c. Primary repair undertaken with sutures. Horizontal mattress sutures are used to pass underneath coronary arteries; use pledgetted sutures on the thin-walled right ventricle to prevent erosion of sutures through wall.
10. Tracheobronchial injury may be secondary to blunt or penetrating injury.
    a. May demonstrate a massive air leak upon chest tube placement. Consider tracheobronchial injury if pneumothorax persists despite appropriate placement of two chest tubes. Up to 60% may have subcutaneous emphysema, and 70% may have pneumomediastinum.

17

THORACIC TRAUMA

   b. Adequate ventilation must be ensured. This may require advancement of endotracheal tube distal to the injury or into the contralateral mainstem bronchus.

   c. Sensitivity of CT scanning for diagnosis is approaching 100%; however, diagnostic bronchoscopy remains the gold standard for diagnosis of a tracheobronchial injury.

   d. Treat with debridement and primary repair with end-to-end anastomosis and pedicled tissue flap, such as an intercostal muscle flap sutured in place around the anastomosis.

   e. Distal airway injuries may be managed conservatively with a chest tube. Endoscopic management may be appropriate if an air leak persists.

11. **Pulmonary laceration uncommonly requires operative management; however, persistent bleeding parenchymal edges may be treated with wedge resection or tractotomy with ligation of individual airways and bleeding vessels.**

   a. Stapled pulmonary tractotomy is effective for up to 85% of all pulmonary injuries requiring surgery.

   b. More severe injury may necessitate lobectomy.

   c. If injury is severe enough to warrant pneumonectomy, mortality is extremely high due to associated postoperative right ventricular failure (reportedly 50%–100% mortality).

12. **Esophageal injury is usually associated with penetrating injury to tracheobronchial tree.**

   a. If injury is suspected due to mechanism and/or subsequent CT imaging

      (1) Patient should undergo soluble contrast esophagram followed by thin barium esophagram to evaluate for perforation. This may miss small injuries, in one series diagnosing only 62% of injuries whereas follow-up rigid esophagoscopy diagnosed 100%.

      (2) Patient should undergo esophagoscopy if swallow studies are equivocal to rule out injury.

   b. Treat by early debridement and primary repair.

   c. Larger injury or delayed diagnosis may require wide drainage and diverting esophagostomy or formal esophagectomy.

VII. RESUSCITATIVE THORACOTOMY

Although this procedure can be life-saving in the appropriate patient, it remains highly controversial due to limited survival, the potential for survival with neurologic devastation (anoxic encephalopathy), and the potential risk of exposure to blood-borne disease in health care providers who perform the procedure.

Reported survival varies widely, owing to variation in its application to differing patient situations. One recent study showed up to 41.7% of resuscitative thoracotomies were performed outside of the traditionally published indications, with neurologically intact survival most likely when following the published guidelines.

1. Outcomes:
   a. A recent single-institution study demonstrated a survival-to-discharge of 8.3% (37/448), and 75% of the survivors who were surveyed reported normal cognition and daily functioning.
   b. A major review of the literature by the American College of Surgeons Committee on Trauma revealed a survival rate of 11.2% with penetrating trauma and only 1.6% for blunt trauma.
      (1) Overall survival rate of 13% in penetrating trauma in a series of 2400 patients, which is an optimistic figure that excludes those with neurologic catastrophes; gunshot wounds—7% survival rate; stab wounds—18% survival rate
      (2) Survival in the pediatric population—stab wounds, 9%; gunshot wounds, 4%; blunt trauma, 2%
2. Principles of resuscitative thoracotomy:
   a. Evacuation of pericardial tamponade
   b. Control of massive hemorrhage from the heart, lungs, or great vessels
   c. Performance of internal cardiac massage
   d. Cross-clamping of the descending aorta to improve cerebral and coronary blood flow
   e. Evacuation of bronchovenous air in air embolism
3. Traditional indications for resuscitative thoracotomy:
   a. Penetrating trauma with loss of vital signs in the trauma bay; or less than 15 minutes of cardiopulmonary resuscitation (CPR) en route
   b. Blunt trauma with loss of vital signs in the trauma bay; or less than 5 minutes, CPR en route
   c. 2015 EAST Recommendations:
   After an evidence-based review of 72 studies (10,238 patients), EAST made the following recommendations based on the likelihood of survival with intact neurologic function.
      (1) Patients who present pulseless after penetrating thoracic trauma *with* signs of life (strong recommendation)
      (2) Patients who present pulseless after penetrating thoracic trauma *without* signs of life (conditional recommendation)
      (3) Patients who present pulseless after penetrating extrathoracic trauma *with* signs of life (conditional recommendation)
      (4) Patients who present pulseless after penetrating extrathoracic trauma *without* signs of life (conditional recommendation)
      (5) Patients who present pulseless after blunt trauma *with* signs of life (conditional recommendation)
      (6) Patients who present pulseless after blunt trauma *without* signs of life (conditionally *against*)
   Note that only pulseless penetrating trauma patients *with* signs of life are strongly recommended to undergo resuscitative thoracotomy. Only pulse-

17

THORACIC TRAUMA

less blunt trauma patients *without* signs of life are conditionally recommended against undergoing resuscitative thoracotomy.

4. **Traditional contraindications to resuscitative thoracotomy**
   a. No signs of life in the field
      (1) Signs of life: pupillary reactivity, spontaneous respiration, palpable pulse, cardiac electrical activity, or spontaneous movement
   b. Penetrating trauma with greater than 15 minutes of CPR en route
   c. Blunt trauma with greater than 5 minutes of CPR en route

5. **Technique of emergency department thoracotomy**
   a. Place patient in supine position with left side elevated 15 degrees on a towel roll.
      (1) Left-sided thoracotomy for resuscitation
   b. Arms are positioned overhead in "taxi-cab hailing" position to provide optimal exposure to chest.
   c. Anterolateral incision at fifth intercostal space is made with a scalpel from sternum to the table (inframammary fold). The intercostal muscles are incised with curved Mayo scissors.
   d. The rib spreader is inserted, spreading the rib interspace (handle toward the axilla).
   e. Grasp the pericardium with toothed pickups and incise the pericardium anterior to the phrenic nerve; incise cranial to caudal.
      (1) This relieves tamponade, allows direct cardiac massage, and allows access to the heart for any direct injuries.
         (a) Internal cardiac massage: hinged clapping motion of the hands with wrists apposed
         (b) Internal defibrillation: 15–30 J
         (c) Sutures or skin staples may be used to close cardiac injuries before definitive repair.
   f. The descending aorta or the pulmonary hilum may also be cross-clamped or the lung twisted to stem hemorrhage. Take down the inferior pulmonary ligament to gain appropriate mobilization and exposure.
      (1) Aortic cross-clamping should not exceed 30 minutes.
      (2) Aortic declamping is associated with sudden reperfusion.
         (a) Release of inflammatory mediators into the cardiopulmonary system
   g. The thoracotomy may be extended across the sternum to the right side using a Lebsche knife (clamshell thoracotomy), allowing better access to the heart and the opposite chest cavity.
   h. Factors leading to discontinuation of resuscitation during thoracotomy; that is, "when to stop"
      (1) Systolic blood pressure is less than 70 mm Hg after 15 minutes despite fluid resuscitation.
      (2) Self-sustaining rhythm is not achieved within 15 minutes of thoracotomy.
      (3) Aortic cross-clamping is unable to increase blood pressure proximal to cross-clamp and unable to restore coronary and cerebral perfusion.

(4) There is cardiac asystole when pericardium is opened and tamponade evacuated.

(5) There is evidence of other devastating injuries (such as massive head injury) with independently poor prognoses.

VIII. OTHER THORACIC PROCEDURES IN THE FACE OF TRAUMA

A. FOCUSED ASSESSMENT WITH SONOGRAPHY FOR TRAUMA EXAMINATION

1. Able to detect pericardial or peritoneal fluid
2. Allows expeditious surgical intervention
3. No ionizing radiation, so may repeat as many times as necessary
4. May give false negative results, for example, in large hemothorax or if a cardiac injury is decompressing into the left chest

B. PERICARDIOCENTESIS

1. Useful in a stable patient
2. Beck's triad—distended neck veins, muffled heart sounds, hypotension
3. Take off the cervical collar to examine the neck; muffled heart sounds may be difficult to appreciate in the trauma bay.
4. If pericardial effusion or tamponade, the patient likely requires a pericardial window (Trinkle procedure) or pericardial exploration.
5. Able to transport to the operating room for urgent thoracotomy/sternotomy
6. May benefit from at least partial relief of an acute pericardial tamponade, especially if operative capabilities are not available

C. SUBXIPHOID PERICARDIOTOMY

1. Also suitable in the stable patient with suspected pericardial tamponade or pericardial blood
2. More easily able to evacuate clotted pericardial blood
3. Disadvantage—It releases the tamponade without adequate control of the injury.

D. THORACOSCOPY

1. Assessment and examination of thoracic structures in elective procedures and stable patients
   a. Evacuation of clotted hemothoraces
   b. Assessment of injuries to the diaphragm
   c. Examination of the pericardium
   d. Control of chest wall or intrathoracic bleeding

IX. POSTOPERATIVE CARE OF THE PATIENT WITH A CHEST INJURY

A. CHEST TUBE MANAGEMENT

1. Chest tubes remain on suction (-10 to -20 cm H_2O) for at least 24–48 hours and until the resultant air leak has resolved. This may take hours to days.
   a. This is dependent on the nature of the injury, such as a simple pneumothorax versus large parenchymal injury.

2. Chest tube may be placed to water seal after air leak has resolved.
3. Chest radiograph is obtained 4 hours after water seal to identify recurrent pneumothorax; if a pneumothorax recurs, then the chest tube is placed back on suction.
4. Chest tube output should be less than 100 mL/shift for 24 hours.
5. If these criteria are met, then it is usually safe to remove the chest tube.
6. A chest radiograph is not necessary after the chest tube is removed, unless the patient decompensates clinically.

X. COMPLICATIONS OF THORACIC TRAUMA

Of blunt and penetrating thoracic trauma

1. Persistent air leak
   a. This may require video-assisted thoracoscopic surgery (VATS) to staple off the injured portion of lung or bronchus in an effort to seal the air leak.
   b. Interventional pulmonology consultation can also be considered for placement of an endobronchial valve.
2. Bronchopleural fistula
   a. This may eventually require drainage via thoracic window (Clagett procedure), as well as resection and stapling of leak.
   b. Bronchopleural fistulas often become a chronic problem.
3. Empyema
   a. Empyema is often a result of the gross contamination from an open chest wound.
   b. This may also be a result of chest tubes placed in an emergent situation where sterile technique may have been broken.
   c. Always try to give prophylactic antibiotic coverage before chest tube placement.
   d. Empyema may also result from retained hemothorax.
   e. Treat with adequate chest tube drainage and antibiotics. If multiloculated, drainage may improve with instillation of fibrinolytics (tissue plasminogen activator [TPA]). This may ultimately require thoracoscopic drainage.
4. Retained hemothorax
   a. Results from inadequate chest tube drainage (clotted chest tube, loculation, etc.). Up to 33% may proceed to empyema if there is radiographically demonstrable retained hemothorax after chest tube drainage.
   b. EAST guidelines demonstrate that early VATS drainage of retained hemothorax results in decreased time of chest tube drainage and shorter hospital stays. This should be undertaken within 72 hours.
   c. This may be treated with TPA instillation via the chest tube to cause fibrinolysis on the retained clot in patients too unstable for surgery.
      (1) A protocol of four doses of TPA over a 48-hour period has been shown to produce good results.
      (2) If TPA fails, then VATS versus open thoracotomy for drainage and decortication is necessary.

5. Acute respiratory distress syndrome (ARDS)—acute onset within 1 week of apparent insult, patchy bilateral infiltrates on chest radiograph, PaO_2:FiO_2 ratio (P:F) less than 300 on a minimum positive end-expiratory pressure (PEEP) of 5 cm H_2O, and noncardiogenic origin of respiratory failure

  a. ARDS may result from the systemic inflammatory response to significant injury.

  b. Significant pulmonary contusions may also evolve into ARDS.

  c. ARDS results in significantly reduced lung compliance.

    (1) Low tidal volume (6–8 mL/kg of ideal body weight) ventilation strategy with goal plateau pressures less than 30 cm H_2O

    (2) May require increased PEEP and FiO_2 to maintain oxygenation

    (3) Placing the patient in a prone position may also be beneficial. Inhaled nitric oxide may also help gas exchange.

RECOMMENDED READINGS

Brunicardi FC, Andersen DK, Billiar TR, Dunn DL, Hunter JG. *Schwartz's Principles of Surgery*. 10th ed. New York: McGraw-Hill Education; 2015.

Cameron JL, Cameron AM. *Current Surgical Therapy*. 11th ed. Philadelphia: Elsevier; 2014.

Challoumas D, Dimitrakakis G. Blunt thoracic aortic injuries: new perspectives in management. *Open Cardiovasc Med J*. 2015;9:69–72.

Esme H, Solak O, Sahin DA, Sezer M. Blunt and penetrating traumatic ruptures of the diaphragm. *Thorac Cardiovasc Surg*. 2005;54:324–327.

Ganie FA, Lone H, Lone GN, et al. Lung contusion: a clinico-pathologic entity with unpredictable clinical course. *Bull Emerg Trauma*. 2013;1(1):7–16.

Hunt PA, Greaves I, Owens WA. Emergency thoracotomy in thoracic trauma—a review. *Injury*. 2006;37:1–19.

Parry NG, Moffat B, Vogt K. Blunt thoracic trauma: recent advances and outstanding questions. *Curr Opin Crit Care*. 2015;21:544–548.

Petrone P, Asensio JA. Surgical management of penetrating pulmonary injuries. *Scand J Trauma Resus Emerg Med*. 2009;17:8.

Rabinovici R, Bugaev N. Resuscitative thoracotomy: an update. *Scand J Surg*. 2013;103:112–119.

Seamon MJ, Haut ER, Van Arendonk K, et al. An evidence-based approach to patient selection for emergency department thoracotomy: a practice management guideline from the Eastern Association for the Surgery of Trauma. *J Trauma Acute Care Surg*. 2015;79(1):159–173.

17

THORACIC TRAUMA

Extremity Trauma

Ryan M. Boudreau, MD

Investigation for extremity injuries is a critical portion of the trauma evaluation. During these examinations, the surgeon must look for fractures, dislocations, soft tissue damage, vascular injuries, and neurologic deficits. Upon completion of the tertiary survey, the patient should have undergone a complete and systematic evaluation of every body part. This chapter outlines the keys to diagnosing and managing common extremity injuries seen in the trauma patient.

I. EVALUATION OF THE INJURED LIMB

A. GENERAL POINTS

1. Examination should proceed, if possible, by comparing injured side to uninjured side.
2. Immediate reduction of fractures and dislocations improves pain and limits neurovascular injury.

B. EVALUATION OF FRACTURES AND DISLOCATIONS

Each identified fracture can be classified by the following scheme. The following descriptors determine the prognosis of a given fracture and are extremely useful when orthopedic consultation is required.

1. Open or closed fracture
2. Name of fractured bone
3. Location of fracture
   a. Diaphyseal (shaft) versus metaphyseal (near the articular surface)
   b. Intraarticular versus extraarticular
4. Status of the soft tissue
   a. Presence of any bullae, ecchymosis, swelling, or multiple abrasions ("road rash")
   b. Laceration or degloving injury overlying fracture (suggests an open fracture)
   c. Associated neurovascular deficits
5. Descriptors (tell about the energy of injury)
   a. Pattern (transverse, oblique, spiral, comminuted; Fig. 18.1)
   b. Displacement or angulation
   c. Rotation
   d. Length (presence of limb shortening)

II. OPEN FRACTURES

A. DEFINITION

1. Fracture in which a break in the skin communicates directly with a fractured bone or the surrounding hematoma. An archaic synonym is a "compound fracture."

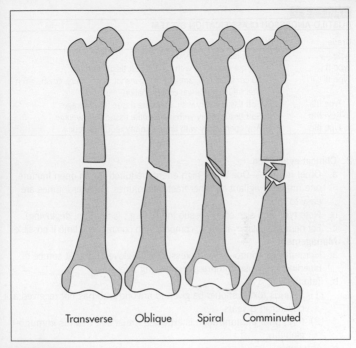

Transverse   Oblique   Spiral   Comminuted

FIG. 18.1
Fracture patterns.

18

EXTREMITY TRAUMA

B. COMPLICATIONS OF OPEN FRACTURES
1. Delayed union or nonunion
2. Infection (soft tissue or osteomyelitis)
   a. All open fractures are contaminated.
3. Compartment syndrome
4. Amputation
5. Death (sepsis, multiple organ dysfunction syndrome [MODS], effects of polytrauma)

C. GUSTILO-ANDERSON CLASSIFICATION SYSTEM (TABLE 18.1)
1. Determined by size of skin defect, mechanism, and presence of contamination. Increasing score correlates with higher rates of complications.

D. EMERGENCY DEPARTMENT MANAGEMENT OF OPEN FRACTURES
1. History—mechanism of trauma and geographic location of open injury
   a. Important to note if gunshot, crush, or farm work related
   b. Duration of time since injury (>8 hours since mechanism is an automatic Gustilo type III fracture)

TABLE 18.1	
GUSTILO-ANDERSON CLASSIFICATION SYSTEM	
Grade	Wound
Type I	<1 cm laceration, clean
Type II	1–10 cm laceration with limited soft tissue damage
Type III	>10 cm laceration, amputation, gunshot, farm injury, crush, >6 h after injury or marked contamination
Type IIIa	Soft tissue injury with adequate tissue for coverage
Type IIIb	Soft tissue injury with inadequate tissue for coverage
Type IIIc	Any open injury with arterial injury requiring repair

2. Clinical evaluation
   a. Other injuries—Due to the high energy required for an open fracture, one must be vigilant for other fractures/injuries. Smaller injuries are easy to miss.
   b. Note type and size of soft tissue injury (e.g., laceration, degloving).
   c. For neurovascular evaluation, compare with contralateral limb if possible.
3. Management
   a. Hemorrhage control—direct pressure with gloved hand at source of bleeding (may use compression dressing if feasible)
   b. Tetanus
      (1) Tetanus toxoid should be given to anyone who has not received a booster in 5 years.
      (2) If no prior immunization is expected, must add tetanus immunoglobulin.
   c. Antibiotics
      (1) Gustilo I and II—Use systemic gram-positive coverage (first-generation cephalosporin).
      (2) Gustilo III—Add gram-negative coverage (first-generation cephalosporin with aminoglycoside).
      (3) Fecal or potential clostridial contamination (i.e., farm-related injury)—Use first-generation cephalosporin, aminoglycoside, and high-dose penicillin G.
      (4) Suggested dosages:
         (a) Cefazolin—2 g every 4 hours preoperatively or every 8 hours postoperatively (3 g if patient over 120 kg)
         (b) Gentamicin—2.5 mg/kg twice daily or 6 mg/kg daily
         (c) Penicillin G—2–4 million units every 4 hours
      (5) Avoid fluoroquinolones because they may have a negative impact on fracture healing.
      (6) Antibiotics should be discontinued within 24 hours of soft tissue coverage to minimize complications from their use.
   d. Initial irrigation and debridement
      (1) All visible debris should be removed from the wound.
      (2) Irrigation with 3 L normal saline should be performed.
      (3) Provide provisional reduction and stabilization with splints or traction.

(4) Wound should be covered with saline-soaked gauze, which is left in place until operating room (manipulation associated with increased infection rate).

e. Formal irrigation and debridement in operating room should be performed as early as possible (classically <6 hours) without increasing overall risk to polytrauma patients.

(1) When possible, attain wound closure (primary, flap, negative pressure wound dressing) before leaving operating room.

(2) Low-pressure normal saline irrigation with a minimum of 3 L for type 1, 6 L for type 2, and 9 L for type 3 open fractures.

f. Operative fixation after patient is stable—external versus internal depending on clinical status, soft tissue coverage

III. COMPARTMENT SYNDROME

A. DEFINITION

1. A clinical condition marked by elevated pressure within a closed tissue space, resulting in venous obstruction, tissue ischemia, and—potentially—necrosis of compartment contents

a. Pressure increases secondary to either swelling or space-occupying lesion (e.g., hematoma).

b. Amount of tissue damage is proportional to the *amount of pressure* and the *duration of exposure* at a given pressure.

c. Necrosis can lead to permanent loss of motor/sensation in the affected limb, as well as the systemic effects of myonecrosis (arrhythmia, acute kidney injury [AKI]).

B. CAUSES OF COMPARTMENT SYNDROME

1. Fracture
2. Intracompartmental or extracompartmental hematoma
3. Cast or external compressive dressings
4. Crush injury
5. Reperfusion injury secondary to ischemia, vascular injury
6. Burns—increased fluid load and capillary permeability
7. Intravenous (IV) infiltration

C. SIGNS AND SYMPTOMS

1. Progressive, severe pain uncontrolled by pain medications (nonspecific, but only symptom where meaningful intervention is possible)
2. Tense, swollen compartment—when palpated, reproduces pain
   a. Possible to miss a deep compartment syndrome with this test
3. Pain on passive stretch test
4. Late findings (associated with poor prognosis for functional outcome)—"The Five *P*s"
   a. *P*aresthesia and *p*aralysis
   b. *P*ulselessness
   c. *P*allor
   d. *P*oikilothermia—limb cold to touch

18

EXTREMITY TRAUMA

5. Pearls
   a. Palpable pulses can be present with clinically significant compartment syndrome and should not be considered reassuring if present.
   b. Distinguishing between compartment syndrome and injury to nerves or vessels is difficult and may require compartment pressure measurement.
   c. Presence of open fractures does not rule out compartment syndrome.

D. DIAGNOSIS OF COMPARTMENT SYNDROME
1. A compartment's perfusion pressure (ΔP) is the difference between the diastolic pressure and the compartment pressure.
2. $\Delta P \leq 30$ mm Hg is diagnostic of compartment syndrome and is an indication for fasciotomy.
3. When to measure compartment pressures:
   a. Equivocal findings on examination with suspicion for compartment syndrome
   b. Unconscious patient with injury pattern concerning for compartment syndrome
4. How to measure compartment pressures:
   a. Solid-state transducer intracompartmental catheter (Stryker) is a handheld device that allows quick, simple measurements.
   b. Arterial line setup is easily accessible in all surgical intensive care units and most emergency departments.
   c. Measurements should be taken at or close to fractures (<5 cm) with distal joints in anatomic position.

E. SURGICAL TREATMENT OF ACUTE COMPARTMENT SYNDROME
1. Fasciotomy, which fully decompresses all at-risk compartments, is the only treatment for compartment syndrome.
2. Indications for fasciotomy
   a. Clearly positive examination findings
   b. Perfusion pressure less than 30 mm Hg
   c. Mangled or crushed limb
   d. Associated vascular injuries with significant ischemia time (>6 hours) or combined arterial and venous injuries
3. Fasciotomy of lower leg
   a. Must open all four compartments of the lower leg.
      (1) Anterior compartment (deep peroneal nerve, anterior tibial artery; tibialis anterior, extensor digitorum longus, hallucis longus)
      (2) Lateral compartment (superficial peroneal nerve, fibularis longus and brevis)
      (3) Superficial posterior compartment (medial sural cutaneous nerve, gastrocnemius, soleus, plantaris)
      (4) Deep posterior compartment (tibial nerve, posterior tibial artery; tibialis posterior, flexor hallucis longus, flexor digitorum longus)

b. Two-incision technique
   (1) Use two vertical incisions separated by skin bridge of at least 7 cm.
   (2) Lateral incision is made midway between the edges of the fibula and tibia starting two fingerbreadths below the tibial tuberosity and extending to two fingerbreadths above the lateral malleolus.
      (a) Lateral incision is used to decompress anterior and lateral compartments.
   (3) Medial incision is placed 2 cm posterior to posteromedial border of tibia and extends from two fingerbreadths below the tibial tuberosity to two fingerbreadths above the medial malleolus.
      (a) Medial incision is used to decompress the superficial and deep posterior compartments.
   (4) The soleus must be taken down from the posterior tibia to expose the fascia and allow adequate decompression of the deep posterior compartment.
   (5) Deficient understanding of relevant anatomy or attempts to make small incisions will result in inadequate decompression.
c. Complications of fasciotomy
   (1) Failure to completely release all at-risk compartments (most common: deep posterior)—Look for soft, mobile, bulging muscle bellies.
   (2) Inability to close incisions due to tissue retraction—Can close as early as 48 hours postoperative if wound is clean and swelling is resolved.

IV. PELVIC FRACTURES

Pelvic fractures are generally associated with high-energy mechanisms and can result in significant bleeding leading to hemodynamic instability. A pelvic x-ray during the patient's initial evaluation can help to quickly identify pelvic fractures that would benefit from pelvic binder placement as well as alert the treating physician to a potential source of hemorrhage.

A. EVALUATION OF PELVIC RING FRACTURES
1. History and physical examination
   a. These frequently result from high-energy blunt trauma (~10% of all blunt trauma).
      (1) These patients have a high incidence of polytrauma.
      (2) Leading causes of death are pelvic hemorrhage (~50%) and intracranial hemorrhage.
   b. Rule out open fracture (perineal, vaginal, and digital rectal examinations on all applicable patients).
   c. Inspect for hematoma, hemorrhage, and contusions over perineum and flanks.

    d. Rule out bladder injury with evaluation for gross hematuria. Gross hematuria requires a cystogram.

    e. Note leg length or rotational discrepancies.

    f. Assess pelvic stability (done by one person, gently, once).

      (1) With hands on anterior superior iliac spine (ASIS), move hands anterior and posterior; also compress across ASIS toward midline.

2. **Classification systems: Most are retrospective and of limited clinical use in trauma bay.**

    a. Key is to recognize that disruption of the pubic symphysis greater than 2.5 cm or vertical fractures of ipsilateral rami ("open book fracture") or combined anterior and posterior fractures ("vertical sheer") are unstable, at increased risk for significant hemorrhage, and require fixation.

3. **Imaging**

    a. Anteroposterior pelvis—blunt trauma, especially with hypotension; examination suspicious for pelvic fracture

    b. Chest radiograph—to rule out associated intrathoracic injury, especially if hypotensive

    c. Focused assessment sonography in trauma (FAST)—when negative in unstable patient with suspected pelvic fracture, suspect retroperitoneal/pelvic hemorrhage

      (1) Consider supraumbilical diagnostic peritoneal aspirate to rule out intraabdominal hemorrhage if necessary. Ten milliliters of gross blood on aspiration should trigger a laparotomy in an unstable patient.

    d. Computed tomography (CT) for abdomen and pelvis—obtained only in the stable patient; provides detail on hemorrhagic sources, fractures

B. MANAGEMENT OF PELVIC HEMORRHAGE—GRAVEST COMPLICATION OF PELVIC FRACTURE

1. **TPOD Pelvic Stabilization Device**—must place across greater trochanters under clothing; decreases transfusion requirements in unstable patients; risk of skin necrosis if left long term

2. **Angiography**

    a. Indications

      (1) Patients with persistent instability despite resuscitation after ruling out of other sources of bleeding

      (2) Patients with prior embolization who have recurrent bleeding or instability

      (3) Evidence of contrast extravasation on CT

3. **Consider preperitoneal packing (PPP) or resuscitative endovascular balloon occlusion of the aorta (REBOA) for hemodynamically unstable patients with pelvic fractures and a negative FAST examination.**

    a. PPP—placement of packs on each side of bladder to provide effective tamponade of the internal iliac vessels

    b. REBOA—if available, can be used in emergency department via percutaneous arteriotomy.

4. Associated injuries
   a. Open fractures—mortality approaches 50%; evidence of perineal or rectal wound mandates diverting colostomy.
   b. Urologic injuries (bladder rupture, urethral injury)
      (1) Urethral injury—classically presents with blood at the meatus. Diagnosed with retrograde urethrogram
      (2) Bladder injury—classically presents with gross hematuria. Diagnosed with cystogram. Most bladder injuries are extraperitoneal and resolve with Foley drainage alone for 14 days. Intraperitoneal bladder rupture mandates laparotomy for repair.
   c. Neurologic injury—chronic unstable gait, sexual dysfunction, incontinence/retention

V. VASCULAR INJURY IN EXTREMITY TRAUMA

A. HISTORY AND PHYSICAL

1. Mechanism
   a. Penetrating trauma (>80%)
   b. Orthopedic injury secondary to blunt trauma
      (1) Brachial artery—secondary to distal humerus fracture or elbow dislocation
      (2) Popliteal artery—proximal tibial fracture or posterior knee dislocation
2. Assess for hard and soft signs of vascular injury (Table 18.2).
3. Ankle-brachial indices (ABIs): normal = 1.0; however, greater than 0.9 is acceptable if no evidence of peripheral vascular disease.

B. MANAGEMENT OF EXTREMITY TRAUMA

1. It is crucial to document as thorough a neurologic examination as patient condition permits to avoid needless reoperation in case of postoperative deficit.
2. Never explore wound in trauma bay.
3. Direct pressure with gloved hand should be adequate for hemostasis; if not, place a tourniquet.

TABLE 18.2
HARD AND SOFT SIGNS OF VASCULAR INJURY

Hard Signs	Soft Signs
Absent distal pulse	Diminished pulses
Pulsatile bleeding	Significant prehospital hemorrhage
Expanding hematoma	Peripheral nerve deficit
Audible bruit	Injury near major artery (e.g., dislocation, wound)
Palpable thrill	
Ischemic limb	

18

EXTREMITY TRAUMA

4. All patients with hard signs of arterial injury require surgical exploration immediately.
   a. These patients should be monitored closely postoperatively for compartment syndrome or undergo fasciotomy during index surgery.
5. Patients without hard signs of arterial injury should undergo ABI determination (use manual cuff and handheld Doppler).
   a. ABI greater than 0.9—no further work-up
   b. ABI less than 0.9 or soft signs of injury—should undergo CT angiography (contrast angiography if shotgun/shrapnel wound)
6. Postoperative care—Perform frequent neurovascular checks; trend creatine kinase (CK) and serial examinations to assess for compartment syndrome if no fasciotomy is performed.

C. COMPLICATIONS OF VASCULAR INJURIES

1. Arteriovenous fistula is a result of injury to both artery and a nearby vein.
   a. Leads to edema, pain, steal syndrome, and congestive heart failure (CHF) as flow across increases
2. Pseudoaneurysm is a partial injury to artery that is contained by surrounding tissue.
   a. Risk of embolic events or compression increases with increased size
3. Thrombosis—Consider missed injury or technical error if early postoperative thrombosis (after vascular repair).
4. Infection at repair site—Minimize risk with adequate soft tissue coverage.

VI. AMPUTATION IN TRAUMA

1. The decision to perform amputation is often multifactorial and represents an attempt to balance the potential handicap of amputation with the risks of salvage, which may include exsanguination, sepsis/MODS, or nonfunctional limb.
   a. The surgeon must weigh the likelihood of amputation with the probability of salvage attaining meaningful functional status.

RECOMMENDED READINGS

Cullinane DC, et al. Pelvic fracture hemorrhage—update and systematic review. *J Trauma*. 2011;71:1850–1868.

Jones CB, Wenke JC. Open fractures. In: Browner BD, ed. *Skeletal Trauma: Basic Science, Management, and Reconstruction*. 5th ed. Philadelphia: Elsevier Saunders; 2015.

Sise MJ, Shakford SR. Peripheral vascular injury. In: Mattox KL, ed. *Trauma*. 7th ed. New York: McGraw-Hill Companies, Inc; 2013.

Stahel PF, Smith WR, Hak DJ. Lower extremity. In: Mattox KL, ed. *Trauma*. 7th ed. New York: McGraw-Hill Companies, Inc; 2013.

Burn Care

Lauren M. Baumann, MD

The most difficult thing of all to see is that which is right in front of your eyes.

—Johan Wolfgang von Goethe

Each year, approximately 1 million people in the United States sustain burn injuries. Sadly, more than 90% of these injuries are preventable, many of which are related to smoking and substance abuse. Fortunately due to advances in burn care, as well as the establishment of large burn centers, the number of burn deaths has been steadily decreasing every year. Treatment with a multidisciplinary, multispecialty team approach to burn care results not only in improved survival but also better cosmetic and functional outcomes.

I. CAUSATIVE FACTORS

A. SCALDS
1. Most common type of burn injury
2. Usually from hot water
   a. Exacerbated by overlying garments that prolong contact
3. Common burn injury seen in child abuse—distribution exhibits a "dip" line pattern

B. FLAME
1. Second most common type of burn injury
2. Full-thickness burns—common given the flammability of overlying garments

C. FLASH
1. Related to the explosion of flammable liquids and gases

D. CONTACT
1. Result from contact with heated or cooled objects
2. Seen frequently in industrial and trauma-related accidents

II. INDICATIONS FOR HOSPITAL ADMISSION

A. OUTPATIENT SETTING
1. Select burn cases can be managed as outpatients, usually those with less than 5% total body surface area (TBSA) injured.
2. Must be seen and examined by an experienced practitioner
3. Availability of close follow-up care
4. Adequate social support for wound care

5. Burn wounds greater than 5%–10% TBSA should be referred to a burn center for evaluation.

B. BURN UNIT SETTING

Referral to a burn center is indicated in the following situations based on the guidelines of the American Burn Association injury severity grading system:

1. Partial-thickness burns of more than 10% TBSA in all patients
2. Burns that involve the face, hands, feet, genitalia, or major joints
3. Full-thickness burns in any age group
4. Electrical, chemical, or inhalation injury
5. Burn injury in patients with preexisting medical conditions that may complicate management, prolong recovery, or affect mortality
6. Any patient with burns and concomitant trauma in which the burn injury poses the greatest risk or morbidity and mortality
7. Children in hospitals without qualified personnel or equipment for appropriate pediatric care
8. Patients who will require special social, emotional, or rehabilitation intervention, including victims of abuse or neglect

III. INITIAL MANAGEMENT

Initial management is immediately directed toward resuscitation, stabilization, and a thorough evaluation of all potential injuries. This process should be conducted in a systematic fashion according to the Advanced Trauma and Life Support protocols.

A. HISTORY

1. Ascertain the circumstances associated with the injury.
   a. History of unconsciousness, arrest, and the report given by the first responders
      (1) Avoid immediate concentration on the burn injuries alone.
2. Identify burn agent—flame, scald, chemical, electrical.
3. Open versus closed space—Assess the possibility of inhalation injury.
4. Time of burn is important for calculating adequate resuscitation.
5. Prehospital treatment administered and vital signs during transport— Patients are often found to be overresuscitated or underresuscitated.
6. Take medical history—allergies, immunizations, current medications, and concomitant medical problems.

B. AIRWAY/BREATHING

1. Ensure adequacy of the airway.
   a. Prophylactic intubation/tracheostomy is indicated for the following conditions:
      (1) Loss of consciousness or decreased mental status with inability to protect airway
      (2) Extensive burns greater than 60% TBSA

      (3) Increasing stridor or hoarseness

      (4) Evidence of posterior pharyngeal burn or injury

  b. Injury to the airway may be difficult to assess, often resulting in over-aggressive intubation. *The presence of singed nose hairs alone is not indicative of airway injury and does not necessitate intubation.*

2. **Inhalation injury is the major contributor to mortality.**

  a. Carbon monoxide (CO) poisoning—CO displaces oxygen and binds hemoglobin, forming carboxyhemoglobin. Results in poor oxygen delivery.

    (1) Diagnosis—signs and symptoms of hypoxia (nausea, headache, confusion) and/or serum carboxyhemoglobin level greater than 10% (nonsmokers) or greater than 20% (smokers) are diagnostic.

    (2) Levels of 40%–50% are not uncommon in survivors with aggressive care.

    (3) *Oxygen saturation levels are normal despite high levels of carboxyhemoglobin.*

    (4) Treatment—100% O_2 reduces half-life of CO.

      (a) Follow with carboxyhemoglobin levels and continue to treat until levels are 10%–15%.

      (b) Persistent metabolic acidosis despite adequate volume resuscitation implies CO poisoning of cellular respiration.

    (5) Carboxyhemoglobin levels greater than 50% are potentially lethal.

    (6) CO has a 200-time greater affinity for hemoglobin than does oxygen.

  b. Thermal injury

    (1) Usually limited to upper airway due to heat absorptive capacity of oropharynx. Steam burns are the exception that may affect lower airways.

    (2) Upper airway obstruction may occur up to 72 hours post injury. Maximal edema is seen between 12 and 24 hours.

  c. Chemical pneumonitis

    (1) Mucosal injury and pulmonary edema are caused by exposure to products of combustion and noxious gases.

    (2) Tracheobronchial mucosal injury leads to decreased immune defenses, bronchoconstriction and obstruction, and loss of ciliary clearance mechanisms.

    (3) Patients with chemical pneumonitis are at high risk of pneumonia, pulmonary edema, and acute respiratory distress syndrome (ARDS).

  d. Diagnostic modalities

    (1) Suspect inhalation injury if the following are present:

      (a) Closed-space injury (e.g., house fire)

      (b) Presence of facial burns, singed nasal hairs, bronchorrhea, carbonaceous sputum, wheezing and rales, tachypnea, progressive hoarseness, and difficulty clearing secretions

    (2) Upper airway—Perform direct laryngoscopy looking for carbon deposits, airway edema, and oropharyngeal burns.

19

BURN CARE

(3) Lower airway—Perform fiberoptic bronchoscopy looking for gross airway edema, carbon deposits in tracheobronchial tree, and mucosal erythema and necrosis.

e. Treatment—Implement immediate O_2 supplementation, ventilatory assistance, aggressive pulmonary toilet, O_2 saturation monitor, placement of an arterial line for serial arterial blood gases, bronchodilators, and bronchioalveolar lavage to remove debris.

C. BURN EVALUATION

The patient should be totally exposed, and any burned clothing and constricting jewelry removed.

1. Depth of the burn wound
   a. First degree—Only the epidermal layer is involved.
      (1) Painful to palpation
      (2) Pink in appearance without blistering
   b. Second degree (partial thickness)—The dermal layer is only partially involved, classified as superficial and deep partial thickness.
      (1) Painful to palpation
      (2) White to pink in appearance; blebs and blisters may be present.
      (3) Epithelialization occurs from epithelial cells surrounding hair follicles or sweat glands (skin appendages) and from the wound edges and is markedly delayed with deeper injury.
      (4) Deeper burns result in the destruction of epidermal appendages in reticular dermis and often require excision.
         (a) Spontaneous reepithelialization is markedly delayed (similar to third-degree injury).
   c. Third degree (full thickness)—The entire dermal layer is affected.
      (1) All dermal appendages destroyed
      (2) Insensate area
      (3) White, black, or red in appearance with a dry and leathery (inelastic) texture
   d. Fourth degree—The underlying fascia, muscle, and/or bone is involved.
2. *The estimate of the TBSA of the burn injury is the sum of second- and third-degree burns only.*
3. Size estimation (Fig. 19.1).
   a. The "rule of 9s" approximates the size of the affected area.
      (1) Head and neck: 9%
      (2) Each upper extremity: 9%
      (3) Each lower extremity: 18%
      (4) Anterior trunk: 18%
      (5) Posterior trunk: 18%
      (6) Perineum: 1%
   b. Children have a proportionally larger head and trunk with a smaller lower body (see Fig. 19.1 for percentages).

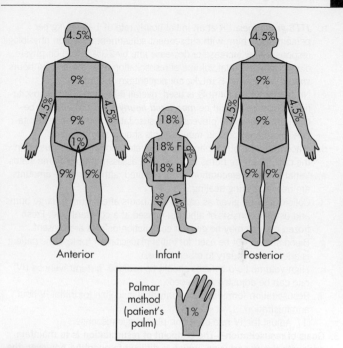

Anterior | Infant | Posterior

Palmar method (patient's palm) 1%

FIG. 19.1

Estimation of burn surface area by rule of 9s.

19

BURN CARE

D. FLUID RESUSCITATION

1. Access

a. Initially, two large-bore (>18-gauge) peripheral catheters can be used even if the access site has been burned.

b. Central venous access is more suitable than peripheral catheters for long-term use and if vasopressors are needed for hemodynamic instability.

c. Central venous pressure or pulmonary catheters are used in patients with cardiac or pulmonary disease, questionable fluid status, or hemodynamic instability.

   (1) Catheter sites should be changed routinely (every 3–7 days) to decrease the risk of infection.

2. Formulas for fluid resuscitation—Multiple formulas and resuscitation schemes have been devised; the Parkland formula is the most widely used. Other formulas include the modified Brook or the military Joint Theater Trauma Systems (JTTS) resuscitation.

a. *Parkland formula:* This resuscitation scheme uses lactated Ringer (LR) solution at 3–4 mL/kg/% burn, with half the total volume given over the first 8 hours (calculated from the time of burn), and the other half over the following 16 hours.

b. *JTTS guidelines:* LR at an initial hourly rate of 1–2 mL/kg per percentage of burn with subsequent adjustment based on physiologic response. May increase or decrease rate by 20% based on physiologic markers. Total volume of resuscitation after the first 24 hours *should not* exceed 6 mL/kg per percentage of burn.

c. No matter which formula is used, overall fluid status and resuscitation endpoints should be *monitored hourly* and fluids should be carefully adjusted to prevent overresuscitation and underresuscitation. Maintenance fluid requirements should also be added.

d. Placement of a pulmonary artery catheter should be considered in the case of severe burns to assist with assessment of volume status.

e. Initial K^+ supplementation is not required, although large amounts are needed during healing.

f. Colloid may be given as early as 12 hours after injury in large burns and usually consists of albumin infused at a constant rate. Fresh frozen plasma may be given if coagulation deficits are present.

g. Blood should not be used for initial resuscitation (unless the patient is anemic secondary to other injuries).

h. High-volume fluid boluses should be avoided, but intravenous (IV) rate can be adjusted as needed.

i. Resuscitation formulas serve only as a guideline for initial IV fluid administration.

   (1) Adjust the IV rate based on physiologic response.

3. Goals of resuscitation—The endpoint of resuscitation is to maintain adequate tissue perfusion, which is difficult to quantify; however, the following parameters can be used:

   a. Adequate urine output (UOP)—adults, 30 mL/h; children, 1–1.5 mL/kg per hour

   b. Blood pressure—goal mean arterial pressure (MAP) ≥60 mm Hg

   c. Normal mentation

   d. Well-perfused extremities (warm, good capillary refill)

   e. Normal arterial pH, lactate levels, and base excess

   f. Mixed venous O_2 saturations greater than 70%

   g. Inadequate volume restoration—manifested by oliguria, tachycardia, and persistent or worsening base deficit

E. INITIAL PROCEDURES

1. Foley catheterization—required for accurate UOP measurements during resuscitation in patients with more than 20% TBSA burns

2. Nasogastric tube—gastric ileus occurs frequently after burns; also a useful route for oral medications

3. Nasojejunal feeding tube—placed under fluoroscopy beyond the ligament of Treitz, with immediate initiation of enteral feedings

   a. *Early enteral feeding has been shown to decrease sepsis-related complications. All patients with greater than 20% TBSA burn should be considered for enteral feedings.*

4. Escharotomies—may be required for burns to extremities and chest to prevent compartment syndrome and respiratory compromise
   a. Compartment syndrome—The symptoms are the *5 Ps (pain, pallor, poikilothermia, pulselessness, and paresthesias)* exhibited by loss of motor and sensory nerve function, diminished peripheral pulses, decreased capillary refill, *pressure greater than 30 mm Hg by direct measurement (causes collapse of the capillary beds).*
      (1) Decompression is achieved by incising the lateral and medial aspects of the extremity while in anatomic position.
      (2) If symptoms are unrelieved, then fasciotomy may be required to relieve compartment syndrome.
      (3) Extremity burns should be managed with elevation of the affected extremity.
      (4) Compartment syndrome is especially important to look for with electrical burns.
   b. Circumferential chest burns reduce compliance of chest wall, but escharotomies are rarely needed.
      (1) Escharotomies should be performed in the presence of increased peak pressures, increased partial pressure of carbon dioxide ($Paco_2$), and decreased compliance.

F. INITIAL TESTS
1. Baseline weight
2. Laboratory tests—complete blood cell count, electrolytes, arterial blood gas with carboxyhemoglobin (for large burns or suspected inhalation injury), coagulation studies
3. Chest radiograph and electrocardiogram (history of cardiac problems or electrical burns)
4. Urinalysis

G. MEDICATIONS
1. Tetanus prophylaxis—unless received booster within last 5 years
2. Ulcer prophylaxis—may use proton pump inhibitor or H_2 blocker, should attempt at enteral administration as soon as is safe for the patient and a route for enteral administration has been established
3. Multivitamins (particularly vitamin C and the other antioxidants) in tube feedings
4. Hemoglobinuria/myoglobinuria— If myoglobinuria is present, aim for UOP greater than 100 mL/h for clearance and renal protection. If there is no improvement, may give mannitol 12.5 g IV, and alkalinize urine with 1 ampule $NaHCO_3$ in IV fluids to keep urine pH greater than 7.0 to prevent precipitation. If not adequately treated, renal failure can occur. Watch K^+ levels as well.
5. *Prophylactic antibiotics are contraindicated.*

19

BURN CARE

IV. PATHOPHYSIOLOGIC CHANGES ASSOCIATED WITH BURN INJURIES

A. EDEMA

1. Maximal at 18–24 hours after the burn for the following reasons:
   a. Generalized increase in microvascular permeability secondary to release of inflammatory mediators in affected tissue (histamine)—involves nonburned tissue if burns more than 20% TBSA
   b. Generalized impairment in cell membrane function—increased intracellular volume drawn in by increased intracellular Na^+ with concomitant loss of K^+

B. HEMODYNAMICS

1. Relatively predictable pattern is seen in large burn injuries.
2. Initial hypodynamic state has decreased cardiac output/contractility and increased vascular resistance with profound capillary leak.
   a. This usually resolves with adequate resuscitation.
3. By days 2–3, a hyperdynamic state exists with increased cardiac function and decreased vascular resistance.
4. Metabolism—There is a state of wound–, central nervous system–, and stress hormone–induced hypermetabolism.
   a. Begins at 48 hours after burn
   b. Caloric needs increased 1.3–2 times normal
   c. Characterized by increased oxygen consumption, heat production, increased body temperature, hypoproteinemia caused by catabolism and wound exudate, gluconeogenesis, and hyperglycemia
   d. Gradually returns to normal after wound is closed and the inflammation is resolved
5. Immunocompromised
   a. All aspects of the immune function are initially depressed, including:
      (1) Cellular-mediated immunity (T cells), humoral-mediated immunity (B cells), opsonization caused by decreased complement and antibodies, decreased phagocytosis and bactericidal activity by macrophages and neutrophils, and loss of natural barrier function of the skin
   b. Predisposes the patient to infections and multiorgan failure

V. BURN WOUND CARE

A. GOALS OF BURN WOUND CARE

1. Cover wound.
2. Decrease infection.
3. Allow for optimal reepithelialization of partial-thickness burns.
4. Burns (second or third degree) that do not heal by 2–3 weeks produce more scarring; thus these wounds require early excision and grafting for best cosmetic and functional results.
5. The mortality of large burns has been reduced by the early excision of the burn wound followed by coverage with autograft or allograft.

TABLE 19.1

TOPICAL ANTIMICROBIAL AGENTS

Agent	Antimicrobial Coverage	Usage	Disadvantages
Bacitracin	Gram-positive bacteria	Useful for partial-thickness burns; good for use on face; use with petroleum gauze	Can be nephrotoxic in large doses when used in triple antibiotic formula
Mupirocin (rare use, primarily in infants <2 years old)	MRSA	Wound infection with MRSA organisms	Expensive
Silver sulfadiazine (Silvadene)	Broad spectrum, includes *Candida* and *Pseudomonas*	No pain with application; good for use as prophylaxis or treatment	Does not penetrate eschar; not good when infection already established; patient may have allergy; risk of **neutropenia**
Mafenide acetate (Sulfamylon)	Broad spectrum including *Clostridium* and *Pseudomonas*	Full-thickness burns; penetrates eschar; used as soak or irrigation dressing 2.5% or 5%	Burns on application; metabolized to a carbonic anhydrase inhibitor which can lead to **metabolic acidosis**
Silver nitrate (historical interest only; rarely used)	Broad spectrum	Used as wet dressing, 0.5% irrigations every 4 h	Poor eschar penetration; electrolyte leaching and hyponatremia; can cause methemoglobinemia; stains black

MRSA, Methicillin-resistant *Staphylococcus aureus.*

19

BURN CARE

B. TOPICAL AGENTS
Goal is to decrease wound sepsis, not prevent colonization of eschar (Table 19.1).

C. LOCAL CARE
1. First-degree burns—Treat with minor care and symptomatic pain control.
2. Partial-thickness burns—Initially wash with antiseptic soap (e.g., chlorhexidine gluconate), remove debris, unroof vesicles.
   a. Apply topical agents (bacitracin/Silvadene/Sulfamylon) wrapped with a nonadherent dressing.
3. Deep partial-thickness, full-thickness burns—Initially treat as for partial-thickness burns.
   a. If there is no healing after 2 weeks, grafting is required.

D. EARLY EXCISION AND GRAFTING
1. Tangential excision of eschar in layered fashion to the point of capillary bleeding

2. Perform within 2–7 days of admission for obvious deep second- and third-degree burns. Should not be performed less than 24 hours after admission due to interference with resuscitation and wound evolution.
3. Graft immediately or cover temporarily with allograft or biologic dressing.
4. Can perform staged excision and grafting the next day (decreases operative blood loss)
   a. Advantages include early removal of eschar and coverage, improved joint function, shortened hospitalization, earlier mobilization and rehabilitation, improved immune status, and decreased wound sepsis.

E. GRAFTING
1. Grafting decreases evaporation, desiccation, and pain and protects neurovascular tissue and tendons.
2. Superficial partial-thickness wounds should heal spontaneously by day 14.
3. Without immediate physiologic coverage, fascial desiccation and subsequent infection may occur.
4. Sheet versus mesh graft
   a. Sheet grafts are optimal for cosmetic appearance but do not expand to cover a large surface area.
   b. Mesh grafts are better for nonoptimal recipient beds.
   c. Sheet grafts are preferred for hands, feet, and face.
5. Grafts are usually 0.010–0.014 inches thick (split thickness).
   a. Thicker grafts have less scarring but slightly increased risk for graft failure and increased scarring of donor sites.
   b. Full-thickness grafts include the entire dermis.
6. Types of grafting material
   a. Autograft (from self)—optimal; split thickness versus full thickness, sheet versus mesh
   b. Allograft (same species, e.g., cadaver). The following are indications for use of allograft:
      (1) Insufficient autologous skin available
      (2) Temporary wound coverage before autologous grafting
      (3) Speeds epithelialization—promotion of vascularization
      (4) Prevents infection
   c. Xenograft (different species, e.g., porcine)—infrequently used because of the establishment of skin banks; can be used as coverage in superficial partial-thickness wounds until epithelialization occurs
   d. Dermal substitutes
      (1) Provides dermal replacement in areas where split-thickness graft would be inadequate for elasticity and durability; also can use as temporary coverage in superficial partial-thickness wounds
         (a) Dermal allograft
         (b) Collagen glycosaminoglycan
         (c) Products include Biobrane, TransCyte, Dermagraft, Integra, AlloDerm, and Dermatrix.

7. Priority of sites to be grafted are hands, feet, joints, extremities, and face first, then trunk.
8. Graft care
    a. Donor site—covered with absorbent dressing (calcium alginate [Kaltostat]) and/or nonadherent dressing (Xeroform) with or without topical antimicrobial (bacitracin) or an occlusive dressing.
    b. Graft site
        (1) Wet—dressings irrigated with antibiotic solution to be kept constantly damp
            (a) Mixture of Sulfamylon with double antibiotics alternating every 2 hours
        (2) Dry—nonstick gauze (Adaptic) with a silver-based (e.g., Acticoat) pressure dressing over graft
        (3) Nonadherence of graft is due to avascular or infected graft bed, hematoma, seroma, or graft movement.

VI. SUPPORTIVE CARE
A. NUTRITION
The importance of starting early nutritional support cannot be emphasized enough given the hypermetabolic state that exists secondary to a burn injury and the risk for sepsis.
1. The metabolic rate is proportional to burn size up to 40%–50% TBSA burns.
2. Total body O_2 consumption and water loss are proportional to burn size.
3. Nutrient requirements need to be determined.
    a. Caloric needs are based on the Harris-Benedict equation using a multiplier.
    b. Indirect calorimetry is often used.
    c. Nitrogen losses may be as great as 150–200 g/day and are calculated with 24-hour urine blood urea nitrogen (BUN) measurements, as well as estimates for insensible losses.
4. Route
    a. Enteral (nasoduodenal) route is preferred and should be started during first 12 hours after injury.
        (1) Leads to decreased infection, complication rates, and decreased cost
        (2) Lower rates of stress ulcers and ileus
    b. Total parenteral nutrition is associated with an increased rate of sepsis in burn patients.
    c. Exogenous albumin supplementation for hypoalbuminemia has not been seen to affect complication or mortality rates.

B. PHYSICAL AND OCCUPATIONAL THERAPY
1. Aggressive physical therapy and occupational therapy are necessary to prevent contracture and maintain joint function.
2. Positioning of limbs and joints begins on day 1. Immobility leads to increased swelling and may worsen the extent of injury and increase infection.

19

BURN CARE

3. Splinting may be necessary to prevent contractures after grafts are applied.
4. Active exercise program with stretching is greatly superior to passive range of motion.
5. Involve occupational therapy early for long-term rehabilitation planning.

C. ANALGESIA

1. Three types of pain—background, breakthrough, and procedural
   a. Long-term, baseline pain management is essential; use methadone or other long-acting medications.
   b. Breakthrough pain control with short-acting oxycodone. If patient is needing breakthrough pain medications more frequently, consider increasing the baseline dose.
   c. Procedural/wound care pain control—Use IV medications such as Dilaudid, morphine, or fentanyl.
      (1) Patients often have a significant amount of anxiety around wound care that may be interpreted as pain. Consideration of short-acting anxiolytics during wound care may be warranted in select patients.

VII. MANAGEMENT OF INFECTION IN THE BURN PATIENT

A. THE MOST COMMON INFECTION IN BURN PATIENTS IS PNEUMONIA.

1. Early pneumonia—commonly the result of gram-positive organisms
2. Later pneumonia (>7 days after hospitalization)—typically the result of gram-negative organisms
3. May occur in up to 50% of burn patients. More common in intubated patients, although can occur in nonintubated patients

B. PATHOGENESIS OF WOUND SEPSIS IN AN UNTREATED BURN WOUND

1. Surface bacteria proliferate, migrate through nonviable tissue, pause at the subeschar space, and when microbial invasiveness "outweighs" host defense capability, invade viable tissue with microvascular involvement and systemic dissemination.
2. Avascularity and ischemia of full-thickness burn wound allow microbial proliferation and prevent delivery of systemic antibiotics and cellular components of host defense.

C. CLINICAL SIGNS

1. Conversion of a partial- to full-thickness injury
2. Rapidly spreading ischemic necrosis

D. DIAGNOSIS OF INVASIVE BURN WOUND SEPSIS

1. Cultures of burn wound surface do not accurately predict progressive bacterial colonization or incipient burn wound sepsis.

2. Bacterial growth is best monitored by semiquantitative burn wound biopsy.
   a. Calculate the precise number of organisms per gram of tissue.
   b. If biopsy cultures reveal more than 10^5 organisms per gram of tissue, or if there is a 100-fold increase in the concentration of organisms per gram of tissue within a 48-hour period, then the organisms have escaped effective control by the topical chemotherapeutic agent.
   c. Wound colonization of dead tissue must be differentiated from invasion of viable tissue.
      (1) Best evaluated by clinical diagnosis
      (2) Biopsy will find organisms in viable subeschar tissue on histologic examination.
      (3) Microvascular invasion connotes possible hematogenous dissemination and mandates systemic antibiotic therapy.
   d. Wound is often dry, crusted, black, or violaceous color, or it may be unchanged.
   e. Clinical picture of sepsis—fever, hypoxia, mental status changes, leukocytosis, new-onset ileus, tachypnea, thrombocytopenia, hypotension, oliguria, acidosis, tachycardia, hyperglycemia

E. BACTERIOLOGY OF NOSOCOMIAL BURN INFECTION
1. Know your hospital's flora and antibiotic sensitivities of species.
2. Most common pathogens are *Staphylococcus aureus, Pseudomonas aeruginosa, Acinetobacter baumannii,* other gram-negative rods, *Enterococcus* spp., and *Candida albicans.*

F. PREVENTION OF BURN INFECTION
1. Daily dressing changes and application of topical agents
2. No indication for prophylactic antibiotics
3. Strict hand washing

G. TREATMENT OF BURN INFECTION
1. Remove all devitalized tissue.
2. Surgically drain closed-space abscesses.
3. Apply diffusible topical agent.
4. Empiric antibiotic therapy should be broad spectrum.
   a. Always cover initially for *Pseudomonas* spp.; rarely need anaerobic coverage

H. NONBACTERIAL INFECTION
1. Viral infection—usually improves with time
   a. Virucidal agent recommended for systemic involvement
2. Fungal infection—topical application of nystatin effectively clears fungi and yeast and may be used prophylactically before eschar excision
   a. Amphotericin B is used for systemic involvement.
   b. Fungal infection is associated with increased mortality, independent of age or size of burn.

VIII. ELECTRICAL INJURIES

A. TISSUE DESTRUCTION

1. The points of entry and exit have most severe destruction (the points at which the electrical current is most concentrated).
2. *Deep tissue damage often greatly exceeds skin injury.*
   a. Not obvious at the time of initial injury
   b. Electrical resistance of tissues—(from least to most) nerve, blood, blood vessel, muscle, skin, tendon, fat, and bone

B. TREATMENT

1. Cardiopulmonary resuscitation—high-voltage currents usually cause cardiac arrest, whereas low-voltage (<440 volts) currents usually produce ventricular fibrillation.
2. Protect against neurologic damage caused by fractures of the spine.
   a. Place in cervical spine collar and on a long backboard to immobilize the entire spine.
   b. Tetanic contraction of muscle may cause fractures of the cervical and lumbosacral spine and long bones.
      (1) Perform screening radiographs.

C. FLUID RESUSCITATION

1. This cannot be calculated from percentage of skin burns.
2. Give sufficient volume to establish UOP of 1.5 mL/kg per hour.
3. High incidence of muscular injury causes hemoglobinuria/myoglobinuria.
   a. May need mannitol (25 g/h) and $NaHCO_3$ to prevent precipitation of myoglobin/hemoglobin in the renal tubules
4. Progressively severe metabolic acidosis occurs with electrical injuries and massive tissue destruction.
   a. Use IV sodium bicarbonate to temporarily correct base deficit.

D. EARLY DEBRIDEMENT

1. Of grossly necrotic tissue; amputation may be needed if unable to control acidosis.

E. IMMEDIATE EXTREMITY FASCIOTOMY

1. Frequently required; check compartment pressures.

IX. CHEMICAL INJURIES

A significant problem in the management of chemical injuries is the failure to recognize ongoing destruction of tissue.

A. MANAGEMENT

1. Initially dilute with copious amounts of water.
2. *Do not neutralize a chemical burn because the heat of neutralization can extend the injury.*

3. Avoid hypothermia.
4. Special precautions
   a. Lithium—Remove particles before irrigation.
   b. Hydrofluoric acids—Apply 10% calcium gluconate cream in most cases; calcium gluconate can be injected subcutaneously for severe burns.
   c. Phenol—Irrigation must be vigorous (shower) because absorption increases when spread over a large area.
   d. Tar/asphalt—Use bacitracin or other petroleum-based product.

X. OUTPATIENT AND CLINIC TREATMENT

A. SELECTION
1. If the patient does not meet admission criteria, he or she can be treated as an outpatient.

B. TREATMENT
1. Perform tetanus prophylaxis.
2. Wash wounds with mild soap.
3. Debris and blisters should be debrided.
4. Apply antibiotic ointment (bacitracin, Neosporin, Polysporin) and nonstick porous gauze (Adaptic), and wrap with gauze.
5. Manage pain.

C. FOLLOW-UP CARE
1. Dressing care twice daily—Wash with mild soap (to remove debris and fibrinous exudate), and reapply dressing.
2. Perform vigorous range-of-motion exercises and massage of post-burn scar.
3. Patient should return to clinic and/or physical therapy as needed.

D. WOUNDS
If the wounds are deep partial- or full-thickness burns, the patient may be treated as an outpatient until excision and grafting are required.
1. If the wound is not reepithelialized by 2 weeks, it should undergo excision and grafting.
2. Longer healing time increases scarring.
3. If hypertrophic scarring is a problem, the patient should be fitted for pressure garments and wear them 23 hours a day until wounds no longer blanch.
4. Use moisturizing cream on healing skin.
5. As long as the healed wound is hyperemic and blanches, the patient should vigorously put pressure on the wound daily to help prevent scarring.
6. Avoid sun exposure to graft or burn because it may cause hyperpigmentation.

19

BURN CARE

7. Pruritus is treated with moisturizing cream and oral diphenhydramine (Benadryl) or hydroxyzine (Vistaril) as needed.

XI. COMPLICATIONS OF BURN INJURIES

A. GASTROINTESTINAL

1. Adynamic ileus has gastric and colonic involvement.
   a. Generally resolves within 24 hours with IV hydration and nasogastric suction
2. Ulcers—"Curling ulcer" generally involves stomach, duodenum, and jejunum.
   a. Cause is unknown but may be due to hypovolemia or hypoperfusion.
   b. Incidence is rare now with early antacids and H_2 blockers and with early enteral feeding.
3. Acalculous cholecystitis is uncommon but diagnosed with a hydroxy iminodiacetic acid (HIDA) scan or ultrasound.
   a. Treat with antibiotics and either percutaneous drainage or cholecystectomy.

B. OCULAR

1. Keep eyes moist using artificial tears or ointments.
2. Corneal abrasions—associated with facial burns
   a. Treatment includes topical antibiotics and release and grafting of ectropion.
3. Cataracts (especially with electrical injury)

C. CUTANEOUS

1. Wound contracture—may result in cosmetic or functional problems, limiting range of motion
   a. Contractures may be released surgically with grafting or Z-plasty.
2. Hypertrophic scar
   a. Occurs with wounds that take more than 2 weeks to heal
   b. Increased incidence with deep burns and extended exposure of ungrafted burn wound
   c. Treatment
      (1) Pressure-fitted masks, garments, and massage are used for the first year to reduce scar formation.
      (2) Resurface with graft later.
      (3) Laser treatment with pulsed dye laser and fractional CO_2 laser is showing promising results for decreasing volume, redness, and pruritus of burn scars.
3. Keloids—variant of hypertrophic scarring that extends beyond the original wound
   a. Difficult to treat, but steroid injections have been used. Often recur after excision. Best outcomes include external beam radiation therapy after excision.

D. MISCELLANEOUS
1. Heterotopic calcification
   a. Elbow—most common joint affected
   b. May be related to vigorous occupational/physical therapy and frequent microtrauma to the affected joint
2. Chondritis—secondary to *S. aureus* and *Pseudomonas* spp., involving the ear and joint
3. Hyperpigmentation—Avoid sun exposure for at least 1 year. Use sun-blocking agents (>15 sun protection factor).

RECOMMENDED READINGS

Herndon DN, et al. A comparison of conservative versus early excision. Therapies in severely burned patients. *Ann Surg.* 1989;209:547.

Joint Theater Trauma System Clinical Practice Guidelines for Burn Care. Available at: http://www.usaisr.amedd.army.mil/cpgs/Burn_Care_11May2016.pdf

Mulholland M, Lillemoe K, Doherty R, Simeone D, Upchurch G. Burns. In: *Greenfield's Surgery: Scientific Principles and Practice*. 5th ed. Philadelphia, PA: Lippincott Williams & Wilkins; 2010: chap 11.

19

BURN CARE

Neurosurgical Emergencies

Christopher P. Carroll, MD

Care of the neurotrauma patient involves evaluation of injuries to the cranium, spine, peripheral nerves, or often a combination thereof. Rapid evaluation and decisive intervention are essential to significantly reduce the risk of morbidity and mortality. After stabilizing the airway, breathing, and circulation in a patient with suspected neurotrauma, attention then must turn to the rapid assessment of level of consciousness and systematic evaluation for neurologic deficits of cranial nerve (CN), motor, or sensory function. It cannot be overstated that intracranial injuries leading to herniation syndromes are an imminent threat to life and can be fatal over the course of minutes. Initial findings on systematic nervous system examination will inform early clinical maneuvers, guide appropriate triage, inform the choice of imaging modalities, and save lives. A high index of suspicion for spinal column or spinal cord injury is essential in the trauma patient to prevent exacerbation of injury and further morbidity. This chapter outlines the essential principles needed to identify and care for the patient sustaining neurotrauma in concert with neurosurgical consultants.

I. EVALUATION AND MANAGEMENT OF THE NEUROTRAUMA PATIENT

A. INITIAL ASSESSMENT

1. Ensure stability of airway, ventilation, and circulatory status before a rapid survey for neurologic deficit suggestive of intracranial or spinal injury.
   a. Depressed level of consciousness in traumatic brain injury (TBI), particularly severe TBI, impairs ability to ventilate and protect airway.
      (1) Ideally the neurologic assessment is performed before administration of sedative or paralytic medications that would confound examination.
      (2) Fast-acting, short-duration paralytics are preferred to facilitate neurologic assessment (e.g., succinylcholine, rocuronium if depolarizing agent cannot be used).
   b. Robust scalp bleeding must be controlled to prevent hypotension; however, intracranial hemorrhage—except in select pediatric patients—is rarely a cause of hypotension.
      (1) Hypotonic fluids can exacerbate cerebral edema and should be avoided in fluid resuscitation of the neurotrauma patient.
      (2) Cerebral perfusion pressure (CPP) = mean arterial pressure (MAP) − intracranial pressure (ICP); goal is to maintain MAP ≥60 mm Hg because CPP <60 mm Hg can confound assessment of level of consciousness.

B. UNCONSCIOUS PATIENT

1. Impaired consciousness implies a deficit in thought content, arousal, or both.

   a. Impairment of consciousness can vary from mild (disorientation) to severe (coma).

   b. An "unconscious" state implies bilateral dysfunction of the cerebral hemispheres; bilateral dysfunction of diencephalon; depression of the reticular activating system (midbrain and pons); or a combination thereof.

2. Structural causes of impaired consciousness include traumatic, vascular (hemorrhagic and ischemic), neoplastic, infectious, congenital, and inflammatory etiologies.

   a. Supratentorial mass lesions
      (1) Direct compression of brain and, eventually, brainstem
      (2) Progressive deterioration of level of consciousness
      (3) Symmetric deterioration suggests central herniation syndrome, whereas asymmetric decline suggests uncal or subfalcine herniation.

   b. Infratentorial mass lesions
      (1) Direct compression of reticular activating system resulting in rapid onset and progression to coma

   c. Often accompanied by CN deficits

3. Toxic or metabolic etiologies of coma result in a gradual, symmetric decline in neurologic status with preserved CN function, often characterized by physical and laboratory signs (tremor, asterixis, myoclonus, acid-base disturbance) that suggest a toxic or metabolic cause.

   a. Electrolyte or endocrine imbalance: hyponatremia, hypoglycemia, hyperammonemia, diabetic ketoacidosis, myxedema, kernicterus

   b. Intoxication or poisoning (intentional, accidental, or iatrogenic): ethanol, drug overdose, lead poisoning, carbon monoxide poisoning

   c. Central nervous system infection or systemic infection: meningitis, encephalitis, systemic inflammatory response syndrome (SIRS)/sepsis

   d. Nutritional deficiency: B12 deficiency, thiamine deficiency

   e. Inherited metabolic disorders: porphyria

   f. Global ischemia or hypoxia

   g. Seizure: generalized seizures, status epilepticus, nonconvulsive status epilepticus

   h. Organ failure: uremia, hyperammonemia, hepatic encephalopathy

4. A focused history can suggest possible etiologies for impaired consciousness.

   a. Important features include an abrupt versus subacute versus insidious onset; the presence of lucid intervals; recent neurologic complaints; and progression of any neurologic deficits with time (e.g., leg to arm to face, unilateral to bilateral).

20

NEUROSURGICAL EMERGENCIES

TABLE 20.1

GLASGOW COMA SCALE (3–15)

Points	Best Eye Opening	Best Verbal Response	Best Motor Response
6	—	—	Follows verbal commands
5	—	Fluent, fully oriented	Localizes to pain
4	Spontaneous	Fluent, disoriented/confused	Withdraws to pain
3	To verbal stimuli	Inappropriate speech	Flexor posturing
2	To painful stimuli	Incomprehensible, guttural noises	Extensor posturing
1	No response	No verbalizations/intubated	No response

   b. Review medical record, and ask family about any medical and surgical history, allergies, social or sexual habits (especially alcohol or drug use/abuse), possible occupational exposures, and recent travel that could explain the decline.
   c. Take medication history, with focus on possible sedative, narcotic, or psychotropic drugs that directly impair consciousness, as well as anticoagulant and antiplatelet agents that could suggest increased risk of hemorrhage (intracranial or otherwise).

C. PHYSICAL EXAMINATION
1. General examination
   a. Vital signs
   b. Respiratory pattern with attention to disturbance of rate and/or rhythm
   c. Outward signs of trauma: track marks of IV drug abuse; Battle sign (mastoid, postauricular ecchymoses); raccoon eyes (periorbital ecchymoses); hemotympanum; clear fluid rhinorrhea or otorrhea; deformity of spinal curvature or extremities
   d. Nuchal rigidity
2. Level of consciousness
   a. Level of consciousness is defined across a spectrum.
      (1) Awake and alert: eyes open, responds to verbal stimuli
      (2) Somnolence/lethargy: sleepy but arouses easily to a full wakeful state
      (3) Obtundation: can be fully aroused to wakeful state with effort but returns to sleeplike state in absence of continuous stimulation
      (4) Stupor: responds to physical stimulus but never fully aroused to wakeful state
      (5) Coma: unarousable despite physical stimuli
   b. Glasgow Coma Scale (GCS)—Use for age ≥4 years (Table 20.1).
      (1) Widely used assessment of ability to open eyes, communicate verbally, and provide motor response
      (2) Score ranges from 3 to 15, with "T" often added to denote a patient who is intubated
      (3) Does not replace neurologic assessment but provides a rapid, reproducible survey of level of consciousness and neurologic impairment with a high degree of interrater reliability

TABLE 20.2

CHILDREN'S COMA SCALE (3–15)

Points	Best Eye Opening	Best Verbal Response		Best Motor Response
6	—	—		Follows verbal commands
5	—	Smiles, orients to sound, tracks objects, interactive		Localizes to pain
4	Spontaneous	Crying Consolable	Interaction Inappropriate	Withdraws to pain
3	To verbal stimuli	Inconsistent Inconsolable	Moaning	Flexor posturing
2	To painful stimuli	Inconsolable	Restless	Extensor posturing
1	No response	No verbalizations / intubated		No response

    (4) Categorizes TBI as mild (GCS 13–15), moderate (GCS 9–12), or severe (GCS ≤8)

  c. Children's Coma Scale—Use for age less than 4 years (Table 20.2).

  d. If appropriate, perform Mini–Mental Status Examination.

3. **Comprehensive neurologic evaluation**

  a. CN examination

    (1) Response to visual threat—CNs II, VII

    (2) Pupillary light response—CNs II, III

    (3) Corneal reflex—CNs V, VII

    (4) Extraocular movements, including assessment of conjugate gaze, gaze deviation, and presence/absence of roving eye movements—CNs III, IV, VI

    (5) Oculocephalic reflex (doll's eye reflex)—CNs VI, VIII

    (6) Oculovestibular reflex (cold calorics test)—CNs VI, VIII

    (7) Gag reflex—CNs IX, X

    (8) Cough reflex—CN X, C3–5 (diaphragm)

  b. Motor examination

    (1) Check tone and bulk.

    (2) Perform formal graded motor evaluation (if possible).

      (a) 0 = no visible or palpable contraction, paralysis

      (b) 1 = no gross movement but visible or palpable muscle contraction

      (c) 2 = movement with gravity eliminated, incomplete range of motion (ROM)

      (d) 3 = movement through full ROM against gravity

      (e) 4 = movement through full ROM against resistance (4– = slight resistance, 4 = moderate resistance, 4+ = strong resistance overcome by examiner)

      (f) 5 = full movement against resistance, full strength

    (3) Decorticate (flexor) posturing indicates lesion above the level of the red nucleus (midbrain).

20

NEUROSURGICAL EMERGENCIES

(4) Decerebrate (extensor) posturing indicates lesion above the lateral vestibular nucleus but below the red nucleus.

c. Sensory examination

(1) Evaluate response to pain (spinothalamic), temperature (spinothalamic), vibration (dorsal column), and light touch (dorsal column).

(2) Difficult to assess in an unconscious patient; can evaluate response to supraorbital, sternal, or temporomandibular joint pressure—this tests general integrity of both motor and sensory tracts of the brainstem in those patients who cannot follow commands.

(3) In an unconscious patient, check response to central and peripherally painful stimuli—localizes to painful stimulus, withdraws from painful stimulus, or posturing with painful stimulus.

d. Reflex examination

(1) Check superficial and deep-tendon reflexes.

(2) Check for the presence or absence of pathologic reflexes: Hoffmann, Babinski, sustained clonus, frontal release signs

(3) Check for rectal sphincter tone

e. Cerebellar examination

(1) Assess stability of finger-to-nose movements bilaterally.

(2) Check rapid alternating movements bilaterally.

(3) Assess presence or absence of extremity drift.

f. Gait examination

(1) Assess stance and gait with attention to stride, cadence, and stability.

(2) Evaluate tandem walking.

D. RADIOLOGIC EVALUATION

After patient is clinically stabilized from standpoint of ABCs, imaging can be performed using findings on neurologic examination to guide the selection of imaging modalities.

1. Plain radiographs (XRs)

a. Anteroposterior and lateral cranial XRs can be used to evaluate the presence of intracranial foreign bodies (particularly in cases of penetrating trauma or prior cranial surgery) and skull fractures but have been supplanted by the use of head computed tomography (CT) in evaluating cranial trauma.

b. Anteroposterior and lateral spine XRs are useful in the evaluation of spinal trauma that can be rapidly performed in the trauma bay or centers with limited or no capacity for CT; however, this modality has largely been supplanted by the use of spinal CT in evaluating spinal trauma.

(1) Deformity of the vertebral body, pedicles, and facets can be identified, although many fractures may be missed with XRs alone.

(2) Particular attention should be paid to alignment along the craniocervical junction, anterior vertebral margin, posterior vertebral margin, sublaminar margin, and posterior spinous margin because misalignment is suggestive of discoligamentous injury or fracture.

2. CT
   a. In cases of suspected cranial trauma, noncontrast head CT (CTH) is the imaging modality of choice for both blunt and penetrating cranial trauma and should not be delayed except for stabilization of the patient's ABCs and treatment of life-threatening injuries.
      (1) Noncontrast CTH can be used to evaluate for skull fractures, intracranial hemorrhage, parenchymal injuries, cerebral edema, cerebral compression/elevated ICP (loss of sulcal-gyral pattern), hydrocephalus, and herniation syndromes—especially subfalcine herniation ("midline shift"), uncal herniation, and tonsillar herniation—affecting both the supratentorial and infratentorial compartments.
      (2) A negative CTH in an awake, alert, and oriented patient without neurologic deficit can effectively rule out intracranial trauma.
      (3) Typically performed with 5-mm axial cuts and gantry to reduce radiation exposure to the orbits
   b. Spinal CT has a higher sensitivity for spinal fractures in blunt trauma patients than do XRs alone.
      (1) In most trauma centers a CT cervical spine is performed with the CTH.
      (2) CT reconstructions of the thoracic and lumbar spine can often be made from CT abdomen and pelvis.
      (3) Imaging of thoracic and lumbar spine is often based on neurologic examination.
      (4) Attention should be paid to alignment of the craniocervical junction, atlantoaxial interval, and longitudinal axis of the spine, as previously noted, with additional attention to compromise of canal diameter and the presence of any fracture or facet joint abnormalities.
   c. CT angiography (CTA) can be used to evaluate for blunt cerebrovascular injury (BCVI).
      (1) CTA should be considered in patients with blunt or penetrating neck trauma and should be performed in patients found to have fractures of the cervical spine involving the lateral vertebral body or transverse process/transverse foramen.
      (2) CTA is often performed concurrently with CTA head in the event of arterial dissection or thrombus that extends intracranially.
3. Magnetic resonance imaging (MRI)
   a. MRI of the head is not used as a first-order imaging modality in cranial trauma because of the relatively long time needed for image acquisition, which may be prohibitive in trauma patients.
      (1) Can be used as an adjunct after patients are clinically stable to evaluate for posttraumatic stroke, venous sinus thrombosis/occlusion, and diffuse-axonal injuries that are often difficult to image with CT
      (2) Of particular value for the evaluation, after clinically stable, of patients with neurologic deficit or depressed mental status in setting of negative CTH

20

NEUROSURGICAL EMERGENCIES

b. MRI of the cervical, thoracic, or lumbar spine should be performed urgently in any patient with incomplete or complete spinal cord injury not explained by findings on XR, CT, or both.

(1) Provides much better resolution of the spinal cord (e.g., cord compression, cord contusion, myelitis); soft tissue injuries (e.g., traumatic disc herniation); and traumatic spinal hemorrhages (epidural hematoma, subdural hematoma [SDH])

(2) May be performed when CT or XR do provide satisfactory explanation of clinical findings as supplement for operative planning

II. CRANIAL TRAUMA

A. TRAUMATIC BRAIN INJURY

TBI results in approximately 50,000 patient deaths and 80,000–90,000 patients with new, permanent disability each year in the United States.

1. Mild TBI—GCS score 13–15

a. The most common form of TBI, accounting for 70%–80% of TBI burden

b. Clinical findings may include headache, dizziness, memory loss, scalp laceration, or bruising; TBI may be clinically asymptomatic.

c. Cranial imaging may be normal ("concussion") or may demonstrate a small contusion, SDH, or traumatic subarachnoid hemorrhage (SAH).

d. Patients with abnormal imaging should be monitored for neurologic deterioration with serial neurologic examinations.

(1) Repeat imaging should be performed 6–24 hours after initial imaging to establish stability of intracranial injuries.

(a) Chemoprophylaxis for deep vein thrombosis should be held until stability of intracranial injury is established; it is often implemented 24–72 hours after stable CTH.

(2) Perform urgent repeat CTH if patient undergoes neurologic deterioration.

(3) Patient may be discharged home with stable imaging and examination.

2. Moderate head injury—GCS score of 9–12

a. Relatively small proportion of injuries compared with mild TBI and severe TBI

b. Depressed level of consciousness after resuscitation with patients usually amnesic to events

c. Often associated with skull fractures and/or multiple traumatic intracranial injuries

d. Full trauma evaluation necessary to rule out other traumatic abnormalities confounded by depressed mental status

e. Admission necessary because of risk of injury progression

3. Severe head injury—GCS score ≤8

a. This represents 10%–25% of TBI burden but disproportionately accounts for TBI mortality, the highest rate of which is seen in severe penetrating TBI.

b. Severe TBI patients are comatose postresuscitation by definition (GCS ≤8) and have a high likelihood of both focal neurologic deficit and intracranial injury on CTH.

c. CT scan often demonstrates radiographic injury(s), and injuries are multiple in more than 70%.

  (1) Extraaxial hemorrhage (epidural hematoma and SDH)

  (2) Traumatic SAH (often in diffuse cortical distribution)

  (3) Intraparenchymal hemorrhage(s), parenchymal contusion(s), and/or hemorrhagic parenchymal contusion(s)

  (4) Cerebral edema, cerebral compression, and herniation (e.g., uncal, subfalcine, transtentorial, or tonsillar)

  (5) Diffuse axonal injury (characterized by petechial ["shear"] hemorrhages in central structures such as corpus callosum, subcortical white matter, thalamus, pons, and brainstem)

  (6) Complex, comminuted, and/or depressed skull fracture(s)

  (7) Penetrating TBIs

d. The majority of severe TBI patients (50%–60%) sustain multisystem trauma, and 5% will have comorbid spinal injury.

e. Sustained GCS score ≤8 warrants invasive intracranial monitoring of ICP and directed ICP.

f. Seizure prophylaxis decreases the incidence of early posttraumatic seizures and is recommended for 7 days post injury; it does not reduce the incidence of late posttraumatic seizures.

B. ELEVATED INTRACRANIAL PRESSURE

1. Clinical manifestations:

a. Classic signs are headache, oculomotor palsies, and Cushing triad (hypertension, *bradycardia*, and respiratory irregularities).

b. Suspicion for elevated ICP should increase in the presence of new or progressive focal neurologic deficit; deterioration in neurologic examination; or decline in GCS score to ≤8.

c. Normal ICP ranges from 0 to 15 mm Hg, with sustained ICP greater than 20 mm Hg considered abnormal, although physiologic spikes may occur.

  (1) Treatment is indicated when ICP is greater than 20–25 mm Hg for sustained period, often 15–30 minutes.

  (2) Sustained elevation of ICP is associated with increased TBI mortality.

2. Indications for invasive ICP monitoring

a. GCS score ≤8 unexplained by other factors that could account for depressed level of consciousness after resuscitation (e.g., alcohol or drug intoxication, seizure, sedative or narcotic medication administration) and an abnormal CTH (hematomas, contusions, swelling, herniation, or compressed basal cisterns)

b. GCS score ≤8, normal CTH, and two or more of the following:

  (1) Age older than 40 years

    (2) Unilateral or bilateral motor posturing

    (3) Systolic blood pressure less than 90 mm Hg

c. Relative indications for monitoring include multisystem trauma in which other therapies may have adverse effect on the ICP or confound the ability to follow serial neurologic examination (e.g., paralytics, heavy sedations, frequent trips to operating room [OR]) in the presence of head injury.

d. Invasive monitoring can include placement of extraventricular drain (EVD), ICP monitor, multimodality monitor, microdialysis catheters, subdural electrodes, or combination thereof.

    (1) Invasive monitoring may include monitors of brain tissue oxygen tension, cerebral perfusion, brain temperature, intracranial electroencephalogram (EEG), and/or microdialysis in addition to ICP.

    (2) Ventriculostomy is superior to parenchymal, subarachnoid, epidural, or subdural ICP monitors in that it is the only monitoring modality that provides a therapeutic potential (e.g., cerebrospinal fluid [CSF] diversion); many parenchymal monitors cannot be calibrated once in situ.

3. Other modes of monitoring of head-injured patients may include:

a. Cerebral blood flow monitor

b. Jugular venous oxygen saturation ($S_{jv}O_2$)

4. Management of elevated ICP can be divided into three tiers of therapeutic intervention.

a. Tier I treatments

    (1) Optimize positioning by elevating head of bed to 30 degrees.

        (a) This can be performed in reverse Trendelenburg with head of bed flat in cases of spine precautions.

        (b) Elevating the head of bed ≥30 degrees may negatively affect CPP (CPP = MAP − ICP).

    (2) Maintain head in neutral position (not rotated or flexed) and ensure cervical collar is not compressing anterior neck to promote jugular venous outflow.

    (3) Ensure adequate sedation with short-acting agents that allow frequent neurologic examination (e.g., propofol, fentanyl).

    (4) Maintain normothermia and treat fevers; there is currently limited level III evidence for improved outcomes with prophylactic hypothermia such that it remains controversial and under active investigation.

    (5) Avoid hypotension by maintaining systolic blood pressure ≥90 mm Hg and MAP ≥65 mm Hg.

    (6) Avoid hypoxia by maintaining oxygen saturation (SaO_2) ≥90%; minimize positive end-expiratory pressure (PEEP) as clinically feasible to promote jugular venous drainage by decreasing intrathoracic pressure.

b. Tier II treatments

    (1) Osmotic therapy

    (a) Mannitol 1 g/kg bolus (avoid hypotension) *if* signs of increasing pressure and herniation; prolonged use is not supported by evidence.

    (b) Hypertonic (3% or 23.4%) saline can be given as bolus (150–500 mL and 30 mL, respectively) in cases of elevated ICP or suspected herniation or as continuous infusion protocol to increase serum sodium to goal of 150–155 mmol/L (higher if refractory).

(2) CSF diversion via EVD for elevation of ICP to reduce volume of ventricular system

(3) Maintain CPP greater than 50–60 mm Hg.

    (a) Aggressive attempts to maintain CPP greater than 70 mm Hg are associated with increased incidence of acute respiratory distress syndrome.

(4) Hyperventilation

    (a) Results in cerebral vasoconstriction thereby decreasing intracranial intravascular volume and decreasing cerebral perfusion

    (b) Used only as an emergent temporizing measure to reduce ICP by hyperventilating to partial pressure of carbon dioxide ($Paco_2$) of 30–35 mm Hg while preparing for operative intervention or other Tier III treatments; evidence does not support prophylactic hyperventilation.

(5) Glucocorticoid administration is contraindicated.

    (a) Evidence does not support role in reduction of ICP or improvement of TBI outcomes.

    (b) Associated with increased mortality in moderate and severe head injury (level I evidence, Corticosteroid Randomization After Significant Head injury [CRASH] trial 2004)

c. Tier III treatments

(1) Barbiturate-induced coma; performed in conjunction with continuous EEG monitoring of burst suppression. Avoid hypotension.

(2) Nondepolarizing paralytics

(3) Operative decompression (e.g., hemicraniectomy)

C. SPECIFIC TRAUMATIC CRANIAL INJURIES

1. Epidural hematomas (Fig. 20.1A)

a. They are reported in 1% of patients with head trauma but may be underreported.

b. Classic presentation is brief loss of consciousness followed by a lucid interval and then progressive neurologic decline to obtundation, ipsilateral pupillary dilation ("blown pupil"), and contralateral hemiparesis (seen in 60% of cases).

(1) Other clinical presentations include headache, nausea, vomiting, seizure, unilateral hyperreflexia, and Babinski sign.

c. They are often associated with skull vault fractures, although clinically significant epidural hematomas often result from laceration of branches of meningeal arteries (85%); they can also be produced by laceration of a dural venous sinus.

d. On CT, epidural hematomas appear as lenticular, biconcave hyperdense to isodense mass lesions overlying the brain.

   (1) Hematomas generally will not cross suture lines because of interdigitation of dura into suture.

e. For clinically significant lesions the optimal treatment is surgical evacuation.

   (1) In isolated epidural hematoma, rapid implementation of optimal treatment results in a low mortality rate (5%–10%) even for large lesions.

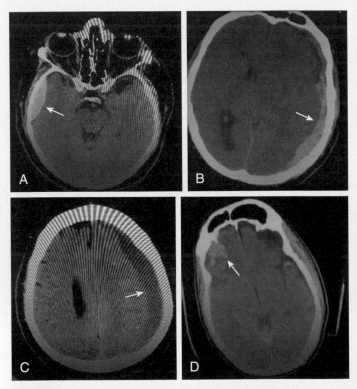

FIG. 20.1

Pathologies seen in traumatic brain injury. (A) Acute right temporal epidural hematoma; (B) acute left frontotemporal subdural hematoma (SDH), note hyperacute blood (hypodense) anteriorly; (C) chronic SDH; (D) acute right frontal contusions;

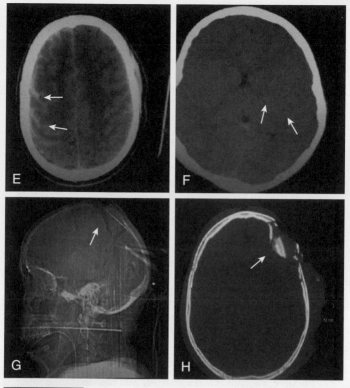

FIG. 20.1, cont'd
(E) right frontal convexity traumatic subarachnoid hemorrhage; (F) petechial hemorrhages of left subcortical white matter *(arrows)* characteristic of shear injury/diffuse axonal injury; (G) lateral radiograph demonstrating complex open skull vault fracture; and (H) CT demonstrating open, depressed, complex skull vault fracture.

2. SDH

a. More frequent than epidural hematoma, with higher morbidity and mortality (50%–90%) due to increased incidence of comorbid parenchymal injuries; often associated with venous bleeding, although it can also be arterial

b. On CT, SDH appears as a crescent-shaped mass overlying the cerebral convexity; will cross suture lines

c. Classified as acute, subacute, or chronic, although mixed lesions are common

    (1) Acute: 0–48 hours; hyperdense on CT, although fresh uncoagulated blood may appear hypodense (see Fig. 20.1B)

      (2) Subacute: 2–21 days; isodense on CT

      (3) Chronic: ≥3 weeks; hypodense on CT (see Fig. 20.1C)

  d. Acute SDH often results from a cortical venous, arterial, or parenchymal injury and is frequently associated with underlying cortical injury.

  e. Chronic SDHs develop from asymptomatic acute SDHs, which may have been clinically occult.

      (1) After the acute stage a gradual accumulation of subdural fluid results in progressive cerebral compression and neurologic deterioration.

      (2) Classic clinical symptoms at presentation are confusion, incontinence, ataxia, and unilateral weakness; it is often asymptomatic.

  f. Surgical management is dependent on type of SDH.

      (1) Symptomatic acute SDH is often a neurosurgical emergency; because of the thick nature of acutely clotted blood, craniotomy is required to evacuate the lesion and hemicraniectomy may be needed to decompress any underlying injured brain.

      (2) Chronic SDH is rarely a neurosurgical emergency; due the motor oil to watery consistency of chronic blood, symptomatic lesions can often be evacuated through a small burr hole or trephine. This can be performed under local anesthetic alone if needed.

3. Other types of intracranial injury

  a. Hemorrhagic contusions (see Fig. 20.1D)

      (1) Most commonly found in temporal, frontal, and occipital lobes where brain collides with bony prominences of floor of anterior fossa, sphenoid wing, and petrous ridge during acceleration and deceleration

      (2) Frequently progress or "blossom" for 24–72 hours after presentation

      (3) Generally managed nonoperatively with neurologic observation and treatment of elevated ICP as indicated

        (a) Surgical intervention is entertained when conservative medical management fails: decompressive craniectomy with or without resection of damaged brain.

      (4) Patients with isolated temporal lobe contusion can proceed to herniation and death without clinical evidence of elevated ICP and must be monitored closely for neurologic decline.

        (a) Local temporal swelling results in uncal herniation.

  b. Traumatic SAH (see Fig. 20.1E)

      (1) Frequently seen in CT-positive TBI of any severity but rarely of immediate clinical consequence because of lack of mass effect

      (2) Low risk of cerebral vasospasm

      (3) Large quantities of traumatic SAH may portend risk of posttraumatic communicating hydrocephalus.

  c. Diffuse axonal injury (see Fig. 20.1F)

      (1) Results from shearing of long descending fibers within white matter tracts due to rotational forces at the time of impact

(2) Can be visualized on MRI and, less often, CT as punctate hemorrhages in centrum semiovale, corpus callosum, pons, or brainstem

(3) Generally not associated with increases in ICP but can result in profound depression of consciousness or coma

(4) Extremely poor prognosis for functional recovery if brainstem is affected

d. Skull fractures (see Fig. 20.1G–H)

(1) They are categorized as open or closed; linear, complex, or comminuted; nondisplaced, compound, or depressed; single or multiple.

(2) They can involve the cranial vault, skull base, bones of the face and orbit, or combination thereof.

  (a) Skull base fractures can result in CSF leak; look for a "ring" sign if CSF leak is suspected and fluid is blood-tinged.

(3) Raccoon eyes are highly suggestive of fracture of the skull base at the floor of the anterior fossa or midfacial fractures.

(4) Basilar skull fractures can be suspected clinically in the presence of Battle sign (retroauricular hematoma), CSF otorrhea, or CSF rhinorrhea.

(5) Linear nondisplaced skull fractures rarely require intervention; depressed skull fractures may require elevation if:

  (a) Depressed greater than 8–10 mm or, generally, if the outer table of the skull is depressed below the inner table

  (b) Deficit related to compression of the underlying brain

  (c) CSF leak from wound due to dural laceration

  (d) Open, depressed skull fracture due to risk for intracranial infection

D. PENETRATING TRAUMATIC BRAIN INJURY

1. Gunshot wounds (GSWs) to the head account for the majority of penetrating TBIs in the United States.

a. Leading cause of TBI mortality: approximately 20,000/50,000 TBI deaths per year due to firearms versus 18,000 due to motor vehicle crashes (MVCs)

(1) Majority are due to assault by handguns with most deaths occurring in the first 24 hours.

b. Often characterized by multiple traumatic injuries including skull fracture, cerebrovascular injury, traumatic SAH, epidural hematoma, SDH, and parenchymal injury (Fig. 20.2A–B)

(1) Higher risk for vasospasm (20%–30%), posttraumatic seizures (30%–50%), infection, and traumatic aneurysm formation than blunt TBI

(2) Infection risk increases with CSF leak and impaled bone fragments.

c. Initial management: ABCs and aggressive resuscitation before postresuscitation neurologic reevaluation

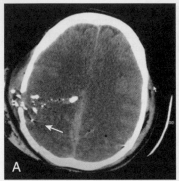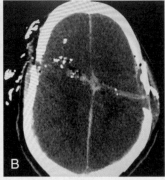

FIG. 20.2

Penetrating traumatic brain injury. (A) Axial computed tomography (CT) demonstrating retained bullet fragments (note "starburst artifact" *[arrow]*), diffuse traumatic subarachnoid hemorrhage (tSAH), and skull vault fracture with depressed bone fragments (note absence of "starburst" artifact); (B) axial CT of different patient demonstrating bihemispheric gunshot wounds with depressed bone fragments at entry wound, subdural hematoma, tSAH and hemorrhagic projectile trajectory hemorrhage crossing midline to contralateral skull fracture at exit wound.

(1) If postresuscitation GCS ≤5, mortality rate is reported as high as 92%–99%; care is generally supportive.
   (a) Poor prognosis associated with: low admission and postresuscitation GCS scores; bihemispheric GSW, transventricular GSW, thalamic or brainstem GSW; and unilaterally fixed or dilated pupil
(2) Operative intervention should be considered on case-by-case basis for those with postresuscitation GCS >5 or GCS >3 with compressive hematoma and intact papillary examination.
(3) All patients should be managed as with blunt severe TBI, with the addition of empiric antibiotic prophylaxis, aggressive wound irrigation, and closure.
   (a) Most authors recommend third-generation cephalosporin or amoxicillin-clavulanic acid and metronidazole for 3–5 days.

E. TRAUMATIC BRAIN INJURY PROGNOSIS

1. Approximately 20% of blunt TBI patients with presentation GCS = 3 will survive, but only 8%–10% will have a functional recovery (Glasgow Outcome Scale score 4–5).
   a. Age is a strong independent predictor of outcome, with a significant increase in poor outcome in patients older than 60 years.
   b. A single episode of hypotension (systolic blood pressure <90 mm Hg) during the acute care of a patient with head injury doubles the mortality rate.

    c. A strong correlation exists between the severity of abnormal findings on initial CT scan and outcome.

2. **Penetrating TBI patients with postresuscitation GCS ≤5 have a very low prospect of survival.**

    a. Mortality remains high for those with postresuscitation GCS ≤8; those who survive often do so with severe disability.

    b. Patients with postresuscitation GCS >8 have a good prospect for survival (mortality <25%) and improved prospect of recovery without disability (40%–85%, depending on intracranial injuries).

III. SPINAL TRAUMA

A. GENERAL

"Spinal emergencies" encompass multiple clinical situations but mostly include injuries involving the spinal cord, vertebrae, or soft tissues (ligaments, discs). Nerve roots are occasionally also affected. The level and degree of involvement of each one of the elements determine the clinical picture associated with a particular injury. It is important for all surgeons to be familiar with presentation and basic early management of spinal injuries because they commonly occur in the polytrauma patient.

1. **Prehospital immobilization and stabilization (collar, backboard) are essential in trauma patients.**

    a. In the past, 10% of quadriplegics did not become so at impact but rather at some point thereafter (1957).

    b. Trauma patients with loss of consciousness or injury above the clavicle must be assumed to have an associated cervical spine injury until proven otherwise clinically and radiographically.

    c. If in doubt, maintain cervical immobilization (collar) and spinal precautions with neutral spine position (flat) until full spinal assessment, clearance, or specialist consultation.

    d. The majority of patients with spinal injuries have normal peripheral neurologic findings.

B. ASSESSMENT

Clinical assessment follows a standard approach as for all patients; however, the patient's level of consciousness will dictate level of patient cooperation and frequently depressed consciousness increases the need for and reliance on imaging for spinal clearance or identifying spinal injury. The following usually occurs simultaneously with and in accordance with Advanced Trauma Life Support guidelines.

1. **History**

    a. Mechanism and modifiers, for example: MVC (velocity, seat belt use, ejection); fall (height, surface fallen upon, body area striking); assault (with what object(s), GSW)

    b. Symptoms at time of injury, onset, duration, evolution, and new symptoms since injury (e.g., pain, numbness, tingling, weakness or paralysis, incontinence)

2. **Examination**
   a. ABC principle applies to all patients, including those with spinal injury, but additional clinical vigilance must be maintained for spinal shock that may cause hypotension in the trauma patient, particularly those with cervical spine injuries (see later).
   b. Maintain strict spinal precautions during the assessment.
      (1) Mechanical assessment involves log roll of patient for inspection and palpation of the entire spine, as well as performance of the rectal examination.
      (2) Look for any obvious deformities, open wounds, or so-called step-offs (prominent, unequal spinous processes).
      (3) Feel for tenderness, deformities, and step-offs.
   c. Neurologic examination is guided by the level of consciousness; a detailed assessment helps guide treatment and prognosis. It must include motor, sensory, and sphincter function assessment. The following questions should be answered in an expeditious manner:
      (1) Is there a neurologic deficit (weakness, paralysis)?
      (2) If so, what is the level of injury?
      (3) Is the injury complete or partial? This determines the urgency of subsequent intervention and imaging.
   d. Incomplete spinal cord injury is a neurosurgical emergency. It includes patients with the following conditions:
      (1) *Any* motor or sensory function below the level of injury
      (2) Sacral sparing of sensation (to pinprick)
         (a) Presence of anal wink or bulbocavernosus reflex does not represent sacral sparing.
      (3) Preservation of voluntary sphincter function
   e. The level of spinal cord injury is determined by sensory and motor examinations (Fig. 20.3A) and described using the American Spinal Injury Association (ASIA) impairment scale (see Fig. 20.3B).
   f. High cervical spine injuries (above C6) may be accompanied by respiratory compromise.
         (a) Phrenic nerve (C3-4-5) innervates the diaphragm.
   g. Assess and document rectal tone, as well as the presence of pathologic reflexes (Babinski, Hoffmann) or absence of normal deep tendon reflexes.
   h. Spinal shock—Abrupt loss of sympathetic tone results in a distributive shock.
      (1) Usually occurs in complete spinal cord injuries; injury level usual in cervical or high thoracic spine
      (2) Characterized by *hypotension with bradycardia*; warm extremities (peripheral vasodilation), loss of reflexes, and flaccid paralysis
   i. Absence of the bulbocavernosus reflex (anal sphincter contraction in response to glans penis pinch or Foley catheter tug) in a patient with spinal shock has prognostic value and its return may signify resolution of the shock period.

3. Radiographic assessment

a. This may include one or a combination of plain XR (dynamic flexion/extension should be avoided until ruling out bony abnormality or misalignment), CT, and/or MRI.

b. Imaging review should include assessment of alignment, presence of fractures, and identification of soft tissue abnormalities (swelling, hematoma, etc.).

c. Patients with incomplete spinal cord injury not explained by findings on XR, CT, or both warrant urgent MRI to identify injury and guide any intervention.

(1) Compressive spinal epidural hematoma, spinal SDH (rare), and traumatic disc herniation are often radiographically occult on XR or CT and require emergent surgical intervention (Fig. 20.4A and B).

d. Decreased level of consciousness or history of loss of consciousness confounds assessment of spinal cord integrity.

(1) Adequate plain films of cervical, thoracic, and lumbar patient are essential.

(a) CT cervical spine is commonly obtained concurrently with CTH in trauma patients with altered mental status; thoracolumbar CT can often be reconstructed from CT of chest and abdomen if already obtained.

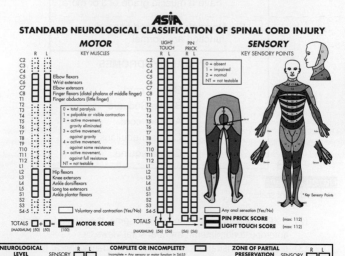

FIG. 20.3

American Spinal Injury Association impairment scale. (A) Motor and sensory examination guide;

ASIA IMPAIRMENT SCALE

☐ **A = Complete:** No motor or sensory function is preserved in the sacral segments S4-S5.

☐ **B = Incomplete:** Sensory but no motor function is preserved below the neurological level and includes the sacral segments S4-S5.

☐ **C = Incomplete:** Motor function is preserved below the neurological level, and more than half of key muscles below the neurological level have a muscle grade less than 3.

☐ **D = Incomplete:** Motor function is preserved below the neurological level, and at least half of key muscle below the neurological level have a muscle grade of 3 or more.

☐ **E = Normal:** Motor and sensory function are normal

CLINICAL SYNDROMES

☐ Central cord
☐ Brown-Séquard
☐ Anterior cord
☐ Conus medullaris
☐ Cauda equina

B

FIG. 20.3, cont'd
(B) impairment scale.

(2) If XRs are obtained of the cervical spine, they should include anteroposterior, lateral, and transoral views.
(3) If unable to visualize cervicothoracic or craniocervical junction on plain films, obtain CT scan (Eastern Association for the Surgery of Trauma [EAST] guidelines).
e. If there is no history of loss of consciousness and the patient has GCS = 15
(1) Mechanism of injury and clinical examination should guide radiographic evaluation.

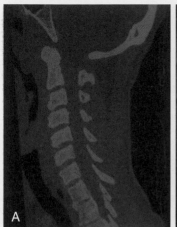 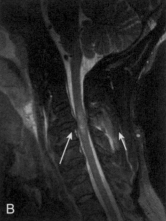

FIG. 20.4

Traumatic cervical disc herniation in patient who presented as C4 American Spinal Injury Association (ASIA) A spinal cord injury. (A) Computed tomography cervical spine without evidence of fracture, misalignment, or canal compromise; (B) T2 magnetic resonance imaging cervical spine demonstrates acute C4–5 disc herniation *(long white arrow)* impinging on cord with cord contusion (hyperintense T2 signal). Also note posterior ligamentous injury *(short white arrow)* (hyperintense T2 signal).

20

NEUROSURGICAL EMERGENCIES

        (2) Patients with no spinal tenderness on palpation and no pain on movement are unlikely to have sustained significant spinal injuries and may not require any imaging.
        (3) Obtain imaging of areas with abnormal examination findings.
    f. If a spinal fracture is identified, completion spinal films must be obtained (XR or CT); identification of a spinal fracture carries approximately 20% risk of additional, clinically occult fracture.
4. Spinal clearance
    a. "Clearance" of spine in a trauma patient involves clinical and/or radiographic assessment depending on mechanism of injury, altered mental status, or history of unconsciousness.
        (1) When in doubt, maintain full spinal precautions, cervical immobilization, and consult spine specialist for assistance.
    b. Clinical criteria for cervical spine stability (National Emergency X-Radiography Utilization Study [NEXUS]—five *N*s):
        (1) No mental status change
        (2) No intoxication (drugs, alcohol)
        (3) No neck pain or tenderness
        (4) No distracting injury/pain
        (5) No neurologic deficits

     (a) If one of the above is present, the patient cannot be clinically cleared and should remain immobilized and undergo imaging studies.

     (b) Canadian C-spine Rule can be used or a combination of both.

  c. Radiographic assessment as previously described

     (1) A 2-week interval assessment with dynamic (neutral, flexion, extension) XR or MRI with fat-suppression sequences may be needed in patients with negative imaging who cannot be clinically cleared to exclude ligamentous injury (institution dependent, evidence not clear).

     (2) Accordingly, unconscious patients should not have their collar removed at the initial assessment, even with negative imaging.

  d. Absence of thoracolumbar tenderness and neurologic symptoms renders those regions clinically clear.

  e. Remove backboard as soon as possible to prevent unnecessary pressure ulcers.

C. SPECIFIC SPINAL INJURIES

1. Spinal cord injury

  a. Generally due to injury above L1–2; it is more frequent in males and most commonly results from MVC (40%) and assault (25%).

  b. Urgent assessment is essential to avoid delay in treatment and preserve neurologic function.

  c. High cervical cord injuries may require intubation (or tracheostomy) because of impairment of phrenic nerve function.

  d. Spinal shock may require intravenous fluids and the use of vasopressors (sympathomimetics).

     (1) Dopamine is historically agent of choice.

     (2) Phenylephrine used despite theoretical risk for reflexive exacerbation of bradycardia; use alternative agent if this occurs.

     (3) Goal is to maintain MAP ≥85 for first 7 days after injury to provide for adequate perfusion of spinal cord; hypotension may further injure the spinal cord.

  e. It is essential to determine whether the neurologic injury is complete or incomplete (see Fig. 20.3B).

     (1) Incomplete spinal cord injury requires an urgent MRI and spine service consultation.

  f. The use of high-dose methylprednisolone is not recommended for treatment of acute spinal cord injury based on level I evidence.

     (1) Associated with increased morbidity, particularly in polytrauma patients, those with medical comorbidities, and older adults

     (2) No class I or II evidence for benefit available; class I, II, and III evidence of detrimental effects is available.

     (a) National Acute Spinal Cord Injury Study (NASCIS) trial demonstrated only mild motor improvement; it has not been reproduced.

g. Expedient spine team consultation is necessary for all spinal cord injuries.

h. Immobilization and/or realignment of obvious deformities may be achieved through the use of cervical traction.

i. Postoperative care requires appropriate skin care, bowel and bladder training, and involvement of rehabilitation units as soon as possible.

2. **Traumatic cauda equina syndrome**

a. Compression or injury of the cauda equina (distal to spinal cord); injury level will generally be below L1–2.

b. Characterized by bilateral paraparesis of the lower extremities, areflexia alternating or bilateral radiculopathy, saddle (rectal, perineum, genital) anesthesia, and disturbance of bowel and bladder function (urinary retention, rectal sphincter incompetence)

c. Suspected cauda equina syndrome warrants urgent MRI and, in the presence of surgical pathology, emergent treatment.

   (1) Spine specialist consultation is mandatory.

3. **Cervical spine fractures (Fig. 20.5A–F)**

a. They must be suspected with any injury above the clavicle, and implement cervical immobilization until clearance or diagnosis possible.

   (1) In the event of unstable fractures or dislocations, spinal traction may be applied by a spine specialist for immobilization or reduction.

b. Fractures amenable to nonoperative treatment may require cervical immobilization for 8–12 weeks.

   (1) Fractures of subaxial spine (C3–C7) often require rigid cervical collar (e.g., Aspen, Miami J).

   (2) Fractures of craniocervical junction, atlas (C1), or axis (C2) may require rigid cervical collar or halo-vest.

   (3) Fractures at cervicothoracic junction (C7 and distal) may require extension of bracing to stabilize the thorax (e.g., Minerva brace).

c. Have suspicion for BCVI of the vertebral artery in cervical fractures involving the transverse foramina.

   (1) Can evaluate with CTA, MR angiography, or diagnostic angiogram

d. Be familiar with some specific cervical trauma pathologies:

   (1) Atlantooccipital dislocation is compromise of the ligamentous atlantooccipital joint.

      (a) Usually fatal when severe but commonly missed in survivors; must assess for widening of craniocervical junction

   (2) Jefferson fracture is a burst fracture of the atlas.

      (a) It is considered stable if transverse ligament is uncompromised and can be evaluated with "rule of Spence."

      (b) Lateral masses overhanging C2 is a clue suggesting compromise of transverse ligament and instability.

   (3) Odontoid/dens fractures of axis (C2)

      (a) Type I: odontoid tip fracture/avulsion—stable, generally treated with external immobilization

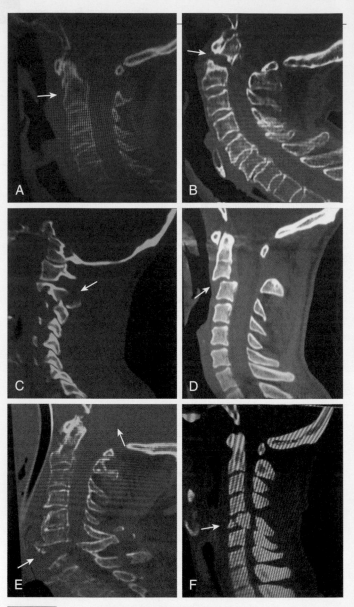

FIG. 20.5

Acute cervical spine fractures. (A) Minimally displaced type II dens (C2) fracture *(arrow)*; (B) distracted type II dens fracture; (C) patient with bilateral C2 facet fractures *(arrow)*; (D) resulting in anterolisthesis of C2 on C3 *(arrow)*; (E) fracture-dislocation of C6–7 *(arrow)*; (F) tear drop–type burst fracture of C5 resulting in canal compromise *(arrow)*.

(b) Type II: fracture of the shaft of the dens—high rate of malunion, must be evaluated for surgical treatment, although may be treated with immobilization

(c) Type III: fracture of C2 vertebral body—usually stable, generally treated with external immobilization

(4) "Hangman's fracture" is fracture of bilateral pars interarticularis of axis (C2) that disrupts C2–3, often resulting in subluxation.

(a) Historically it is due to judicial hanging (hyperextension with distraction).

(b) Fracture is unstable and generally treated with cervical fixation and fusion.

(5) Perched or jumped facets are due to ligamentous injury and considered unstable.

(a) Spine specialist may attempt closed reduction with cranial tongs and traction.

(b) Generally treated with either closed or open reduction then fixation and fusion

(c) Carries risk of vertebral artery injury (distraction) and traumatic disc herniation

4. **Thoracolumbar fractures (Fig. 20.6)**

a. Thoracolumbar fractures can be classified as compression fractures, burst fractures, chance fractures, flexion-distraction injuries, or fracture dislocations (Fig. 20.7; Table 20.3).

b. Spine specialist consultation is indicated, and assessment of stability and neurologic compromise determines need for operative intervention.

c. Many are managed nonoperatively with the use of external bracing, for example

(1) Fracture above T6 may be treated with Minerva brace.

(2) Fracture T7 and below may be treated with thoracolumbosacral orthosis (TLSO).

d. Unstable fractures are treated with open reduction, internal fixation, and fusion.

(1) Neurologic compromise may be treated with decompression alone or in addition to those aforementioned.

e. Isolated fractures of bony prominences (e.g., thoracolumbar spinous process or transverse process fractures) do not compromise the stability or neurologic function.

(1) Do not require operative intervention or spine specialist involvement but hint at amplitude of traumatic force and may raise possibility of intraabdominal, retroperitoneal, or rib injury

5. **GSW to the spine**

a. Most are due to assault

(1) Cervical: 20%–40%; thoracic: 50%–60%; and lumbar: 10%–30%

(2) Spinal cord injury is usually due to direct injury from the bullet in civilian environments.

20

NEUROSURGICAL EMERGENCIES

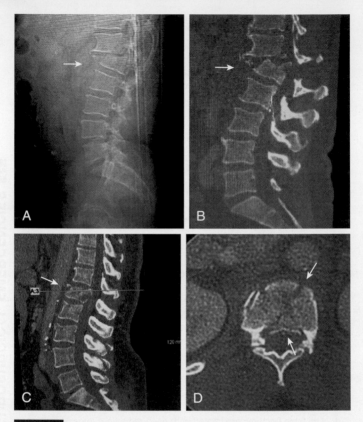

FIG. 20.6

Thoracolumbar spine fractures. (A) Plain radiographs demonstrating traumatic wedge deformity of L1 with translation and canal compromise; (B) computed tomography (CT) lumbar spine of same patient demonstrating characteristic pattern of flexion-distracture fracture *(arrow)*; (C) sagittal and (D) axial CT lumbar spine demonstrating L1 burst fracture with canal compromise *(arrows)*.

    b. High-dose steroids are not indicated for spinal cord injury due to penetrating trauma.

    c. Fractures caused by isolated GSW to the spine are generally considered stable.

    d. In general, management is supportive, but indications for surgery include

        (1) Neurologic deterioration suggesting spinal epidural hematoma; often difficult to assess on CT because of metal artifact

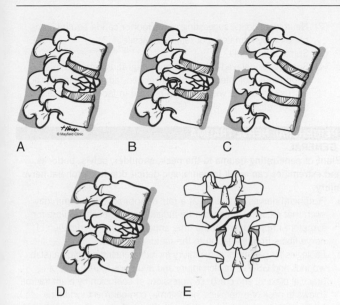

20

NEUROSURGICAL EMERGENCIES

FIG. 20.7

McAfee classification of thoracolumbar spine fractures (A) Compression; (B) burst; (C) chance; (D) flexion-distraction; (E) translational/fracture-dislocation.

TABLE 20.3

MCAFEE CLASSIFICATION OF THORACOLUMBAR SPINE FRACTURES

Fracture Type	Pathology
Wedge compression	Isolated failure of anterior column; flexion injury
Burst fracture, stable	Anterior and middle-column compression failure, posterior column intact
Burst fracture, unstable	As above but anterior vertebral height compressed >50%, spinal canal compromised >50%, or kyphosis >20 degrees; spinal cord injury requires decompression
Chance fracture	Horizontal vertebral avulsion injury with center of rotation anterior to anterior longitudinal ligament, hyperflexion injury (e.g., seat belt injury)
Flexion-distraction injury	Compressive failure of anterior column, ligamentous failure of posterior column, center of rotation is posterior to anterior longitudinal ligament
Translational injury/ fracture-dislocation	Disruption of spinal canal alignment in transverse or horizontal plane, commonly due to shear mechanism; involves all three columns and ligamentous disruption

(2) Neurologic deficit suggesting nerve root or cauda equina compression by hematoma or retained missile
(3) Spinal fluid fistula
(4) Surgery for delayed complications: migrating retained missile, debridement of infection, copper-related radiculitis, lead toxicity (risk increases with retained missile in facet joint or disc space), etc.

IV. PERIPHERAL NERVE TRAUMA
A. GENERAL
1. Blunt or penetrating trauma to the neck, shoulder, pelvis, buttocks, and extremities can result in neurologic deficit due to peripheral nerve injury.
   a. Peripheral nerves regenerate at a rate of approximately 1 mm/day such that recovery timing can be judged with respect to failure for symptom improvement in the time anticipated for regeneration of nerve fibers from the lesion to the motor end plate.
   b. Etiologies for peripheral nerve injury include penetrating trauma (stab wounds and GSWs); traction injury and avulsions (particularly of brachial plexus); and crush, compression, or contusion by blunt trauma (blows to neck or extremities, hematoma, compartment syndrome, etc.).
   c. Injuries are commonly classified with Sunderland or Seddon classification systems (Table 20.4).

B. EVALUATION
1. Evaluation includes spinal examination and focused peripheral nerve evaluation including assessment of both sensory and motor function
   a. Frequently occult on imaging, although some findings should raise suspicion if neurologic deficit is present: displaced fracture of first rib; extraforaminal or transverse foramen pseudomeningocele on MRI; hematoma of posterior triangle of neck; hematoma along ala of ilium; large gluteal hematoma
      (1) Must maintain high index of suspicion in stabbing and GSW victims with neurologic deficit not explained by cranial or spinal injury
   b. Suspicion of injury often warrants specialty consultation to plastic surgery, orthopedics, or neurosurgery (institution dependent).
   c. Findings on examination that suggest a preganglionic injury (not amenable to surgical repair) include:
      (1) Horner syndrome: injury to preganglionic white rami
      (2) Neuropathic pain: may suggest nerve root avulsion, MRI may show CSF pseudomeningocele at level of avulsed nerve root
      (3) Winged scapula: long thoracic nerve injury
      (4) Rhomboid palsy: dorsal scapular nerve injury
   d. Familiarity with common brachial plexus injury syndromes can help to localize the level of injury.

TABLE 20.4

CLASSIFICATION OF PERIPHERAL NERVE INJURIES

Seddon Classification	Sunderland Classification	Anticipated Recovery
Neurapraxia	Type I	—
Nerve in continuity, no axonal violation. Contusion, compression, or ischemia leads to focal block of nerve impulse. No wallerian degeneration present.		Often complete recovery in 4–12 weeks
Axonotmesis	Type II	
Nerve in continuity	Injury to axons and myelin sheath	Axons regenerate at 1 mm/day with new axons following endoneurium to target.
Violation of axons and supporting tissues	Endoneurium, perineurium, and epineurium preserved	Degree of recovery depends on distance new axons must grow to target end plate
Wallerian degeneration present		Proximal deficits recover before distal deficits.
	Type III	
	Type II + endoneurium injury	Axonal regeneration <1 mm/day due to scarring
	Epineurium and perineurium preserved	Recovery minimal to complete, depends on degree of scarring and number of nerve fascicles involved
	Type IV	
	Type III + perineurium violated	Robust scarring blocks axonal regeneration.
	Epineurium preserved	Surgical intervention to remove scarred segment and reconnect clean nerve endings
Neurotmesis	Type V	—
Nerve in discontinuity, transection of entire nerve	Type IV + epineurium violated	Surgical repair needed for recovery
	Type VI	—
Wallerian degeneration present	Mixed features of type I–IV	—

(1) Erb-Duchenne palsy: internal rotation of shoulder, elbow extension, wrist flexion (also known as "waiter's tip")
    (a) Due to upper brachial plexus injury: C5–6, superior trunk, may additionally involve C7
    (b) Commonly seen as a birth injury, after motorcycle crashes, or as an athletic injury; due to downward force on shoulder
    (c) Often a traction injury though nerve root avulsions may occur
(2) Klumpke palsy: paralysis of the intrinsic hand muscles (claw hand deformity) and loss of sensation along medial aspect of arm
    (a) Due to lower brachial plexus injury: C8–T1, inferior trunk, occasionally involves C7

(b) Commonly seen resulting from traction on the upper extremity while shoulder abducted (e.g., grasping for railing while falling)

(c) Involvement of T1 preganglionic rami can result in Horner syndrome.

c. Examination can be supplemented with electromyogram (EMG) at 3–4 weeks if deficit persists and is unexplained; earlier evaluation may miss injury.

C. TREATMENT

1. Urgent operative intervention in first 24–48 hours is indicated for fresh laceration, non-GSW penetrating injuries, including operative exploration and direct nerve repair.

2. Closed blunt or traction injuries will usually recover within 8–12 weeks.
   a. Conservative management with physical therapy and EMG should be performed at 4–6 weeks to assess degree of injury.
   b. If no improvement in function by 3 months, EMG is repeated—if no improvement, surgical exploration and repair should be considered.

3. Birth brachial plexus injuries are typically observed until at least 3 months of age, at which point motor evaluation is repeated.
   a. Exploration may be performed if there is marked weakness, less than 3 out of 5 motor score, in major muscle groups.
   b. Positive EMG or MRI findings may lead to exploration, repair, or nerve transfer surgery for reanimation.

4. Compartment syndrome is an emergency treated with emergency fasciotomy.
   a. If performed promptly, recovery is often rapid and complete.

5. GSW injuries are typically due to blast effect and compression by hematoma rather than laceration.
   a. The majority (~70%) will recover with conservative management.
   b. Operative intervention is entertained if there is no improvement clinically or on repeat EMG at ≥3 months from injury.
      (1) Operative intervention may include exploration, repair, and/or reanimation.

V. TRAUMATIC CEREBROVASCULAR INJURIES

A. TRANSECTION DUE TO PENETRATING TRAUMA REQUIRES EMERGENT HEMOSTASIS AND OPEN SURGICAL REPAIR OR EVALUATION FOR ENDOVASCULAR OCCLUSION.

B. BLUNT CEREBROVASCULAR INJURY

Traumatic transaction, dissection, occlusion, or compression of the internal carotid or vertebral arteries

1. BCVI is seen in approximately 2%–3% of trauma patients.
   a. Risk factors include high-energy trauma (e.g., skull base fracture involving carotid canal); severe TBI, cervical fracture; hangings; and seat belt–type injuries to the neck.

(1) Suspicion should be high in high cervical fractures (C1–C3) and cervical fractures involving transverse foramen.

(2) Medical risk factors are primarily connective tissue disorders; patients may have BCVI with seemingly minor trauma.

C. EVALUATION

1. Examination findings could include focal neurologic deficit (e.g., Horner syndrome), stroke/ transient ischemic attack (TIA) symptoms, expanding cervical hematoma, carotid bruit in young patients, or neurologic deficit not explained by CTH.

   a. BCVI is often clinically occult.

2. Radiographic evaluation

   a. Urgent CT or diagnostic angiography is indicated in patients with symptomatic BCVI.

      (1) Expanding cervical hematoma

      (2) Arterial bleeding from nasopharynx

      (3) Symptoms of stroke or TIA

   b. Asymptomatic patients should be evaluated whenever risk factors are present.

      (1) CTA is modality of choice and has similar predictive value to diagnostic cerebral angiography.

      (2) MR angiography and ultrasound are often inadequate for evaluation of BCVI; a negative result does not exclude BCVI.

   c. Injury grading is based on angiographic features.

      (1) Grade I: luminal filling defect, less than 25% luminal stenosis

      (2) Grade II: luminal filling defect, ≥25% luminal stenosis *OR* luminal intimal flap or thrombus (Fig. 20.8A)

      (3) Grade III: pseudoaneurysm present

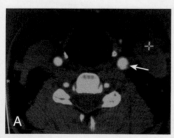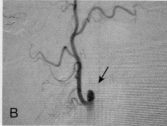

FIG. 20.8

Blunt cerebrovascular injury (A) Grade II blunt cerebrovascular injury (BCVI) of the left internal carotid artery; note small intimal flap at arrow; (B) lateral angiogram of carotid artery demonstrating grade IV BCVI of internal carotid artery just distal to the carotid bifurcation.

20

NEUROSURGICAL EMERGENCIES

    (4) Grade IV: complete luminal occlusion (see Fig. 20.8B)

    (5) Grade V: transection with active extravasation

D. TREATMENT

1. **Most grade I and II will not progress and will ultimately resolve with antiplatelet therapy.**
   a. Antiplatelet therapy reduces risk of progression; patients without contraindication are generally treated with aspirin.
   b. Grade II injuries frequently progress, but antiplatelet therapy reduces risk of stroke.
2. **Grade III injuries will persist.**
   a. Often treated with heparin drip and then reevaluated at 7–14 days
      (1) If lesion regresses on follow-up imaging, anticoagulation can be discontinued.
      (2) If pseudoaneurysm persists, patient may be considered for endovascular stent sequestration and transition from heparin to aspirin with follow-up imaging at 6–12 weeks.
3. **Grade IV injuries have high risk of embolization.**
   a. Often treated with antiplatelet regimen, and symptomatic embolic events treated with endovascular evaluation for occlusion to prevent further embolic events
4. **Grade V injuries have high mortality rate and are neurosurgical emergencies.**
   a. Surgically accessible lesions should be taken for emergent surgical repair or ligation.
   b. Inaccessible lesions can be evaluated for endovascular stent sequestration or occlusion.

RECOMMENDED READINGS

Aarabi B, Tofighi B, Kufera JA, et al. Predictors of outcome in civilian gunshot wounds to the head. *J Neurosurg*. 2014;120:1138–1146.

American Spinal Injury Association (ASIA) (includes links to ASIA spinal cord injury worksheet and examination guide). <www.asia-spinalinjury.org/>; Accessed 12.01.17.

Benzel EC, Hadden TA, Coleman JE. Civilian gunshot wounds to the spinal cord and cauda equina. *Neurosurgery*. 1987;20:281–285.

Brain Trauma Foundation, Brain Injury Guidelines (includes surgical and pediatric guidelines. <www.braintrauma.org/coma/guidelines/>; Accessed 12.01.17.

Carvalho GA, Nikkhah G, Matthies C, Penkert G, Samii M. Diagnosis of root avulsions in traumatic brachial plexus injuries: value of computerized tomography myelography and magnetic resonance imaging. *J Neurosurg*. 1997;86:69–76.

Denis F. The three column spine and its significance in the classification of acute thoracolumbar spinal injuries. *Spine*. 1983;8:817–831.

Edwards NM, Fabian TC, Claridge JA, Timmons SD, Fischer PE, Croce MA. Antithrombotic therapy and endovascular stents are effective treatment for blunt carotid injuries: results from longterm follow-up. *J Am Coll Surg*. 2007;204:1007–1113.

Guidelines for the management of acute cervical spine and spinal cord injuries. *Neurosurgery*. 2013;72(suppl 2):S1–S259.

Guidelines for the management of severe traumatic brain injury, 3rd ed. *J Neurotrauma*. 2007;24(suppl 1):S1–S116.

Guidelines for the surgical management of severe traumatic brain injury. *Neurosurgery*. 2006;58:S2–S62.

Hoffman JR, Mower WR, Wolfson AB, Todd KH, Zucker MI. Validity of a set of clinical criteria to rule out injury to the cervical spine in patients with blunt trauma. *N Engl J Med*. 2000;343:94–99.

Indications for intracranial pressure monitoring. *J Neurotrauma*. 2000;17:479–491.

Joseph B, Aziz H, Pandit V, et al. Improving survival rates after civilian gunshot wounds to the brain. *J Am Coll Surg*. 2014;218:58–65.

Kline DG, Hudson AR. *Operative Results for Major Nerve Injuries, Entrapments and Tumors*. Philadelphia: Saunders; 1995.

Resuscitation of blood pressure and oxygenation. *J Neurotrauma*. 2000;17:471–478.

Stiell IG, Wells GA, Vandemheen KL, et al. The Canadian C-spine rule for radiography in alert and stable trauma patients. *JAMA*. 2001;286:1841–1848.

Vaccaro AR, Lehman Jr RA, Hurlbert RJ, et al. A new classification of thoracolumbar injuries: the importance of injury morphology, the integrity of the posterior ligamentous complex, and neurologic status. *Spine*. 2005;30:2325–2333.

20

NEUROSURGICAL EMERGENCIES

PART V

Gastrointestinal Surgery

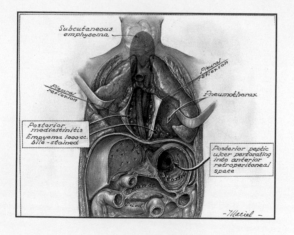

Acute Abdomen

Ben Huebner, MD

*There are many who do not appreciate the full significance of the
earlier and less flagrant symptoms of acute abdominal disease
...or find it hard to believe that a patient with a non-distended
abdomen and normal pulse and pressure can be the victim of a
perforated gastric ulcer.*

—Zachary Cope, 1921

The acute abdomen is defined as undiagnosed pain that develops suddenly
and is less than 7 days in duration.

I. PHYSIOLOGY OF ABDOMINAL PAIN

A. VISCERAL PAIN

Visceral or intestinal contraction, spasm, stretching, distention, or chemical
irritation results in visceral afferent nerve fiber stimulation.

1. Location—Pain experienced in the midline corresponds to the embryonic anatomic origin with subsequent descent during organogenesis.
   a. **Foregut**—stomach to second portion of duodenum, pancreas, gallbladder, and liver
      (1) Pain transmitted via celiac plexus.
      (2) Pain experienced in the **epigastrium**.
   b. **Midgut**—third part of duodenum to first two-thirds of the transverse colon
      (1) Pain transmitted via celiac plexus
      (2) Pain experienced in the **periumbilical** region
   c. **Hindgut**—last third of transverse colon to rectum
      (1) Pain transmitted via the inferior epigastric plexus
      (2) Pain experienced in the **suprapubic** region

B. SOMATIC PAIN

Caused by direct parietal peritoneal irritation perceived by segmental somatic
nerve fibers.

1. Precisely localized areas
   a. Anterior abdominal wall
   b. Causes reflex muscle rigidity of overlying musculature (rectus and
      oblique involuntary guarding)
2. Poorly localized areas
   a. Pelvis and central portion of posterior abdominal wall
   b. No reflex muscle rigidity
   c. May elicit indirect signs such as psoas sign or ureteral colic

Clinical Pearl: *A pelvic or retrocecal inflamed appendix may not generate somatic or
rebound tenderness. Hence "beware of the retrocecal appendix."*

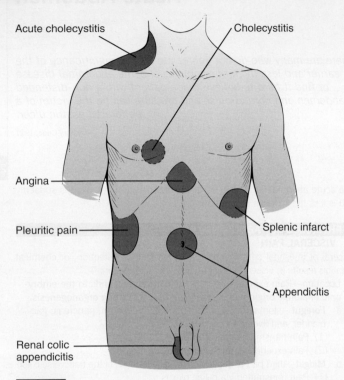

Acute cholecystitis

Cholecystitis

Angina

Pleuritic pain

Splenic infarct

Appendicitis

Renal colic
appendicitis

FIG. 21.1
Diagram of referred pain.

C. REFERRED PAIN

Abdominal pain may be referred to distant locations. This is the result of mapping of visceral afferent impulses to the level of embryonic organogenesis. This mapping results in "interpretation" of the pain to the corresponding somatic dermatome within the central nervous system (Fig. 21.1).

II. HISTORY

In the overwhelming majority of cases, a diagnosis can be made from a thorough history and careful physical examination.

A. PAIN

1. Onset
   a. Timing—sudden or gradual
      (1) Sudden suggests perforation of viscus (gut, ovary, etc.) as a result of a precipitous and discrete event

   b. Mode—Did the pain develop immediately after an event?
     (1) Trauma may be associated with solid organ injury.
     (2) Severe abdominal pain may be associated with ruptured abdominal aortic aneurysm, perforated duodenal ulcer, acute pancreatitis, or ruptured ectopic pregnancy (severe rapid peritoneal irritation by blood).
     (3) Pain following meals may be associated with intestinal colic or mesenteric ischemia.
     (4) Pain that awakens patient in the middle of the night—Think peptic ulcer disease.

2. **Location-based differential diagnosis:** Location of pain may lend information about the cause; however, pain may be referred. Pain may be diffuse or localized. Diffuse pain is more commonly associated with visceral pain or diffuse peritonitis.
   a. Right upper quadrant—biliary colic, acute cholecystitis, acute cholangitis, sphincter of Oddi dysfunction, acute hepatitis, liver abscess, Budd-Chiari syndrome, portal vein thrombosis, Fitz-Hugh–Curtis syndrome
   b. Left upper quadrant—likely splenic in origin—splenomegaly, splenic abscess, splenic infarct, splenic rupture
   c. Epigastric—myocardial infarction, peptic ulcer disease, acute/chronic pancreatitis, gastroesophageal reflux disease, gastritis, biliary colic or acute cholecystitis
   d. Lower abdomen—appendicitis, diverticulitis, nephrolithiasis, pyelonephritis, acute urinary retention, cystitis, infectious colitis, gynecologic

3. **Character**
   a. Burning pain is associated with perforated gastric ulcer or acute pancreatitis, as well as acute peritonitis.
   b. Sharp, constricting pain is associated with biliary colic.
   c. Tearing pain is associated with dissecting aneurysm.
   d. Gripping pain is associated with intestinal obstruction.
   e. Constant, dull, fixed pain is associated with an abscess.
   f. Colic—Waves of peristalsis are associated with intestinal obstruction

4. **Exacerbating or ameliorating factors**—movement, eating, breathing, vomiting

Clinical Pearl: *Abdominal pain associated with driving over bumps/lying rigid suggests peritonitis.*

B. VOMITING

Usually caused by irritation of the nerves of the peritoneum or obstruction of an involuntary muscle tube with concomitant attempts to evacuate/relieve pressure (bile duct, ureter, intestine, or appendix)

1. **Relation of pain to vomiting**
   a. Acute obstruction of the bile duct or ureter causes pain followed shortly by vomiting.

21

ACUTE ABDOMEN

b. Vomiting occurs late in abdominal pain secondary to bowel obstruction. The more proximal the source of intestinal obstruction, the more voluminous the vomiting. Distal small bowel and colonic obstruction may not result in vomiting.

2. **Character**
   a. Bilious—nonspecific or early obstruction
   b. Food particles—proximal obstruction
   c. Feculent—caused by bacterial overgrowth in small bowel caused by prolonged distal small bowel obstruction; rare in colonic obstruction (especially with competent ileocecal valve)
3. **Frequency**—increased in proximal bowel obstruction

C. BOWEL FUNCTION
1. Constipation (absence of bowel movements)/obstipation (absence of bowel movements or gas)—obstruction, paralytic ileus, acute appendicitis
2. Diarrhea—gastroenteritis, early or partial small bowel obstruction
3. Blood/mucus—intussusception in children, colitis, proctitis in adults

Clinical Pearl: *When hypogastric pain and diarrhea are followed by hypogastric tenderness and constipation, suspect pelvic abscess.*

D. MEDICAL HISTORY
May give clues about the cause of abdominal pain
1. Previous abdominal surgery
2. History of peptic ulcer disease, cardiovascular disease, gallstones, inflammatory bowel disease, or diverticular disease
3. Immunocompromised (transplant, steroids, chemotherapy)—consider blunting of signs/symptoms secondary to immune status.

Clinical Pearl: *Older adult patients do not present with the same signs/symptoms and may not have abnormal lab values. A high index of suspicion is required for this group of patients.*

E. MEDICATION
1. Steroids
   a. Can decrease symptoms produced by inflammation
   b. Can cause atypical perforations of the colon and small intestine
2. Analgesics, antibiotics, and antipyretics—may mask pain and fever
   a. Nonsteroidal antiinflammatory drugs (NSAIDs)—peptic ulcer disease, gastritis
   b. Antibiotics—*Clostridium difficile*

III. PHYSICAL EXAMINATION
A. GENERAL APPEARANCE
1. Facial expression
2. Attitude in bed
   a. Restlessness suggests colic.
   b. Immobility in patients with peritonitis

   c. Knees drawn up to relieve abdominal wall tension in peritonitis (also may reflect psoas inflammation, i.e., retrocecal appendix)

   d. Pain out of proportion to examination suggests mesenteric ischemia.

3. Dull eyes and ashen countenance in patients with sepsis
4. Skin tenting and dry mucosa associated with volume loss and dehydration from proximal bowel obstruction
5. Pale conjunctiva in patients with anemia
6. Jaundice-biliary disease

B. VITAL SIGNS

1. Temperature
   a. Severe shock: 95°F–96°F
   b. Early inflammation, usual in acute appendicitis: 99°F–100°F
   c. Intraabdominal abscess or urinary source: 104°F–105°F
2. Pulse
   a. Tachycardia may be seen in fever, anemia, agitation, dehydration, or pain.
      (1) May be absent in patient on beta-blocker or similar cardiac medications
   b. Bradycardia can be seen in advanced sepsis or metabolic disturbances (i.e., hypothyroidism).
3. Respiratory rate
   a. Kussmaul respirations are present with diabetic ketoacidosis.
   b. If respiratory rate is increased to twice the normal rate, the cause is likely thoracic in origin.
4. Blood pressure
   a. Hypotension may be associated with anemia, sepsis, or volume depletion.
   b. Hypertension may be associated with severe pain.

C. ABDOMINAL EXAMINATION

1. Observation, inspection

Clinical Pearl: Be sure that clothing and bedding do not interfere with the THOR-OUGH visualization and examination of all aspects of the abdomen. More than one sheepish intern has been "burnt" by the occult and incarcerated groin hernia. Examine the patient and abdomen in the same sequence and from the same side of the patient whenever possible.

   a. Scaphoid, flat, obese, distended

   b. Movement with respiration—Note limitation of movement indicating rigidity of the abdominal muscles or diaphragm.

   c. Have patient localize area of pain (exact point in somatic pain, location in visceral pain).

   d. Inspect all potential sites for hernias, especially the inguinal and femoral region.

   e. Stethoscope is a great tool for palpation in anxious patients.

21

ACUTE ABDOMEN

2. Auscultation
    a. Absent or hypoactive bowel sounds—peritonitis or ileus
    b. High-pitched bowel sounds with rushes, hyperactive—distention of lumen (obstruction or ileus)
    c. Aortic and renal artery bruits—Absence of a bruit never excludes the presence of an aortic aneurysm.
3. Palpation/percussion—Gentleness is essential.
    a. Evaluate presence and extent of muscular rigidity.
    b. Percussion—Pain with gentle percussion may indicate peritonitis; you can also use percussion to identify ascites/hepatomegaly (dullness) or distended bowel (tympany).
    c. Palpate four quadrants of abdomen and costovertebral angles to assess tenderness (mild, moderate, or severe). Palpate for abdominal masses, abnormal pulsations, and hernial orifices. **Begin away from point of maximal pain**. See Table 21.1 for signs and findings in abdominal examination. When all else fails, ask the patient to palpate his or her own abdomen, indicating the site of maximal tenderness.
    d. Rocking the bed can also cause worsening of pain with peritonitis.
4. Muscle rigidity or guarding
    a. **Involuntary guarding**—reflex flexion of abdominal muscles secondary to **peritonitis**
    b. Voluntary guarding—flexion on abdominal muscle in anxious and tender patients; can be relieved by encouraging relaxation and flexing the knees

D. EXAMINATION OF PELVIC CAVITY
1. Suprapubic palpation and percussion
2. Rectal examination: A gloved, lubricated finger should be inserted 3–4 inches into the rectum. The rectal canal should be palpated in all directions.
    a. Pressing forward: In male patients, the examiner can detect a distended bladder, an enlarged prostate, or diseased seminal vesicles. In female patients, pain and swelling in Douglas pouch or an enlarged uterus can be detected.
    b. Passing the finger more proximal can detect a rectal stricture, polyps, or metastatic implants.
    c. Pressing laterally: Tender, inflamed appendix or pelvic sidewall abscess can be identified.
    d. Pressing anteriorly: Pelvic abscess or a Blumer shelf (carcinomatous implants) can be detected.
3. Digital examination of stomas: Assess for strictures, parastomal hernias, or foreign bodies.
4. Bimanual pelvic and speculum examination
    a. Palpate bilateral adnexal regions.
    b. Examine cervix.
    c. Obtain cultures for sexually transmitted diseases.

TABLE 21.1

SIGNS AND FINDINGS ON PHYSICAL EXAMINATION

Signs/Findings	Description	Associated Clinical Condition(s)
Charcot triad	Intermittent right upper quadrant abdominal pain, jaundice, and fever	Choledocholithiasis
Courvoisier sign	Palpable, nontender gallbladder in presence of clinical jaundice	Periampullary neoplasm
Cullen sign	Periumbilical darkening of skin from blood	Hemoperitoneum (especially in ruptured ectopic pregnancy)
Cutaneous hyperesthesia	Increased abdominal wall sensation to light tough	Parietal peritoneal inflammation secondary to inflammatory intraabdominal pathology
Fothergill sign	Abdominal wall mass that does not cross midline and remains palpable when rectus muscle is tense	Rectus muscle hematoma
Grey Turner sign	Local areas of discoloration around umbilicus and flanks	Acute hemorrhagic pancreatitis
Iliopsoas sign	Elevation and extension of leg against pressure of examiner's hand causes pain	Appendicitis (retrocecal) or inflammatory mass in contact with posts
Kehr sign	Left shoulder pain when patient is supine or in the Trendelenburg position (pain may occur spontaneously or after application of pressure to left subcostal region)	Hemoperitoneum (especially ruptured spleen)
Murphy sign	Palpation of right upper abdominal quadrant during deep inspiration results in right upper quadrant abdominal pain and cessation of inspiration	Acute cholecystitis
Obturator sign	Flexion of right thigh at right angles to trunk and external rotation of same leg in supine position results in hypogastric pain	Appendicitis (pelvic appendix); pelvis abscess, inflammatory mass
Rovsing sign	Pain referred to McBurney point on application of pressure to descending colon	Acute appendicitis

21

ACUTE ABDOMEN

IV. LABORATORY EXAMINATION

Laboratory tests may be useful; however, they can be misleading, and the clinical evaluation should have the most weight when making the diagnosis. For example, with acute appendicitis, a patient may have a normal white blood cell count, and patients with acute intraabdominal hemorrhage may have normal hemoglobin. Laboratory tests should be ordered as an adjunct to the history and physical examination. They should also be ordered to evaluate specific organ systems.

A. WHITE BLOOD CELL COUNT
1. Determines the degree of leukocytosis and the differential

B. HEMATOCRIT

1. The hematocrit can indicate anemia, whether chronic (microcytic or macrocytic) or acute.
2. Hemoconcentration may indicate hypovolemia.

C. PLATELET COUNT

1. Thrombocytopenia is consistent with severe sepsis.

D. ELECTROLYTES

1. Electrolytes are indicative of volume status and may demonstrate gastrointestinal losses from diarrhea or protracted vomiting (e.g., hypochloremic hypokalemic metabolic alkalosis or "contraction alkalosis").
2. Hyperglycemia can be observed in diabetic ketoacidosis or sepsis-induced glucose intolerance.

E. ARTERIAL BLOOD GAS

1. Arterial blood gases measure metabolic acidosis or alkalosis. Metabolic acidosis in the presence of generalized abdominal pain in older adults is ischemic gut until proven otherwise.

F. LIVER FUNCTION TESTS

1. Bilirubin (direct and total) and alkaline phosphatase concentration increases in biliary obstruction and increased transaminase concentration in hepatocellular injury or hepatitis.

G. AMYLASE LEVEL INCREASE

1. Amylase level increases are seen in pancreatitis, although it is relatively nonspecific. It may be increased in mesenteric ischemia, perforated duodenal ulcer, ruptured ovarian cyst, and renal failure. The serum lipase determination is more sensitive.

H. URINE STUDIES

1. Urinalysis—may be of limited value in patients with chronic indwelling catheters
2. Pregnancy test

I. TROPONINS

Cardiac ischemia can manifest as upper abdominal pain.

V. RADIOGRAPHIC EVALUATION

The radiographic evaluation may be helpful; however, in most patients, the diagnosis can be made from a thorough history and physical examination.

A. UPRIGHT CHEST RADIOGRAPH

1. Look for pneumonia.
2. Look for free air under the diaphragm, suggestive of a perforated viscus.

B. ABDOMINAL RADIOGRAPH

Look for bowel distention and air (in general, **air in small bowel is abnormal**) and fluid levels consistent with ileus or obstruction, as well as bowel gas cutoff versus air through to rectum.

1. Localized ileus ("sentinel loop") may indicate location of inflammatory process (i.e., pancreatitis).
2. Abnormal calcifications—chronic pancreatitis, 10% of gallstones, 90% of renal calculi
3. Pneumatosis coli (air in the bowel wall) and air in the biliary tree (pneumobilia) are ominous signs of dead gut.
4. Mass effect from tumor or abscess
5. Volvulus can also be identified on plain film.
   a. Cecal volvulus is identified by a distended loop of colon in a comma shape (coffee bean).
   b. Sigmoid volvulus looks like a bent inner tube (apex in right upper quadrant).

Clinical Pearl: *The best opportunity to see free air under the diaphragm is in an upright chest radiograph or in the left lateral decubitus position after the patient has been upright or in the decubitus position for at least 10 minutes before the radiograph.*

C. ULTRASONOGRAPHY

Ultrasonography is of value in visualizing the hepatobiliary tree, pancreas, vascular structures, kidneys, pelvic organs, and intraabdominal fluid collections. It is inexpensive and noninvasive, but operator dependent.

D. COMPUTED TOMOGRAPHY SCAN

Computed tomography (CT) scan is beneficial in some cases of acute abdominal pain but is costly, takes time, and can cause allergic reactions and nephropathy. However, CT is helpful for some causative agents. When ordering a CT scan, the clinician must understand and consider the value and/or risks of oral contrast and the period of time allowed for transit of contrast before scanning. The addition of oral contrast in the patient with high-grade or complete bowel obstruction may be hazardous secondary to the osmotic load and volume.

1. Acute pancreatitis—helpful in distinguishing among pancreatic necrosis, abscess, or pseudocyst
2. Blunt trauma—can diagnose solid organ injuries
3. Ruptured aortic aneurysm
4. Acute appendicitis—usually a clinical diagnosis. In certain cases, CT can be helpful.
   a. For symptom duration longer than 4 days, CT can demonstrate a perforation and abscess that may be amenable to nonoperative percutaneous drainage.
   b. CT may be used for obese patients for whom a reliable examination cannot be obtained.
   c. Patients with acute appendicitis who get a CT scan as part of their work-up do not have a greater incidence of rupture.
   d. There is a lower negative appendectomy rate in female patients.

ACUTE ABDOMEN

21

VI. INITIAL TREATMENT AND PREOPERATIVE PREPARATION

A. ASSESSMENT
1. Prompt work-up and differential diagnosis (see pain location for differential diagnosis)

B. DIET
1. Keep the patient NPO (nothing by mouth) until the diagnosis is firm and the treatment plan is formulated.

C. INTRAVENOUS FLUIDS
1. Intravenous fluid administration should be started early and based on expected fluid losses; large volumes may be required.
2. Correct electrolytes.
3. Central access may be needed.

D. HEMODYNAMIC MONITORING
1. May be required in cases in which fluid status and cardiac status are in question or when septic shock is present

E. NASOGASTRIC TUBE
1. Should be inserted for bleeding, vomiting, or signs of obstruction, or when urgent or emergent laparotomy is planned in a patient who has not been NPO

F. FOLEY CATHETER
1. Use to monitor fluid resuscitation.

G. TREATMENT
1. Immediate surgery
   a. Obtain consent of patient.
   b. In the face of sepsis, fluid resuscitation should precede surgery.
   c. Use appropriate preoperative antibiotics based on suspected pathology.
   d. Develop a primary operative plan.
2. Admit and observe patient for possible operation.
   Serial examinations should be performed every 2–4 hours during the first 12–24 hours in cases without definite diagnosis and clearly documented in the medical record. Use narcotics and sedatives minimally to avoid masking physical signs and symptoms until treatment plan has been established. Monitor vital signs frequently.

RECOMMENDED READING

Silen W. *Cope's Early Diagnosis of the Acute Abdomen*. 21st ed. New York: Oxford University Press; 2005.

Abdominal Wall Hernias

Richard S. Hoehn, MD

I tried to contain myself ... but I escaped!

—Gary Paulsen

I. HISTORICAL PERSPECTIVE

Numerous surgeons and anatomists have participated in the development of the modern-day herniorrhaphy. Several warrant particular interest because of their major contributions to early hernia surgery.

A. HENRY MARCY (1837–1924)
1. Boston surgeon who described anterior approach to hernia repair with high ligation of the hernia sac in 1871

B. EDOARDO BASSINI (1844–1924)
1. In 1887 he wrote "Nuevo Metodo Operativo per la Cura Radicale dell'Ernia Inguinale." In this landmark article, he described the "triple layer" consisting of the internal oblique muscle, transversus abdominis muscle, and transversalis fascia.

C. SIR ASTLEY COOPER (1768–1841)
1. Published his description of inguinal anatomy and repair, which included a description of the superior pubic ligament, in 1804. He himself had a right indirect hernia as a teenager and wore a truss for 5 years.

D. CHESTER MCVAY (1911–1987)
1. Submitted his thesis on groin anatomy in 1939 for a doctorate at Northwestern University, asserting that normal groin anatomy involved Bassini's "triple layer" inserting on Cooper's ligament, not the inguinal ligament. In 1942, while a resident at the University of Michigan, he reported his technique of groin hernia repair, which included the critical "relaxing incision."

E. EDWARD EARLE SHOULDICE (1890–1965)
1. His interest in treatment of inguinal hernias developed in 1930s. The Shouldice Hospital opened in 1945 and has performed more than 300,000 hernia repairs since.

F. IRVING LICHTENSTEIN AND PARVIZ AMID
1. Revolutionized hernia surgery with their "Lichtenstein open 'tension-free' mesh repair of inguinal hernias." They reported four recurrences in more than 4000 patients.

II. TERMINOLOGY

A. HERNIA

1. Protrusion of a part or structure through the tissues normally containing it; from the Latin for "rupture"

B. REDUCIBILITY

1. Contents of the hernia sac can be returned to their normal location.

C. INCARCERATION

1. Nonreducible hernia sac contents that, in the acute setting, may present with obstructive symptoms and pain, among other symptoms. This may also occur chronically and be essentially asymptomatic.

D. STRANGULATION

1. Incarcerated hernia with vascular compromise of contents of the sac leading to gangrene and perforation of hollow viscus if left untreated. This is a surgical emergency and is often accompanied by obstructive symptoms (exception is Richter hernia), pain (potentially focal peritonitis), leukocytosis, fever, and skin changes (e.g., warmth, erythema).

III. NATURAL HISTORY

A. INCIDENCE

1. Approximately 5% of all people will develop a hernia in their lifetime.
   a. Lifetime risk reported variably in the literature: males 5%–24%; females 1%–2%
2. Likelihood of strangulation increases with age.
   a. Only 1%–3% of all hernias will strangulate.
   b. Femoral hernias have a significantly greater rate of strangulation at 15%–20%.
3. Inguinal hernias make up 75% of all abdominal wall hernias.
   a. Indirect hernias are the most common type of hernia regardless of sex and outnumber direct hernias 2:1 in men.
   b. Right-sided hernias are more common than left because of the slower descent of the right testicle and the delay in atrophy of the processus vaginalis.
4. Femoral hernias account for 10% of abdominal wall hernias, yet upward of 40% will present as surgical urgency or emergency in the form of an incarcerated or strangulated hernia.
   a. Predominance of right-sided femoral hernias is thought to be due to the occluding effect of the sigmoid colon on the left femoral canal.

IV. ANATOMIC CONSIDERATIONS

A. LAYERS OF THE ABDOMINAL WALL

1. The layers of the abdominal wall in order of encounter while performing groin hernia surgery are skin, subcutaneous fat (Camper), Scarpa fascia, external oblique muscle laterally and aponeurosis medially, internal oblique muscle, transversus abdominis muscle, transversalis fascia, and peritoneum.

B. INGUINAL CANAL

1. It is a fibrous canal that contains the spermatic cord, the ilioinguinal nerve, the genital branch of the genitofemoral nerve, and hernia sac, if present.
2. The canal is bordered inferiorly by the inguinal ligament, superiorly by the conjoint tendon and the reflections of the transversus abdominis and the internal oblique muscle, anteriorly by the external oblique aponeurosis, and posteriorly by the transversalis fascia.

C. SPERMATIC CORD

1. Complex of structures exiting the abdomen, traversing the inguinal canal, and entering the scrotum
2. Composed of the testicular artery, pampiniform plexus of veins, vas deferens, cremasteric muscle fibers, genital branch of genitofemoral nerve, and hernia sac (if indirect hernia present, sac typically lies anteromedial to the cord structures)

D. PROCESSUS VAGINALIS

1. Diverticulum of parietal peritoneum that descends from the abdomen along with the testicle and comes to lie adjacent to the spermatic cord. This structure subsequently obliterates in normal development to remain as the tunica vaginalis.

E. DEEP (INTERNAL) INGUINAL RING

1. Composed of fibers of the internal oblique muscle superiorly, and transversalis fascia and inferior epigastric vessels inferomedially

F. SUPERFICIAL (EXTERNAL) INGUINAL RING

1. Composed of a medial and lateral crus of the external oblique aponeu-rotic fibers that is traversed by the spermatic cord (in male individuals) or round ligament (in female individuals), as well as branches of the ilioinguinal and genitofemoral nerves

G. HESSELBACH TRIANGLE

1. Site of direct inguinal hernia. Formed by lateral border of the rectus abdominis muscle medially, inferior epigastric vessels laterally, and the inguinal ligament inferiorly

H. INGUINAL (POUPART) LIGAMENT

1. Fibrous band formed by the thickened inferior border of the external oblique aponeurosis that inserts laterally on the anterior superior iliac spine of the ileum and medially on the pubic tubercle
2. Forms the inferior wall of the inguinal canal

I. ILIOPUBIC TRACT

1. Thickening of transversalis fascia inferiorly leading in to inguinal (Poupart) ligament, only 7–8 mm

22

ABDOMINAL WALL HERNIAS

J. LACUNAR (GIMBERNAT) LIGAMENT

1. Medial reflection of the inguinal ligament that reflects inferiorly from the pubic tubercle to the pectineal line of the pubis. Acts as the medial border of the femoral canal

K. PECTINEAL (COOPER) LIGAMENT

1. Fibrous band that joins the lacunar ligament medially and runs laterally along the pectineal line of the pubis

L. FEMORAL CANAL

1. Serves as the location for femoral hernias and is defined anatomically by the lacunar ligament medially, the femoral vessels laterally (namely the femoral vein), the inguinal ligament anteriorly, and the Cooper ligament posteriorly

Surgical Pearl: *Femoral canal contents from lateral to medial are NAVEL—nerve (femoral nerve), artery (femoral artery), vein (femoral vein), empty space (site of femoral hernia), and lymphatics.*

M. INFERIOR LUMBAR (PETIT) TRIANGLE

1. Site of Petit hernia formed by the lateral border of latissimus dorsi medially, posterior/medial margin of the external oblique laterally, and by the iliac crest inferiorly

N. SUPERIOR LUMBAR (GRYNFELTT) TRIANGLE

1. Site of Grynfeltt hernia formed by 12th rib superiorly, the sacrospinous muscle medially, and the lateral border of the internal oblique muscle inferiorly

V. CLASSIFICATION OF HERNIAS

A. GROIN HERNIAS (FIG. 22.1)

1. Indirect inguinal hernia—the sac exits through internal ring, lateral to the inferior epigastric vessels. Hernia sac is found anteromedial to the spermatic cord in males and the round ligament in female individuals.
2. Direct inguinal hernia—the sac exits through Hesselbach triangle, medial to the inferior epigastric vessels.
3. Pantaloon hernia—inguinal hernia that involves both indirect and direct components straddling the inferior epigastric vessels
4. Femoral hernia—the sac exits through the femoral canal, medial to the femoral vein.

B. VENTRAL HERNIAS

1. Umbilical hernia—This may be congenital or acquired.
2. Epigastric hernia—the sac exits in the midline through the linea alba, above the umbilicus.

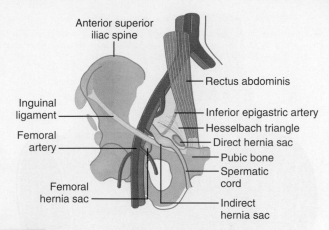

FIG. 22.1

Groin hernias.

3. Incisional hernia—defect of the fascia resulting at the site of a previous fascial closure, most commonly after a midline laparotomy; however, it may develop in the setting of any fascial repair, including those from laparoscopic surgical procedures.
4. Rectus diastasis—not a true hernia but is often mistaken for one. Represents a weakening of the linea alba and stretching of the rectus abdominis muscles away from each other. There is no sac and no true herniation of abdominal contents through this weakened layer.

C. MISCELLANEOUS HERNIAS
1. Amyand hernia—Inguinal hernia contents include appendix, described first in the setting of acute appendicitis.
2. Grynfeltt hernia—the sac exits through the superior lumbar triangle.
3. Littre hernia—Inguinal hernia contents include Meckel diverticulum.
4. Obturator hernia—the sac exits through the obturator foramen and compresses the obturator nerve and vessels.

Surgical Pearl: *Howship-Romberg sign is pain along medial thigh exacerbated by abduction, extension, and medial rotation of the thigh. This is secondary to compression on the obturator nerve whose anterior branch supplies sensory fibers to the distal medial thigh. This finding is present in only 50% of patients.*

5. Parastomal hernia—This hernia is at an ostomy site, more commonly occurring at colostomy sites, in particular, those stomas through the semilunar line.

22

ABDOMINAL WALL HERNIAS

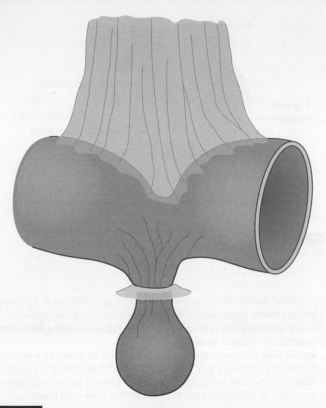

FIG. 22.2
Richter hernia.

6. Petit hernia—the sac exits through the inferior lumbar triangle.
7. Richter hernia—condition in which one sidewall of a viscus is incorporated into hernia sac, thus the hernia contents may incarcerate and strangulate without causing bowel obstruction symptoms (Fig. 22.2). Bowel may also reduce after incarceration, leading to intraabdominal perforation with peritonitis.
8. Sciatic hernia—the sac exits through the greater or lesser sciatic foramen.
9. Sliding hernia—the wall of the hernia sac is composed of a viscus (commonly sigmoid colon, cecum, or bladder) (Fig. 22.3).
10. Spigelian hernia—This abdominal hernia is through the semilunar line of Spigelius (lateral to the rectus abdominis), most commonly

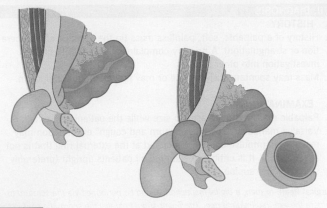

FIG. 22.3
Sliding hernia.

22

ABDOMINAL WALL HERNIAS

at the junction of the semilunar line and the semicircular line of Douglas (the point at which the posterior rectus sheath terminates).

VI. CAUSATIVE FACTORS

A. INDIRECT INGUINAL HERNIA
1. Persistence of a patent processus vaginalis is the primary causative factor in pediatric population; in adults, the cause is likely multifactorial.

B. DIRECT INGUINAL HERNIA
1. Considered to be an acquired phenomenon related to chronic increases in intraabdominal pressure, placing stress in the area of Hesselbach triangle, as well as inguinal floor weakness

C. FEMORAL HERNIA
1. Similar to the causes of direct inguinal hernias involving chronic increases in abdominal pressure together with anatomic variability. Femoral hernias are particularly at risk for incarceration and subsequent strangulation, given the relative rigidity of the structures that make up the femoral canal.

D. CONTRIBUTING FACTORS
1. Contributing factors include obesity, smoking, chronic cough, connective tissue disorders, chronic straining from constipation/obstipation, prostatism, pregnancy, and ascites.

VII. DIAGNOSIS

A. HISTORY

1. History of a palpable, soft, painless mass (in the absence of incarceration or strangulation). A primary complaint of pain should prompt investigation into other sources.
2. Mass may spontaneously reduce or may require manual reduction.

B. EXAMINATION

1. Palpable mass that increases in size while the patient performs the Valsalva maneuver. The classic "turn and cough" examination may result in an impulse being appreciated at the external ring that is not a true hernia. It is critical to examine all patients upright (preferably standing) and supine.

Surgical Pearl: *In men, a digital inspection should be performed via the scrotum to palpate the external inguinal ring. The finger should parallel the spermatic cord in the scrotum to follow it up to its exit point at the external ring.*

2. Examination should focus on location of hernia relative to inguinal ligament.
3. Hernias below inguinal ligament may be a femoral hernia.
4. Femoral hernias may reflect above inguinal ligament as well, making it difficult to distinguish between an inguinal and a femoral hernia.
5. Obesity may make it difficult to appreciate small hernias.
6. Obturator, lumbar, sciatic, Spigelian, and small femoral hernias may be easily missed on physical examination.
7. Computed tomography or ultrasound may demonstrate hernias not appreciated on physical examination and serve as a useful adjunct to the physical examination.

C. SMALL BOWEL OBSTRUCTION

1. May be the first manifestation of a hernia. A thorough examination for any hernias should always be included in the work-up for obstructive symptoms.

D. DIFFERENTIAL DIAGNOSIS OF GROIN MASS

1. Inguinal/femoral hernia, hydrocele, varicocele, inguinal lymphadenitis, ectopic testes, lipoma, epithelial inclusion cyst, neoplasms, arterial aneurysm/pseudoaneurysm

E. REDUCTION OF INCARCERATED HERNIA

1. Position the patient in steep Trendelenburg position, use adequate sedation, and place ice on hernia. Taxis (process of reducing hernia) requires paradoxical traction on the hernia sac while applying gentle pressure at the neck of the hernia to reduce the contents. This is thought to decrease edema of intestinal contents and also decrease the volume of sac contents being reduced at any one time.

2. Significant tenderness, induration, erythema, or leukocytosis suggests possible strangulation and should prompt urgent surgical exploration; if these signs/symptoms are present, no reduction should be attempted.

F. REDUCTION EN MASSE
1. Reduction of the hernia sac and contents without exploration of the sac or freeing of the contents within. Patients should be observed after reduction for any signs or symptoms of strangulation.

VIII. PREOPERATIVE CONSIDERATIONS
A. PATIENT COMORBIDITIES AND RISK FACTORS
1. Characteristics that predispose patients to wound complications and hernia recurrence
   a. Smoking
   b. Diabetes
   c. Chronic obstructive pulmonary disease (COPD) (poor oxygenation + chronic cough)
   d. Obesity
   e. Chronic steroid use
2. Patient selection/risk modification
   a. Smoking cessation or reduction for 4 weeks before hernia repair has demonstrated reduced complications.
   b. Weight loss programs, as well as bariatric surgery before or during hernia repair, have demonstrated reduced risk of recurrence.
   c. Optimize nutrition to ensure proper healing.

B. LAPAROSCOPIC VERSUS OPEN REPAIRS
1. Approach and choice of repair should be based on surgeon expertise, experience, and the anatomy of each hernia defect.
2. Ventral and umbilical hernias
   a. For defects less than 3–4 cm in size, open primary repair is adequate.
   b. For larger ventral and incisional hernias, laparoscopic repair may offer fewer complications, decreased length of stay, and reduced risk of recurrence compared with open repair.
      (1) Open repair with mesh: 10%–25% recurrence
      (2) Laparoscopic repair with mesh: 3%–11% recurrence
   c. Laparoscopic repair may offer technical advantages for smaller hernias in obese patients.
3. Inguinal and femoral hernias
   a. Open mesh repairs have been the standard for several decades. As a result, most surgeons have more experience with these techniques. There is no consensus regarding open versus laparoscopic repairs for primary inguinal hernias.
      (1) Open techniques have been shown to have shorter operating time, lower costs, and slightly lower recurrence rates.

22

ABDOMINAL WALL HERNIAS

b. Laparoscopic repairs are recommended for recurrent or bilateral inguinal hernias.
   (1) May offer less chronic pain and earlier return to normal daily activities
c. Some suggest reserving laparoscopic repairs for bilateral or recurrent inguinal hernias, but this remains controversial.

IX. INGUINAL/FEMORAL HERNIA REPAIR

A. OPEN REPAIR

1. Considerations for all anterior repairs
   a. Current acceptable recurrence rates are 1%–2%.
      (1) Tissue repairs have generally fallen out of favor because of their high recurrence rate (>10%).
      (2) Many favor tissue repairs in the setting of strangulated hernias to avoid mesh infection.
   b. Uniformly, a transverse/oblique skin incision is made, and the external oblique aponeurosis is incised, revealing the contents of the inguinal canal.
   c. Key to success is a tension-free reapproximation of the tissues.
2. Bassini repair: Bassini described an interrupted suture repair of his "triple layer"—the internal oblique muscle, transversus abdominis, and transversalis fascia to iliopubic tract/inguinal ligament.
   a. Repair is flawed because of tension.
3. McVay (Cooper ligament) repair: This is the only anterior tissue repair approach that treats all three groin hernia types—indirect, direct, and femoral.
   a. Standard tissue repair for groin hernias in which mesh is contraindicated (e.g., strangulated hernia contamination). This repair relies on approximation of the conjoined tendon to Cooper ligament medially and the inguinal ligament laterally.

Surgical Pearl: *The "relaxing incision" on the anterior rectus sheath allows this operation to be relatively tension free.*

Surgical Pearl: *The "transition" stitch is critical to this repair and is the suture placed just medial to the femoral vein transitioning from approximation to Cooper ligament to approximation to the inguinal ligament. If this suture is placed too far laterally, compression of the femoral vein may occur, which increases the risk for venous thrombosis.*

4. Shouldice repair: This technique expanded on the Bassini repair and has essentially replaced it as a tissue repair. The critical difference is the use of a continuous, nonabsorbable suture that sequentially reinforces the inguinal floor.
   a. This repair will treat inguinal hernias but not femoral hernias.
   b. The Shouldice Clinic reports a recurrence rate of 0.5%. In appropriate settings, this is a suitable repair option.

5. Lichtenstein repair: This is considered the current standard for open inguinal herniorrhaphy because it is a tension-free repair.
   a. This involves securing a piece of synthetic mesh (classically polypropylene) medially to the pubic tubercle, inferiorly to the shelving edge of the inguinal ligament (iliopubic tract), and superiorly to the rectus abdominis, internal oblique, and transversus abdominis.
   b. This repair recreates the floor of the inguinal canal and the deep (internal) inguinal ring, with the spermatic cord passing through the lateral portion of the mesh.
   c. Resection of the ilioinguinal nerve appears to decrease the long-term incidence of groin pain.
6. Plug-and-patch repair: involves placing a cone-shaped mesh plug into the inguinal or femoral defect, with the outer rim of mesh sutured to the edge of the defect. For inguinal hernias, an onlay mesh is also placed over the entire inguinal floor.

B. FEMORAL HERNIAS

1. Given the high propensity relative to other hernia types for femoral hernias to incarcerate and strangulate, all femoral hernias should be repaired when diagnosed.
2. McVay (Cooper ligament) tissue repair
3. Nyhus repair: This is a posterior, preperitoneal tissue repair advocated for repair of indirect, direct, and femoral hernias. The presence of a satisfactory iliopubic tract is necessary for this repair.
   a. Of note, the Nyhus approach to repair of the femoral hernia involves suturing of the iliopubic tract to Cooper ligament, thus obliterating the femoral canal.

C. LAPAROSCOPIC REPAIR

1. Anatomy of the preperitoneal space (Fig. 22.4)
   a. "Triangle of doom"—bounded medially by the vas deferens and laterally by the gonadal vessels. The external iliac vessels run in this triangle.
   b. "Triangle of pain"—bounded by gonadal vessels medially, iliopubic tract superiorly, and the pelvic sidewall inferolaterally. The genitofemoral nerve and lateral femoral cutaneous nerve are at risk for injury if mesh is tacked down in this area.
2. Transabdominal preperitoneal (TAPP) approach
   a. General anesthesia, the patient supine with arms tucked
   b. Intraabdominal laparoscopy with three ports: a 10-mm angled camera in infraumbilical port, and bilateral lower quadrant ports for dissection
   c. Hernia contents are reduced into the abdomen.
   d. Incision of peritoneum lateral to medial umbilical fold and entry into preperitoneal space, peeling peritoneum inferiorly. This exposes the

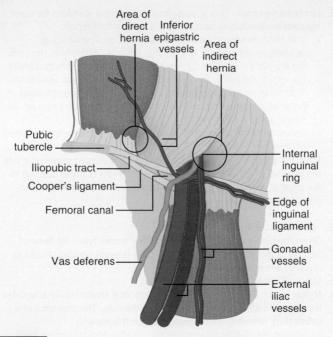

FIG. 22.4

Key landmarks of the inguinal anatomy in the preperitoneal space and typical locations of direct, indirect, and femoral hernias. From Geis WP, Crafton WB, Novak MJ, Melago M. Laparoscopic herniorrhaphy: results and technical aspects in 458 consecutive procedures. *Surgery.* 1993;114:765.

inferior epigastric vessels, the pubic symphysis, Cooper ligament, and the iliopubic tract.

   (1) Avoid the "triangle of doom."

  e. Reinforcement of posterior abdominal wall with mesh, thereby closing the hernia defect. It is critical to secure mesh to Cooper ligament and pubic symphysis medially, rectus sheath superiorly, and transversalis fascia laterally.

   (1) Mesh can be placed directly on the cord or "key-holed" around the cord.

   (2) All tacks should remain above the iliopubic tract to avoid neurovascular structures. Avoid lateral abdominal wall to prevent nerve entrapment.

  f. Peritoneum is then reapproximated over mesh, thereby preventing direct contact between mesh and bowel.

g. Advantages
   (1) Reduction of hernia sac may be technically easier, and hernia sac contents can be directly visualized, particularly if concern for viability exists.
h. Disadvantages
   (1) Procedure traverses abdominal cavity, incurring attendant risks for visceral and vascular injury.
   (2) If the peritoneum is inadequately closed, there is risk of contact between bowels and mesh, which may increase risk for small bowel adhesions or fistulization, or both.

3. Total extraperitoneal preperitoneal (TEPP) approach
   a. General anesthesia, the patient supine with arms tucked. Ten-millimeter skin incision in infraumbilical position with incision of the anterior rectus sheath lateral to the midline on the affected side. A dissecting balloon is then inserted in the preperitoneal space and used to dissect this plane, then insufflated.
   b. Two 5-mm ports are placed in the midline between the pubis and the camera port.
   c. Dissection and repair of the hernia are the same as for TAPP.
   d. Advantages
      (1) Because the peritoneum is not disrupted, ideally there is no contact between intraabdominal contents and mesh.
   e. Disadvantages
      (1) TEPP is more difficult than TAPP to reduce a large hernia sac.
      (2) If peritoneum is unintentionally violated, loss of pneumoperitoneum may make dissection difficult.

X. VENTRAL/UMBILICAL/INCISIONAL HERNIA REPAIR

A. OPEN REPAIR

1. Primary suture herniorrhaphy for small hernia defects
2. Suture repair with mesh for larger defects
   a. Mesh may be placed as underlay (intraperitoneal), inlay (preperitoneal/retrorectus), or onlay.
3. Component separation
   a. External oblique aponeurosis is incised 1 cm lateral to the rectus sheath and separated from the internal oblique.
      (1) For hernias less than 15 cm in transverse diameter, this may be achieved by inserting a laparoscope in between the oblique tissue plains, inferior to the 11th rib.
   b. Successful component separation allows up to 10-cm medial mobilization of the rectus sheath for primary suture repair.
      (1) Mesh underlay or onlay should be considered to reinforce the repair.
4. Rives-Stoppa repair (giant prosthetic reinforcement of the visceral sac): This is a preperitoneal approach to hernia repair that is useful for treating recurrent groin hernias (in particular, incisional hernia),

bilateral hernias, or high-risk hernias (those likely to recur). The basic principle is using a large synthetic mesh to either reinforce or replace the transversalis fascia placed in the preperitoneal plane.

5. Transversus abdominis release (TAR)
   a. TAR involves modified Rives-Stoppa repair with posterior component separation and retrorectus mesh placement.
   b. Posterior rectus sheath is mobilized and then incised laterally to allow division of transversus muscle.
   c. Posterior sheath is then reapproximated in the midline, mesh is placed in the retromuscular space, and the midline anterior rectus sheath is closed.
   d. Early data from this approach are very promising.

B. LAPAROSCOPIC REPAIR

1. Laparoscopic or robotic intraperitoneal repair
   a. Initial laparoscopic entry is usually preferred in the subcostal region.
      (1) Use 5- or 10-mm angled laparoscope.
      (2) Use 3–4 trocars for lateral aspects of the hernia defect.
   b. Adhesiolysis, the most challenging part of the case, is performed with a combination of sharp, blunt, and cautery dissection.
      (1) Cold scissors should be used in proximity to bowel to avoid delayed cautery injury.
   c. Measure the hernia defect—Mark all four cardinal positions after complete release of carbon dioxide from the abdomen.
   d. Roll and insert mesh through trocar or trocar site.
      (1) For defects less than 5 cm, absorbable tacks may be sufficient for fixing mesh to the abdominal wall.
      (2) For larger defects, preplace 2–4 transfascial sutures on mesh and affix with transabdominal laparoscopic suture passer.
      (3) Release insufflation as much as visualization will allow.
      (4) Absorbable tacks will then be placed in between sutures.
   e. Mesh should overlap the defect by at least 5 cm on all aspects.

2. Laparoscopic or robotic preperitoneal repair
   a. Rectus sheath and peritoneum dissected from the overlying abdominal wall
   b. Mesh placed in the preperitoneal space
   c. May be combined with TAR

XI. POSTOPERATIVE COMPLICATIONS

A. RECURRENT HERNIA

1. This may be related to missed hernia intraoperatively or failure of repair. Repairs under tension are most likely to recur. Mesh inguinal repairs most commonly fail medially.

2. Recurrence rates are greater in patients with chronic cough, constipation, smoking, and obesity. Attempts should be made before surgery to correct these conditions if at all possible.

3. Technical errors
   a. Excessive suture line tension
   b. Failure to adequately reconstruct internal ring
   c. Failure to identify indirect hernia or femoral hernia sac during initial operation
   d. Failure to repair laxity in the inguinal floor

B. INFECTION

1. Infection rates were thought to be greater among mesh repairs; however, this has never been demonstrated in the literature, and the repairs likely share a similar rate of infection when similar elective cohorts are compared.

C. BLEEDING

1. Bleeding may occur in the preperitoneal space and track retroperitoneally, as well as into the scrotum. A significant amount of bleeding may occur before recognition, and a high index of suspicion must be maintained after surgery in any patient with tachycardia, hypotension, or orthostasis.

Surgical Pearl: *If worsening scrotal hematoma occurs, reexploration should be performed via inguinal incision to identify and ligate the source of bleeding.*

D. DYSEJACULATION

1. This is seen in male patients after hernia repair and was initially reported by the Shouldice Clinic, citing an incidence rate in long-term follow-up of 0.25%. Patients may develop a searing pain with ejaculation, and this is thought to be related to constriction of the vas deferens.

E. TESTICULAR ATROPHY

1. This is a long-term complication resulting from chronic testicular ischemia. This is seen more commonly in recurrent hernia repairs.

F. DIFFICULTY VOIDING

1. This is more common in older men. A thorough history before surgery should focus on symptoms of prostatism, and if the hernia is stable, adequate treatment should be sought before hernia repair.

G. NEUROMA/NEURITIS

1. Usually results from entrapment of sensory nerve fibers, in particular the ilioinguinal nerve. Symptoms may resolve; however, persistence of symptoms may require reexploration and ligation of the nerve.

H. PAIN

1. Scrotal swelling may result from inadequate hemostasis intraoperatively or impairment of testicular venous return after surgery.

22

ABDOMINAL WALL HERNIAS

I. URINARY RETENTION

1. Most common complication, particularly in men

RECOMMENDED READINGS

Montgomery A. The battle between biological and synthetic meshes in ventral hernia repair. *Hernia*. 2013;17:3–11.

Pisanu A, et al. Meta-analysis and review of prospective randomized trials comparing laparoscopic and Lichtenstein techniques in recurrent inguinal hernia repair. *Hernia*. 2015;19:355–366.

Rogmark P, et al. Short-term outcomes for open and laparoscopic midline incisional hernia repair: a randomized multicenter controlled trial: the ProLOVE (prospective randomized trial on open versus laparoscopic operation of ventral eventrations) trial. *Ann Surg*. 2013;258:37–45.

Gastrointestinal Bleeding

Richard S. Hoehn, MD

The only weapon with which the unconscious patient can immediately retaliate upon the incompetent surgeon is hemorrhage.

—William Stewart Halsted

Gastrointestinal (GI) bleeding can be characterized and managed by its location. Upper GI bleeding is defined as bleeding originating proximal to the ligament of Treitz, whereas lower GI bleeding occurs distal to the ligament of Treitz.

I. HISTORY

History and physical examination can elucidate the cause of GI bleeding. This assessment should be conducted simultaneously with resuscitation.

A. CHARACTERIZATION OF BLEEDING

1. Hematemesis (bright red or coffee-ground emesis): usually indicates an upper GI source
2. Hematochezia (bloody stool): usually a lower GI source but may also be caused by brisk upper GI bleeding
3. Melena (black tarry stool): caused by gradual bleeding, usually from an upper GI source
4. Occult blood (guaiac positive stool): may be an upper or a lower GI source
5. Avoid mistaking massive pulmonary, upper airway, or nasopharyngeal hemorrhage for GI source.

B. CAUSATIVE FACTORS

1. Iatrogenic: GI instrumentation (nasogastric tube, colonoscopy, esophagogastroduodenoscopy [EGD])
2. Ulcerogenic agents: steroids, aspirin, nonsteroidal antiinflammatory drugs, alcohol, and tobacco
3. Severe stress: major trauma or massive burns (Curling ulcer), intracranial pathology (Cushing ulcer)
4. Blunt or penetrating trauma

C. ADDITIONAL MEDICAL HISTORY

1. Painless bleeding: varices, angiodysplasia, diverticulosis, or cancer
2. Epigastric pain: ulcer disease, gastritis, or esophagitis
3. Cramping abdominal pain: diverticulitis, inflammatory bowel disease, colitis, or partially obstructing cancer

4. Severe, acute, sudden onset of pain: usually indicates perforated viscus
5. Pain out of proportion to examination: hallmark for bowel ischemia
6. Prior surgical interventions: marginal ulcers, arterioenteric fistulae
7. Chronic alcohol or drug use: risk factors for liver disease precipitating gastric varices
8. Fevers and chills: infectious or inflammatory causative agent
9. Weight loss, anorexia, and fatigue: malignancy
10. Dizziness, orthostatic symptoms: indicate large, acute volume loss or severe anemia

II. PHYSICAL EXAMINATION

A. GENERAL APPEARANCE
1. Pallor, diaphoresis, anxiety all concerning for hemorrhagic shock

B. VITAL SIGNS
1. Blood pressure: hypotension or orthostatic changes (decline in systolic blood pressure >20 mm Hg on standing)
2. Pulse: tachycardia (>110 beats/min indicates >15% blood loss)
3. Temperature: may be increased with infection or falsely low or normal with dehydration

C. SKIN
1. Jaundice, palmar erythema, and spider angiomata are associated with cirrhosis and portal hypertension

D. HEAD AND NECK
1. Inspection may reveal sclera icterus or an oropharyngeal source of hemorrhage

E. ABDOMEN
1. Abdominal distention, caput medusae, scars from prior vascular surgery
2. Bowel sounds: usually increased with upper GI bleeding
3. Palpation to localize abdominal tenderness, masses, ascites, hepato-splenomegaly

F. DIGITAL RECTAL EXAMINATION
1. Attention should be paid to presence of hemorrhoids, anal fissures, fistula, or rectal mass.
2. Include stool guaiac.

III. INITIAL MANAGEMENT

A. ASSESS THE MAGNITUDE OF HEMORRHAGE.
1. Is the patient stable or unstable?

B. **STABILIZE HEMODYNAMIC STATUS.**
1. Use two large-bore intravenous lines.
2. If patient is stable, begin resuscitation with isotonic crystalloid solution.
3. For patients in hemorrhagic shock, initiate a balanced blood component resuscitation.
   a. Plasma (fresh frozen plasma [FFP]), platelets, and packed red blood cells (pRBCs) in 1:1:1 ratio
4. Place Foley catheter to facilitate monitoring of intravascular volume status.
5. Place nasogastric tube to protect against aspiration, as well as aid in diagnosis (see later).

C. **MONITOR FOR CONTINUED BLOOD LOSS.**
1. For unstable patients or those with continued, unidentified bleeding, transfer them to intensive care unit.
   a. Continuously monitor vital signs with hourly urinary output.
   b. Transfuse for active bleeding or to maintain hemoglobin greater than 7 g/dL.
   c. Pulmonary artery catheter use should be limited to patients with unclear cardiac function or pulmonary hypertension.
2. Pursue diagnostic work-up (Fig. 23.1).

IV. LABORATORY EVALUATION
A. **TYPE AND CROSSMATCH**
B. **HEMOGLOBIN/HEMATOCRIT/RED BLOOD CELLS CHARACTERISTICS**
1. Hemoglobin/hematocrit (H/H): may underestimate the volume in cases of acute blood loss before resuscitation because equilibration has not yet occurred
2. Hypochromia or microcytosis: chronic blood loss
3. Megaloblastosis: nutritional abnormalities caused by alcohol abuse

C. **PLATELET COUNT**
1. Thrombocytopenia: result of massive hemorrhage, cirrhosis secondary to hypersplenism

D. **PROTHROMBIN AND PARTIAL THROMBOPLASTIN TIMES**
1. Screen for coagulation defects or abnormalities.

E. **THROMBOELASTOGRAPHY**
1. This measures the speed and strength of clot formation.
   a. Time to clot, clot firmness, platelet aggregation, clot lysis
2. Determine which blood components or therapy to administer during resuscitation.
   a. Prolonged activated clotting time (ACT) or reaction (R) time: FFP
   b. Prolonged kinetic (K) time or decreased α angle: cryoprecipitate
   c. Decreased maximum amplitude (MA): platelets
   d. Elevated clot lysis (LY30): tranexamic acid

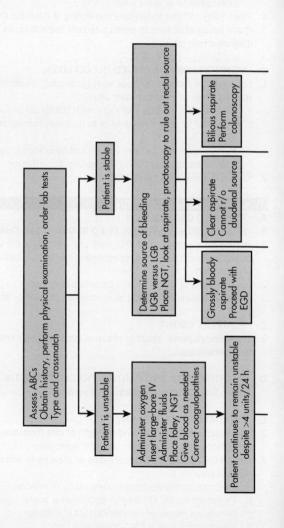

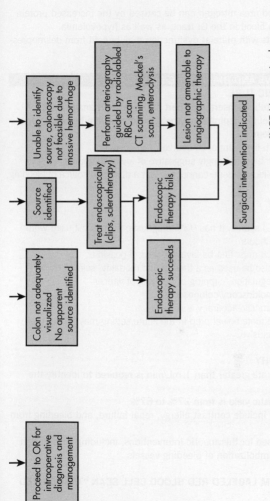

FIG. 23.1

Algorithm for evaluation of a patient with gastrointestinal bleeding. *CT,* Computed tomography; *EGD,* esophagogastroduodenoscopy; *IV,* intravenous; *LGB,* lower gastrointestinal bleeding; *NGT,* nasogastric tube; *UGB,* upper gastrointestinal bleeding.

23

GASTROINTESTINAL BLEEDING

F. RENAL PROFILE

1. Renal failure and electrolyte disturbance may be secondary to volume loss.
2. Increased blood urea nitrogen can be caused by the increased protein absorbed from blood in the GI tract, as well as hypovolemia.
3. Uremic patients with platelet dysfunction may benefit from desmopressin (DDAVP).

V. INVESTIGATIVE AND DIAGNOSTIC PROCEDURES

A. NASOGASTRIC TUBE

1. A nasogastric tube is inserted as part of the initial management.
2. The character of the aspirate may help to differentiate between upper and lower GI source.
   a. Gross blood: likely upper GI source
   b. Bile, but no blood: strongly suggestive of lower GI source
   c. Clear nonbilious effluent: cannot rule out a duodenal source of bleeding

B. ENDOSCOPY

1. EGD
   a. For upper GI source, it has 95% diagnostic accuracy if used within the first 24 hours.
   b. The stomach must first be lavaged clear, if possible.
   c. EGD may also be used as a therapeutic modality: sclerotherapy, thermal coagulation, clipping or banding of varices
2. Anoscopy/sigmoidoscopy/colonoscopy
   a. Overall diagnostic accuracy is up to 97%.
   b. Lack of adequate bowel prep in the acute setting may render these tests inconclusive.

C. ANGIOGRAPHY

1. Bleeding at a rate greater than 1 mL/min is required to identify the source.
2. Overall diagnostic yield is from 27% to 67%.
3. Complications include contrast allergy, renal failure, and bleeding from puncture site.
4. This can be used for therapeutic interventions, including vasopressin infusion and embolization of bleeding vessels.

D. TECHNETIUM-LABELED RED BLOOD CELL SCAN "TAGGED RED CELL SCAN"

1. More sensitive and less invasive but less specific
   a. Bleeding at a rate of 0.1 mL/min is required to identify source.
   b. No therapeutic interventions can be performed.
2. Best used to confirm a non–life-threatening lower GI bleed before angiography

E. COMPUTED TOMOGRAPHY
1. Radiographic contrast studies are rarely useful and may interfere with other diagnostic procedures.

VI. NONSURGICAL TREATMENT

A. ENDOSCOPIC
1. Injection of alcohol (sclerotherapy) or epinephrine
2. Often used for bleeding varices

B. ELECTROCAUTERY
1. Control of bleeding vessels from peptic ulcer disease
2. Can be used for high-risk patients during endoscopy

C. VASOPRESSIN INFUSION
1. This can be given systemically or by selective arterial infusion.
2. Selective infusion may be started at the time of the diagnostic angiogram and may minimize the systemic effects of the drugs.
3. Recent myocardial infarction or significant coronary artery disease is relative contraindication.
4. Dosage:
   a. Loading dose: 20 units over 20–30 minutes
   b. Infusion dose: 0.2–0.4 units/min

D. EMBOLIZATION
1. Embolization of colonic bleeds carries a higher risk for ischemia with perforation.

VII. DISEASE-SPECIFIC THERAPY

A. ACUTE HEMORRHAGIC GASTRITIS
1. Stress gastritis
2. It occurs after multiple traumatic injuries, massive transfusion, complicated sepsis, burns (Curling ulcer), central nervous system injury (Cushing ulcer), and steroid use.
3. Treatment includes prompt initiation of proton pump inhibitor (PPI) or H_2 blocker, possibly with adjuncts (i.e., sucralfate).
4. Targeted resuscitation of shock and coagulopathy
5. Bleeding commonly stops after lavage.
6. If unstable or with refractory bleeding, rarely requires total or near total gastrectomy; however, the mortality rate in this setting is quite high.

B. PEPTIC ULCER DISEASE
1. Bleeding in this setting is usually self-limited and responds to targeted resuscitation.
2. Treat with nasogastric decompression and PPIs (scheduled or continuous infusion).

3. Endoscopy for targeted hemostatic control
   a. For gastric ulcer, biopsy should always be performed to rule out malignancy.
   b. Pulsatile bleeding or visible vessel is indicative of high rebleeding risk.
   c. Giant duodenal ulcer (ulcer >2 cm) will most likely require surgical intervention.

4. Treatment for *Helicobacter pylori*
   a. More than 85% of ulcer patients are colonized, and treatment is crucial to preventing recurrence.
   b. Diagnose with urea breath test, stool studies, serologic studies, or surgical pathology.
   c. Use triple therapy: PPI, metronidazole, clarithromycin/amoxicillin.

5. Surgery for failure of medical therapy

C. ESOPHAGOGASTRIC VARICES

1. Primary management is with pharmacologic therapy and endoscopic banding.
   a. Pharmacologic therapy: vasopressin infusion, beta-blockers
   b. Endoscopy (banding, sclerotherapy)
   c. Success rate at controlling bleeding: 90%

2. If the bleeding cannot be controlled endoscopically, balloon tamponade is indicated.
   a. Sengstaken-Blakemore tube
   b. Four-port Minnesota tube: This tube has a gastric balloon, an esophageal balloon, and aspiration ports for the esophagus and the stomach. The gastric balloon is inflated first and placed on traction. If the bleeding is not controlled, the esophageal balloon is then inflated. Pressure in the balloon is released in 24–48 hours to prevent necrosis.

3. Surgical management to prevent rebleeding:
   a. Transjugular intrahepatic portosystemic shunt (TIPS)
      (1) If the patient is a candidate for transplant, surgical shunting should be avoided.
      (2) If the patient is not a transplant candidate, surgical shunts are an option.
         (a) Total decompressive shunts: side-to-side portocaval anastomosis
         (b) Partial decompressive shunts: 8-mm portocaval graft
         (c) Selective shunts: mesocaval superior mesenteric vein–inferior vena cava (SMV-IVC) graft, distal splenorenal shunt (most widely used)
         (d) All carry a risk of encephalopathy.

D. MALLORY-WEISS TEAR

1. This is a linear mucosal tear at the gastroesophageal junction secondary to violent retching or vomiting.
   a. Most heal spontaneously with supportive measures alone.

2. VATS drainage and repair may be indicated for significant leakage and contamination.
3. Endoscopic stenting can be considered.

E. DIEULAFOY LESION (EXULCERATIO SIMPLEX)
1. Rupturing of a 1- to 3-mm bleeding vessel through the gastric mucosa without any surrounding ulceration
2. It is usually found high on the lesser curvature of the stomach.
   a. No mucosal or vascular abnormalities are noted.
3. Managed endoscopically with either coagulation or mechanical application of clips or rubber bands. Endoscopic therapy has 95% success rate with excellent long-term control.
4. Operative treatment may be required if this fails (resection of lesion vs. ligation of vessel).
5. Embolization may be used in patients too ill to tolerate surgical intervention.

F. NEOPLASM
1. Benign tumors (leiomyomas, hamartomas)—hemorrhage may be controlled with wedge resection.
2. Malignant tumors—bleeding should be controlled initially with endoscopic measures.
   a. Resection of mass after stabilization

G. DIVERTICULOSIS
1. In Western societies, this affects 30% of individuals by age 60 and 60% by age 80.
   a. Lifetime risk of bleeding from diverticular disease is 25%.
      (1) A total of 10%–20% will require surgery.
   b. Half of lower GI bleeds may be from colonic diverticulum.
2. Up to 80% of hemorrhages stop spontaneously.
3. Mesenteric angiography will detect bleeding greater than 1 mL/min.
4. Coiling or direct vasopressin infusion is successful in 80% of cases.
5. Surgical therapy is rarely necessary; it is indicated for unstable patients or refractory bleeding.
   a. Exploratory laparotomy, on-table enteroscopy
   b. If no bleeding identified and colon highly suspected, total colectomy

H. ARTERIOVENOUS MALFORMATIONS
1. Incidence of colonic arteriovenous (AV) malformations is 2%–30% in older patients and less than 1% in healthy, asymptomatic adults.
   a. Can occur throughout the GI tract, commonly in the right colon
2. Diagnosis is made at the time of angiography or colonoscopy.
   a. Typically, the bleeding is chronic, slow, and intermittent.
   b. Bleeding stops spontaneously in 85%–90% of cases.

3. Treat surgically for massive acute bleeding or chronic intermittent bleeding.
   a. Segmental resection of localized segment is preferred.

I. MECKEL DIVERTICULUM

1. This is the most common congenital abnormality of the small bowel.
   a. Remnant of the proximal omphalomesenteric duct
2. Ileal ulceration may occur secondary to Meckel diverticulum containing gastric mucosa.
3. The lesion can be localized before surgery with a nuclear medicine scan.
4. Treated with segmental resection and end-to-end anastomosis or wedge resection

J. BENIGN ANORECTAL DISEASE

1. An estimated 11% of lower GI bleeding can be attributed to benign anorectal pathology.
   a. Anorectal varices caused by portal hypertension, congestive heart failure, splenic vein thrombosis
   b. Does not eliminate the possibility of a more proximal cause for hemorrhage
2. In general, patients with hemorrhoids on examination should still undergo thorough endoscopic evaluation of the colon to rule out other pathologic conditions.

K. AORTOENTERIC FISTULA

1. This occurs after abdominal aortic aneurysm repair.
2. Patients will present with a small herald bleed, usually more than 6 months after abdominal aortic aneurysm repair.
   a. Triad consists of massive GI hemorrhage, pulsatile mass, and infection.
3. It is usually found in the third or fourth portion of the duodenum at the proximal aortic suture line.
4. Computed tomographic scanning is the diagnostic procedure of choice.
   a. Air around the aorta or the aortic graft is diagnostic.
5. Resection of the graft with extraanatomic bypass is the preferred surgical treatment of choice.

RECOMMENDED READINGS

Gralnek IM, et al. Diagnosis and management of nonvariceal upper gastrointestinal hemorrhage: European Society of Gastrointestinal Endoscopy (ESGE) guideline. *Endoscopy*. 2015;47:1–46.

Lau JY, et al. Omeprazole before endoscopy in patients with gastrointestinal bleeding. *N Engl J Med*. 2007;356:1631–1640.

Villanueva C, et al. Transfusion strategies for acute upper gastrointestinal bleeding. *N Engl J Med*. 2013;368:11–21.

Intestinal Obstruction

Drew D. Jung, MD

Every day some new fact comes to light—some new obstacle which threatens the gravest obstruction. I suppose this is the reason which makes the game so well worth playing.

–Robert Falcon Scott

I. TERMINOLOGY

A. ILEUS
1. Mechanical or functional obstruction, usually caused by failure of movement of luminal contents secondary to poor motility

B. MECHANICAL OBSTRUCTION
1. Partial or complete physical blockage of lumen

C. SIMPLE OBSTRUCTION
1. Occlusion at one area of the bowel

D. CLOSED-LOOP OBSTRUCTION
1. Afferent and efferent bowel limb blockage
2. Occasionally seen with strangulation

E. STRANGULATION
1. Ischemic damage to obstructed area of bowel
2. Usually secondary to restricted circulation, can be seen with closed-loop obstruction, or caused by increased intraluminal pressure

II. CAUSATIVE FACTORS

A. SMALL BOWEL OBSTRUCTION
1. Adhesions
   a. Most common cause of small bowel obstruction (SBO) (80%)
   b. Most often as a result of prior abdominal surgery
2. Hernia
   a. Second most common cause of SBO overall; most common cause in patients who have not had previous abdominal surgery
3. Intraluminal
   a. Neoplasia
   b. Inflammation
      (1) Enteritis, Crohn disease
      (2) Radiation enteritis or stricture
   c. Gallstone ileus (older adults)—gallstone usually stuck at ileocecal valve
   d. Foreign bodies
   e. Meconium ileus

    f. Intussusception

    g. Congenital lesions

      (1) Small bowel atresia, stenosis, webs

      (2) Small bowel duplications or mesenteric cysts

      (3) Meckel diverticulum

4. **Extraluminal/mass effect**

    a. Carcinomatosis/adjacent tumor compressing bowel wall

    b. Intraabdominal abscess

    c. Hematoma

    d. Malrotation/volvulus

    e. Annular pancreas (duodenal obstruction)

    f. Endometriosis

    g. Superior mesenteric artery syndrome

      (1) Superior mesenteric artery compression of third portion of duodenum

      (2) More commonly seen in thin patients who have experienced recent dramatic weight loss

B. LARGE BOWEL OBSTRUCTION

1. **Intraluminal**

    a. Colon cancer—most common cause (60%) of large bowel obstruction

    b. Inflammation with subsequent stricture

      (1) Ulcerative colitis, Crohn disease

      (2) Diverticulitis

      (3) Radiation enteritis

    c. Congenital

      (1) Imperforate anus

    d. Ischemic colitis

    e. Foreign bodies

    f. Meconium ileus

    g. Intussusception

    h. Fecal impaction

2. **Extraluminal/mass effect**

    a. Adhesions

    b. Hernia (particularly sliding type)

    c. Volvulus

      (1) Sigmoid—60%–80% of cases

      (2) Cecal—20%–40% of cases

      (3) Transverse colon—less than 5% of cases

C. OFTEN MISDIAGNOSED AS SMALL OR LARGE BOWEL OBSTRUCTION

1. **Adynamic ileus (see later)**

2. **Vascular insufficiency**

    a. Nonocclusive mesenteric ischemia

    b. Mesenteric thrombosis
    c. Mesenteric embolism
3. Hirschsprung disease

D. ILEUS
1. Metabolic
    a. Hypokalemia, hypomagnesemia, hyponatremia
    b. Ketoacidosis
    c. Uremia
    d. Porphyria
    e. Heavy metal poisoning
2. Medications
    a. Narcotics
    b. Dopaminergics
    c. Antipsychotics
    d. Anticholinergics
    e. Ganglionic blockers
    f. Diuretics
    g. Polypharmacy
3. Infection
    a. Sepsis
    b. Peritonitis
    c. Localized process—appendicitis, cholecystitis, diverticulitis, pyelone-
       phritis, abscess, urinary tract infection
4. Retroperitoneal process
    a. Pancreatitis
    b. Hematoma
    c. Vertebral or pelvic fracture
5. Neuropathic process
    a. Diabetes mellitus
    b. Multiple sclerosis
    c. Scleroderma
    d. Lupus erythematosus
    e. Hirschsprung disease
6. Bed rest
7. Postoperative (after abdominal surgery)
    a. Return of small bowel function: 48 or fewer hours after surgery
    b. Return of gastric motility: 48 hours after surgery
    c. Return of colonic motility: 3–5 days after surgery
8. Ogilvie syndrome
    a. Pseudo-obstruction of the colon
    b. Typically older adults, institutionalized, bedridden, presence of
       retroperitoneal process, narcotic use, antipsychotics, polypharmacy
    c. Cecal dilation—more than 12 cm increases perforation risk; 23% at
       14 cm

INTESTINAL OBSTRUCTION

24

d. Treatment—decompression
   (1) Enema
   (2) Colonoscopic decompression if enema unsuccessful or if patient has significant cecal dilation—40% recurrence
   (3) Intravenous (IV) neostigmine—20% recurrence. Caution in cardiac patients (bradycardia). Should only be pursued in a monitored setting
   (4) Partial colectomy if perforated, ischemic, or colonoscopy unsuccessful; try to avoid operation, given that multiple comorbidities are typically present in this patient population.

III. PRESENTATION

A. HISTORY

1. Signs and symptoms
   a. Nausea/emesis, abdominal fullness, *decreased flatus,* constipation/obstipation
      (1) Proximal obstruction—bilious emesis early in course, minimal distention unless prolonged course. May still have bowel movements while moving bowels distal to obstruction—Patient will eventually stop passing flatus and stool.
      (2) Distal obstruction—obstipation and distention; feculent emesis if prolonged course—may see fecalization of small bowel. Obstipation is characteristic of complete obstruction.
   b. Abdominal pain
      (1) Proximal obstruction—cramping pain referred to periumbilical region; caused by bowel distention from continued peristalsis against the obstructed point. The pain may decrease after large emesis.
      (2) Distal obstruction—cramping pain referred to lower abdomen. When succeeded by continuous severe pain, suspect strangulation and peritonitis. Immediate torsion and vascular compromise of a segment of bowel can cause early obstruction and ischemia.
   c. Duration of symptoms—onset very important, quality of pain, tolerance of oral intake (liquids and solids), recent unintentional weight loss

2. Surgical and medical history
   a. Previous abdominal operations
   b. Suspicion of intraabdominal neoplasia or previous radiation for cancer
   c. History of ventral/incisional/inguinal hernia
   d. Review of medications
   e. Atherosclerotic disease, previous myocardial infarction, arrhythmia history
   f. History of inflammatory bowel disease or diverticulitis
   g. History of chronic biliary colic

3. Age
   a. Adhesions can be a source of obstruction at any age, given a history of previous intraabdominal surgery.
   b. Neonate
      (1) Meconium ileus, Hirschsprung disease, intestinal atresias, malrotation, volvulus
   c. Two to 24 months
      (1) Intussusception, Hirschsprung disease
   d. Young adult
      (1) Inflammatory bowel disease, hernia
   e. Adult
      (1) Inflammatory bowel disease, hernia, neoplasm, diverticulitis
   f. Older adult
      (1) Hernia, neoplasm, diverticulitis, Ogilvie syndrome, sigmoid/cecal volvulus

B. **PHYSICAL EXAMINATION**
   1. Fever—can suggest infectious/inflammatory process or strangulation. Patient may be afebrile if uncomplicated disease.
   2. Bowel sounds are initially active with intermittent rushes and borborygmus but decrease with time.
   3. Hiccups or belching is a sign of gastric distention.
   4. Abdominal tenderness—If localized or if patient is guarding, there is increased probability of strangulation or perforation. Tenderness may also be mild.
   5. Abdominal distention—There is tympany on percussion.
   6. Note any surgical abdominal scars.
   7. Presence of mass/hernia. You may be able to palpate fixed distended bowel loop, carcinoma, or inflammatory mass.
   8. Digital rectal examination—Note empty rectal vault versus stool impaction.
      a. Extrinsic pelvic masses and colonic lesions can sometimes be palpated on digital rectal examination.
   9. Guaiac-positive stool—cancer/inflammatory process/diverticulitis/strangulation
   10. Tachycardia—may be secondary to dehydration and hypovolemia, but can be an early indicator of strangulation, especially if patient also has increased white blood cell (WBC) count and localized tenderness

C. **LABORATORY TESTS**
   1. Leukocytosis—There may be mild increase in uncomplicated obstruction.
   2. Increased hemoglobin, hematocrit, blood urea nitrogen, and creatinine imply hemoconcentration and dehydration.
      a. Alternatively, anemia in the setting of SBO or colonic obstruction may indicate carcinoma of the colon.

24

INTESTINAL OBSTRUCTION

3. Electrolyte imbalances (particularly hypokalemia)
4. Metabolic alkalosis—usually seen in proximal SBO or pyloric obstruction. Emesis causes loss of hydrogen ion from the gastric secretions.
5. Metabolic acidosis, base deficit—typically seen late in obstruction. Normal pH does not rule out bowel infarction. Lactic acid level is nonspecific finding suspicious for ischemia.
6. Urinalysis—Rule out urinary tract infection as cause of SBO-like symptoms, especially in older adults.
7. Amylase—may or may not be increased in SBO.
8. Of note, lab values may be normal in setting of volvulus/strangulation. Collapse of venous system at level of strangulation can prevent return of products of ischemia into normal circulation. In this case, laboratory and metabolic derangements may not be seen until after reduction of hernia or resolution of volvulus.

IV. IMAGING
A. PLAIN FILMS
1. Basic principle of imaging for obstruction
   a. Determine the presence of colonic (distal) gas. Gas in the rectum favors a diagnosis of ileus, not SBO.
2. Abdominal series versus upright and flat versus supine and left lateral decubitus (Fig. 24.1)
   a. Abdominal series—upright abdominal, supine abdominal, upright chest films
   b. Air-fluid levels are seen best in upright or decubitus positions.
      (1) "Stair-step" or "ladder pattern" of air-fluid levels in distended bowel, proximal to an obstruction, can be seen progressing down the abdomen. More pronounced in obstructive disease than in ileus
   c. Distention of bowel with no stool or air in rectal vault
   d. Identification of closed loops (U shaped, "bird's beak") can indicate bowel strangulation or volvulus.
   e. Bowel gas may be seen distally with partial obstruction, in early complete obstruction, or if air has been introduced during rectal examination or enema.
   f. Note diameter of distention. **(law of Laplace: tension = pressure × radius)**
      (1) Colonic obstruction or ileus—increased risk for perforation if cecal diameter is larger than 12 cm. Consider emergent decompression.
      (2) When cecal diameter dilates acutely to 12–14 cm, wall tension exceeds perfusion pressure and focal areas of necrosis can develop. Necrosis may progress even after decompression. This can lead to bowel perforation.
   g. Sigmoid volvulus—"omega" or "bent inner tube" appearance of large, dilated bowel loop. Apex in left lower quadrant and convexity in right upper quadrant

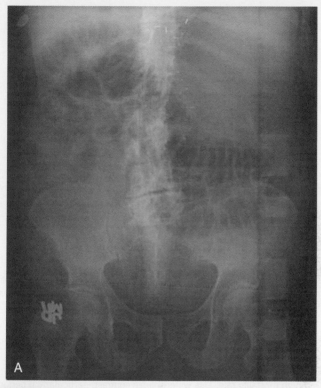

FIG. 24.1

(A) Supine abdominal plain film showing multiple loops of dilated small bowel. The plicae circulares of the small bowel are well defined secondary to the distention, helping to differentiate it from the haustral markings of the large bowel. Plicae circulares traverse the entire diameter of the small bowel; haustra extend one-half to two-thirds the diameter of the colon. This patient's small bowel obstruction was secondary to an incarcerated inguinal hernia.

    h. Cecal volvulus—large, dilated, ovoid, air-filled cecum in the upper abdomen. Caused by rotation of hypermobile cecum around the ileocolic vessels. Apex in right lower quadrant
3. Upright chest radiograph can help to rule out free air.

B. CONTRAST STUDIES
1. Contrast enema
    a. To identify the site of obstruction, not define mucosal detail. It is useful when diagnosis is uncertain.

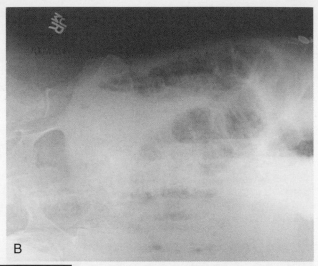

B

FIG. 24.1, cont'd

(B) Left lateral decubitus plain film from same patient as in *A*. Note the ability to define air-fluid levels with the patient in this position. (A and B, Courtesy Susan Sharp, MD, and Doan Vu, MD, Department of Radiology, University of Cincinnati.)

    b. It is most commonly used to rule out colonic (distal) obstruction.
    c. Conduct under low pressure. Free barium in peritoneal cavity has high mortality rate. Use water-soluble contrast, particularly if perforation could be present.
    d. Do not force contrast beyond partial obstruction; this can create complete obstruction.
    e. Can do before upper gastrointestinal series if distal SBO suspected. Reflux through ileocecal valve can identify a collapsed terminal ileum, confirming SBO.
    f. If intussusception is suspected in children, perform hydrostatic or air contrast barium enema. Functions as diagnosis and treatment (reduction); 60%–70% of pediatric intussusceptions reduce with enema alone. No hydrostatic reduction in adults: There is a high likelihood of neoplasm as the lead point.
    g. In sigmoid or cecal volvulus, see bird's-beak pattern at volvulus point.
2. **Upper gastrointestinal series with small bowel follow-through**
    a. This is useful if diagnosis is uncertain or to visualize a partially obstructing lesion.
    b. If colonic obstruction is suspected, rule out by performing contrast enema first.

(1) Great care must be taken when administering contrast above an obstruction; additional volume above a fixed obstruction point may exacerbate proximal bowel distention without a means for relief.

(2) However, in setting of partial SBO, administration of contrast can be both diagnostic and therapeutic.

c. This is study of choice when investigating possible malrotation.

C. COMPUTED TOMOGRAPHY

1. Sensitivity of 85% and specificity of 80% for identifying SBO; less than 50% sensitivity for identifying partial SBO

   a. If unable to find transition point on computed tomography (CT), upper gastrointestinal series with small bowel follow-through may be more sensitive.

2. Preferably oral and IV contrast

   a. Oral contrast may worsen distention in the setting of a true SBO. Can administer through nasogastric tube if patient unable to tolerate oral intake

   b. Better to give isotonic, not hypertonic, oral contrast solution to minimize osmotic distension of potentially obstructed bowel

3. Identification of transition point

   a. Dilated proximal bowel, collapsed distal bowel

   b. Inability to identify oral contrast past the point of dilation

   c. Identification of closed-loop or vascular compromise

   d. Identification of intraabdominal or intraluminal mass

V. MANAGEMENT

A. EXPECTANT/PREOPERATIVE MANAGEMENT (FIG. 24.2)

1. Early versus late postoperative obstruction

   a. Early postoperative SBO typically resolves on its own. If symptoms occur during postoperative days 1–14, the obstruction will likely resolve with bowel rest, nasogastric tube decompression, and IV hydration.

   b. After 14 days from surgery, surgical intervention is more likely required to resolve a fixed point of obstruction.

2. True complete bowel obstruction is a surgical emergency; patients should undergo exploration with few exceptions.

   a. Exceptions include partial obstruction; patient with history of previous laparotomies for bowel obstruction and now with a hostile abdomen; and severely medically debilitated patients who would have high postoperative complications and for whom the team would want to give a trial of expectant management.

   b. Partial or early SBO (patient still passing gas or stool) may also be caused by an exacerbation of inflammatory bowel disease, like Crohn disease, that may resolve. If partial SBO is the diagnosis, continue to resuscitate and evaluate.

24

INTESTINAL OBSTRUCTION

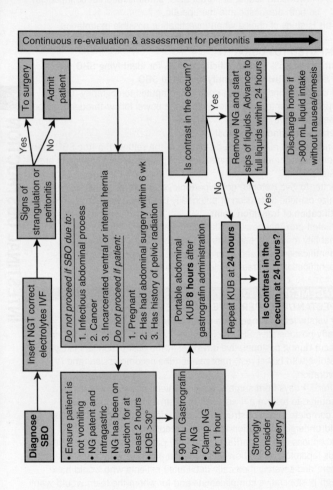

FIG. 24.2

Flow diagram for management of small bowel obstruction.
HOB, Head of bed; *IVF*, intravenous fluid; *KUB*, kidney, ureter, bladder; *NG*, nasogastric; *NGT*, nasogastric tube; *SBO*, small bowel obstruction. (Data from Azagury D. Small bowel obstruction: a practical step-by-step evidenced-based approach to evaluation, decision making, and management. *J Trauma Acute Care Surg.* 2015;79:661–668.)

3. NPO (nothing by mouth)
   a. IV hydration
   b. Correction of electrolyte imbalances
   c. Need for total parenteral nutrition if patient expected to remain NPO for longer than 7 days
4. Nasogastric tube (14 Fr at least) to continuous low suction
   a. Prevents vomiting with aspiration
   b. Partially decompresses small bowel
   c. Prevents further stomach distention due to swallowed air
5. Foley catheter to monitor urine output and success of resuscitation
6. Treatment with Gastrografin
   a. This is useful in patients with history of abdominal surgery and persistent signs and symptoms of obstruction. It is not for patients with active inflammatory bowel disease, obstructed hernias, history of hostile abdomen, hyperthyroidism, iodine allergy, or patients with signs of intestinal ischemia.
      (1) Gastrografin is a water-soluble, hyperosmolar contrast. Will draw fluid out of bowel wall, increase fluidity of succus, and may increase the likelihood of resolution of obstruction
   b. Decompress with nasogastric tube for 2 hours.
   c. If prior CT scan with contrast, obtain kidney, ureter, bladder (KUB) radiograph to determine if contrast in colon. If so, obstruction has resolved.
   d. Administer 8 mg ondansetron IV. After 30 minutes, administer 120 mL Gastrografin via nasogastric tube. Flush with 20 mL water.
   e. Keep nasogastric tube clamped for 4 hours.
   f. Obtain KUB in 24 hours. If contrast in colon, obstruction likely to resolve with nonoperative management. If no contrast in colon, consider exploratory laparotomy.

B. OPERATIVE MANAGEMENT
1. Indicated when no improvement or when worsening of patient condition during expectant management for initial diagnosis of partial obstruction
2. Antibiotic coverage of gram-negative aerobes and anaerobes
3. Operative treatment of SBO
   a. If patient exhibits signs of peritonitis, leukocytosis, fever, and tachycardia with a diagnosis of SBO, take to operating room after resuscitation. It is appropriate to presume that the patient has ischemic or necrotic bowel.
   b. If patient has complete SBO but no ischemic or necrotic bowel, resuscitate and take to operating room as soon as possible when optimal operative resources are available.
   c. Lysis of all adhesions or resection of the involved segment is recommended. Limit manipulation and surgical intervention if obstruction is caused by radiation enteritis; injured bowel may be "revascularized" by the adhesions.

24

INTESTINAL OBSTRUCTION

   d. If SBO is due to malignancy, the involved segment may need to be bypassed.

   e. If SBO is due to hernia, resect any necrotic bowel and repair hernia with autologous tissue (e.g., McVay repair with relaxing incision; lateral release for large defect). Mesh in this setting is associated with increased infection.

   f. Operative approach may be via laparoscopy or laparotomy.

4. **Operative treatment of colonic obstruction**

   a. Ischemic colon typically treated with resection and end colostomy with mucous fistula or rectal (Hartmann) pouch

   b. Obstructive right colon carcinoma

     (1) Resection and primary anastomosis if no fecal contamination, massive edema, shock, or long-standing peritonitis. Otherwise, perform resection with decompressive ileostomy and mucous fistula.

   c. Obstructive left colon carcinoma

     (1) Primary resection with colostomy and mucous fistula or Hartmann pouch

     (2) If patient is debilitated or unstable but has no abscess or perforation, perform diverting colostomy to allow decompression and stabilization. Patient should return later for resection, then colostomy closure.

     (3) Controversial data have been reported regarding success of primary anastomosis with on-table bowel preparation. This is also difficult to perform neatly, and the risk-to-benefit ratio should be carefully considered in the setting of a patient who may benefit from chemotherapy.

     (4) Colonic stenting has been described as a bridge to surgery in those not medically fit for operation, or as palliation.

   d. Obstructing diverticulitis

     (1) Resect involved segment and perform primary anastomosis or end colostomy with Hartmann pouch.

     (2) See Chapter 28 for more details.

   e. Cecal volvulus

     (1) Treat with operation. Do not attempt endoscopic reduction.

     (2) Standard of care is right hemicolectomy/ileocecectomy.

   f. Sigmoid volvulus

     (1) First, attempt decompression via sigmoidoscopy, placing rectal tube past obstruction. Immediate reduction in 80% of cases. Inspect mucosa for viability.

     (2) Greater than 50% recurrence rate; therefore recommend elective or urgent sigmoid resection after the first episode.

     (3) If you cannot endoscopically reduce it (no stool or flatus), suspect strangulation and resect emergently.

5. **Determining bowel viability: color, motility, arterial pulsation**

   a. Resect anything obviously nonviable.

b. If questionable, release adhered segment, place in warm saline-soaked gauze for 15–20 minutes, then reexamine. If bowel has normal color and motility, may be returned safely. If any further question of viability, can perform second-look laparotomy at 24–48 hours.

c. Tools to help determine viability are IV fluorescein dye and Wood lamp, Doppler examination

C. POSTOPERATIVE CARE
1. Nasogastric decompression until bowel activity returns
2. Postoperative antibiotic coverage if patient is septic or if there is gross contamination or preoperative long-standing peritonitis
3. If bowel function does not return within 7 days or if the total NPO time (including the preoperative course) is longer than 7 days, consider total parenteral nutrition.

D. PARALYTIC ILEUS
1. Common in the immediate postoperative period from intraabdominal procedure. Typically resolves after 2–3 days
2. Nasogastric decompression, IV fluids
3. Correction of electrolytes
4. Long-tube or colonoscopic decompression for severe distention
5. Exclude obstructive processes if ileus persists without an obvious cause.

VI. OUTCOMES
A. RECURRENCE
1. Ten percent of patients having undergone lysis of adhesions will obstruct in the future.
2. Incidence of recurrence increases with each subsequent operative intervention.

B. OPERATIVE MORTALITY
1. SBO
   a. Occurs in 0%–5% of cases
   b. Occurs in 4.5%–31% of cases if gangrene develops
2. Colonic obstruction
   a. Occurs in 1%–5% when caused by diverticulitis
   b. Occurs in 5%–10% when caused by carcinoma
   c. Occurs in 40%–50% in cases of bowel necrosis secondary to volvulus

RECOMMENDED READINGS
Azagury D. Small bowel obstruction: a practical step-by-step evidenced-based approach to evaluation, decision making, and management. *J Trauma Acute Care Surg.* 2015;79:661–668.

Ceresoli M. Water soluble contrast agent in adhesive small bowel obstruction: a systematic review and meta-analysis of diagnostic and therapeutic value. *Am J Surg.* 2016;211:1114–1125.

Frago R. Current management of acute malignant large bowel obstruction: a systemic review. *Am J Surg.* 2014;207:127–138.

Person B, Wexner SD. The management of postoperative ileus. *Curr Probl Surg.* 2006;43:6–65.

Vogel J. Clinical practice guidelines for colonic volvulus and acute colonic pseudo-obstruction. *Dis Colon Rectum.* 2016;59:589–600.

Peptic Ulcer Disease

Ben Huebner, MD

If anyone should consider removing half of my good stomach to cure a small ulcer in my duodenum, I would run faster than he.

—Charles H. Mayo (1865–1939)

In the era of Helicobacter pylori *doing a gastrectomy for peptic ulcer is like doing a lobectomy for pneumonia.*

—Asher Hirshberg

I. OCCURRENCE

1. Lifetime risk—10%
2. US prevalence—2%
3. Age
   a. Duodenal ulcers are more common in younger patients.
   b. Gastric ulcer incidence peaks at age 55–65 years.
4. Male predominance for both types
5. Risk factors
   a. Nonsteroidal antiinflammatory drug (NSAID) use
      (1) Chronic users have 25% prevalence rate of peptic ulcer.
      (2) Risk for adverse gastrointestinal events is three times that of healthy control subjects (>60 years, risk increases to five times normal).
   b. Cigarette smokers are twice as likely to experience development of peptic ulcer disease as nonsmokers.
   c. Stressful life events
      (1) Burn injury—Curling ulcer, can be in stomach, duodenum, or jejunum
      (2) Head injury—Cushing ulcer

II. PRESENTATION AND EVALUATION

Differential: pancreatitis, celiac disease, gastric malignancy, biliary disease, gastroparesis

A. SYMPTOMS

1. Abdominal pain (80% of cases)—epigastric, burning, may radiate to the back (uncommon)
   a. Gastric ulcer—with eating
   b. Duodenal ulcer—2–3 hours postprandial, relieved by food; also at night
2. Nausea, bloating
3. Weight loss
4. Complicated disease—worsening abdominal pain, hematemesis, melena

Erosion   Acute ulcer   Chronic ulcer

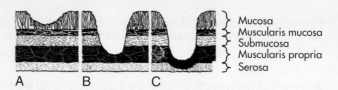

} Mucosa
} Muscularis mucosa
} Submucosa
} Muscularis propria
} Serosa

A   B   C

FIG. 25.1

Diagram of gastric erosions and ulcers. (From Dempsey DT. Stomach. In: Brunicardi FC, ed. *Schwartz's Principles of Surgery*. 8th ed. New York: McGraw-Hill; 2004:953.)

B. PHYSICAL EXAMINATION

1. Epigastric tenderness
2. Complicated disease—tachycardia, hypotension, peritonitis, older patient, persistent vomiting, jaundice, palpable mass

C. LABORATORY STUDIES

1. Positive *Helicobacter pylori* tests
2. Complicated disease—decreased hemoglobin, acidosis, or metabolic alkalosis (gastric outlet obstruction with vomiting)

D. DEFINITIVE DIAGNOSIS

Differential diagnosis: nonulcerative dyspepsia, gastric neoplasia, biliary disease, inflammatory/neoplastic disorder of pancreas

1. Esophagogastroduodenoscopy (EGD)—90% sensitivity, direct visualization of ulcer; the gold standard
2. Upper gastrointestinal series (with air and barium contrast)—75%–80% accurate, filling defect in wall

E. MODIFIED JOHNSON CLASSIFICATION

1. Type I—lesser curvature (60% of gastric ulcers)
2. Type II—synchronous ulcers in gastric body and duodenum (most common in first portion of duodenum)
3. Type III—prepyloric
4. Type IV—near gastroesophageal junction
5. Type V—related to NSAIDs, can be located anywhere, but typically greater curvature

III. PATHOGENESIS

1. Focal defect in gastric or duodenal mucosa, extending to submucosa or deeper (Fig. 25.1)

2. Increased gastric acid production
   a. Acid produced by parietal cells, located mostly in corpus of stomach
      (1) Stimulated by **acetylcholine** from branches of vagus nerve in response to smell, taste, and sight of food (cephalic phase of acid secretory response)
      (2) Stimulated by **gastrin** from G cells in antrum in response to amino acids in lumen (gastric phase)
          (a) Gastric distension also stimulates acetylcholine and gastrin release.
      (3) **Histamine**, released from enterochromaffin-like cells (basal acid secretion), mediates large portion of parietal cell stimulation in response to acetylcholine and gastrin release.
      (4) Inhibited by somatostatin, released from D cells in response to antral acidification
   b. Zollinger-Ellison syndrome is characterized by pancreatic, duodenal, or nodal gastrinoma, leading to increased gastrin secretion.
      (1) Cases are 80% sporadic and 20% inherited (most common tumor associated with multiple endocrine neoplasia type 1, tend to be multiple tumors; see Chapter 62).
      (2) Diarrhea is most common symptom.
      (3) Peptic ulcer disease is present in 90% of patients with Zollinger-Ellison syndrome.
      (4) It is diagnosed by increased gastrin levels (can be falsely increased with proton-pump inhibitor [PPI] use) and confirmed by secretin stimulation test (increase of 200 pg/mL serum gastrin after 2 units/kg intravenous secretin bolus)
      (5) Fifty percent are malignant.
      (6) Surgical enucleation of gastrinoma is curative in 60% of patients.
      (7) Most are found in gastrinoma triangle (junction of second and third portions of duodenum, junction of cystic and common bile ducts, junction of head and neck of pancreas).
      (8) Preoperative localization is by computed tomography scan, transabdominal ultrasound, endoscopic ultrasound, or octreotide scan (gastrinoma cells contain type 2 somatostatin receptors, which bind radiolabeled somatostatin analogue with high affinity). In rare situations, angiography with selective venous sampling may be used.
      (9) Intraoperative localization—exploration of gastrinoma triangle/pancreas, longitudinal duodenotomy, sampling of lymph nodes (portal, peripancreatic, celiac). Intraoperative ultrasound is helpful in identifying the lesion.
   c. Duodenal ulcers, concurrent duodenal and gastric ulcers (Johnson type II), and prepyloric gastric ulcers (Johnson type III) are associated with increased acid production.
3. Weakened mucosal defenses
   a. Defenses consist of mucosal barrier, bicarbonate secretion, and healthy epithelial cell barrier.

b. Mediators of defense system include prostaglandins and nitric oxide.
   (1) NSAIDs inhibit prostaglandin production.
   (2) Cigarette smoking inhibits prostaglandin and bicarbonate production.
c. Gastric outlet obstruction causes increased exposure of gastric mucosa to acid and can overwhelm defenses.
d. Gastric ulcers along the lesser curvature (Johnson type I), near the gastroesophageal junction (Johnson type IV), and those associated with pills (Johnson type V) are associated with weakened defenses.

IV. HELICOBACTER PYLORI

1. **Characteristics**
   a. Oxidase-positive, catalase-positive, microaerophilic gram-negative rod
2. **Associations**
   a. Associated with 90% of duodenal ulcers and 70%–90% of gastric ulcers (85% of peptic ulcers overall)
3. **Fifty percent of adults worldwide and 33% of adults in the United States are infected.**
4. **Associated, although not causally, with gastric cancer and mucosa-associated lymphoid tissue lymphoma**
5. **Predisposes to ulcer formation by both increasing acid production and weakening defenses**
   a. Local alkalinization of antrum leading to increased acid production
      (1) To survive in acidic environment, *H. pylori* possesses urease, which converts urea to ammonia and bicarbonate.
      (2) Increased bicarbonate → inhibition of D cells → decreased somatostatin production → less inhibition of G cells → hypergastrinemia → increased acid in stomach
   b. Colonization of duodenum leading to decreased bicarbonate production
      (1) Antral epithelial metaplasia of the duodenum secondary to increased acidity
      (2) Leads to further decrease in bicarbonate production
   c. Production and release of toxins (vacA, CagA) and cytokines (interleukin-8)
6. **Diagnosis of infection**
   a. Endoscopic biopsy, if endoscopy is otherwise indicated
      (1) Histologic analysis to directly visualize organisms (gold standard)
         (a) Benign features: smooth, regular, rounded edges
         (b) Concerning features (suggestive of malignancy): ulcerated mass protruding into lumen, thickened/irregular ulcer margins
      (2) Rapid urease test (CLOtest)—sensitivity of 80%–95%, specificity of 95%–100%; do not use if patient taking PPI/antibiotics
   b. Serologic test—test of choice when endoscopy not indicated; "scar" remains after eradication following treatment; sensitivity of 80%, specificity of 90%

   c. Fecal antigen test—for active infection and to confirm cure
   d. Urea breath test—gold standard to confirm cure after 4 weeks of treatment
      (1) Ingest urea labeled with ^{13}C, which is converted to CO_2 by urease and exhaled as $^{13}CO_2$
   e. Culture only with treatment failure, when antibiotic resistance is suspected, or when ulcer has concerning features
7. Treatment of known infection
   a. "Triple therapy" (amoxicillin, clarithromycin, and PPI) for eradication of infection
      (1) Adequate for eradication in 90%
      (2) May substitute metronidazole for amoxicillin
      (3) Levofloxacin for resistant strains

V. TREATMENT OF UNCOMPLICATED DISEASE

A. PREVENTION
1. High-risk NSAID users (>60 years, before gastrointestinal event, concomitant steroid use or anticoagulation, high NSAID dose) should take a PPI.

B. EMPIRIC MEDICAL THERAPY
For peptic ulcer if patient younger than 45 years, no alarm symptoms (weight loss, recurrent vomiting, dysphagia, bleeding/anemia)
1. Smoking cessation
2. Avoidance of NSAIDs
3. Acid-reducing medication alone
   a. PPIs (omeprazole, pantoprazole), OR
   b. Selective histamine H_2 receptor blockers (ranitidine, famotidine)
4. Continue treatment for 3 months.
5. Consider testing for *H. pylori* if infection is suspected, and change to eradication therapy for positive test.
6. If no improvement in symptoms, change to *H. pylori* eradication therapy, even with no test or with negative results.

C. CONCERN FOR GASTRIC CANCER
1. If patient older than 45 years, or with alarm symptoms (weight loss, >65 years at diagnosis)—EGD with test for *H. pylori* and biopsy of edges of gastric ulcer

D. SURGICAL THERAPY
1. Indicated for bleeding, perforation, obstruction, or intractability

VI. TREATMENT OF COMPLICATED DISEASE

A. CONCERN FOR GASTRIC CANCER
With complicated disease:
1. All gastric ulcers visualized during surgical procedure should undergo biopsy (ulcer edges).

25

PEPTIC ULCER DISEASE

B. BLEEDING PEPTIC ULCER

1. Most common complication
   a. Present with nausea, hematemesis (either red or coffee ground), or melena
   b. Most common location in the duodenum is posteroinferior from the gastroduodenal artery.
2. Most common cause of death for peptic ulcer (10%–20% mortality rate), greater with bleeding gastric ulcers because patients are typically older with more comorbidities
3. Initial treatment—nothing by mouth (NPO) and PPI drip; 75% stop bleeding with this therapy
4. EGD to control bleeding by cauterization, epinephrine injection, or clipping
5. Early surgical therapy (without prior EGD) indicated for patients presenting in shock, requiring greater than 4 units of blood in 24 hours, in patients older than 60 years, or in patients with recurrent bleeding ulcer disease
6. Surgical therapy after EGD indicated with failure of endoscopic control of bleeding, rebleeding after endoscopy, ulcer location on lesser curvature, or posterior duodenal bulb (because of risk for erosion into large vessels)
7. Surgical options
   a. Unstable patient—oversewing to control bleeding
   b. Stable patient—vagotomy and drainage or vagotomy and antrectomy depending on patient history, characteristics, and location of ulcer

C. PERFORATED PEPTIC ULCER

1. Second most common complication
   a. Sudden onset severe diffuse abdominal pain
   b. Duodenal most common (60%) followed by antral (20%) and gastric body (20%)
2. Surgery always indicated, unless patient is stable with radiographic demonstration of sealed perforation
3. Surgical options—laparoscopic comparable with open approach
   a. Unstable patient or significant peritoneal contamination—omental patch
   b. Stable patient (duodenal ulcer)—patch with PPI therapy, highly selective vagotomy (HSV), or vagotomy and drainage
   c. Stable patient (gastric ulcer)—removal of ulcer by excision and primary repair of stomach; antrectomy is ideal, or patch with PPI and *H. pylori* therapy

D. OBSTRUCTION

1. Acute (caused by inflammation) or chronic (caused by cicatrix)
2. Ulcers located in the pyloric channel or duodenum
3. Symptoms: early satiety, bloating, indigestion, nausea, vomiting, epigastric pain, weight loss

4. Acute obstruction—can be managed by nasogastric decompression
5. Endoscopic balloon dilation associated with 50% recurrence rate
6. Surgical options (patients typically stable, or resuscitated from acute obstructive event)—vagotomy and antrectomy, vagotomy and drainage, or HSV with gastrojejunostomy

E. INTRACTABILITY—CURRENTLY RARE
1. Differential diagnosis—gastric cancer, noncompliance with PPI therapy, gastric motility disorder, Zollinger-Ellison syndrome
2. Surgical options—HSV; HSV and wedge resection

VII. DETAILS OF SURGICAL OPTIONS

A. HIGHLY SELECTIVE VAGOTOMY (OR PROXIMAL GASTRIC OR PARIETAL CELL)
1. Surgical technique—ligation of vagus nerve branches to proximal two-thirds of stomach
   a. Vagal innervation to pylorus controls relaxation of the pyloric sphincter, and thus denervation of pylorus may require a drainage procedure.
   b. May be performed laparoscopically
2. Mortality rate: approximately 0.5%, which is the highest of procedures discussed
3. Decreases acid production by 65%–75% (similar to PPI therapy)

B. OMENTAL (GRAHAM) PATCH
1. Surgical technique: patch of greater omentum loosely placed over perforated portion of duodenum, with or without (true Graham patch) underlying primary closure of duodenum
2. Low mortality; recurrence rate unchanged unless acid-reducing procedure performed in addition to patch
3. Historically described for duodenal perforation but may also be used for perforation of gastric ulcer

C. VAGOTOMY AND DRAINAGE
1. Surgical technique—truncal vagotomy (denervates pylorus), plus drainage of stomach by pyloroplasty or gastrojejunostomy
   a. Heineke-Mikulicz pyloroplasty—close longitudinal incision in transverse fashion
   b. Gastrojejunostomy—loop of proximal jejunum sutured to dependent part of greater curvature, antecolic or retrocolic fashion
2. Low mortality; 10% recurrence rate
3. Ten percent of patients experience dumping or diarrhea after pyloroplasty.

D. VAGOTOMY AND ANTRECTOMY
1. Surgical technique—excision of antrum, leaving 60%–70% gastric remnant, with reestablishment of continuity with either gastroduodenostomy (Billroth I), loop gastrojejunostomy (Billroth II), or Roux-en-Y gastrojejunostomy

2. Greater mortality rate; should be avoided in hemodynamically unstable patients
3. Low recurrence rate
4. Gastrojejunostomy side effects possible

E. DISTAL GASTRECTOMY

1. Surgical technique—excision of antrum and portion of stomach affected by ulcer, leaving 40%–50% gastric remnant, with Billroth I, Billroth II, or Roux-en-Y reconstruction
2. Similar mortality, recurrence, and side-effect profile as vagotomy and antrectomy

F. POSTOPERATIVE COMPLICATIONS

1. Early dumping (5%–10% of patients)—occurs after pyloroplasty or gastrojejunostomy
   a. Postprandial diaphoresis, weakness, light-headedness, tachycardia, followed by diarrhea
   b. Caused by abrupt delivery of hyperosmolar load into small bowel, leading to peripheral and splanchnic vasodilatation
   c. Relieved by supine position
   d. Treated initially by dietary modification (small, frequent, low-fat, low-carbohydrate, high-protein, low-liquid meals), octreotide
   e. Most patients improve with time, after months or years.
   f. Reoperation in rare patients—Roux-en-Y gastrojejunostomy to slow gastric emptying
2. Late dumping—occurs after pyloroplasty or gastrojejunostomy
   a. Similar symptoms to early dumping, occurring 2–3 hours postprandial
   b. Due to hypoglycemia from release of large amount of insulin
   c. Treat by eating carbohydrates when symptoms occur; acarbose
3. Diarrhea (5%–10% of patients)—occurs after vagotomy, pyloroplasty, or gastrojejunostomy
   a. Differentiate from dumping by lack of other symptoms.
   b. Mechanism caused by accelerated transit, bile acid or fat malabsorption, or blind loop syndrome (see later).
   c. Treatment options include loperamide, cholestyramine, pancreatic enzymes, and trial of empiric antibiotics.
4. Delayed gastric emptying—occurs after gastrojejunostomy
   a. Characterized by emesis, epigastric distension or pain, and weight loss
   b. Evaluate objectively by gastric emptying scan (nuclear medicine)—liquid transit is typically normal, and solid transit is delayed.
   c. Must rule out mechanical obstruction by EGD, upper gastrointestinal series.
   d. Treat with promotility agents (erythromycin, metoclopramide).
   e. Reoperation in rare patients—more extensive gastrectomy accompanied by Roux-en-Y gastrojejunostomy

5. Afferent loop syndrome—occurs after Billroth II
   a. Characterized by bilious emesis (sometimes 1–2 hours postprandial), epigastric distension or pain, weight loss
   b. Caused by obstruction of afferent intestinal limb (containing duodenum and coming toward stomach), either acutely by postoperative edema or chronically by intermittent obstruction
   c. Malabsorption caused by bacterial overgrowth in afferent limb, leading to deconjugation of bile salts ("blind loop syndrome")
   d. Treat with antibiotics if blind loop syndrome is suspected; reoperation (conversion to Roux-en-Y gastrojejunostomy)

6. Efferent loop syndrome
   a. Primarily associated with internal hernia but may also be due to adhesive disease
   b. Present with symptoms of small bowel obstruction: colicky abdominal pain, nausea, vomiting

7. Roux stasis syndrome
   a. Believed to be due to dysmotility due to disconnection of transected Roux limb from duodenal pacemaker
   b. Present with early satiety, postprandial vomiting, and epigastric pain
   c. Initial treatment with promotility agents (metoclopramide, erythromycin), dilation by endoscopy
   d. Surgical therapy consists of subtotal gastrectomy with reconstruction.

8. Marginal ulcer—occurs after gastrojejunostomy
   a. Presents with abdominal pain, bloating, vomiting
   b. Diagnose with EGD, usually on intestinal side of anastomosis
   c. Usually responds to medical therapy with PPI; refractory cases require reoperation

9. Bile reflux gastritis—occurs most often after Billroth II
   a. Symptoms include nausea, epigastric pain, bilious vomiting.
   b. May occur years after initial operation
   c. Treat with PPI or sucralfate and rarely reoperation (Roux-en-Y gastrojejunostomy with long Roux limb).

10. Cholelithiasis—caused by vagotomy with disruption of vagal branches to gallbladder, leading to bile stasis

11. Nutritional deficiencies after gastrojejunostomy
    a. Weight loss may be caused by insufficient intake (due to early satiety or dietary modifications to treat dumping or diarrhea) or malabsorption.
    b. Iron deficiency: Iron absorption requires acidic environment.
    c. Vitamin B12 deficiency: Parietal cells synthesize intrinsic factor, which is necessary for vitamin B12 absorption.
    d. Calcium deficiency: This is caused by poor absorption of calcium (which occurs in duodenum) or vitamin D (fat-soluble vitamin).

25

PEPTIC ULCER DISEASE

RECOMMENDED READINGS

Behrman SW. Management of complicated peptic ulcer disease. *Arch Surg.* 2005;140: 201–208.

Dempsey DT. Stomach. In: Brunicardi FC, ed. *Schwartz's Principles of Surgery.* 8th ed. New York: McGraw-Hill; 2004:933–995.

Marshall BJ, Warren JR. Unidentified curved bacilli in the stomach of patients with gastritis and peptic ulceration. *Lancet.* 1984;1:1311–1315.

Inflammatory Bowel Disease

J. Leslie Knod, MD

The state of the health of the individual is equivalent to the state to the health of the colon.

—Woody Harrelson

I. INFLAMMATORY BOWEL DISEASE

A. ULCERATIVE COLITIS
1. Diffuse inflammatory disease limited to mucosa of colon and rectum
2. Operative therapy is almost always curative; indicated for refractory disease, toxic distension, or dysplasia

B. CROHN DISEASE
1. Chronic, relapsing, transmural, usually segmental, and often granulomatous inflammatory disorder involving any portion of the gastrointestinal (GI) tract from mouth to anus; most common in the terminal ileum
2. Surgical intervention reserved for treatment of complications or intractable disease

C. INDETERMINATE COLITIS
1. A total of 15% of cases are indistinguishable between ulcerative colitis (UC) and Crohn disease (CD).

D. ETIOLOGY
Etiology is unknown, likely multifactorial. Theories include:
1. Environmental factors include diet or infection (viral and bacterial), as well as smoking (smoking in CD exacerbates disease flares; may be therapeutic in UC), alcohol, and oral contraceptives.
2. Genetics may play a role considering 10%–30% of inflammatory bowel disease (IBD) patients report a family history of disease, incidence is higher in white United States and Northern European populations, and it is associated with human leukocyte antigen phenotypes.
3. Immunologic factors including the interaction between the intestinal immune system, mucosal barrier of the gut, and infectious agents are involved in the pathophysiology. Because of similarity between extraintestinal manifestations and rheumatologic disorders, autoimmune defects are also a theory.

II. EXTRAINTESTINAL MANIFESTATIONS

A. CUTANEOUS
Often correspond to disease severity and should improve with treatment of affected bowel

1. Erythema nodosum is present in 5%–15% of IBD patients.
   a. Women are affected 3–4 times more frequently than men.
   b. Characteristic lesions are red, raised, and predominately located on lower legs.
2. Pyoderma gangrenosum is uncommon.
   a. Begins as erythematous plaque, papule, or bleb generally located on pretibial region of leg or occasionally near a stoma. May progress to ulcerated, painful, and necrotic wound

B. OCULAR
1. Occurs in up to 10% of IBD patients and often arises during acute flare
2. Includes uveitis, iritis, conjunctivitis, and episcleritis

C. MUSCULOSKELETAL
1. Arthritis
   a. Incidence 20 times greater than in general population
   b. Often improves with treatment of colonic disease
2. Sacroiliitis, ankylosing spondylitis
   a. Unaffected by medicosurgical treatment of colonic disease
3. Associated with human leukocyte antigen-B27

D. HEPATOBILIARY
Liver common site for extracolonic disease
1. Fatty infiltration of liver
   a. Occurs in 40%–50% of patients with IBD and may be reversed by treatment of colonic disease
2. Cirrhosis
   a. Develops in 2%–5% of patients with IBD and is irreversible
3. Primary sclerosing cholangitis
   a. A total of 40%–60% with primary sclerosing cholangitis have UC.
   b. Progressive disease is characterized by strictures of intrahepatic and extrahepatic bile ducts.
   c. It is not reversed by colectomy; the only treatment is liver transplantation.
4. Pericholangitis
5. Bile duct carcinoma
   a. It is a rare complication of long-standing disease.
   b. Generally, patients are 20 years younger than the average patient with bile duct carcinoma.

III. ULCERATIVE COLITIS
A. PATHOPHYSIOLOGY AND DISTRIBUTION
1. Inflammation is limited to the mucosa and submucosa, not transmural. The rectum is always (95%) involved, and disease spreads contiguously throughout the colon only. "Backwash ileitis" may be present in the terminal ileum but is related to proximal colonic disease, not primary small bowel disease.
2. Crypt abscesses may be present or inflammatory pseudopolyps.

B. **EPIDEMIOLOGY**
1. There is a bimodal age at onset, in third and seventh decades.
2. Incidence is 8–15 per 100,000 people in United States and Northern Europe.

C. **CLINICAL MANIFESTATIONS**
1. Signs and symptoms
   a. Characterized by exacerbations and remissions. Related to degree and extent of mucosal inflammation
   b. Most common: *bloody* diarrhea, rectal bleeding, tenesmus (proctitis)
   c. Less common: cramping abdominal pain, weight loss, fever, malnutrition
   d. Rare: vomiting, perianal disease, abdominal mass
   e. Clinical spectrum ranges from (1) inactive (quiescent) phase, to (2) low-grade active disease, or (3) fulminant disease.
   f. Onset may be insidious or acute and fulminant.
      (1) Fulminant colitis (toxic megacolon) develops in 10% of cases with additional symptoms of severe abdominal pain and fever.

D. **DIAGNOSIS**
1. Laboratory findings
   a. Anemia, leukocytosis, increased erythrocyte sedimentation rate
   b. Ensure negative stool cultures for infection, ova, and parasites
   c. Severe disease leading to hypoalbuminemia, dehydration, electrolyte/vitamin depletion, and steatorrhea
2. Serologic markers
   a. Perinuclear antineutrophil cytoplasmic antibody (pANCA+)
3. Radiographic findings
   a. Plain films
      (1) Abdominal radiographs will evaluate colonic distension during acute phase to exclude toxic megacolon.
      (2) Upright chest radiograph will rule out pneumoperitoneum due to perforation.
   b. Barium enema
      (1) Less sensitive than colonoscopy and may not detect early disease
      (2) Mucosal irregularity, "collar-button" ulcers, and pseudopolyps
      (3) Chronic disease leading to foreshortened colon that lacks haustral markings, "lead pipe" colon
      (4) Strictures: uncommon and should raise suspicion for malignancy
4. Endoscopy ± biopsy
   a. Essential for diagnosis and determination of disease extent
   b. Findings
      (1) Early: mucosal edema with loss of normal vascular pattern, confluent erythema, and rectal involvement
      (2) Moderate:
         (a) Granularity, friable mucosa with contact bleeding, multiple inflammatory pseudopolyps
         (b) Pus and mucus present

26

INFLAMMATORY BOWEL DISEASE

      (3) Late: foreshortened colon, discrete ulcers, mucosa replaced by scar

  c. Do not perform colonoscopy during acute colitis flare because of risk of perforation.

5. Pathology

  a. During acute phase, biopsy often shows only nonspecific inflammation.

  b. In the chronic phase, depletion of mucosal goblet cells, mucosal atrophy, and crypt abscesses are noted.

  c. Inflammatory polyps may be present in the healing stage.

E. COMPLICATIONS

1. Rectal or colonic strictures

  a. Highly uncommon because disease is limited to the mucosa

  b. Presumed to be malignant until proved otherwise

2. Toxic colitis with or without megacolon (10% of cases)

  a. May be initial presentation of UC in 30% of cases

  b. Greatest risk for perforation with initial attack of toxic megacolon

  c. Clinical findings—fever, abrupt onset of bloody diarrhea, abdominal pain, nausea, vomiting, abdominal distention, systemic toxicity

  d. Radiographic findings—transverse colon >6 cm in diameter on plain abdominal films

  e. Perforation can lead to localized abscess or generalized peritonitis.

  f. Mortality

    (1) With perforation: 40%

    (2) With surgery before perforation: 2%–8%

  g. Treatment

    (1) Treat with aggressive intravenous fluid resuscitation, electrolyte repletion, and broad-spectrum intravenous antibiotics.

    (2) Bowel rest with nasogastric tube decompression; consider total parenteral nutrition.

    (3) Avoid colonoscopy, barium enema, and antidiarrheal agents.

    (4) Medical treatment includes high-dose intravenous steroids and/or immunosuppression.

    (5) Rule out infectious causes of toxic distension, such as *Clostridium difficile* and cytomegalovirus (CMV).

    (6) Surgery is indicated if conservative therapy fails after 24 hours, patient clinically deteriorates, or free perforation, peritonitis, or massive hemorrhage develops.

      (a) Perform total abdominal colectomy with end ileostomy with delayed restorative procedure.

      (b) Proctectomy and ileoanal anastomosis can be performed in delayed fashion.

3. Massive hemorrhage—can occur in toxic colitis, although rare

  a. Treatment is total abdominal colectomy and end ileostomy.

4. Colorectal cancer
   a. Risk is related to severity and extent of disease (i.e., pancolitis).
   b. After 8–10 years, risk of colorectal cancer increases 1%–2% above baseline risk for average American adult annually.
   c. It is more common in patients with initial colitis before 25 years of age.
   d. If a stricture is present, must rule out carcinoma.
   e. Carcinoma often arises from areas of flat dysplasia (in contrast with sporadic colon cancer), which is difficult to diagnose at an early stage. Therefore periodic surveillance with random biopsies is indicated.
   f. Perform surveillance colonoscopy annually in patients with pancolitis after 8 years, or left-sided colitis after 12 years.
      (1) Colonoscopy with four-quadrant biopsies should be obtained every 10 cm from the cecum to the rectum, as well as biopsies of suspicious lesions to identify dysplasia.
         (a) Invasive carcinoma present in up to 20% of patients with low-grade dysplasia.
         (b) Any patient with multifocal low-grade dysplasia, or high-grade dysplasia anywhere, should have proctocolectomy.

5. Malnutrition
   a. Decreased oral intake because of abdominal pain and obstructive symptoms leads to low caloric intake, while diarrhea contributes to protein losses and ongoing inflammation leads to a catabolic physiologic state.
   b. It can result in failure to thrive and poor growth in children.
   c. Nutritional status should be assessed before surgical intervention by nutritional parameters such as prealbumin, transferrin, and retinol-binding protein.

F. MEDICAL MANAGEMENT
1. Treatments are geared to decrease inflammation and alleviate symptoms. Mild-to-moderate flares can often be treated on an outpatient basis, whereas more severe flares require hospitalization.
2. Aminosalicylates—sulfasalazine, mesalamine, olsalazine, balsalazide
   a. First-line agents for mild-to-moderate disease and require direct contact with affected mucosa. They are also good for sustaining remission.
   b. Mechanisms of action are decreases inflammation by inhibiting cyclooxygenase and 5-lipoxygenase in gut mucosa.
      (1) Inhibit prostaglandins and leukotriene production
      (2) Inhibit bacterial peptide-induced neutrophil chemotaxis
      (3) Scavenge reactive oxygen metabolites
   c. Enemas may be used for proctitis and proctosigmoiditis.
   d. Side effects are dose-related toxicity and include oligospermia, inhibition of folate absorption, hemolytic anemia, nausea, vomiting, headaches, abdominal discomfort, and allergic hypersensitivity (10%–15%).

26

INFLAMMATORY BOWEL DISEASE

    e. Sulfasalazine
      (1) Conjugated to prevent small bowel absorption
      (2) Metabolized by bacteria to 5-aminosalicylic acid (the active component) and sulfapyridine, which is responsible for major side effects
    f. Mesalamine
      (1) This has fewer side effects than sulfasalazine at comparable doses.
      (2) Various formulations allow different areas to be targeted.
        (a) Rowasa, Canasa—rectal enemas and suppositories
        (b) Asacol, Salofalk—pH dependent, distal ileum and colon
        (c) Pentasa—time release, most active in small bowel

3. Antibiotics in UC are only used in setting of fulminant colitis or toxic megacolon.

4. Corticosteroids
    a. These are used to control acute exacerbations with no relapse prevention and no proven maintenance benefit.
    b. Nonspecific inhibitors of the immune system. Limit treatment to shortest possible time course.
    c. Improvement is noted in 75%–90% after treatment.
    d. Side effects include adverse effect on growth in children and failure to wean, which is a relative indication for surgery.
    e. Intravenous steroids may be used for severe or fulminant disease. Otherwise oral steroids used for less severe or improving disease.
    f. Enemas or topical preparations for proctitis or proctosigmoiditis have fewer side effects compared with systemic preparations.
    g. Luminal steroids, such as budesonide (Entocort), are nonsystemic corticosteroids with high first-pass metabolism in the liver (90%). Effective at inducing remission for mild-to-moderate UC with proctitis and proctosigmoiditis and are effective in ileal and ileocecal CD

5. Immunosuppressives
    a. Azathioprine (6-mercaptopurine, active metabolite)
      (1) Antimetabolite drugs. Interfere with nucleic acid synthesis, decreasing proliferation of inflammatory cells. Onset of action in 6–12 weeks
      (2) Used for disease refractory to salicylate therapy or corticosteroids and for patients dependent on corticosteroids
        (a) Allows gradual tapering of corticosteroids but may be required up to 6 months
      (3) Adverse side effects—bone marrow suppression, hepatotoxicity, pancreatitis and possible increased risk of lymphoma
    b. Cyclosporine
      (1) It interferes with T-cell function. Long-term use is limited by toxicity.
      (2) It is used in severe, acute toxic colitis that would otherwise need urgent proctocolectomy and is refractory to high-dose corticosteroids.

(3) Up to 80% of patients with an acute flare will improve after treatment within 2 weeks. However, up to 50% of patients will eventually need proctocolectomy within a year.

(4) It is rarely used nowadays.

c. Methotrexate

(1) Folate antagonist

(2) Reports of more than 50% of patients improving after treatment

d. Infliximab (Remicade), Humira, Cimzia—reports of efficacy, although used more commonly in CD

e. Vedolizumab (Entyvio)

(1) Monoclonal antibody used in UC and CD that targets $\alpha4\beta7$ integrin, blocking the interaction with mucosal adhesion molecule and thus inhibits memory T-lymphocyte migration.

G. SURGICAL MANAGEMENT

1. Indications

a. Elective

(1) Chronic, debilitating disease intractable to maximal medical therapy

(2) High risk for development of major complications from medical therapy, such as aseptic necrosis of joints caused by chronic steroids

(3) Growth failure in children

(4) Severe extraintestinal complications

(5) Carcinoma or high risk for carcinoma, such as dysplasia on biopsy

b. Emergent

(1) Perforation, toxic megacolon, massive life-threatening hemorrhage, obstruction

(2) Fulminant colitis that has failed to respond rapidly to medical therapy

(3) Total abdominal colectomy with end ileostomy

(a) Total proctocolectomy is not recommended because of time required for pelvic dissection and increased risk of hemorrhage.

(b) Rarely if the patient is too unstable to undergo colectomy, you can perform loop ileostomy with decompressing colostomy. Definitive surgery can be performed at later date.

2. Surgical procedures

a. Restorative proctocolectomy with ileal pouch-anal anastomosis with diverting loop ileostomy

(1) Curative procedure; elective procedure of choice for most patients. It is sphincter sparing and preserves continence.

(2) Bladder and sexual dysfunction can occur in approximately 5% of patients.

26

INFLAMMATORY BOWEL DISEASE

      (3) Disadvantages include pouch fistulas, frequent soiling, nighttime incontinence, pouchitis (chronic in 15%), anal excoriation, and risk for intestinal obstruction and sepsis.

      (4) Contraindications include CD, diarrhea, preexisting fecal incontinence, lack of psychological stability to withstand complex operation or complications, and distal rectal cancer.

      (5) Pouch (15–20 cm) is created from terminal ileum with anastomosis to anus.

         (a) J pouch or S pouch configuration; the latter provides more length if needed

  b. Total proctocolectomy with standard (Brooke) end ileostomy

      (1) This is gold standard operation against which all other operations must be compared.

      (2) Curative procedure has minimal contraindications, in a single-step operation.

      (3) Disadvantage is permanent ileostomy.

      (4) Complications include peristomal hernia, perineal wound infections, small bowel obstructions, bladder dysfunction, and sexual dysfunction.

      (5) Elective operative mortality rate is 1%–3%.

  c. Total proctocolectomy with continent (Kock) ileostomy

      (1) Rarely performed. Use is now limited to patients who strongly desire continence after total proctocolectomy or sphincter excision/injury.

      (2) Major problem is stability of continent valve within ileal reservoir (40%–50% require reoperation).

  d. Total abdominal colectomy with ileostomy, rectal preservation

      (1) This is reserved for emergency procedures (hemorrhage, toxic megacolon) to decrease operative morbidity and mortality rates (3%–10%).

      (2) Proctectomy and ileal pouch-anal anastomosis can be subsequently performed to control proctitis, reduce cancer risk, and preserve continence.

  e. Total abdominal colectomy with ileorectal anastomosis

      (1) May be performed in the rare patient with rectal sparing

      (2) Must undergo lifelong surveillance of rectum because risk of malignancy remains (10% at 20 years). Also risk of proctitis, which may require proctectomy

      (3) No mesorectal dissection, therefore decreased sexual and urinary function complications.

H. PROGNOSIS
1. Mortality
  a. Mortality rate over 10 years (pancolitis): 5%

  b. Elective surgery (2%)

  c. Emergent surgery (8%–15%)

2. Left-sided colitis and pancolitis
   a. Acute intermittent presentation (60%)—most relapse within first year.
   b. Chronic, unremitting presentation (20%)
   c. Fulminant presentation (10%)
   d. Up to 50% require colectomy in first 10 years.
3. Ulcerative proctitis
   a. Left-sided colitis develops in 20% of patients.
   b. Only 2%–15% are reported to progress to pancolitis.

IV. CROHN DISEASE

A. EPIDEMIOLOGY
1. Bimodal age at onset is 15–30 years to 55–60 years.
2. Incidence is lower than UC, at 1–5 per 100,000 population.

B. PATHOPHYSIOLOGY AND DISTRIBUTION
1. Disease is transmural, affecting any portion of the GI tract from "mouth to anus."
   a. Terminal ileum and cecum—ileocolic CD (55%)
   b. Distal rectum and anal canal—perianal CD (35%)
      (1) Isolated anal CD uncommon (3%–4%)
   c. Small bowel only (30%)
   d. Colon only (15%)
2. Noncaseating granulomas and ulcers that have a "cobblestone" appearance are characteristic.
3. Skip lesions and rectal sparing (40%) are pathognomonic for CD.
4. Chronic inflammation may lead to fibrosis, strictures, and fistulas in small or large bowel.

C. CLINICAL MANIFESTATIONS
1. Characterized by exacerbations and remissions
2. Signs and symptoms
   a. Depend on severity of inflammation or fibrosis, as well as the location of inflammation
   b. Diarrhea present in 90% of cases, usually *nonbloody*
   c. Recurrent abdominal pain, often mild colicky pain, abdominal distention and flatulence
   d. Strictures may cause obstructive symptoms.
   e. Anorectal lesions
      (1) Chronic, recurrent, or nonhealing anal fissures, ulcers, complex anal fistulas, perirectal abscesses
      (2) May precede bowel involvement in 4% of cases
   f. Malnutrition: protein-losing enteropathy, steatorrhea, mineral and vitamin deficiencies, failure to thrive
   g. Acute inflammatory presentation
      (1) This may present similar to acute appendicitis due to terminal ileal disease.

26

INFLAMMATORY BOWEL DISEASE

(2) Acute inflammation can be complicated by fistulas, intraabdominal abscesses, or both.

h. Chronic fibrotic presentation: strictures in any portion of GI tract; fibrotic strictures not likely to improve with medical therapy

3. **Extraintestinal manifestations present in 30% of CD patients (see Section II).**

D. DIAGNOSIS

1. **Diagnosis is more difficult compared with UC because of nonspecific, indolent symptoms.**
   a. Mean time from onset to diagnosis is 35 months.

2. **Laboratory findings**
   a. Anemia caused by iron, vitamin B12, or folate deficiency
   b. Hypoalbuminemia
   c. Tests of bowel function (D-xylose absorption, bile acid breath test)— abnormal with extensive disease

3. **Serologic markers—anti-*Saccharomyces cerevisiae* antibody (ASCA+)**
   a. Present in 60% of patients with CD compared with 5% of patients with UC
   b. Less than 5% in normal population

4. **Radiographic findings**
   a. Upper GI with small bowel follow-through or enteroclysis
      (1) Narrowed terminal ileum (Kantor string sign), fistulas, nodules, sinuses, clefts, linear ulcers
   b. Barium enema
      (1) Thickened bowel wall, longitudinal ulcers, transverse fissures, cobblestone formation, and rectal sparing
      (2) Terminal ileum may contain strictures (string sign).
   c. Abdominal computed tomography
      (1) Findings may include intraabdominal abscesses, thickened bowel wall, and/or fistulas (i.e., enterovesical or enteroenteric).

5. **Endoscopy**
   a. Esophagogastroduodenoscopy
   b. Colonoscopy
      (1) Rectum is normal (rectal sparing) in 40%–50% of patients.
      (2) Random biopsies are required because grossly normal-appearing rectum may have histologic disease.
      (3) Characteristic lesions
         (a) Aphthous ulcers
         (b) Mucosal ulcerations
         (c) Anal fissures
         (d) Cobblestoning
      (4) Chronic inflammation may ultimately lead to fibrosis, strictures, and fistulas in either small or large intestine.
      (5) Segmental (skip) lesions

(6) Annual surveillance with multiple biopsies is recommended for patients with long-standing Crohn colitis (more than 7 years in duration).

E. COMPLICATIONS
1. Intestinal obstruction
2. Abscess formation
3. Fistulas
   a. Internal
      (1) Between segments of bowel, bowel to other viscera (bladder, uterus, vagina) or bowel to retroperitoneal sites
   b. External
4. Anorectal lesions including abscess, fistula, and/or fissure
5. Free perforation and hemorrhage
   a. Rare because of gradual fibrosis and formation of strictures
   b. Adjacent structures generally "wall off" perforation sites causing formation of internal fistulas.
6. Carcinoma
   a. It is less common than UC, but Crohn colitis (particularly pancolitis) has nearly the same risk for malignancy as UC.
   b. Finding of dysplasia on biopsy is indication for total proctocolectomy.
7. Toxic megacolon
   a. Occurs in 5% of patients with colonic involvement
   b. Responds to medical therapy better than does UC
8. Extraintestinal (see Section II)
   a. More common with colonic involvement
   b. Urinary—cystitis, calculi (oxalate), ureteral obstruction
9. Strictures

F. MEDICAL MANAGEMENT (SEE SECTION III.G)
1. Aminosalicylates—oral agent (mesalamine) used for mild-to-moderate disease
2. Antibiotics in CD, decreases the intraluminal bacterial load
   a. Metronidazole—reported to improve Crohn colitis and perianal disease
   b. Fluoroquinolones—may be effective in some cases
3. Corticosteroids—used for acute exacerbations
4. Immunosuppressants
   a. Azathioprine, 6-mercaptopurine, cyclosporine
      (1) Useful during remission to decrease steroid requirements, usually added after 7–10 days of high-dose intravenous steroids. May be required for 2–3 months
      (2) Cyclosporine
         (a) Two thirds of patients will note some improvement with therapy, often after 2 weeks.
   b. Methotrexate—used in steroid-dependent active disease and to maintain remission

    c. Infliximab (Remicade)
      (1) It is an intravenously administered monoclonal antibody against tumor necrosis factor that decreases systemic inflammation.
      (2) More than 50% of patients with moderate-to-severe disease will show improvement.
      (3) It is useful with perianal disease—has some efficacy in healing chronic fistulas.
      (4) Recurrence is common; many patients require lifelong infusions.
    d. Vedolizumab (Entyvio)

5. Acute flare
    a. Management includes antiinflammatory medications as described earlier, bowel reset, and antibiotics and may require parenteral nutrition if patient is malnourished.
    b. Interventional radiology should drain intraabdominal abscess.
    c. Surgical resection of diseased bowel may be necessary, although it can often be performed after patient has been stabilized, nutrition optimized, and inflammation decreased.
    d. If medical management fails, total abdominal colectomy with end ileostomy is recommended. Elective proctectomy may be necessary for refractory Crohn proctitis.

6. Anal and perianal CD
    a. Symptom alleviation
    b. Skin tags and hemorrhoids should not be excised unless extremely symptomatic because of risk for creating chronic, nonhealing wounds.
    c. Fissures may respond to local or systemic therapy. They often occur in atypical locations (lateral rather than anterior or posterior midline).
      (1) Sphincterotomy is contraindicated because of the possibility of creating chronic, nonhealing wound and the increased risk for incontinence in patients with diarrhea from underlying colitis or small bowel disease.
    d. It is imperative that all abscesses be drained before initiation of immunosuppressive therapy.

G. SURGICAL MANAGEMENT
1. Eventually required in 70%–75% of cases over lifetime of disease
2. Indications for surgery
    a. Reserved for treatment of complications only, because surgery is not curative; all at-risk intestine cannot be resected as in UC.
    b. Small bowel obstruction often caused by strictures. Indication in 50% of surgical cases
    c. Fistula
    d. Abscess, although some may be amenable to percutaneous drainage by interventional radiology
    e. Hemorrhage
    f. Perianal disease unresponsive to medical therapy

    g. Disease intractable to medical management
    h. Failure to thrive—chronic malnutrition, growth retardation
    i. Toxic megacolon
    j. Dysplasia seen on biopsy
3. Intraoperative findings
    a. Creeping of mesenteric fat toward antimesenteric border
    b. Serosal and mesenteric inflammation
    c. Bowel wall thickening
    d. Strictures
    e. Shortening of bowel and mesentery
    f. Mesenteric lymphadenopathy
    g. Inflammatory masses, abscesses, adherent bowel loops
4. Surgical procedures
    a. Midline incision should be used because of possible need for stoma. If anticipated, optimal stoma site should be marked preoperatively to ensure the following:
       (1) It is easy for patient to reach (avoid pannus).
       (2) Does not disturb patient's pant line
       (3) Stoma appliance fits easily on skin without leaking (avoid deep skin creases or bend of abdomen).
    b. Conservative resection of diseased or symptomatic bowel segment
       (1) Resect only grossly diseased bowel with short, "normal-appearing" margins; it is unnecessary to get histologically free margins for anastomosis.
       (2) Primary anastomosis can be safely created if patient is medically stable, nutritionally optimized, and on minimal immunosuppressive medications.
       (3) Stomas should be created in patients who are hemodynamically unstable, septic, malnourished, taking high-dose immunosuppressive medications, or with extensive intraabdominal contamination.
       (4) Distal ileum and cecal resection with ileocolostomy is a common procedure. These are most common site for disease.
       (5) Fistulas
          (a) They generally require resection of only bowel segment with active CD.
          (b) Secondary fistula sites are often normal and require only repair of fistula site with simple closure rather than resection.
       (6) Recurrence rate in long-term follow-up: 60%
    c. Stricturoplasty
       (1) Relieves obstruction in chronically scarred/fibrotic bowel without resection; especially useful for multiple symptomatic strictures to conserve bowel length
       (2) Short strictures—bowel opened along antimesenteric surface, then closed transversely (Heineke-Mikulicz)

26

INFLAMMATORY BOWEL DISEASE

  (3) Long strictures—bowel opened along antimesenteric surface, then folded into an inverted U-shape to create a side-to-side anastomosis

 d. Total proctocolectomy

  (1) Indicated for dysplasia seen on biopsy

  (2) Ileal pouch—anal reconstruction not recommended because of high risk for CD developing within the pouch and high risk for complications (fistula, abscess, stricture, pouch dysfunction, pouch failure)

 e. Exclusion bypass—has a greater incidence of recurrence and carcinoma; may be indicated in the following:

  (1) Bypass unresectable inflammatory mass

  (2) Gastroduodenal CD

  (3) Multiple, extensive skip lesions

 f. Continent (Kock) ileostomy and mucosal proctectomy procedures are contraindicated.

 g. Recurrent perianal abscesses or complex anal fistulas

  (1) Local drainage of abscesses if possible

  (2) Sphincter preservation

   (a) Endoanal ultrasound or magnetic resonance imaging is useful to delineate complex anatomy and fistulous tracts.

   (b) Use setons liberally.

   (c) Endoanal advancement flaps should be considered for definitive therapy if the rectal mucosa is uninvolved.

   (d) Intractable perianal sepsis may require proctectomy (10%–15%).

 h. Rectovaginal fistula: If rectal mucosa appears healthy with minimal rectovaginal septum scarring, rectal or vaginal mucosal advancement flap can be used.

H. PROGNOSIS

1. Cure is not possible in chronic disease, and medical therapy does not avoid surgery.

2. Recurrence rates 10 years after initial operation

 a. Ileocolic disease (50%)

 b. Small bowel disease (50%)

 c. Colonic disease (40%–50%)

3. Reoperation rates at 5 years

 a. Primary resection (20%)

 b. Bypass (50%)

4. A total of 80% to 85% of patients who require surgery lead normal lives.

5. Mortality rate is 15% at 30 years.

  See Table 26.1 for a comparison of IBD.

TABLE 26.1		
COMPARISON OF INFLAMMATORY BOWEL DISEASE		
Characteristics	Ulcerative Colitis	Crohn Disease
Epidemiology	15–30 and 50–70 years of age	20–30 and 50–60 years of age
	Females > males	Females = males
Clinical presentation	Bloody diarrhea	Nonbloody diarrhea
	Rectal bleeding	Colicky abdominal pain
	Tenesmus	Anorectal lesions
	Weight loss	Weight loss
Gross pathology	Contiguous disease	Skip lesions
	Friable mucosa	Longitudinal fissures
	Pseudopolyps	Focal strictures
	Stovepipe narrowing	Bowel wall thickening
	Granular irregularity	"Cobblestoning"
Microscopic pathology	Confined to mucosa	Transmural
	Loss of goblet cells	Granulomas
	Crypt abscesses	Mesenteric adenopathy
	Plasma cell infiltrate	
Gastrointestinal distribution	Contiguous from anus proximally	30% small bowel only
	<5% rectal sparing	55% small bowel and colon
	No skip lesions	15% colon only
	10% terminal ileitis	30% rectal involvement
		20% skip lesions
		35% perianal disease
Complications	Toxic megacolon	Abscesses
	Perforation	Fistulas
	Sclerosing cholangitis	Intestinal obstruction
	Extraintestinal less common	Extraintestinal more common
	Colon cancer	Strictures
		Colon cancer
Surgical intervention	Potential for cure	Reserved for complications, not curative
		Conservative bowel resections
Mortality	2%–3% elective surgery	3%–6% elective surgery
	8%–25% emergent surgery	

26

INFLAMMATORY BOWEL DISEASE

V. INDETERMINATE COLITIS

A. **TYPICALLY PRESENT WITH SYMPTOMS SIMILAR TO ULCERATIVE COLITIS**

1. Endoscopic and pathologic findings include features common to both UC and CD.
2. Differential diagnoses—infectious colitis caused by *Campylobacter jejuni*, *Entamoeba histolytica*, *C. difficile*, *Neisseria gonococcus*, *Salmonella* spp., and *Shigella* spp.

3. Indications for surgery
   a. Intractability
   b. Complications of medical therapy
   c. Malignancy or high risk for malignancy
4. Surgical options
   a. Total abdominal colectomy with end ileostomy may be best initial procedure for patients who prefer sphincter-sparing operation.
      (1) Pathology may provide more accurate diagnosis.
         (a) UC can undergo ileal pouch-anal anastomosis.
         (b) If still indeterminate, perform completion proctectomy with end ileostomy.
   b. Abdominal colectomy with ileorectal anastomosis is an option for patients with rectal sparing disease.

RECOMMENDED READINGS

Oakley JR, Jagelman DG, Fazio VW, et al. Complications and quality of life after ileorectal anastomosis for ulcerative colitis. *Am J Surg*. 1985;149:23–30.

Ross H, Steele SR, Varma M, et al. Practice parameters for the surgical treatment of ulcerative colitis. Standards Practice Task Force of the American Society of Colon and Rectal Surgeons. *Dis Colon Rectum*. 2014;57:5–22.

Strong S, Steele SR, Boutrous M, et al. Clinical practice guidelines for the surgical management of Crohn's disease. Clinical Practice Guidelines Committee of the American Society of Colon and Rectal Surgeons. *Dis Colon Rectum*. 2015;58:1021–1036.

Benign Esophageal Disease

Winifred Lo, MD

Be yourself. Everyone else is already taken.

—Oscar Wilde

I. ANATOMY

A. GENERAL DESCRIPTION

1. The esophagus is an approximately 30-cm-long, muscular tube that begins 15 cm from the incisors at the cricopharyngeus muscle and ends at the gastroesophageal junction (GEJ) along the cardia of the stomach. There are three normal areas of anatomic narrowing: (1) the cricopharyngeal muscle (the narrowest point of the esophagus), (2) the aortic arch and left main stem bronchus, and (3) the diaphragmatic hiatus.
2. The cervical esophagus (5 cm) spans the C6 vertebra to T1–2. Recurrent laryngeal nerves lie in the tracheoesophageal groove on either side.
3. The thoracic esophagus (20 cm) begins at the thoracic inlet and lies between the trachea anteriorly and prevertebral fascia posteriorly. The azygous vein lies to the right and the thoracic aorta to the left of the esophagus.
4. The abdominal esophagus (2 cm) enters the abdomen at the esophageal hiatus at T11. Right and left vagal trunks also enter here.

B. BLOOD SUPPLY AND NERVES

1. Arterial supply is segmental from superior and inferior thyroid, aortic, bronchial, and esophageal branches, inferior phrenic, and left gastric arteries (Fig. 27.1).
2. Venous drainage is to the submucosal venous plexus, with subsequent drainage to the inferior thyroid veins, azygos vein, hemiazygos vein, intercostal, gastric, and left and right phrenic veins. All are a potential source of varices if portal hypertension is present.
3. Innervation is from both parasympathetic and sympathetic systems. The cervical esophagus receives innervation from the recurrent laryngeal nerves. Damage to these nerves interferes with the function of the vocal cords, as well as the function of the cervical esophagus, predisposing to pulmonary aspiration with swallowing. The thoracic esophagus has both parasympathetic and sympathetic innervation via the vagus; these form the Auerbach plexus between muscle layers and the Meissner plexus within the submucosal layer. As the vagus nerve enters the abdomen, parasympathetic fibers form the left (anterior) and right (posterior) vagus nerves.

Pearl: *LARP (left vagus lies anteriorly and right vagus lies posteriorly) on the distal esophagus.*

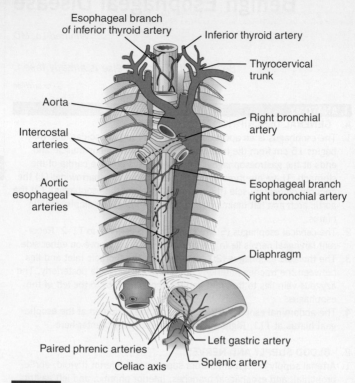

FIG. 27.1

Arterial supply to the esophagus. (From Sabiston D, Townsend C. *Sabiston Textbook of Surgery*. Philadelphia: Elsevier; 2012.)

C. HISTOLOGY

1. Mucosa is squamous epithelium, which becomes columnar epithelium of the stomach at the GEJ.

Pearl: *Squamous to columnar metaplasia is the hallmark of Barrett esophagus.*

2. Submucosa contains glands, arteries, Meissner neural plexus, lymphatics, and veins.
3. Muscularis is composed of two layers, an outer longitudinal and an inner circular layer. Nerves and blood vessels run between the layers. The upper one-third is composed of striated muscle, and the lower two-thirds are smooth muscle.
4. No serosa. The lack of a serosal layer potentially contributes to an increase in anastomotic leaks and early mediastinal invasion by cancer.

II. PHYSIOLOGY

The esophagus functions to transport swallowed material, in a coordinated fashion, from the pharynx to the stomach. Once initiated, swallowing is entirely a reflex act coordinated by the swallowing center of the medulla and involving cranial nerves 5, 7, 10, 11, and 12 and motor neurons of C1–3.

A. SWALLOWING MECHANISM

1. Oropharyngeal phase
   a. Food is chewed and ready for swallowing.
   b. Tongue pushes the food bolus into the hypopharynx.
   c. Simultaneously, the soft palate elevates to prevent regurgitation of food into the nasopharynx and the hyoid bone moves anteriorly and superiorly to open the retrolaryngeal space.
   d. Epiglottis moves over the larynx to prevent aspiration with the movement of the hyoid bone.
   e. Rapid increase in the pressure of the hypopharynx and a subsequent relaxation of the upper esophageal sphincter (UES) (cricopharyngeus muscle) completes this phase.

2. Esophageal phase
   a. Primary peristalsis is initiated by swallowing, relaxing the UES and simultaneous contraction of the posterior pharyngeal constrictors, which propels swallowed material from pharynx to stomach; food bolus is propelled by pressure differential between cervical esophagus and negative pressure of intrathoracic esophagus. Upper esophageal sphincter (UES) closes again to prevent reflux back into pharynx.
   b. Secondary peristalsis is initiated by esophageal distention.

B. SPHINCTERS

1. UES or cricopharyngeal muscle is approximately 3 cm long with resting pressure of 20–60 mm Hg.

2. Lower esophageal sphincter (LES)
   a. The LES is not an anatomically defined sphincter in humans but a zone of high pressure that reduces gastric regurgitation and reflux. Located in the distal 3–5 cm of the esophagus, its normal resting pressure is 10–35 mm Hg.
   b. LES pressure increases with inspiration and drug and/or hormone levels.
      (1) Pressure is increased by gastrin, alpha-adrenergic drugs, bethanechol, and metoclopramide.
      (2) Pressure is decreased by secretin, cholecystokinin, caffeine, glucagon, progesterone, alcohol, nitroglycerin, nicotine, anticholinergics, and beta-adrenergic drugs.

27

BENIGN ESOPHAGEAL DISEASE

III. MOTILITY DISORDERS

A. ACHALASIA

1. Aperistalsis and in complete relaxation of the LES.
2. Etiology can be idiopathic or infectious (i.e., *Trypanosoma cruzi*) degeneration of Auerbach plexus; degeneration can lead to hypertension of LES, failure to relax, and progressive loss of peristalsis.
3. Symptoms include dysphagia, regurgitation, weight loss, retrosternal chest pain, nocturnal coughing, recurrent pulmonary infections. Progressing dysphagia beginning with liquids, then solids. Patient should eat carefully at meals and consume copious amounts of water.
4. Diagnosis: Barium swallow demonstrates "bird's beak" narrowing of distal esophagus with proximal dilation; esophageal manometry is the gold standard for diagnosis—it will show aperistalsis and incomplete relaxation of the LES. LES resting pressure is often hypertensive, but it can be normotensive.
5. Treatment:
   a. Medical management: nitroglycerin, calcium channel blockers, bougie dilation, Botox injection into the LES (symptoms frequently recur)
   b. Surgical management:
      (1) Heller myotomy with partial fundoplication
      (2) Esophagectomy may be needed for sigmoid esophagus, failure after prior myotomy, or stricture refractory to dilation.
      (3) POEM (*per*oral *e*ndoscopic *m*yotomy) is a newer endoscopic treatment modality that creates an opening in the mucosa to access circular muscles, which are divided. No antireflux procedure is performed. Long-term outcomes are unknown at this time.
6. Approximately 1%–10% of patients experience development of squamous cell carcinoma after 15–25 years of disease.

B. DIFFUSE ESOPHAGEAL SPASM

1. More common in women; repetitive, simultaneous contractions
2. Symptoms: chest pain, dysphagia; aggravated by reflux, cold liquids, and periods of emotional stress. Associated with other gastrointestinal (GI) complaints (e.g., irritable bowel syndrome [IBS], peptic ulcer disease [PUD])
3. Diagnosis: esophagram ("corkscrew esophagus"), manometry (simultaneous contractions with multiple peaks or long duration >2.5 seconds)
4. Treatment:
   a. Medical (variable efficacy): elimination of trigger foods/drinks, acid suppression, nitrates, calcium channel blockers, anticholinergics, psychiatric evaluation
   b. Surgical: for refractory dysphagia despite optimized medical therapy; long esophagomyotomy, including LES via left chest approach and partial fundoplication as LES is disrupted.

C. NUTCRACKER ESOPHAGUS

1. Hypermotility disorder: hypertensive peristalsis or high-amplitude peristaltic contractions; exact etiology unclear; commonly associated with gastroesophageal reflux disease (GERD) (>50%)
2. Symptoms: chest pain, dysphagia
3. Diagnosis: manometry—peristaltic esophageal contractions two standard deviations above normal amplitudes (i.e., >40 mm Hg); notably, LES pressure is normal and relaxes with each swallow
4. Treatment: medical management primarily. Treat GERD first. Calcium channel blockers, nitrates, antispasmodics can be used, but efficacy is low.
5. Surgical treatment can be performed in the setting of significant dysphagia. Outcomes poor for symptoms of pain alone

D. HYPERTENSIVE LES

1. Increased LES pressure greater than 35 mm Hg with normal LES relaxation; peristalsis typically normal
2. Symptoms: chest pain, dysphagia
3. Diagnosis: manometry, LES pressure greater than 35 cm with normal LES relaxation, normal peristalsis (50%)
4. Treatment:
   a. Endoscopic management: Botox injection, balloon dilation
   b. Surgical management: for those patients who fail endoscopic therapy and have severe symptoms; laparoscopic Heller myotomy with partial fundoplication

E. SCLERODERMA

1. Fibrous replacement of esophageal smooth muscle and atrophy. LES loses tone.
2. Esophageal manometry reveals hypotensive LES with normal relaxation. Esophageal body has aperistalsis; this results in GE reflux.
3. Medical/surgical treatment should be directed at antireflux measures to decrease esophagitis.
4. Antireflux surgery for severe esophagitis and reflux symptoms must be partial fundoplication.

IV. DIVERTICULA

A. DEFINITION

1. Diverticula are epithelial-lined mucosal pouches that protrude from the esophageal lumen.
2. True diverticula involve all layers of esophageal wall (mucosa, submucosa, muscularis).
3. False diverticula involve only mucosa and submucosa (i.e., Zenker diverticula, epiphrenic diverticula).
4. Traction diverticula result from external inflammatory mediastinal lymph nodes adhering to the esophagus, which is pulled as the lymph nodes heal and contract (true diverticulum).

27

BENIGN ESOPHAGEAL DISEASE

5. Pulsion diverticula result from elevated intraluminal pressures generated from abnormal motility disorders (false diverticulum).

B. PHARYNGOESOPHAGEAL (ZENKER DIVERTICULUM)

1. Most common esophageal diverticulum (false pulsion diverticulum); herniates into Killian triangle between thyropharyngeus and cricopharyngeus muscles
2. More common in older patients (60–70s)
3. Symptoms: asymptomatic, cough, intermittent dysphagia, halitosis, regurgitation of undigested food, aspiration, retrosternal pain. Rarely, aspiration pneumonia.
4. Diagnosis: barium esophagram
5. Treatment:
   a. Diverticulectomy or diverticulopexy with myotomy of the cricopharyngeus muscle via a left cervical incision
   b. Endoscopic transoral stapling: endoscopic division (via stapler) of esophageal wall and diverticular wall
   c. Results similar for diverticula greater than 3 cm in size; open approach superior for diverticula less than 3 cm

C. MIDESOPHAGEAL

1. Usually traction (histoplasmosis, tuberculosis [TB]): large, inflamed adjacent lymph nodes pull on wall of esophagus to form true diverticulum as they heal
2. Symptoms: asymptomatic (most common), dysphagia, chest pain, regurgitation, hemoptysis (rare)
3. Diagnosis: barium esophagram (lateral views needed to lateralize diverticulum), although they tend to present on the right; computed tomography (CT) chest (identify lymphadenopathy), endoscopy (rule out cancer, mucosal abnormalities), manometry (identify if primary motor disorder is present)
4. Rarely symptomatic, tend to be small, and are discovered incidentally

D. EPIPHRENIC

1. False, pulsion diverticula; usually associated with motility disorder (i.e., achalasia, diffuse esophageal spasm, neuromuscular disorders)
2. Located in distal 10 cm of esophagus, preponderance for right side and wide mouthed
3. Etiology: usually due to thickened distal esophageal musculature or increased intraluminal pressure
4. Symptoms: asymptomatic, dysphagia, regurgitation, epigastric pain
5. Diagnosis: barium esophagram (delineates anatomy), manometry (esophageal motility, LES resting pressures), endoscopy (evaluate for mucosal lesions)
6. Treatment: diverticulectomy and treat underlying motility disorder (myotomy performed 180 degrees away from diverticulum). Most epiphrenic

diverticula can be approached laparoscopically, but very large diverticulum or more proximal diverticulum may require left chest approach.

V. GASTROESOPHAGEAL REFLUX

A. ANATOMY

1. LES: not a distinct anatomic structure but a high-pressure zone at the distal end of the esophagus. Acts like a valve with reflex of decreased pressure in association with swallowing. Characterized by resting LES pressure, overall length, and intraabdominal length
2. Acid-protecting mechanisms:
   a. LES prevents gastric reflux into esophagus.
   b. Peristalsis clears gastric acid.
   c. Saliva (1000–1500 mL/day) is bicarbonate rich.

B. PATHOPHYSIOLOGY

1. Decreased LES tone or shortening of intraabdominal portion of esophagus
2. Significant gastric distention (food, air)—shortens LES
3. Hiatal hernia
4. Increased intraabdominal pressure because of obesity and tight garments
5. Motor failure of esophagus with loss of peristalsis (decreases clearance of acid reflux)

C. DIAGNOSIS

1. Symptoms:
   a. Long-standing heartburn (80%, epigastric, retrosternal, stinging)
   b. Regurgitation (54%, digested vs. undigested food)
   c. Dysphagia (solid food → mechanical obstruction, solid/liquid → neuromuscular disorder)
   d. Other symptoms: pain, hoarseness, bloating, belching, wheezing
2. Physical examination: largely noncontributory toward diagnosis
3. Preoperative evaluation:
   a. Endoscopy: exclude other diseases, assess for complications of GERD such as esophagitis, presence of Barrett esophagus, cancer
   b. Manometry: rule out motility disorders
      (1) LES: mean resting pressure (normal: 12–35 mm Hg), total length, location of sphincter, intraabdominal length
      (2) Peristalsis: typically more than 80%; ineffective motility = less than 70% peristalsis OR distal esophageal amplitudes less than 30 mm Hg
   c. pH testing: 24-hour pH test, measures total number of reflux episodes, longest episode of reflux
      (1) DeMeester score: composite score that includes total number of reflux episodes, longest episode of reflux, number of episodes lasting more than 5 minutes, extent of reflux in the upright position/supine position (normal <14.7)
   d. Esophagogram: identifies external anatomy of esophagus, proximal stomach (i.e., identify hiatal hernia).

D. TREATMENT

1. Medical management:
   a. Can initiate presumptive treatment based on history and physical alone. Start with 6 weeks of therapy; if no improvement, can then pursue more evaluations
      (1) Proton pump inhibitors (PPIs): irreversible binding of proton pump on luminal side of stomach parietal cells (common end pathway). Need to hold for 1 week before pH monitoring.
      (2) Histamine (H_2) blockers, antacids also used
   b. Dietary modifications: avoid smoking, chocolate, alcohol, heavy/fatty foods, eating within 2 hours of bedtime
   c. Lifestyle modifications: elevate head of bed (6 inches), lose weight (if obese), eat smaller meals

2. Surgical management:
   a. Indications:
      (1) Severe esophageal injury (ulcer, stricture, Barrett esophagitis)
      (2) Inadequate symptom control while on optimized medical therapy
      (3) Poor compliance or financial burden
      (4) Patient choice
   b. Goals of surgery:
      (1) Restore segment of intraabdominal esophagus.
      (2) Reduce any hernia that is present.
      (3) Close hiatus to normal diameter without compression of esophagus.
      (4) Create new antireflux barrier; avoid increasing the resistance of the relaxed sphincter to level that exceeds peristaltic force of esophagus.
   c. Procedures:
      (1) Nissen fundoplication (360-degree wrap): mobilize esophagus, reapproximate crura, pass posterior fundus behind esophagus to create 2.5–3 cm wrap
      (2) Dor fundoplication (180-degree partial wrap): fundus folded over anterior aspect of esophagus, anchored to hiatus; use in patients with known esophageal dysmotility to prevent dysphagia
      (3) Toupet fundoplication (220–250-degree partial wrap): mobilize esophagus, reapproximate crura, pass posterior fundus behind esophagus
      (4) If unable to restore adequate esophageal length, can perform Collis gastroplasty (stomach is stapled to elongate esophagus and allow a tension-free fundoplication around the neo-esophagus)
      (5) Magnetic sphincter augmentation—newer antireflux device composed of titanium beads with magnets. Placed around the LES to augment the valve. It is noncompressive. Ability to burp and vomit is retained so less chance of gas-bloat syndrome. Short-term outcomes are excellent. Long-term (>10 year) data unknown

    d. Complications (3%–10%)
      (1) Operative complications: pneumothorax, injury to the esophagus, stomach
      (2) Postoperative complications: delayed gastric emptying (secondary to vagal trauma), persistent/recurrent symptoms, recurrent hiatal hernia
      (3) Possible side effects of fundoplication: increased flatulence, bloating, difficulty belching and vomiting, dysphagia

E. HIATAL HERNIA

See Fig. 27.2.

1. Type I (sliding)

    a. GEJ migrates above diaphragm; phrenoesophageal membrane intact; no true peritoneal sac
    b. Most common hiatal hernia—90% of cases
    c. Significant only if reflux symptoms
    d. Causative factors

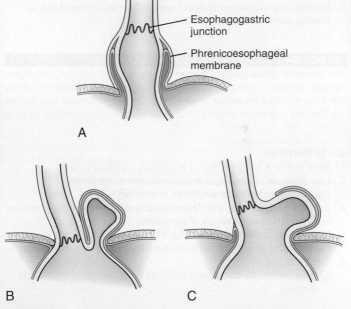

Esophagogastric junction

Phrenicoesophageal membrane

A

B

C

FIG. 27.2

Types of hiatal hernias. (A) Type I, (B) type II, and (C) type III. (Adapted from Fischer JE, Jones DB, Pomposelli FB, et al. *Fischer's Mastery of Surgery.* 6th ed. Philadelphia: Lippincott Williams & Wilkins; 2011.)

(1) Chronically increased intraabdominal pressure, including obesity

(2) Weakness of supporting structures at esophageal hiatus

2. Type II (paraesophageal, rolling)

   a. GEJ anchored in abdomen, fundus of stomach herniates into thorax

   b. Peritoneal sac

   c. Reflux rare

   d. Uncommon type of hernia

   e. Can result in gastric strangulation

   f. All type II hernias should be repaired.

3. Type III (combination of types I and II): GEJ, fundus, and cardia of stomach herniate into chest.

4. Type IV: Stomach and other intraabdominal organs (e.g., spleen, colon) herniate into chest.

F. BARRETT ESOPHAGUS

1. Etiology: Prolonged gastric and biliary juice exposure from reflux causes change in squamous epithelium to columnar epithelium.

2. Diagnosis: Perform endoscopic evaluation (biopsy to confirm intestinal metaplasia, e.g., goblet cells present, and rule out dysplasia).

3. Patients with Barrett esophagus have a 50 times increased risk to develop adenocarcinoma.

VI. BENIGN TUMORS OF THE ESOPHAGUS

The incidence of benign esophageal tumors is rare (<1% of esophageal tumors). Benign tumors and cysts can be categorized as intramural versus intraluminal. Most intramural lesions are leiomyomas. Intraluminal lesions are typically polyps, originating in the submucosa and extending into the lumen.

A. LEIOMYOMA

1. Most common benign tumor of esophagus—75% of cases

2. Less common in esophagus than stomach or small bowel

3. Usually located in distal two-thirds of esophagus

4. Symptoms: dysphagia, pain; hematemesis rare. Size and location have low correlation with severity of symptoms.

5. Diagnosis by barium swallow diagnostic. Do not biopsy; this increases the likelihood of mucosal perforation during subsequent enucleation.

6. Treatment

   a. Enucleation via thoracotomy or VATS (video-assisted thoracoscopic surgery)

B. OTHER BENIGN LESIONS

1. Esophageal cysts—20% of cases

2. Polyps

VII. ESOPHAGEAL RUPTURE AND PERFORATION

A. CAUSATIVE FACTORS

1. Iatrogenic—most common causative factor
   a. Endoscopy
   b. Dilation (balloon or bougienage)
   c. Biopsy
   d. Traumatic intubation (esophageal or endotracheal)
2. Noniatrogenic
   a. Boerhaave syndrome (spontaneous perforation)
   b. Penetrating neck, chest, or abdominal trauma
   c. Foreign body
   d. Caustic ingestion
   e. Erosion by adjacent inflammation
   f. Carcinoma

B. CLINICAL PRESENTATION

1. Presentation can be dramatic and catastrophic with tachycardia, hypotension, and respiratory compromise.
2. Other symptoms include dyspnea, neck or chest pain, fever, subcutaneous emphysema, and pneumothorax.

C. DIAGNOSIS

1. Chest radiograph may reveal pneumothorax, pneumomediastinum, pleural effusion, or sub-diaphragmatic air.
2. Esophagram with water-soluble contrast, then barium (water-soluble less likely to incur mediastinitis in context of perforation, but barium study has significantly greater sensitivity and specificity)
3. CT chest: can identify contained leaks or perforations and fluid collections

D. TREATMENT

1. Early recognition and treatment are essential to survival. The differential diagnosis also must include myocardial infarction, perforated viscus, dissecting aortic aneurysms, and pulmonary embolus.
2. Resuscitation
   a. Operative intervention versus chest tube drainage of pleural effusions
   b. Nothing by mouth
   c. Fluid resuscitation, urine output monitoring
   d. Broad-spectrum antibiotics: coverage of gram-positive, gram-negative, and fungal organisms
   e. Nutritional support in recovery period; parenteral route is preferred
   f. If perforation occurs in the presence of other pathology, the underlying disease must be treated at the time of surgery or the repair will break down.

27

BENIGN ESOPHAGEAL DISEASE

3. Nonoperative management of esophageal perforation
   a. Controversial; applicable only in patients with the following conditions
      (1) Hemodynamic stability
      (2) Small perforation
      (3) Cervical perforation
      (4) A contained leak
      (5) No evidence of sepsis
      (6) Wide drainage back into esophagus on esophagram
   b. Antibiotics and close observation
4. Operative management depends on the location, extent of the perforation, and patient condition.
   a. Cervical esophagus—left-sided neck incision (at anterior border of sternocleidomastoid muscle [SCM]), dissection down to posterior mediastinum, repair (if obvious defect is identified; often it is not), drainage, antibiotics
      (1) Careful not to injure the recurrent laryngeal nerve
      (2) Even if defect is not identified, wide drainage usually facilitates adequate control and healing.
   b. Upper two-third thoracic perforation—
      (1) Fully covered esophageal stent ± percutaneous endoscopic gastrostomy (PEG) tube. Can be combined with drainage procedure for collections (i.e., chest tube or VATS washout). Stent removed 6–8 weeks and perforation reassessed. If healed, stent left out; if still healing, new stent replaced
      (2) Open repair via right thoracotomy (fifth intercostal space); debride perforation, repair in two layers, buttress repair (pleura, pericardium, intercostal muscle flap), irrigate and drain, feeding tube placement
   c. Distal thoracic perforation
      (1) Fully covered esophageal stent, same as previous
      (2) Open repair via left thoracotomy (sixth intercostal space), same as previous
   d. Abdominal perforation—approach via upper midline incision; debride perforation, close primarily, buttress repair (omentum, fundus of stomach)
   e. Special circumstances:
      (1) Perforation with achalasia: perform myotomy on opposite side from perforation and repair
      (2) For perforation with malignancy, options include:
         (a) Stent and drain to control contamination
         (b) Cervical esophagostomy, drainage of collections, esophagectomy (if candidate), and feeding tube placement
         (c) Esophagectomy, if immediate recognition and operative candidate
      (3) If patient unstable, nonstentable perforation, nonoperative candidate–esophagostomy (spit fistula) to completely divert and feeding tube placement
5. Complications of esophageal perforation include sepsis, abscess, fistula, empyema, mediastinitis, and death.

VIII. CAUSTIC INJURY

A. **BACKGROUND**

1. This usually results from ingestion of alkalis, acids, bleach, or detergents (Fig. 27.3).
2. Patients are usually younger than 5 years or adolescent or adult attempting suicide.
3. Alkalis cause liquefactive necrosis that results in greater depth of injury.
4. Must consider early (acute phase) and chronic (late phase) manifestations of injury.

B. **CLINICAL PRESENTATION**

1. Acute phase: pain/burns around mouth, pain on swallowing, hypersalivation, dysphagia, bleeding, vomiting; rarely, laryngeal edema, pulmonary edema with ingestion of strong acids
2. Chronic phase: dysphagia (80% present in first 2 months after incident) secondary to stricture formation

C. **DIAGNOSIS**

1. Perform upper endoscopy to establish severity of the injury.
   a. First degree: hyperemia, edema
   b. Second degree: hemorrhage, exudate ulceration, pseudomembrane formation
   c. Third degree: sloughing of mucosa, deep ulcers, massive hemorrhage, complete edematous obstruction of lumen, esophageal perforation
2. Contrast examination of esophagus can demonstrate injury and suspected perforation.

D. **TREATMENT**

1. Initial therapy
   a. Induction of emesis should be avoided, as should attempts to dilute the caustic agent (damage is nearly instantaneous, and intake of large volumes of fluid may only cause distention and emesis).
   b. Nothing by mouth
   c. Intravenous hydration
   d. Broad-spectrum antibiotics after diagnosis confirmed
   e. Use of steroids remains controversial.
2. Operative intervention
   a. Patients with evidence of esophageal or gastric perforation require immediate operation.
      (1) Best explored through abdominal incision; prep patient from mandible to pubis to allow for possibility of cervical incision
      (2) Insert G-tube to drain stomach and feeding J-tube for enteral nutrition.
      (3) Restoration of alimentary continuity should await resolution of the acute insult.

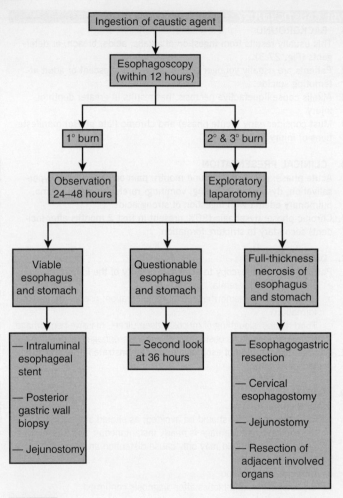

FIG. 27.3

Ingestion of caustic agent. (Data from Brunicardi FC, Andersen DK, Billiar TR, et al. *Schwartz's Principles of Surgery*. 10th ed. New York: McGraw-Hill; 2014.)

b. Stricture formation tends to be the rule.
   (1) Dilation is traditional therapy; early dilation (soon after injury) is controversial.
   (2) Stricture that cannot be dilated or remains refractory to dilation after 1 year requires esophagectomy and reconstruction.

(a) Stomach is the preferred substitute but often is unusable secondary to scarring from original injury.

(b) Colon interposition is an option (left colon typically).

RECOMMENDED READINGS

Anon. <http://www.surgicalcore.org/>; 2016. Accessed 13.07.16.

Pandolfino J, Gawron A. Achalasia. *JAMA*. 2015;313:1876.

Sabiston D, Townsend C. *Sabiston Textbook of Surgery*. Philadelphia: Elsevier; 2012.

Benign Colorectal Disease

J. Leslie Knod, MD

*According to a Public Policy Polling survey, most Americans find
lice and colonoscopies more appealing than Capitol Hill.*

—Ron Fournier

I. ANATOMY

A. RECTUM

1. The rectum is 12–15 cm in length and extends from the sacral prom-
   ontory to the levator ani muscles.
2. The teniae coli splay out at the rectosigmoid junction and fuse to form
   a contiguous smooth muscle layer.
3. The internal rectum is segmented by three horizontal rectal mucosal
   folds (valves of Houston) that help to support its contents.
4. The proximal third of the rectum is covered by peritoneum anteriorly
   and laterally. The anterior peritoneal reflection extends deep into the
   pelvis to 7 cm above the anal verge and lies behind the bladder in
   men and behind the uterus (pouch of Douglas) in women.

B. ANAL CANAL

1. Anatomic anal canal is 3 cm in length and extends from anal verge to
   the dentate line.
2. Surgical anal canal extends from the anal verge to the top of the anorectal ring and is generally 5 cm in length.
3. The rectum is lined by colonic columnar epithelium. The transitional
   zone is lined with cuboidal epithelium that lines the anal canal from
   the columns of Morgagni to the dentate line. Anal glands located in
   the intersphincteric plane drain into the anal crypts that are pockets
   formed between each column. Below the dentate line, the anal canal
   is lined by squamous epithelium.
4. Internal sphincter (involuntary) is a thickened continuation of the
   circular smooth muscle of the rectum under control of the autonomic
   nervous system.
5. External sphincter (voluntary) is an inferior extension of the puborectalis, which is striated muscle with somatic innervation (branch of the
   internal pudendal nerve S2–S4).

C. LEVATOR ANI MUSCLE

1. Composed of iliococcygeus and pubococcygeus muscles, which constitute the pelvic floor with innervation from the fourth sacral nerve

D. BLOOD SUPPLY AND LYMPHATIC DRAINAGE

1. Arterial supply is segmental but with rich anastomoses.
   a. Superior hemorrhoidal—last branch of the inferior mesentery artery

b. Middle hemorrhoidal—branch of the internal iliac artery
c. Inferior hemorrhoidal—branch of the internal pudendal artery

2. **Venous drainage parallels the arterial supply.**
   a. Superior hemorrhoidal—drains the rectum and upper part of anal canal into the portal system
   b. Middle hemorrhoidal—drains rectum and upper anal canal into internal iliac vein (systemic circulation)
   c. Inferior hemorrhoidal vein—drains rectum and lower anal canal into the systemic venous return
   d. The superior, middle, and inferior hemorrhoidal veins—converge to form the inferior hemorrhoidal plexus in the submucosa of the columns of Morgagni

3. **Lymphatic drainage follows the paths of the arteries.**
   a. Superior and middle rectum—drains into the inferior mesenteric artery nodes
   b. Lower rectum and upper anal canal—drain into the superior rectal lymphatics (leading to the inferior mesentery artery) and to the internal iliac nodes
   c. Anal canal distal to the dentate line—has dual drainage to the inguinal nodes and the internal iliac nodes

II. HEMORRHOIDS

1. **The normal anal canal has three fibrovascular cushions that contribute to the resting anal pressure and adjust to aid fecal continence.**
   When a cushion becomes abnormally large it is then termed a hemorrhoid. Direct etiology is unclear but likely secondary to constant straining with defecation.

2. **Location (relative to dentate line)**
   a. Internal hemorrhoids: cushions of dilated submucosal veins of the superior rectal plexus that lie *proximal* to the dentate line and are covered by transitional or columnar epithelium. Typically found in three locations:
      (1) Left lateral
      (2) Right posterolateral
      (3) Right anterolateral
   b. Classification of internal hemorrhoids
      (1) First degree: painless, bleeding without prolapse
      (2) Second degree: prolapse during defecation but spontaneously reduce
      (3) Third degree: prolapse during defecation requiring manual reduction
      (4) Fourth degree: permanently prolapsed
   c. External hemorrhoids—dilated veins arising from the inferior hemorrhoidal plexus *below* the dentate line that are covered with squamous epithelium (anoderm); generally asymptomatic, unless thrombosed

A. SIGNS AND SYMPTOMS

1. Rectal bleeding is most common (usually bright red with spotting on toilet paper or squirting into the commode) ± iron deficiency anemia, pruritus, swelling, prolapse, hygiene problems, and pain.
2. Hemorrhoid prolapse and swelling can cause fecal leakage and skin irritation but not frank incontinence. Clearly document bowel function and anatomy before surgery.
3. Pain is usually associated with *thrombosed* external hemorrhoids and subsides in 48–72 hours, although the hemorrhoid will take longer to resolve; internal hemorrhoids can also cause pain if incarcerated or strangulated.

B. DIAGNOSIS

1. Ensure a thorough examination with visual inspection, digital rectal examination, and anoscopy to develop broad differential, such as perianal Crohn disease, fissure, abscess, condyloma accuminata, rectal/anal neoplasm or polyp, hypertrophied anal papillas, proctitis, or angiodysplasia. Additional endoscopic evaluation may be indicated.
2. Rectal varices are distinct from hemorrhoids. Present in the setting of portal hypertension or rectal varicosities are more proximal in the anal canal and are best treated with reduction in portal hypertension.

C. MEDICAL TREATMENT

1. Medical management is recommended for all hemorrhoids, and grade I–III hemorrhoids often respond.
2. Recommend dietary modifications including increased fiber (25–30 g/day) and fluid intake (6–8 glasses/day), avoiding constipating foods and foods causing diarrhea. Improve anal hygiene, including sitz baths and avoidance of prolonged straining during defecation. Topical steroids may be used with caution as prolonged use will thin perianal skin. Over-the-counter astringent agents (Tucks, Preparation H) can help mitigate discomfort from external hemorrhoids.

D. OFFICE TREATMENT

1. Rubber band ligation is used in the treatment of grade I–III internal hemorrhoids but optimal for grade I–II. Bands must be placed above the dentate line to avoid somatic pain. Depending on provider preference and patient tolerance, typically only one to two hemorrhoids are ligated per session with repeat banding performed at 4 weeks when inflammation has decreased. Band is retained for 2–10 days, while tissue necrosis and scarring occur.
   a. Potential complications (0.5%–8% rate) include vasovagal reaction, severe bleeding after necrotic tissue sloughs off (1–2 weeks postoperatively), and pelvic sepsis (presenting with pelvic pain, fever, urinary incontinence, and perineal cellulitis).

2. Sclerotherapy involves injection of hemorrhoid or its base with sclerosing agent, which obliterates the hemorrhoid by thrombosis then fibrosis. This is the preferred treatment for patients who are on anticoagulation or are immunocompromised.

3. Infrared coagulation involves direct application of infrared light resulting in protein destruction. It is most applicable to grades I and II hemorrhoids without prolapse or thick tissue and requires 2–3 repeat treatments at 2-week intervals.

4. Other therapies include cryotherapy, bipolar diathermy, and direct current therapy.

E. SURGICAL HEMORRHOIDECTOMY

Indicated for large grade III–IV internal hemorrhoids, mixed hemorrhoids, large external hemorrhoids, and patients who failed office procedural management

1. Closed or Ferguson hemorrhoidectomy is most commonly performed for complex/mixed hemorrhoids.
    a. A perianal nerve block is performed by injecting four quadrants around the anus in both superficial submucosa and deep intersphincteric spaces.
    b. The hemorrhoidal bundle is retracted with forceps or hemostat, and the anoderm is excised with an elliptical incision.
    c. The hemorrhoid is then dissected off the external and internal sphincter, sparing muscle, and excised to the proximal anal canal, while leaving enough anoderm for closure without narrowing the anal canal.
    d. If not excised with cautery and hemostatic, the pedicle is suture ligated with a chromic or Vicryl suture followed by approximation of wound edges with a running chromic suture beginning at the apex (using this as a lever) and extending to the anoderm. Up to three hemorrhoidal bundles may be excised in this fashion, permitting enough anoderm remains to prevent the complication of anal stenosis.

2. Procedure for prolapsing hemorrhoids (PPH) is best for patients with large internal hemorrhoids with minimal external component.
    a. Circumferential stapled hemorrhoidectomy (or more accurately hemorrhoidopexy) involves transanal circular stapling of redundant anorectal mucosa with a specialized circular stapling instrument. Redundant mucosa is drawn into the instrument with a circumferential purse-string suture and excised within the device. Care is taken to ensure this is performed well above the dentate line to avoid somatically innervated anoderm and to avoid injury to vaginal canal that may lead to the dreaded complication of a rectovaginal fistula.
    b. Patients often have less postoperative pain and shorter recovery, but there is a higher rate of recurrence.

3. Hemorrhoidal artery ligation (HAL) is a new technique that uses a Doppler transducer to localize the proximal feeding vessels above the dentate line. Often six arteries are located and ligated with 2-0 braided suture.

28

BENIGN COLORECTAL DISEASE

4. Thrombosed external hemorrhoids: These can be extremely painful and should be excised if seen within 48 hours. Beyond this time, texts recommend conservative therapy with analgesics, and sitz baths are appropriate, but clinically if the pain is unrelenting, surgical excision can be offered.

III. ANAL FISSURE

A. OVERVIEW

1. Represents an acute or chronic linear tear in the skin or anoderm distal to the dentate line. Most are located at posterior midline, but 10% are anterior especially in women. Lateral or multiple fissures should raise suspicion of trauma, inflammatory bowel disease, lymphoma, neoplasm, or infection and require further investigation with biopsy and/or endoscopic evaluation.
2. There is equal incidence among men and women, and most are in young adults.
3. Proposed etiology is increased resting anal pressure and hypertonia of internal anal sphincter.

B. SIGNS AND SYMPTOMS

1. These include sharp tearing pain associated with defecation and possible bright red blood on toilet paper.
2. Chronic fissures may be associated with a "sentinel pile" or hypertrophied papilla and external anal skin tag.

C. TREATMENT

1. Nonoperative management is initial treatment and best for acute fissures.
   a. Stool softeners and bulk laxatives relieve straining.
   b. Sitz baths offer symptomatic relief and improve hygiene.
   c. Topical application of compounded calcium channel blockers (nifedipine, diltiazem) has been proven to be the most effective and least symptomatic medical therapy and will achieve healing in 75%–80% of patients who comply with fiber supplementation.
   d. Anesthetic suppositories and nitroglycerin 0.2% cream may be helpful but may cause headache and are associated with increased cost when compared with compounded calcium channel blockers.
   e. Chemical sphincterotomy is achieved with botulinum toxin administered into the internal anal sphincter.
2. Operative therapy is indicated for unsuccessful response to above management. The goal of surgery is to achieve relaxation of internal anal sphincter.
   a. Lateral internal sphincterotomy is the surgical treatment of choice, often performed on right side to avoid left lateral hemorrhoid.
   b. Fissurectomy with advancement flap is an option for patients without hypertonia of internal anal sphincter or with compromised fecal incontinence.

IV. ANORECTAL ABSCESS

Anorectal abscesses typically originate from a cryptoglandular infection. The acute phase of the infection causes an anorectal abscess, whereas approximately 50% become chronic, leading to fistula formation. An anorectal abscess typically forms in the intersphincteric space. Subsequent spread can occur along various paths (Fig. 28.1). Factors implicated in the development of an abscess include constipation, diarrhea, trauma, Crohn disease, tuberculosis, actinomycosis, anorectal malignancy, leukemia, and lymphoma, although most patients will have no antecedent history. The disease is more common in diabetic and immunocompromised patients than in the general public, and the incidence is much greater in men (2:1). Infection is typically polymicrobial (*Escherichia coli, Proteus* spp., *Streptococcus* spp., and *Bacteroides* spp.).

A. CLASSIFICATION (BASED ON LOCATION)

1. Simple perianal abscess is a superficial abscess that lies beneath the skin of the anal canal but does not traverse the sphincters.
2. Ischiorectal abscess occupies the ischiorectal fossa below the levators and lateral to the sphincters. The abscess can cross the midline to form a bilateral abscess called a *horseshoe abscess*, which requires bilateral drainage.
3. Intersphincteric or transsphincteric abscess is located between or through the external and internal sphincter muscle and is most common in the posterior quadrant. It typically exists without evidence of perianal swelling or induration.

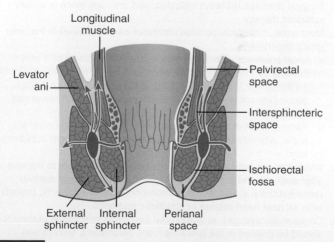

FIG. 28.1
Potential pathways of abscess extension in perianal planes.

Labels: Longitudinal muscle; Levator ani; Pelvirectal space; Intersphincteric space; Ischiorectal fossa; External sphincter; Internal sphincter; Perianal space

28

BENIGN COLORECTAL DISEASE

4. Supralevator abscess occurs above the levators and is more difficult to diagnose and drain; it can mimic intraabdominal pathology.
5. Postanal space abscess originates in the posterior midline and causes an abscess in the deep postanal space anatomically bounded by the levators, anococcygeal ligament, and anal canal. It may extend into the ischiorectal space. Typically, patients present with severe pain without evidence of perianal swelling or induration.

B. SIGNS AND SYMPTOMS

1. They usually present with extreme, local perianal pain, tenderness, and fluctuance. However, a more complex abscess may present with paucity of external examination findings and instead present with deep rectal pain (intersphincteric abscess) or abdominal pain (supralevator abscess).
2. A fullness or bogginess may be felt on rectal examination with high abscesses, whereas erythema and fluctuance are often seen with superficial lesions.
3. Pelvic computed tomography (CT) may be necessary to accurately diagnose complex, deep abscesses or disease in the morbidly obese patient, but it should not be used in routine evaluation of most perianal or perirectal abscesses.
4. Systemic toxicity (e.g., fever, chills, leukocytosis, and cellulitis) warrants urgent surgical decompression.

C. TREATMENT

1. Surgical drainage is always indicated, and drainage alone is usually sufficient therapy.
2. Most small, superficial perianal abscesses can be drained in the emergency department.
   a. Local anesthetic with epinephrine is injected, followed by a generous, cruciate incision over maximally fluctuant aspect of the lesion. Gently explore cavity and bluntly break up loculi to achieve full drainage, taking care not to disrupt pudendal nerve fibers, which can impair continence.
   b. Packing is left in overnight and removed with the institution of sitz baths. Alternatively, an indwelling, mushroom-tip catheter may be used.
3. Antibiotics are indicated for cellulitis, fasciitis, and failure to improve after drainage and in patients with systemic symptoms or complex comorbidities (i.e., diabetic or immunocompromised patients, patients with valvular heart disease or prosthetic implants).
4. Complex disease such as ischiorectal abscesses or multiple abscesses should be drained in the operating room. Necrotizing fasciitis and Fournier gangrene are serious complications if left undrained and require emergent operation.

5. Supralevator abscesses often arise from intraabdominal sources and may require CT-guided drainage and treatment of underlying etiology (e.g., diverticulitis).
6. Horseshoe abscess requires operative drainage initially by accessing the deep postanal space (incision between tip of coccyx and anal verge) and lateral extensions with placement of drains. After 6–8 weeks of drainage, the fistula is then operatively addressed (see Section V).
7. Consider proctosigmoidoscopy to rule out other etiologies.

V. FISTULA IN ANO

A.   GENERAL
1. It is an abnormal communication between epithelialized surfaces, the anal canal (internal opening) at about the level of the dentate line, and the perianal skin (external opening).
2. One must localize the causative primary opening AND establish the relationship of the fistula tract to the sphincter complex.

B.   CLASSIFICATION
1. Intersphincteric fistula is located in the intersphincteric space with external opening typically on the perianal skin near the anal verge.
2. Transsphincteric fistula is the most common type of fistula. It starts in the intersphincteric space and traverses the external sphincter into the ischiorectal fossa, with external opening lateral to the anal verge. Horseshoe fistula falls into this category.
3. Suprasphincteric fistula starts in the intersphincteric space, passes above the puborectalis muscle, and tracks laterally between the levator and the puborectalis muscle.
4. Extrasphincteric fistula is a complicated fistula. It passes from the perianal skin through the ischiorectal fossa and levator ani muscles and subsequently through the rectal wall.

C.   GOODSALL RULE
1. This predicts internal opening of fistula based on external opening. Divide the pelvis into anterior and posterior segments with an imaginary transverse line through anal verge.
2. Fistulas with external openings *anterior* to a transverse line have a fistula tract that extends directly to the dentate line anteriorly, in a *radial* fashion.
3. Fistulas with external openings *posterior* to the transverse line have a tract that *curves* and have their internal opening in the posterior midline.
4. Exceptions to Goodsall rule include horseshoe fistula, inflammatory bowel disease, long tracts distant from anal verge, and women with anterior openings.

28

BENIGN COLORECTAL DISEASE

D. SIGNS AND SYMPTOMS

1. Chief complaint is typically intermittent or constant drainage. A history of recurrent perianal abscess may be present.
2. The external opening may be represented by a red cluster of granulation tissue, and a cordlike tract may be palpated on rectal examination.

E. TREATMENT

1. Delineation of the fistula tract must be achieved under anesthesia by gentle probing with a fistula probe and, if needed, injected hydrogen peroxide via external opening to localize the internal opening.
2. Imaging studies such as ultrasound ± hydrogen peroxide or magnetic resonance imaging (MRI) may be of use in complex patients.
3. Fistulotomy: preferred for intersphincteric and low transsphincteric, simple fistulas. The skin overlying the tract is divided followed by fibers of the internal sphincter to the intersphincteric plane. It is generally safe to divide the distal one-third of the external sphincter without compromising continence. The tract is curetted and allowed to heal secondarily.
4. Complex fistulas may be managed by setons, endoanal advancement flap, ligation of the intersphincteric fistula tract (LIFT) procedure, or, less successfully, fibrin glue or anal fistula plug (AFP).
   a. Sphincter-sparing surgery (AFP, LIFT) is recommended in select patients with current fecal incontinence, prior fistula surgery, complex fistula, and anterior fistula in women.
   b. Seton placement: may be either *cutting* or *drainage* seton based on tension applied at placement. Setons are often used as the initial drainage procedure in staged planning for previously mentioned sphincter-sparing operations. They are also used for drainage of abscesses or fistulas in the setting of Crohn disease because simple fistulotomy is prone to complication and prolonged healing in the setting of Crohn disease (Fig. 28.2). A heavy suture or vascular loop is passed through the tract to improve drainage and stimulate fibrosis and closure of the tract. The seton may be sequentially tightened to *cut* through sphincter complex slowly, although this has produced similar rates of incontinence when compared with simple fistulotomy.
   c. Horseshoe fistulas as described in Section III require complex management, including initial drainage followed by modified Hanley procedure (cutting seton around posterior midline sphincter complex) or AFP.

VI. PILONIDAL DISEASE

A. GENERAL

1. This disease of the sacrococcygeal region is now thought to be from obstructed hair follicles in the subcutaneous tissue at the intergluteal cleft that leads to acute abscess or chronic sinus.

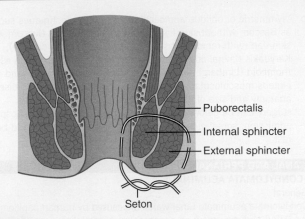

- Puborectalis
- Internal sphincter
- External sphincter

Seton

FIG. 28.2

Use of a seton in a high fistula.

2. It is often seen between ages 20 and 35 years and is more common in men.
3. Midline pits in the gluteal cleft on physical examination are a classic finding. Rule out other diagnoses, such as perianal abscess/fistula, hidradenitis suppurativa, granulomatous disease, and osteomyelitis with draining sinus tracts.
4. Nonoperative treatment includes weekly shaving (or laser hair removal), sitz baths, and possibly phenol injections into sinuses. Indications for surgery include chronic pain, recurrent abscesses, or chronic drainage.

B. TREATMENT

1. Acute abscess: incision (off-midline by at least 1 cm) and drainage with curettage of the cavity and removal of impacted hair. The wound is left open to drain and heal. Up to 40% of patients experience development of chronic draining pilonidal sinuses, which will require further treatment.
2. Chronic pilonidal sinus: Several options exist, depending on the severity of disease and weight of potential complications.

   a. Midline approach:

   Unroof: Probe sinus and open tract, plus curettage. Can partially close with marsupialization to reduce wound healing time (possibly 6 weeks).

   Sinus excision: Completely excise sinus tracts, possibly down to presacral fascia. There is prolonged healing of approximately 2 months. Wound can be primarily closed (40% recurrence), left open, or marsupialized, or a vacuum suction dressing is applied.

b. Asymmetric or oblique approach: more complex techniques such as Bascom without skin flap (lateral approach), cleft Bascom with skin flap (with removal of skin that includes midline disease), Karydakis (lateral advancement flap), and formal flaps such as rhomboid (Limberg) flap, V-Y advancement flap, Z-plasty, and gluteus musculocutaneous flap. Choice of flap is based on disease anatomy and size of defect created with excision. Extensive surgery can be deforming cosmetically and often requires hospital admission, sometimes with several days for pain control and bed rest.

VII. ANAL AND PERIANAL INFECTIONS

A. CONDYLOMATA ACUMINATA

1. General

Condylomata acuminata (anal warts) are caused by human papillomavirus (HPV) and may occur on perianal skin, anorectal mucosa, or genital region. Anogenital HPV is strongly associated with anal intraepithelial neoplasia (AIN) and squamous cell cancer (SCC). Examination should include anoscopy to evaluate potential intraanal lesions. Transmission is often by direct contact or sexually transmitted but can occur in vapors after cauterization. Lesions appear cauliflower-like, exophytic, or sessile.

2. Treatment—excision/cauterization and topical agents

   a. Excision/cauterization under anesthesia for extensive involvement. Be mindful of anal stenosis as a complication with large, treated areas.

   b. Podophyllin, cryotherapy, and trichloroacetic acid (TCA) are routine office treatments. Biopsy should be performed before chemical treatment.

   c. Podofilox, 5-fluorouracil, and imiquimod are home treatments, with variable frequency of application.

   d. A giant condyloma (Buschke-Löwenstein tumor) is often locally invasive, and half contain SCC. Major morbidity is due to local invasion and recurrence.

B. ANORECTAL HERPES

1. Presenting symptom is severe pain.

2. Characteristic herpetic lesions are seen on examination and confirmed by Giemsa (Tzanck prep) stain, viral culture, and biopsy.

3. Treatment: Antiviral agents such as valacyclovir shorten the clinical course and frequency of recurrence.

C. GONOCOCCAL PROCTITIS

1. Presenting symptoms include pain and discharge.

2. Anoscopy reveals mucosal erythema and purulence from the anal crypts. It is confirmed by Gram stain and culture.

3. Treatment: Because of the increase in prevalence of penicillinase-producing *Neisseria gonorrhoeae,* ceftriaxone 250 mg intramuscularly (IM) (single dose) followed by doxycycline 100 mg orally twice daily for 7 days is recommended.

VIII. PRURITUS ANI

Primary (idiopathic) pruritus ani accounts for 50%–90% of cases and is most often in males and patients aged 40–70 years. It is a diagnosis of exclusion, and a thorough, detailed history and physical are paramount.

A. ETIOLOGY

Conditions that lead to perianal moisture, drainage, or soiling
1. Hemorrhoids, fissures, fistula, polyps, skin tags, diarrhea, constipation, rectal prolapse, sphincter weakness
2. Other causes: fungal dermatitis, pinworms, sexually transmitted infections, and other infectious agents; may also relate to dermatologic conditions, such as psoriasis or lichen planus
3. Other underlying disease such as diabetes, hyperbilirubinemia, Crohn disease
4. Topical (soaps or perfumes) or dietary sensitivities
5. Neoplasm, such as carcinoma, melanoma, Paget disease of bone, Bowen disease

B. DIAGNOSIS

1. A detailed history is important and should include dietary and detailed bowel habits, hygiene practice, menopausal state, systemic diseases, prior anorectal surgeries, and previous radiation.
2. A careful examination of the perianal skin and anorectum is required and possibly anoscopy. Biopsy and specimens for cultures are obtained when indicated.

C. TREATMENT

1. Therapy is directed at achieving clean, dry, intact skin. Certainly, if a secondary cause is identified, it should be treated accordingly.
2. Reassure patient to reduce anxiety, and educate patient regarding hygiene, including sitz baths and warm tap water enema to clear rectum and maintain dry anus. Other treatments include elimination of irritants (such as soaps, wet wipes, synthetic or dyed undergarments), smoking cessation, and diet modifications.
3. Topical agents, such as mild topical drying agents, antiinflammatory agents, and inert skin barrier such as a zinc oxide ointment or steroid cream, can be used, although relief is temporary.
4. Treatment often requires patience of both patient and physician and good follow-up.

28

BENIGN COLORECTAL DISEASE

IX. ANAL NEOPLASM

Malignancies of the anal canal are relatively uncommon and represent only 2%–3% of all colorectal carcinomas. The location of the tumor in the anal canal relative to the dentate line is important with regard to the behavior of the tumor, particularly its lymphatic drainage that follows venous drainage. Most tumors spread by direct extension and lymphatic drainage, not hematologically. Anal tumors are classified into two groups based on location: (1) anal canal tumors and (2) anal margin tumors.

A. TUMORS OF THE ANAL CANAL

1. **AIN is a precursor to invasive SCC.**
   a. It is subdivided into grade I (low-grade), II (moderate-grade), and III (high-grade) dysplasia.
   b. It is associated with HPV infections, especially types 16 and 18.
   c. Affected areas may include anal canal and/or perianal skin. Disease is often multifocal and may be microscopic or macroscopic with warts, ulcers, plaques, or tumors.
   d. Risk factors include HPV infection, multiple sexual partners, anoreceptive intercourse, cervical dysplasia or cancer, smoking, immunosuppression, and HIV infection.
   e. AIN has low risk of progression to cancer. Grade III AIN risk of progression is approximately 5%–10%, but in immunosuppressed patients risk is approximately 50%.
   f. Treatment is not standardized. Microscopic disease in an immunocompetent patient can be followed conservatively with periodic physical examination with anoscopy, whereas macroscopic lesions should be resected. Imiquimod has been used for microscopic AIN.
   g. High-risk, immunosuppressed patients should have anal Pap smears every 3–6 months. If positive, follow by thorough physical examination and high-resolution anoscopy with acetic acid and/or Lugol iodine ± biopsy, ablation, and/or local excision of macroscopic disease.

2. **SCC/epidermoid carcinomas include subtypes: squamous, basaloid, cloacogenic, or transitional carcinomas. Although each has different histologic features, they exhibit similar biologic behavior and are thus grouped together.**
   a. Location of SCC is vital to determine optimal treatment. If SCC on the perianal skin *(anal margin)*, it is treated as its respective skin cancer, often with wide local excision for T1 tumors or with chemoradiation for T2 or larger tumors.
   b. Examination of SCC of anal canal includes inguinal lymph node evaluation, anoscopy, and biopsy of tumor. Prognosis correlates with size of primary tumor and status of lymph nodes. Obtain CT chest/abdomen/pelvis for staging ± positron emission tomography (PET) scan.

   c. Treatment: chemoradiation, not surgical excision. Use mitomycin C and 5-fluorouracil combined with concomitant radiation (Nigro protocol). If inguinal lymph nodes are positive, additional radiation is indicated.

   d. After chemoradiation alone, 5-year survival is 70%–90%.

   e. Abdominoperineal resection (APR) is indicated for failure to regress after 12 weeks or recurrence thereafter, in the absence of metastatic disease. Survival for salvage APR is approximately 50%.

3. **Malignant melanoma is rare.**

   a. Anal canal is the third most common site after skin and eyes.

   b. Rectal bleeding is the most frequent complaint. It is often not pigmented and may not resemble malignancy, so diagnosis is difficult.

   c. Treatment: wide local excision with negative margins if possible. If lesion is too large, consider APR.

   d. Disease-free survival is 30% at 5 years.

   e. Benefit of adjuvant radiation, chemotherapy, or interferon is unclear.

4. **Adenocarcinoma of anal canal is treated as rectal adenocarcinoma.**

X. RECTAL PROLAPSE

A. CLASSIFICATION

1. **False prolapse or mucosal prolapse:** redundant prolapsed rectal mucosa with radial folds in orientation

2. **Incomplete prolapse:** rectal intussusception

3. **True prolapse or complete prolapse:** protrusion of the entire rectal wall through the anal orifice with herniation of the pelvic peritoneum or cul-de-sac; circular mucosal folds are seen.

B. CLINICAL FEATURES

1. Majority of patients are women (6:1) and older (>50 years old). Risk increases with multiparity and vaginal delivery.

2. Etiology is unknown but likely related to chronic constipation and straining. Fecal incontinence is present in up to 70% and constipation in 15%–65%.

3. Anatomic findings include deep cul-de-sac, redundant sigmoid or lack of normal rectal fixation, weak pelvic floor muscles, pudendal neuropathy, or anal sphincter weakening.

4. It must be distinguished from obstructive defecation with etiologies such as rectocele or nonrelaxing puborectalis muscle.

5. Initial evaluation addresses duration of symptoms, specific bowel habits, and associated symptoms (e.g., urinary incontinence or uterine prolapsed), including alleviating factors, such as laxatives (may point to colonic inertia) and manual digitation (may suggest rectocele).

   a. Note specific bowel habits (i.e., constipation, fecal incontinence, tenesmus, frequency of bowel movements).

   b. If prolapse is reported, inquire regarding amount of tissue prolapsed, triggers (exertion, coughing, sneezing), and what is required to reduce it.

6. Perform physical examination with patient in lateral decubitus position or prone or sitting on commode and straining.
   a. Demonstrate prolapse during Valsalva maneuver.
   b. Digital rectal examination assesses resting tone and squeeze and sphincter defects with evaluation of puborectalis muscle.
   c. Excoriation or circumferential inflammation of midrectum on anoscopy or proctosigmoidoscopy. Also evaluate degree of prolapse during Valsalva (i.e., mucosal, hemorrhoidal, or full thickness).

C. EVALUATION

1. Endoscopic evaluation and defecography should be considered in all patients with prolapse. Reduce the prolapse and perform sigmoidoscopy or proctoscopy to determine the condition of the bowel and the presence of any associated lesions, which may serve as a lead point for prolapse.
2. Manometry assesses sphincter tone when clinically indicated based on associated symptoms. Electromyography and defecography may diagnose paradoxic puborectalis muscle contraction, and the latter also assesses for pelvic floor disorders. Diagnosing a nonrelaxing puborectalis will aid planning additional therapy such as biofeedback.
3. Colonic transit studies document colonic inertia, which, if left uncorrected, will result in the patient having persistent, chronic constipation and straining, despite correction of rectal prolapse. Obtain when clinically indicated based on associated symptoms.
4. False prolapse:
   a. Common in young children. Conservative therapy is often successful. Gently replace the prolapsed rectum after each defecation or straining. Excision of redundant mucosa is rarely necessary.
   b. In adults, hemorrhoidectomy with excision of redundant mucosa is effective. Circumferential stapled hemorrhoidectomy may be used with similar results. Fiber and laxatives will minimize straining and constipation, and biofeedback and pelvic floor exercises are also helpful.
5. True prolapse: typically a progressive disorder that is not responsive to nonsurgical therapy. Basic features of the repairs include correction of the following anatomic characteristics:
   a. Abnormally deep or wide cul-de-sac
   b. Weak pelvic floor with diastasis of the levators
   c. Patulous anal sphincter
   d. Redundant rectosigmoid
   e. Lack of fixation of the rectum to the sacral hollow with abnormal mobility and loss of the normal horizontal position of the lower rectum
   f. Associated incontinence is not treated initially because it may resolve after treatment of the prolapse.

D. TREATMENT OPTIONS

1. Abdominal approaches
   a. Abdominal suture rectopexy ± sigmoid resection: Rectum is dissected to level of middle hemorrhoidal vessel, to preserve pelvic nerves, then pulled out of the pelvis and anchored to presacral fascia with sutures. This is a treatment option in young, healthy patients and can be performed laparoscopically.
   b. Rectopexy with mesh: The rectum is fixed to the sacrum using a sling of synthetic mesh either anteriorly (Ripstein procedure or ventral mesh rectopexy) or posteriorly. Possible complications include mesh erosion and infection. Concomitant resection poses increased infection risk with mesh.
2. Perineal approach (useful in debilitated patients who would not tolerate an abdominal procedure or general anesthesia)
   a. Perineal rectosigmoidectomy (Altemeier procedure): resection of the prolapsing bowel. Evert prolapse and incise full thickness, 1 cm proximal to dentate line. After gaining access to the abdominal cavity, divide the mesentery to mobilize sigmoid colon, and then divide redundant bowel and perform primary anastomosis. Perform levatorplasty if needed.
   b. Delorme procedure: Mucosal stripping of the rectum begins with circumferential mucosal incision 1 cm above dentate line and mucosal dissection to apex of prolapse. Then circular muscle is plicated and redundant mucosa is excised followed by mucosal anastomosis.

XI. ANOSCOPY

A. GENERAL

1. Examine the lower rectum and anal canal.
2. Bowel prep is not necessary, but an enema may improve the examination, depending on the clinical situation.

B. TECHNIQUE

1. Positioning
   a. Using examination table that provides prone jackknife positioning is ideal.
   b. Alternatively, place patient in lateral decubitus position with hips and knees flexed.
2. Inspection: Note the presence of fissures, hemorrhoids (with and without Valsalva), skin tags, blood, or pus.
3. Palpation: Digital examination with lubricant must be done before anoscopy.
   a. Note masses, induration, spasm, sphincter tone with Valsalva, tenderness, or discharge.
   b. Palpate normal structures, including prostate.
   c. Inspect examining finger for blood, pus, stool, or mucus. Stool may be analyzed for occult blood.

4. Anoscopy
   a. Lubricate generously and insert obturator.
   b. Introduce anoscope pointing in direction of umbilicus. After the upper end of the anal canal is reached, redirect the anoscope posteriorly, toward sacrum.
   c. Note the character of mucosa and the presence of lesions or foreign body.
   d. Slowly withdraw scope, while observing the passing mucosa.

XII. RIGID SIGMOIDOSCOPY

A. GENERAL
1. Evaluation of distal 25–30 cm
2. Enema improves examination of mucosa

B. TECHNIQUE
1. Position as for anoscopy.
2. Inspect the perianal area and perform a digital examination, as in anoscopy.
3. Insert the scope into the anus directed toward the umbilicus.
4. When the rectum is entered, remove the obturator and close the window. The scope should be advanced farther only under direct visualization of the lumen. Insufflation is used as needed.
5. Slowly advance the scope through the lumen of the bowel. Movements are initially posterior into the sacral hollow.
6. After the scope is fully inserted, it is slowly withdrawn to carefully examine the sigmoid and rectal mucosa.
7. Biopsy should be performed last so that blood does not obscure the remainder of the examination.
8. Before the scope is removed, evacuate insufflated air for the patient's comfort.

RECOMMENDED READINGS

Fleshner PR, Chalasani S, Change GJ, et al. Practice parameters for anal squamous neoplasms. *Dis Colon Rectum*. 2008;51:2–9.

Kaidar-Person O. Hemorrhoidal disease: a comprehensive review. *J Am Coll Surg*. 2007; 204:102–117.

Madiba TE, Baig MK, Wexner SD. Surgical management of rectal prolapse. *Arch Surg*. 2005;140:63–73.

Appendix

Anthony J. Hayes, MD

When I am dying, I should like my life taken out under general anaesthetic, exactly as if it were a diseased appendix.

—Richard Dawkins

I. OVERVIEW

A. ANATOMY
1. The appendix develops as a protuberance of the base of the cecum.
   a. The base is located at the convergence of the teniae coli, and the tip is variably located (e.g., retrocecal, pelvic).
   b. Blood supply is via a terminal branch of the ileocolic artery, a branch of the superior mesenteric artery (SMA).

B. FUNCTION
1. The appendix participates in immune function via secretion of immunoglobulin A (IgA).
   a. Studies have demonstrated a decreased risk of development of ulcerative colitis in patients with a previous appendectomy. The relationship between prior appendectomy and the risk of Crohn disease is inconclusive.

II. EPIDEMIOLOGY

A. GENERAL
1. Appendicitis is the most common cause of acute abdomen requiring surgery, with approximately 300,000 cases per year in the United States affecting 7% of the population.
2. Peak incidence occurs between 10 and 30 years of age, with a slight male predominance.
3. The incidence rate of perforation is 12%.
4. Overall incidence rate of normal appendices after appendectomy is 10%–15%.

B. MORBIDITY AND MORTALITY
1. Overall mortality is 0.1% for nonperforated cases and 5% for perforated cases.
2. Infants and older adults have much greater morbidity and mortality rates—approximately 85% for infants and approximately 28%–60% for older adults because of an increase in the perforation rate.
3. The greater morbidity and mortality rates in infants and older adults are due to atypical and late presentations.

III. PATHOPHYSIOLOGY

A. GENERAL

1. Obstruction of the appendiceal lumen is thought to be the initiating event in two-thirds of cases, most commonly secondary to a fecalith in adults and lymphoid hyperplasia in children.
2. With continued mucosal secretion, luminal pressure increases and eventually exceeds capillary venous and lymphatic pressures, causing venous infarction in watershed areas (middle and proximal antimesenteric regions).
3. Bacterial overgrowth occurs in the inspissated mucus.
4. Polymicrobial infection with anaerobes: aerobes 3:1
5. *Escherichia coli, Bacteroides fragilis,* and *Pseudomonas* spp. present in 80%, 70%, and 40% of cases, respectively.

B. COMPLICATIONS

1. Worsening edema, high luminal pressure, and bacterial proliferation lead to occlusion of arterial blood flow and gangrenous appendicitis.
2. Transmural necrosis and bacterial penetration into the appendiceal wall are associated with perforation, which may either be walled off by omentum or spread throughout the abdomen, inducing diffuse peritonitis.
3. Overall incidence rate is 12% for perforation.

IV. PRESENTATION

A. HISTORY

1. Pain usually begins as vague midabdominal (periumbilical) discomfort caused by appendiceal distention and referred pain along lesser splanchnics.
2. Anorexia and nausea occur almost uniformly after the pain. Almost all adults have anorexia, whereas children with appendicitis may remain hungry.
3. Pain localizes to the right lower quadrant (RLQ) as the parietal peritoneum in that area becomes irritated.
   a. If the appendix lies in the pelvis or retrocecal area, the location of the pain (and tenderness) will be positioned over the area of peritoneal inflammation.
   b. If perforation occurs, diffuse peritonitis may ensue with pain throughout the abdomen, although some may "wall" off the perforation, localizing the symptoms.
4. Patients may have constipation, diarrhea, or no change in bowel habits.
   a. A history of late onset of loose stools may indicate pelvic peritonitis after perforation.

B. PHYSICAL EXAMINATION

1. Low-grade fever may be present: temperature is rarely greater than 38°C (101°F), unless perforation, abscess formation, or both have occurred.

2. When the appendix lies anteriorly, tenderness is present at McBurney point (one-third the distance between the anterior superior iliac spine and the umbilicus).
3. Abdominal wall muscular rigidity may be present.
4. With peritoneal irritation, guarding, rebound, and indirect rebound tenderness may occur.
   a. There are several described physical examination findings associated with appendicitis that are neither sensitive nor specific.
      (1) Rovsing sign is pain in RLQ with palpation of the lower left quadrant.
      (2) The psoas sign is pain occurring with extension of the right thigh and indicates an irritative focus overlying that muscle.
      (3) The obturator sign is pain with passive internal rotation of the flexed right thigh and indicates inflammation overlying that muscle.
5. Rectal examination elicits suprapubic pain if the inflamed appendix tip lies in the pelvis.
6. Male patients may have pain in the right, left, or both testicles because both are innervated by T10.

C. LABORATORY AND RADIOLOGIC FINDINGS

1. The diagnosis of appendicitis is largely a clinical one; however, some objective data may be useful.
2. White blood cell (WBC) count increase from 10,000 to 18,000/mm^3 is expected, although not always present, with a left shift on differential.
   a. WBC count is normal in approximately 10% of patients.
   b. Patients who are human immunodeficiency virus–positive have the same symptoms, but usually the WBC count is normal.
3. Urinalysis may be normal or reveal few red blood cells or WBCs only, especially in retrocecal or pelvic appendix.
   a. All female patients of reproductive age should have a urine pregnancy test.
4. Computed tomography scan has been shown to be superior to ultrasound in diagnosing acute appendicitis in both pediatric and adult populations.
   a. Both are helpful when pain is associated with an RLQ mass to rule out phlegmon versus abscess.
   b. Computed tomography scan should be used to aid diagnosis in patients with atypical presentation.

V. DIFFERENTIAL DIAGNOSIS

1. Gastroenteritis
2. Diverticulitis (adults)
3. Acute mesenteric adenitis (children)

APPENDIX

29

4. Meckel diverticulitis
5. Intussusception (infants and children)
6. Regional enteritis
7. Perforated peptic ulcer
8. Perforating carcinoma of cecum or sigmoid colon
9. Urinary tract infection
10. Ureteral stone
11. Gynecologic disease (e.g., pelvic inflammatory disease, ectopic pregnancy, ovarian cyst)
12. Male urologic disease (e.g., testicular torsion, epididymitis)
13. Epiploic appendagitis
14. Spontaneous bacterial peritonitis
15. Henoch-Schönlein purpura
16. Yersiniosis

VI. COMPLICATIONS

A. PERFORATION
1. This occurs more in patients older than 50 and younger than 10 years.
2. It is associated with more diffuse pain after localized tenderness.
   a. Initially, pain may be relieved, followed by peritonitis.
3. It is uncommon for perforation to occur within 24 hours of onset of abdominal pain.

B. PERITONITIS
1. This occurs after perforation.
2. Localized peritonitis refers to peritonitis that is microscopic and contained by surrounding viscera or omentum, whereas generalized peritonitis refers to gross spillage into the peritoneal cavity.
3. It is associated with high fever and may lead to sepsis.

C. ABSCESS
1. This may be associated with an RLQ mass on physical examination.
2. Computed tomography scan should be performed together with percutaneous drainage.
3. The patient is treated with antibiotics, and an interval appendectomy is performed.
4. If present at the time of operation, the appendix should be removed if it is possible to do so safely and drains placed.
5. It recurs in 10% of patients treated with antibiotics and drainage alone.

VII. TREATMENT

A. GENERAL
1. The treatment of appendicitis is surgical and requires removal of the inflamed appendix, except in cases of appendiceal perforation, in which treatment can vary (drainage and antibiotic treatment).

2. Appendectomy can be performed either open or laparoscopically.
3. Perioperative antibiotics have been shown to be beneficial in decreasing infectious complications.
   a. A single dose of perioperative antibiotics is adequate for uncomplicated appendicitis.
   b. Antibiotic therapy for perforated or gangrenous appendicitis should continue for 5–7 days after appendectomy.

B. TECHNIQUE

1. With the open technique, use a McBurney (or Rockey-Davis) incision over McBurney point with a muscle-splitting technique (Fig. 29.1).
2. If there is reasonable doubt about the diagnosis, some surgeons prefer a midline incision.
3. After resection of the appendix, the ligated stump may be inverted and/or the mucosa may be cauterized.
4. In the case of a perforated appendix with phlegmon formation (or significant cecal inflammation), an "interval" (or delayed) appendectomy is usually performed. Drains are placed to drain discrete collections only, and the fascia is closed while the skin and subcutaneous tissue are left open.

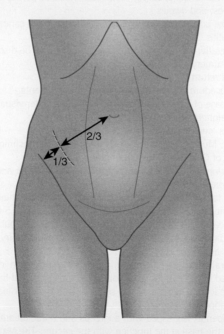

FIG. 29.1
Diagram of method used to locate McBurney point.

5. Patients with a walled-off abscess may be managed by ultrasound-guided or computed tomography–guided percutaneous drainage, followed by interval appendectomy 6–8 weeks later.
6. If no appendiceal inflammation is present, a careful search for other causes of the symptoms should be undertaken.
   a. Examination of pelvic organs
   b. Inspection of gallbladder and gastroduodenal area
   c. Gram stain of any peritoneal exudate
   d. Inspection of the mesentery for lymph nodes
   e. Thorough examination of the small bowel to rule out regional enteritis and Meckel diverticulum
   f. Palpation of the colon and kidneys

C. LAPAROSCOPY

Laparoscopic appendectomy has no major differences in results when compared with open appendectomy.

1. **Advantages**
   a. Evaluate the abdomen/pelvic structures when the diagnosis is in question.
      (1) Women in childbearing years—can visualize pelvis, fallopian tubes, and ovaries
      (2) Older adults—can evaluate for perforated cecal cancer or diverticulitis
   b. Postoperative stay is less, and some patients may be discharged the day of surgery.
   c. Time of return to normal activity is shorter.
   d. The procedure is technically easier in obese patients.
   e. In the case of a perforated appendix, there is better visualization of the peritoneum, allowing more adequate drainage.
   f. There is lower incidence of wound infections.

2. **Procedure: Multiple variations exist. In general, the technique at the University of Cincinnati Medical Center is as follows:**
   a. It is performed under general anesthesia with bladder and stomach decompression.
   b. Access to peritoneum is obtained via the Hasson technique and an infraumbilical 12-mm trocar is placed. Two additional 5-mm trocars are placed in the left lower quadrant (LLQ) and suprapubic positions under direct visualization, with care taken to avoid injury to epigastric vessels and bladder.
   c. Preoperative cross-sectioning imaging, if available, can identify the expected location of the appendix. The convergence of the teniae coli and the fold of Treves can also serve as landmarks for identification of the appendix.
   d. The appendix is grasped with a forceps and retracted anterior to expose the base at the junction with the cecum. The Maryland dissector is then used to create a window between the base of the appendix and the mesoappendix.

e. Using a vascular stapler, commercial energy device, or clips, the mesoappendix is ligated and divided.

f. The appendix can either be amputated with a linear stapler or excised after endoloops have been placed at its base.

g. The appendix is placed in a bag and removed through the 12-mm trocar, with care taken not to contact the subcutaneous tissue with the inflamed appendix.

D. FUTURE RESEARCH

1. Recent studies have attempted to demonstrate the efficacy and safety of antibiotic therapy alone for UNCOMPLICATED appendicitis.

2. Antibiotic Therapy versus Appendectomy for Treatment of Uncomplicated Appendicitis (APPAC Trial)

   a. Randomized controlled, noninferiority trial: Results did indicate noninferiority of antibiotic therapy versus appendectomy.

   b. A total of 27% of patients initially treated with antibiotics required appendectomy; however, these patients had a reduced rate of complications compared with patients treated with initial appendectomy.

VIII. SPECIAL CIRCUMSTANCES

A. OLDER ADULTS

1. They account for nearly 50% of the deaths from appendicitis.

2. Greater mortality rate is due to delay of definitive treatment, uncontrolled infection, and a high incidence of coexistent disease.

3. Constellation of symptoms is usually much more atypical.

   a. Abdominal pain may be minimized.

   b. Fever and leukocyte count are less reliable signs.

4. Perforation rates reach 50%–75%.

5. Morbidity and mortality rates are much greater because of the delay in accurate diagnosis.

B. INFANTS

1. Similarly high rates of rupture and secondary complications as in older adults because of delayed or atypical presentation.

2. Accurate diagnosis is made more difficult by the fact that infants are unable to give a history, the index of suspicion is usually lower, and progression of disease is usually faster.

3. The ability of the infant to wall off perforated appendicitis is inefficient and results in rapid, diffuse peritonitis and distant abscesses.

C. PREGNANCY

1. Although appendicitis is the most common extrauterine surgical emergency in pregnant patients, in 1 in every 1500–2000 pregnancies (1 in 766 births), it occurs with the same frequency in pregnant women as it does in nonpregnant women.

29

APPENDIX

    a. There is a higher negative appendectomy rate among pregnant females.

2. It does occur more frequently in the first two trimesters than in the third trimester.

3. Diagnosis is obscured by the lateral and superior displacement of the appendix by the gravid uterus, with an accompanying change in the point of maximum tenderness.

    a. The appendix is in its "normal" position until 12 weeks, when it is displaced upward and laterally.

    b. It reaches the umbilicus by 20 weeks and the iliac crest at 24 weeks.

4. Diagnosis is also made more difficult by the fact that abdominal pain, nausea, vomiting, and an increased WBC count are normal findings during pregnancy.

    a. An increased neutrophil count is not a normal finding.

    b. Magnetic resonance imaging (MRI) is a useful imaging modality that poses no risk of radiation to the fetus. MRI has greater than 90% sensitivity and specificity for the diagnosis of acute appendicitis in pregnancy.

5. Laparoscopy is as safe as laparotomy in the first and second trimesters.

    a. There is a significant risk of fetal loss and early delivery associated with operative intervention for appendicitis. Risk is 2%–6% for fetal loss and 4%–11% for early delivery.

6. Although maternal mortality rates are low, early operative intervention is essential because perforation and peritonitis result in fetal mortality rates as high as 20%–25%.

IX. APPENDICEAL TUMORS
Tumors are found in almost 5% of removed appendices.

A. CARCINOID
1. Carcinoid tumors are most commonly located in the appendix and are usually benign.

2. Appendectomy is the treatment of choice if the tumor is less than 2 cm, involves the tip of the appendix, and there is no nodal involvement.

3. Right hemicolectomy is the treatment of choice if there is nodal involvement, the tumor is greater than 2 cm, or the mesoappendix or base of cecum is involved.

B. ADENOCARCINOMA
1. Adenocarcinoma of the colon can arise in the appendix.

2. Most of these cases present as acute appendicitis.

3. A right hemicolectomy should be performed.

C. PSEUDOMYXOMA

1. Pseudomyxoma arises in the appendix in 50% of patients with pseudomyxoma peritonei.
2. Appendiceal mucocele or fluid-filled cyst can be seen on imaging and may be associated with gelatinous ascites.
3. Both ovaries should be examined for secondary disease in female patients.
4. In a patient with a preoperative diagnosis of pseudomyxoma peritonei, surgical debulking of all gross disease is the treatment, together with adjuvant chemotherapy after tissue diagnosis of pseudomyxoma.
5. Patients with undiagnosed disease should undergo a right hemicolectomy without penetration of the tumor. After the diagnosis is confirmed, further cancer work-up and treatment are then performed.

RECOMMENDED READINGS

McGory ML, Zingmond DS, Tillou A, Hiatt JR, Ko CY, Cryer HM. Negative appendectomy in pregnant women is associated with a substantial risk of fetal loss. *J Am Coll Surg*. 2007;205:534–540.

Salminen P, Paajanen H, Rautio T, et al. Antibiotic therapy vs appendectomy for treatment of uncomplicated acute appendicitis: the APPAC randomized clinical trial. *JAMA*. 2015;313:2340–2348.

APPENDIX

29

Benign Pancreatic Disease

Brent T. Xia, MD

Physiology has, at last, gained control over the nerves which stimulate the gastric glands and the pancreas.

—Ivan Pavlov, 1904

I. ANATOMY

A. EMBRYOLOGY

1. The pancreas begins as dorsal (from duodenum) and ventral (from hepatic diverticulum) budding from the foregut endoderm at approximately the fifth week of gestation.
2. Both the dorsal and ventral portions of the pancreas possess a main duct and fuse when the two pancreatic buds join. However, the portion of the dorsal duct between the anastomosis and the duodenum regresses. The main duct of the ventral pancreas leading to the duodenum is thus the definitive pancreatic duct (duct of Wirsung).
   a. If the two ducts do not fuse, the majority of the pancreas will drain via the dorsal bud duct (**duct of Santorini**), which is termed pancreas divisum.
   b. If the dorsal bud duct (**duct of Santorini**) fuses with the ventral bud duct (**duct of Wirsung**) but does not regress, then it will either persist as a blind accessory duct or drain via the lesser papilla.
3. Anomalies of pancreatic development include:
   a. Annular pancreas: a ring of pancreatic tissue that encircles the duodenum and rarely can cause duodenal obstruction
   b. Heterotopic pancreatic tissue: found most commonly in the duodenum, stomach mucosa, and in approximately 6% of Meckel diverticulum

B. HISTOLOGY

1. Endocrine
   a. Islets of Langerhans—originate from embryonic ductal epithelium and migrate toward capillaries to form isolated islands of cells within the pancreatic exocrine tissue (acini)
      (1) Alpha cells—cells within the islets that produce glucagon; first cells to develop (8–9 weeks)
      (2) Beta cells—cells within the islets that produce insulin
      (3) Delta cells—cells within the islets that produce somatostatin
      (4) Gamma cells—cells within the islets that produce pancreatic polypeptide

2. Exocrine
   a. Acini—develops in three stages from pancreatic "founder" cells to become differentiated cells that store inactive digestive enzymes as zymogen granules
      (1) Endopeptidases (trypsinogen, chymotrypsinogen, proelastase)
      (2) Exopeptidases (procarboxypeptidase A and B)
      (3) Others (amylase, lipase, phospholipase, colipase)
   b. Ductal—develops from the same pancreatic cellular cords as acinar cells. Originates from the centroacinar cells of each acinus and terminates into the main pancreatic excretory duct

C. GROSS ANATOMY
1. Basics
   a. Retroperitoneal location posterior to the stomach at the level of L1–2 that is nested in the C-loop of the duodenum and lies obliquely to meet the splenic hilum.
   b. Access gained via separating the gastrocolic omentum from the transverse mesocolon to enter the lesser sac. The body and tail of the pancreas will be visible on the floor of the lesser sac.
2. Regions
   a. Head is positioned within the C-loop of the duodenum and posterior to the transverse colon. The head is anterior to the inferior vena cava, right renal artery, and bilateral renal veins.
   b. Uncinate process is the portion of the pancreatic head that projects to the right and posterior to the superior mesenteric vein. It terminates posterior to the superior mesenteric artery (SMA) and vein but anterior to the inferior vena cava and aorta. The tissue connecting the uncinate to the SMA is what is termed the retroperitoneal margin and is an important margin during pancreatectomy for pancreatic cancer.
   c. Neck divides the pancreas into near equal halves and is adjacent to the L1–2 vertebral bodies, making it susceptible to injury during blunt trauma. At the inferior edge of the neck, the splenic vein and superior mesenteric vein join to form the portal vein, which travels directly posterior to the neck of the pancreas on its way to the porta hepatis.
   d. Body lies directly anterior to the splenic artery and vein, with the artery running superior to the vein. Lies directly anterior to the aorta at the takeoff of the SMA, a good landmark to note on abdominal computed tomography (CT) scans.
   e. Tail extends to the left from the pancreatic body to lie near the splenic hilum anterior to the splenic artery and vein.

D. VASCULAR/LYMPHATIC ANATOMY
1. Arterial (Fig. 30.1)

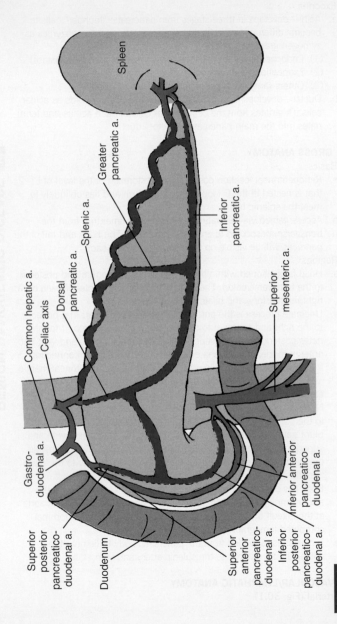

FIG. 30.1
Pancreatic arterial anatomy.

a. Celiac trunk
   (1) The celiac trunk gives rise to the common hepatic artery, the left gastric artery, and the splenic artery. The hepatic artery gives off the gastroduodenal artery (GDA). The GDA divides into the anterior and posterior superior pancreaticoduodenal artery as it passes posterior to the first portion of the duodenum.
   (2) The splenic artery supplies the body and tail of the pancreas as it courses along the superior posterior surface of the pancreas toward the spleen.
b. SMA
   (1) The SMA gives off the inferior pancreaticoduodenal artery. This divides into anterior and posterior branches and forms an anastomosis with the anterior and posterior branches of the superior pancreaticoduodenal artery within the pancreatic parenchyma. This anastomosis not only supplies the head of the pancreas but also the medial aspect of the duodenal C-loop. Therefore any resection of the pancreatic head involves resection of this portion of the duodenum; otherwise it will be devascularized.
   (2) The dorsal pancreatic artery is a branch of the splenic artery that becomes the inferior pancreatic artery and travels parallel to the splenic artery but at the inferior border of the pancreas. Two main arteries run perpendicular to the pancreatic body and create an anastomosis between the splenic and inferior pancreatic arteries. They are the dorsal and greater pancreatic arteries (medial to lateral).

2. **Venous**
   a. Drainage follows similar routes as the arteries, but veins are more superficially located.
   b. The head of the pancreas is drained via veins located anterior and posterior to it.
      (1) The anterior and posterior superior pancreaticoduodenal veins drain directly into the portal vein.
      (2) The anterior inferior pancreaticoduodenal vein drains via the right gastroepiploic and right colic veins into the superior mesenteric vein.
      (3) The posterior inferior pancreaticoduodenal vein drains into the inferior mesenteric vein.
   c. The body and tail of the pancreas drain into the splenic vein.

3. **Lymphatics**
   a. Diffuse drainage likely accounts for early and aggressive metastatic spread of tumor cells.
   b. Communication exists between pancreatic lymphatics and the transverse mesocolon and proximal jejunum mesentery.

E. DUCT SYSTEM
1. Main pancreatic duct (duct of Wirsung) is approximately 2–3 mm in diameter.

30

BENIGN PANCREATIC DISEASE

2. It runs between the superior and inferior borders of the pancreas (one-third of the way up from the caudal margin), closer to the posterior aspect of the organ (two-thirds of the way in from the ventral surface).
3. The main pancreatic duct joins the common bile duct to empty into the second portion of the duodenum (medial aspect) at the ampulla of Vater (9% of the time the main duct and common bile duct [CBD] will be separate and will drain into the duodenum without the presence of an ampulla).
4. An accessory duct may be present approximately 2 cm proximal to the ampulla of Vater if the dorsal bud duct fails to regress during development (see Section I.A).

II. ACUTE PANCREATITIS

A. BASICS
1. Acute inflammatory process of the pancreas. Etiology is multifactorial (see Section II.B).
2. Disease spectrum—Atlanta Classification recognizes two types, edematous interstitial and necrotizing acute pancreatitis (AP), and three severity levels:
   a. Mild: absence of organ failure and local or systemic complications
   b. Moderately severe: transient organ failure (resolves within 48 hours) and/or local or systemic complications
   c. Severe: persistent (multi) organ failure
3. Vast majority of cases (90%) are self-limited, mild AP.
4. AP is responsible for approximately 275,000 hospital admissions. It is the most common reason for hospitalization for a gastrointestinal (GI) disease in the United States.

B. PATHOGENESIS
1. Not mutually exclusive hypotheses, but at the same time may be mutually contradictory. Hypotheses apply to both acute and, over time, chronic pancreatitis.
2. Toxic-metabolic hypothesis
   a. Alcohol may be directly toxic to acinar cells through alterations in cellular metabolism. Acetaldehyde, a toxic metabolite, accumulates and activates pancreatic cells.
   b. Alcohol has been shown to induce lipid accumulation within acinar cells, leading to fatty degeneration and necrosis, as well as inducing fibrosis.
3. Oxidative stress hypothesis
   a. Hepatocytes with overactive mixed-function oxidases lead to the secretion of free radical by-products into the bile which can reflux into the pancreatic duct and induce damage in susceptible acinar and ductal cells.
   b. Fibrosis results after repeat exposure.
   c. Overactivity of mixed-function oxidases may be due to high substrates (i.e., fats) or enzyme inducers (i.e., ethanol).

4. **Stone and ductal obstruction hypothesis**
   a. Long-standing alcohol exposure has been shown to increase the incidence of protein plugs and eventually stones within the pancreatic ducts.
   b. Pressure from lodged stones within the ducts leads to ulceration, obstruction, stasis, and further stone formation, which lead to atrophy and fibrosis.

5. **Necrosis-fibrosis hypothesis**
   a. Periductal scarring and chronic disruption of the glandular architecture leads to repeated inflammation and tissue necrosis.
   b. It represents a step-wise progression of fibrosis, leading to chronic pancreatitis as a result of repeated episodes of acute or subacute pancreatitis.

6. **Primary duct hypothesis**
   a. Immune-mediated destruction of the ductal epithelium, leading to inflammation and fibrosis (similar to primary sclerosing cholangitis)
   b. Helps to explain large duct pancreatitis when alcohol is not a factor

7. **Sentinel acute pancreatitis event (SAPE) hypothesis**
   a. This attempts to combine several of the above hypotheses into one coherent explanation.
   b. Long-term alcohol ingestion leads to metabolic/oxidative stress that, once a "sentinel" event is reached, leads to acinar cell injury and an acute proinflammatory response. Later, with recurrent metabolic stress, the pancreas has already been "primed" by the sentinel event and an antiinflammatory response predominates, leading to fibrosis and chronic pancreatitis.

C. ETIOLOGY/RISK FACTORS

1. **Cholelithiasis**
   a. This is the most common cause of AP (40%) worldwide.
   b. Although mechanical obstruction may lead to pancreatic ductal hypertension with rupture of smaller ductules and leakage of pancreatic enzymes, the exact mechanism is unclear.

2. **Alcohol**
   a. A total of 10%–15% of people who ingest 100–150 g of ethanol daily will develop pancreatitis. Alcohol is responsible for approximately 40% of cases of AP in the United States.
   b. Enzymes may precipitate out with calcium, resulting in ductal obstruction, and continued enzyme release results in ductal hypertension.
   c. Finally, ethanol has been shown to decrease pancreatic blood flow, which may perpetuate pancreatic cellular necrosis.

3. **Obstruction**
   a. Gallstones (as discussed previously), biliary sludge
   b. Periampullary tumors (pancreatic primary tumors, distal cholangiocarcinoma, duodenal cancers, ampullary cancers)
   c. Duodenal ulcer, stricture, or diverticulum
   d. Parasites (*Ascaris* and *Clonorchis*), which can block the pancreatic duct
   e. Pancreas divisum (rare)

4. **Metabolic**
   a. Hypercalcemia may be the cause of pancreatitis in a patient with hyperparathyroidism or multiple myeloma. It likely involves pancreatic hypersecretion with the formation of intraductal calcium stones, resulting in obstruction.
   b. Hyperlipidemia/hypertriglyceridemia: See later (Section II.C.6.a).
5. **Trauma**
   a. Blunt
   b. Penetrating
6. **Hereditary**
   a. Hyperlipoproteinemia syndromes (types I, IV, and V) are responsible for 1%–4% of cases. They are believed to result from obstruction of capillaries from elevated serum chylomicrons, leading to ischemia of pancreatic tissue and release of pancreatic lipases. The reaction of pancreatic lipase and triglycerides yields free fatty acids that propel tissue injury.
   b. *CFTR* gene mutation, affecting cystic fibrosis transmembrane regulator protein expression. This protein is located in the membranes of secretory and absorptive pancreas epithelial cells and modulates ion channels. Dysfunction leads to thick mucus obstruction of the pancreatic ducts and defective secretion of pancreatic enzymes.
   c. *PRSS1* gene mutation, affecting cationic trypsinogen (trypsin-1) protein. Mutations result in loss of fail-safe mechanism to prevent premature activation and autodigestion within the pancreas.
   d. *SPINK1* gene mutation, affecting serine protease inhibitor Kazal-type 1 protein, also known as pancreatic secretory trypsin inhibitor (PSTI). PSTI functions to inactivate prematurely activated trypsinogen within the pancreas. Mutations in PSTI may result in loss of checkpoint inhibition of autoactivated trypsinogen.
7. **Iatrogenic**
   a. Endoscopic retrograde cholangiopancreatography (ERCP)-related pancreatitis occurs in 2%–10% of patients as a result of intraductal hypertension or trauma.
   b. Various surgical procedures near the pancreas (biopsy, ductal cannulation/exploration, gastrectomy, splenectomy)
   c. Cardiopulmonary bypass may result in a pancreatic low-flow state, resulting in ischemia and injury.
   d. Billroth II gastrojejunostomy may allow the reflux of activated pancreatic enzymes into the pancreatic duct, owing to afferent limb obstruction.
8. **Drugs**
   a. Antibiotics (sulfonamides, tetracycline, nitrofurantoin)
   b. Azathioprine
   c. Diuretics (thiazide and furosemide)
   d. Estrogens
   e. Methyldopa
   f. Valproic acid

9. Idiopathic
   a. Responsible for 15% of cases
   b. Third largest group after biliary and alcoholic causes

D. DIAGNOSIS

1. History
   a. First episode is usually the most severe.
   b. A history of alcohol ingestion or cholelithiasis may be elicited.
   c. Onset of epigastric pain (50% with radiation to the back) usually occurs several hours after a meal, is constant in nature, described as sharp or knifelike, and may be relieved by sitting up and aggravated by lying flat or movement.
   d. Nausea/vomiting usually accompany the abdominal pain.

2. Physical examination
   a. Fever, tachycardia, possible hypotension secondary to fluid sequestration (third spacing).
   b. Abdominal pain can range from epigastric to diffuse abdominal tenderness with possible peritoneal signs.
   c. A paralytic ileus can develop, resulting in abdominal distension. Grey Turner sign (left flank ecchymosis) or Cullen sign (periumbilical ecchymosis) may develop in cases of hemorrhagic pancreatitis. This is due to blood-stained peritoneal fluid dissecting through the planes of the abdominal wall to the flank or along the falciform ligament to the umbilicus (very uncommon).

3. Labs
   a. Complete blood count (CBC)—evaluate for possible infectious etiology (including white blood cell count), baseline hematocrit (hemoconcentration may be present because of third spacing in the retroperitoneum)
   b. Basic metabolic profile—evaluate electrolyte status, renal function, and acid/base status.
   c. Prothrombin time/partial thromboplastin time—especially important in cases of hemorrhagic pancreatitis to correct any coagulopathies
   d. Amylase
      (1) Elevated in 90% of cases
      (2) Levels greater than 1000 IU/dL—suggestive of gallstone pancreatitis
      (3) Rises soon after the onset of symptoms and returns to normal in 3–5 days—good marker to follow disease progression
      (4) Sensitive but not specific for pancreatitis; serves a diagnostic and not a prognostic role
   e. Lipase
      (1) Specific but not sensitive for pancreatitis; especially useful 24 hours after presentation
      (2) Remains elevated longer than serum amylase
      (3) Serves a diagnostic and not a prognostic role

f. Hepatic function panel
   (1) Evaluate for possible mechanical ductal obstruction with elevated total bilirubin level.
   (2) Include triglycerides if patient has a history of hyperlipidemia.
g. Electrocardiogram (EKG)—exclude myocardial infarction.

4. Imaging
   a. Chest x-ray
      (1) Findings may include left pleural effusion, elevated hemidiaphragm, or basilar atelectasis.
      (2) It helps to rule out perforated viscus (air under the diaphragm).
   b. Abdominal x-ray
      (1) "Sentinel loop" may be visualized, which represents a loop of distended bowel lying next to an inflamed pancreas.
      (2) Air in the duodenal sweep (C-loop) may be evident.
      (3) The "colon cutoff" sign represents dilation from the proximal colon to the transverse colon with a paucity of gas distal to the splenic flexure.
   c. Ultrasound
      (1) Evaluation for cholelithiasis if gallstone pancreatitis is suspected
      (2) Can determine extrapancreatic ductal dilatation, pancreatic edema, or peripancreatic fluid
      (3) Not used often because bowel gas can prevent an adequate assessment of the pancreas
   d. CT scan with intravenous (IV) contrast (Fig. 30.2)
      (1) This is most common diagnostic imaging modality.
      (2) It can detail pancreatic anatomy, fluid collections, and extrapancreatic ductal dilatation.
      (3) Findings include enlargement of the pancreas with loss of peripancreatic fat planes, fat stranding, and areas of decreased density.
      (4) In noncontrast studies, pancreatic parenchyma has CT attenuation of 30–50 Hounsfield units, which should increase by at least 50 Hounsfield units with IV contrast. A decrease or lack of enhancement is consistent with necrosis.
      (5) Nonenhancement of the pancreas on CT indicates necrosis and, in the face of patient instability, it must undergo fine-needle aspiration (FNA) to rule out infected necrosis.
      (6) Approximately 4 days after presentation, the sensitivity of CT to diagnose necrosis approaches 100%.
   e. ERCP/magnetic resonance cholangiopancreatography (MRCP)
      (1) ERCP is not warranted in cases of AP unless the diagnosis is obstructive gallstone pancreatitis or biliary sepsis, in which case early ERCP has been shown to reduce morbidity when compared with delayed ERCP for severe gallstone pancreatitis (but no difference in mortality).
      (2) ERCP is indicated for recurrent disease after the resolution of an acute attack.

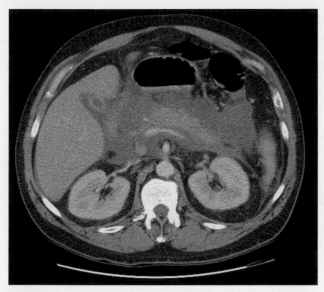

FIG. 30.2

Computed tomography (CT) scan of acute pancreatitis. CT imaging of acute pancreatitis demonstrating an edematous pancreas with peripancreatic fluid and fat stranding. CT is useful in evaluation of potential complications including hemorrhage, pseudocyst formation, abscess formation, and necrotizing pancreatitis.

    (3) MRCP may be useful to diagnose gallstone pancreatitis without subjecting the patient to the complications of ERCP, such as worsening pancreatitis. However, MRCP cannot treat retained stones.

E. TREATMENT

1. If patient is unstable or at high risk, intensive care unit (ICU) monitoring is essential.
2. Restriction of oral intake (food and fluids) with the administration of parenteral fluids and electrolyte replacement is the initial mainstay of treatment.
3. Treat with nasogastric decompression in those patients with nausea/vomiting.
4. Foley catheter is used to monitor urine output.
5. Prophylactic antibiotics are not recommended for interstitial or sterile necrotizing pancreatitis, regardless of disease severity. If infected pancreatic necrosis is suspected, broad-spectrum antibiotics are recommended (imipenem is the drug of choice).

6. Use serial labs (electrolytes, amylase) to guide resuscitation and response.

7. For pain management, meperidine is favored over morphine because it is thought to have less sphincter of Oddi contraction.

8. Alcohol withdrawal prophylaxis in selected patients with the use of benzodiazepine, as well as thiamine (100 mg IV ×1 followed by 50–100 mg IV once daily to prevent Wernicke encephalopathy), folate (400 μg orally [PO] once daily), and multivitamin (1 tab PO once daily) replacement

9. After stabilization, nasojejunal tube feeds can be instituted to avoid stimulating pancreatic exocrine function while maintaining nutrition and normal intestinal bacterial flora. If a patient cannot tolerate feeds (ileus, nausea/vomiting), then total parenteral nutrition should be started.

10. Surgical management varies depending on the presentation, condition, and complications the patient may possess:

    a. Infected pancreatic necrosis based on FNA demands debridement/necrosectomy. Because FNA has a 10% false negative rate, patients with sterile necrosis (i.e., a negative FNA) who continue to deteriorate must be explored for fear of missing an infection.

    b. It is warranted if a definitive diagnosis cannot be made such that intraabdominal catastrophe cannot be ruled out.

    c. In patients whose condition deteriorates despite maximal supportive care

    d. In a single institutional study at the University of Cincinnati, the placement of U-tube drainage catheters (UTDCs) by interventional radiology for necrotizing pancreatitis demonstrated effectiveness in drainage/debridement with low morbidity. For approximately one-third of patients, UTDC was the definitive procedure. Procedural success is operator dependent.

    e. Acute gallstone pancreatitis is best managed by either early cholecystectomy (within 48–72 hours of presentation) or delayed cholecystectomy (after 72 hours but during the same hospitalization) to allow the pancreatitis to resolve.

    f. Pancreatitis secondary to trauma may require surgical intervention to treat a pancreatic ductal injury or hemorrhagic complications.

F. PROGNOSIS

1. Mortality based on severity of disease:

    a. Acute (edematous) pancreatitis (<2%)

    b. Pancreatitis with sterile necrosis (<10%)

    c. Pancreatitis with infected necrosis (50%)

2. Approximately 10%–30% of patients will develop severe pancreatitis that will progress to pancreatic necrosis.

TABLE 30.1		
RANSON CRITERIA		
Initial Presentation	48 Hours After Admission	Calculated Mortality Rate[a]
Age >55 years	Decline in hematocrit ≥10%	0–2 criteria = 0%–3% mortality rate
White blood cell count >16,000/μL	Fluid sequestration >6 L	3–5 criteria = 11%–15% mortality rate
Glucose level >11 mmol/L (>200 mg/dL)	Hypocalcemia (Ca^{2+} <8 mg/dL, <2 mmol/L)	5–6 criteria = 40% mortality rate
Lactate dehydrogenase level >350 IU/L	Hypoxemia (Pao_2 <60 mm Hg)	7–11 criteria = 100% mortality rate
Aspartate aminotransferase concentration >250 IU/L	Blood urea nitrogen increase of >5 mg/dL (>1.98 mmol/L) even after intravenous fluid resuscitation	
	Base deficit of >4 mmol/L	

[a]Sum of the number of criteria at initial presentation and 48 h after admission yields the estimated mortality rate.

3. Ranson criteria (Table 30.1)
    a. Eleven criteria that predict survival, not used very often.
    b. Estimated mortality based on total criteria found at initial presentation and 48 hours after admission
4. Acute Physiology and Chronic Health Evaluation II (APACHE II) score (Table 30.2)
    a. Severity of disease classification system is based on physiologic parameters; higher scores predict higher death rates.
    b. It is more accurate than Ranson criteria.
    c. Special weight can be given to organ system involvement.
5. Bedside Index of Severity in AP (BISAP) score (Table 30.3)
    a. Simplified to five criteria, performed within 24 hours of admission
    b. Validated to have similar performance to Ranson criteria and APACHE II score in predicting mortality

G. COMPLICATIONS
1. Necrotizing pancreatitis
    a. Sterile
        (1) This has a far better prognosis than infected necrosis, with a mortality of near 0% without any other systemic complications.
        (2) It may develop into infected necrosis or chronic pseudocyst, or it may resolve spontaneously.
        (3) Although some studies suggest the use of prophylactic antibiotics even with sterile pancreatic necrosis as this has been shown to

TABLE 30.2

ACUTE PHYSIOLOGY AND CHRONIC HEALTH EVALUATION II SCORING SYSTEM[a]

	Low Abnormal Values				Normal	High Abnormal Values			
	+4	+3	+2	+1	0	+1	+2	+3	+4
Temperature (°C)	<29.9	30–31.9	32–33.9	34–35.9	36–38.4	38.5–38.9		39–40.9	>41
MAP (mm Hg)	<49		50–69		70–109		110–129	130–159	>160
HR	<39	40–54	55–69		70–109		110–139	140–179	>180
RR	<5		6–9	10–11	12–24	25–34		35–49	>50
(A-a)O$_2$, Pao$_2$	<55	55–60		61–70	>70 or <200		200–349	350–499	>500
pH	<7.15	7.15–7.24	7.25–7.32		7.33–7.49	7.5–7.59		7.6–7.69	>7.7
Na (mmol/L)	<110	111–119	120–129		130–149	150–154	155–159	160–179	>180
K (mmol/L)	2.5		2.5–2.9	3–3.4	3.5–5.4	5.5–5.9		6–6.9	>7
Cr (mg/dL, no renal failure)			<0.6 (+4 if renal failure)		0.6–1.4		1.5–1.9 (+4 if renal failure)	2–3.4 (+6 if renal failure)	>3.5 (+8 if renal failure)
Hematocrit (%)	<20		20–29.9		30–45.9	46–49.9	50–59.9		>60
White blood cell count (per liter)	<1		1–2.9		3–14.9	15–19.9	20–39.9		>40
HCO$_3$ (bicarbonate; mmol/L, use if no arterial blood gases)	<15	15–17.9	18–21.1		22–31.9	32–40.9		41–51.9	>52
Score	+0	+2	+3	+5	+6				
Age (year)	<44	45–54	55–64	65–74	>75				
Chronic organ insufficiency?[b]		Elective after surgery		Nonoperative or emergent after surgery					

[a]Tabulate total number of points based on criteria from each row.

[b]Chronic organ insufficiency involves liver (biopsy-proved cirrhosis, portal hypertension [HTN], past upper gastrointestinal bleed, prior encephalopathy/coma), cardiovascular (New York Health Association Class IV), pulmonary disease, exercise restriction, chronic hypoxia, hypercapnia, pulmonary hypertension >40 mm Hg, or respirator dependency), renal (chronic dialysis), or immunosuppression (chemotherapy, radiation, long-term or recent high-dose steroid therapy, disease that suppresses resistance to infection such as leukemia, lymphoma, or acquired immune deficiency syndrome). Predicted death rate calculated as follows: $X = [-3.517 +$ (Acute Physiology and Chronic Health Evaluation [APACHE] II]) $\times 0.146$. Predicted Death Rate $= e^X/(1 + e^X) \times 100$.

Cr, Creatinine; HCO_3, bicarbonate; HR, heart rate; K, potassium; MAP, mean arterial pressure; Na, sodium; RR, respiratory rate.

TABLE 30.3

BEDSIDE INDEX OF SEVERITY IN ACUTE PANCREATITIS SCORING SYSTEM

First 24 Hours of Evaluation

BUN >25 mg/dL (8.92 mmol/L)	0 criteria = 0%–1% mortality rate
Impaired mental status	3–5 criteria = 22% mortality rate
SIRS (2 or more of the following):	

   1. Temperature <36 or >38°C
   2. Respiratory rate >20 breaths/min or Paco$_2$ <32 mm Hg
   3. Pulse >90 beats/min
   4. White blood cell <4000 or >12,000 cells/mm^3 or >10% immature bands

Age >60 years

Pleural effusion detected on imaging

BUN, Blood urea nitrogen; *SIRS,* systemic inflammatory response syndrome.

limit the number of cases that convert to infected pancreatic necrosis, the results of a double-blind placebo study do not concur with these earlier unblinded studies.

b. Infected
(1) This develops in 30%–50% of patients with pancreatic necrosis.
(2) Incidence peaks in the third week of the disease.
(3) High mortality when other systemic complications are present.
(4) Perform FNA of the necrosis to confirm the diagnosis and determine bacterial antibiotic sensitivities.
(5) Most common organisms are enteric: *Enterococcus* (most common), *Escherichia coli*, *Klebsiella*, *Staphylococcus aureus*, *Proteus*, *Pseudomonas*, *Enterobacter*, and *Candida*.
(6) Surgical debridement is necessary for those patients with infected necrosis and thus hemodynamic instability.

2. Pseudocyst (Fig. 30.3)
a. Cystlike space within or near the pancreas that is *not* lined by epithelium, but instead granulated and fibrotic tissue
b. Accounts for the majority of cystic masses of the pancreas and the most common complication of pancreatitis (10% of AP, 20%–40% of chronic pancreatitis)
c. Frequently found in the lesser sac, posterior to the stomach
d. Communicates with the pancreatic ductal system and contains a watery fluid rich in pancreatic enzymes
e. Many pseudocysts will resolve spontaneously without complications, but further intervention may be required if the pseudocyst:
(1) Enlarged—pseudocysts greater than 6 cm are more likely to cause symptoms and less likely to resolve spontaneously.

30

BENIGN PANCREATIC DISEASE

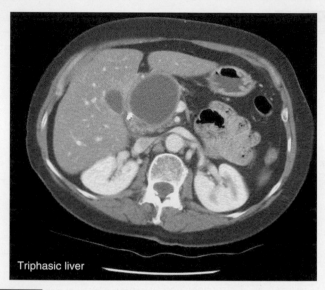

FIG. 30.3

Computed tomography (CT) scan of pancreatic pseudocyst. Complications of pancreatitis include pseudocyst formation (thin-walled collection with water density by CT).

    (2) Causes symptoms (mainly due to size)
        (a) Abdominal pain
        (b) Early satiety (compressed stomach)
        (c) Nausea/vomiting
        (d) Obstructive jaundice (compression of bile duct)
    (3) Creates complications
        (a) Hemosuccus pancreaticus (erosion of the pseudocyst into a neighboring vessel)
        (b) Gastric outlet obstruction (compression of the stomach and/or duodenum)
        (c) Perforation with peritonitis
    (4) Becomes infected and forms an abscess
  f. Ideally treated 4–6 weeks after appearance so that a thick, fibrous wall can mature around the cavity and a drainage procedure (DP) is then performed:
    (1) Pseudocysts are treated only if symptomatic or associated with a complication (infection, obstruction, bleeding), otherwise they are left alone.
    (2) First modality of treatment is endoscopic drainage, either transgastric, transduodenal, or transpapillary.

    (3) Surgical drainage is the next best option and involves internal drainage (cystogastrostomy, cystojejunostomy, or cystoduodenostomy) or percutaneous external drainage (for infected pseudocysts or those with immature walls, reserved for patients who cannot tolerate the endoscopic or surgical drainage).

3. Hemorrhage
   a. It is due to erosion of a pseudoaneurysm from a pseudocyst, abscess, or necrotizing pancreatitis.
   b. Bleeding may be GI, intraperitoneal, or retroperitoneal.
   c. Angiography is used to localize the site of bleeding and possibly embolize the bleeding vessel in an unstable patient. Otherwise, surgical management is necessary when bleeding cannot be controlled by interventional radiology.

4. Splenic vein thrombosis
   a. Because the splenic vein runs posterior to the pancreas, in cases of severe pancreatitis, thrombosis is not unusual.
   b. Gastroesophageal varices can form, with a mortality rate of approximately 20% if they bleed.
   c. Splenectomy can be performed to prevent possible or recurrent gastroesophageal bleeding due to splenic vein thrombosis.

5. Pancreatic ascites
   a. Leakage of pancreatic fluid directly into the peritoneum is caused by rupture of a pancreatic pseudocyst or a leaking pancreatic duct that was never able to form a pseudocyst.
   b. ERCP can be used to identify the area of leak and possibly place a stent across that area.
   c. Octreotide and bowel rest has been shown to be successful in stopping a leak in greater than 50% of patients.
   d. If medical management fails, the site of the pancreatic duct leak dictates the surgical management:
     (1) Body—Roux-en-Y pancreaticojejunostomy
     (2) Tail—distal pancreatectomy or internal DP

6. Pancreaticoenteric fistula
   a. A pseudocyst can erode into various areas of the GI tract, including the stomach, duodenum, small intestine, bile duct, or splenic flexure of the colon.
   b. In some cases, the pseudocyst will decompress via this fistula and no further management is required.
   c. If the fistula does not resolve spontaneously, ERCP is performed to detail the communication and operative management is dictated by the organ(s) involved.

III. CHRONIC PANCREATITIS

A. BASICS
1. Incidence is approximately 10 cases per 100,000 (similar to pancreatic cancer).

30

BENIGN PANCREATIC DISEASE

2. It is characterized by recurrent or persistent chronic abdominal pain with endocrine and exocrine insufficiency.
3. It results in irreversible destruction of the pancreatic parenchyma.
4. Patients with chronic pancreatitis may have attacks of AP superimposed on their chronic pain.

B. ETIOLOGY

1. Alcohol
   a. Most common cause
   b. It usually manifests in middle age (~40 years of age).
   c. Only 5%–15% of patients with heavy drinking habits (50–80 g/day alcohol consumption) develop chronic pancreatitis.
2. Cholelithiasis—Recurrent episodes of gallstone pancreatitis can lead to chronic pancreatitis.
3. Smoking
   a. Smoking prevalence and amount increases alongside alcohol consumption in patients with chronic pancreatitis and has a major impact on the progression of alcoholic pancreatitis.
   b. Association with chronic pancreatitis is dose dependent. Compared with nonsmokers, there is a five-fold risk increase for pancreatic calcifications.
   c. The North American Pancreatitis Study II consortium identified a variant in gene chymotrypsin C *(CTRC)* (protects pancreatic cells from injury from premature activation of trypsin) as a risk factor for tobacco-associated and alcohol-associated chronic pancreatitis.
4. Autoimmune
   a. Associated with primary sclerosing cholangitis and Sjögren syndrome
   b. Responsive to steroid treatment
5. Hypercalcemia
6. Hereditary
   a. Onset is usually during the teenage years.
   b. *PRSS1* (cationic trypsinogen gene) gene mutation (66% of hereditary cases)
   c. *CFTR* (cystic fibrosis transmembrane regulator gene) gene mutation
   d. *SPINK1* gene mutation
7. Pancreas divisum
8. Idiopathic
   a. A total of 10%–25% of cases
   b. Slower rate of pancreatic damage and calcification as compared with alcohol-induced chronic pancreatitis
   c. Early onset: manifestation of first clinical symptoms during the second to third decade of life. Patients tend to have prolonged course of pain.
   d. Late onset: manifestation of first clinical symptoms after the fifth decade of life. Symptoms start with exocrine or endocrine insufficiency, and patients have a milder or painless course as compared with early-onset patients.

9. Tropical pancreatitis (fibrocalculous pancreatic diabetes): early-onset chronic pancreatitis that occurs mainly in the tropics and developing countries, most prevalent in Southern India. It is characterized by main pancreatic duct calcification and ketosis-resistant diabetes.

C. DIAGNOSIS

1. History
   a. Recurrent or chronic abdominal pain with characteristics similar to AP but a more "aching" pain
   b. Weight loss/anorexia: present in 75% of patients
   c. Steatorrhea
      (1) Pale, bulky, malodorous stool that floats
      (2) Exocrine and endocrine insufficiency result in the inability to digest lipids and fat-soluble vitamin deficiency However, 90% of exocrine function must be lost before steatorrhea develops.
   d. Signs/symptoms of endocrine and exocrine insufficiency
2. Physical examination
   a. Cachectic appearance
   b. Pain may be out of proportion to abdominal examination but is usually epigastric in nature.
3. Labs
   a. Usually not very helpful. Indirect pancreatic function tests include measurements of fecal elastase 1 and 72-hour fecal fat estimation. However, fecal elastase 1 test is marred by low sensitivity and specificity and a 10% false positive rate. The fecal fat estimation is cumbersome and not widely available.
   b. Amylase may be normal or only slightly elevated because of destruction of the pancreatic parenchyma.
4. Imaging
   a. Abdominal x-ray may demonstrate calcifications (calcium carbonate) in the pancreas (95% specific; Fig. 30.4).
   b. CT scan typically demonstrates an atrophic pancreas with calcifications and a dilated duct. The presence of calcifications indicates advanced disease.
   c. Endoscopic ultrasound (EUS) demonstrates duct dilation, calcifications, parenchymal fibrosis, and possible pseudocyst with chronic pancreatitis.
   d. ERCP delineates the ductal system and is necessary before any surgical procedure, although EUS, CT, and MRCP may provide as accurate information of the duct system.
   e. The "chain of lakes" is present because of areas of alternating ductal strictures and dilations.

D. TREATMENT

1. Medical—first line treatment
   a. Pain control
   b. Counseling (alcohol abstinence, low-fat meals)

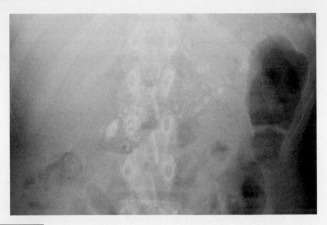

FIG. 30.4
Abdominal x-ray of chronic pancreatitis plain film finding characteristic of chronic pancreatitis includes coarse calcification crossing the midline of the upper abdomen. Also present in the right upper quadrant are surgical clips from prior cholecystectomy.

   c. Acid suppression (to prevent orally administered lipase from being inactivated)
   d. Oral pancreatic enzyme supplementation (coated enzymes for insufficiency, uncoated for pain)
   e. Treatment of diabetes
   f. Steroids (for autoimmune pancreatitis)
2. Surgical—Nearly 50% of patients with chronic pancreatitis will require some form of surgical intervention. Indications include intractable pain not controlled by medical management (most common indication), recurrent flare-ups requiring repeat hospitalization, sequelae of progressive fibrosis (duodenal, CBD, colonic obstructions), effects of ductal rupture (pseudocyst, pancreatic ascites, etc.), and suspected pancreatic cancer. Surgical treatment includes either a DP or resective procedure (RP).
   a. Beger procedure (RP)
     (1) This is a duodenal-sparing pancreatic head resection.
     (2) GI continuity is restored with two pancreaticojejunostomies (one connected to the remaining pancreatic body and another to remnant pancreatic tissue at the duodenal C-loop) and a jejunojejunostomy.
     (3) It is indicated for small duct, head-dominant chronic pancreatitis, but contraindicated if pancreatic cancer is suspected.
     (4) Pancreatic tissue should be sent for frozen sections because of a 5% incidence of occult pancreatic cancer.

b. Berne procedure (RP)
   (1) This is a duodenal-sparing pancreatic head resection *without* division of the pancreas anterior to the portal vein.
   (2) Other aspects are similar to the Beger procedure.
   (3) In a single-institution review (University of Heidelberg), the Berne modification was associated with shorter operation times and hospital stay. There were no differences in quality of life after surgery between the Berne and Berger procedures.

c. Duval procedure (DP)
   (1) Based on the presumption that a single ductal stricture is responsible for the obstructive symptoms
   (2) Involves a distal pancreatectomy with splenectomy and retrograde drainage of the distal pancreatic duct via a pancreaticojejunostomy

d. Frey procedure (RP)
   (1) Subtotal pancreatic head resection ("coring out") with longitudinal decompression of the pancreatic duct in the body and tail
   (2) Originally described for patients with "head dominant" disease

e. Puestow procedure (DP)
   (1) Longitudinal pancreaticojejunostomy allows for decompression of the entire pancreatic duct.
   (2) The entire pancreatic duct is longitudinally opened from the duodenum to the tail, which allows for pain relief in 65%–85% of patients.
   (3) Patients with a pancreatic duct greater than 10 mm, a length of anastomosis greater than 6 cm, and pancreatic calcifications usually respond well to the Puestow procedure.

f. Whipple procedure (RP)
   (1) Pancreaticoduodenectomy
   (2) Three anastomoses involved—pancreaticojejunostomy, choledochojejunostomy, and duodenojejunostomy/gastrojejunostomy (pylorus preserving vs. nonpreserving)
   (3) Indicated for small duct, head-dominant chronic pancreatitis

g. Partial/total pancreatectomy (RP)
   (1) It is indicated for intractable pain or prior failed operations and is usually a last resort procedure that is very rarely used for fear of uncontrolled hypoglycemic attacks.
   (2) It may be reserved for patients with "small duct" disease in which a decompressive procedure cannot be performed.
   (3) Total pancreatectomy can be "near-total," in which a rim of pancreatic tissue is preserved along the duodenal C-loop in addition to preservation of the common bile duct and pancreaticoduodenal vessels. Total pancreatectomy involves removal of the pylorus with reconstruction via a gastrojejunostomy/hepaticojejunostomy. Alternatively, a "pylorus-preserving" procedure is performed with GI continuity restored via duodenojejunostomy.

(4) Complicated by several endocrine and exocrine insufficiencies. In a few select institutions, autologous islet cell transplantation is carried out at the time of the total pancreatectomy.

h. Autologous islet cell transplant

(1) A distal pancreatectomy is performed up to the level of the superior mesenteric vein, and it is this portion that is typically used to harvest the islet cells to limit warm ischemia time.

(2) After the islet cells have been harvested via continuous cold enzymatic perfusion/digestion of the pancreas, 1–2 mL of packed islet cells are injected into a tributary of the middle colic vein or directly into the portal vein.

(3) Postoperative care requires stringent glucose control (levels between 100 and 120 mg/dL) to prevent islet cell "burn-out."

(4) At the University of Cincinnati, 5-year follow-up of patients who underwent total pancreatectomy with islet cell transplant demonstrated 73% narcotic independence rate, stable insulin requirements and glycemic control, and improved quality of life.

i. Celiac plexus blockade

(1) Celiac ganglion innervates the upper abdominal viscera via presynaptic and postsynaptic sympathetics, presynaptic parasympathetics, and pain fibers.

(2) Blockade is used in cases of continued pain after resection or DP for chronic pancreatitis that is not due to an anatomic problem (e.g., biliary stricture, fluid collection).

(3) The celiac plexus is identified after incising the avascular hepatogastric ligament and palpating for a thrill arising from the aorta behind the stomach near the diaphragmatic crura.

(4) The index finger is placed on the splenic artery, the middle finger on the common hepatic artery (the two most anatomically consistent celiac axis branches), and a neurolytic agent is injected into the soft tissue just lateral to the aorta above and below the operator's fingers (this represents the four quadrants where the plexus lies).

(5) A 50% ethanol solution is used with a 22-gauge spinal needle to inject 10 mL into four quadrants around the celiac plexus.

(6) This procedure may also be performed endoscopically with ultrasound assistance.

E. COMPLICATIONS

1. Diabetes mellitus (type I) due to endocrine insufficiency (up to 30% of patients)
2. Malabsorption due to exocrine insufficiency
3. Narcotics abuse
4. Increased risk for pancreatic cancer

RECOMMENDED READINGS

Ahmad SA, Wray CJ, Rilo HR, et al. Chronic pancreatitis: advances and ongoing challenges. *Curr Probl Surg*. 2006;43:135–238.

Dellinger EP, Tellado JM, Soto NE, et al. Early antibiotic treatment for severe acute necrotizing pancreatitis: a randomized, double-blind, placebo-controlled study. *Ann Surg*. 2007;245:674–683.

Janisch NH, Gardner TB. Advances in management of acute pancreatitis. *Gastroenterol Clin North Am*. 2016;45:1–8.

Majumder S, Chari ST. Chronic pancreatitis. *Lancet*. 2016;387:1957–1966.

Nathens AB, Curtis JR, Beale RJ, et al. Management of the critically ill patient with severe acute pancreatitis. *Crit Care Med*. 2004;32:2524–2536.

Stahl CC, Moulton J, Vu D, et al. Routine use of U-tube drainage for necrotizing pancreatitis: a step toward less morbidity and resource utilization. *Surgery*. 2015;158: 919–926.

Wilson GC, Sutton JM, Abbott DE, et al. Long-term outcomes after total pancreatectomy and islet cell autotransplantation: is it a durable operation? *Ann Surg*. 2014;260: 659–665.

30

BENIGN PANCREATIC DISEASE

Surgical Diseases of the Spleen

Teresa C. Rice, MD

Above all things physical, it is more important to be beautiful on the inside—to have a big heart and an open mind and a spectacular spleen.

—Ellen DeGeneres

The spleen is the largest organ of the reticuloendothelial system, responsible for many filtration and host defense mechanisms; however, it is not well understood. It plays a role in many childhood and adulthood hematologic and immunologic disorders and can cause significant morbidity and mortality in blunt and penetrating trauma. Previous management included simple and straightforward guidelines for splenectomy; the indications for surgical management of splenic disease have drastically changed, with more conservative treatment dominating.

I. ANATOMY

A. AVERAGE ADULT SPLEEN
1. Weight: 150 g; length: 7–11 cm

B. ENCAPSULATED
1. Capsule approximately 1–2 mm in thickness

C. SPLENOMEGALY DEFINITION
1. Weight: greater than 500 g; length: greater than 15 cm

D. BLOOD SUPPLY
1. Arterial
   a. Splenic artery off of the celiac trunk
   b. Short gastric arteries
   c. Branch from left gastroepiploic artery, contained in gastrosplenic ligament
2. Venous drainage
   a. Splenic vein, which is posterior and inferior to splenic artery and joins superior mesenteric vein to form the portal vein

E. STRUCTURAL SUPPORT
1. Suspended via four ligaments
2. Splenocolic, gastrosplenic, phrenosplenic, and splenorenal ligaments

F. MICROANATOMY
1. Red pulp
   a. Comprises 75% of splenic volume

    b. Venous sinuses surrounded by reticulum
    c. Site of splenic macrophages responsible for filtration system
2. Marginal zone—narrow interface between red and white pulp
3. White pulp
    a. Comprises 25% of splenic volume
    b. Consists of lymphoid follicles

G. ACCESSORY SPLEENS
1. Present in 20% of the population
2. Most common locations
    a. Approximately 80% in splenic hilum/vascular pedicle
    b. Remainder dispersed in gastrocolic ligament, pancreatic tail, greater omentum, greater curve of the stomach, and mesentery

II. FUNCTION
A. HEMATOLOGIC
1. Pitting
    a. Removal of abnormalities in red blood cell (RBC) membrane
2. Culling
    a. Removal of less deformable or aged RBCs
3. Reservoir for platelets and granulocytes
4. Hematopoiesis
    a. As fetus
    b. In conditions with bone marrow destruction

B. IMMUNOLOGIC
1. Cell-mediated and humoral immunity
2. Clearance of poorly opsonized bacteria
3. Antibody production in germinal follicles
4. Lymphocyte stimulation and proliferation
5. Production of opsonin-tuftsin and properdin

III. GENERAL INDICATIONS FOR SPLENECTOMY
A. TRAUMA
1. Treatment is increasingly more conservative (observation vs. embolization).

B. RED BLOOD CELL DISORDERS
1. Autoimmune hemolytic anemia—warm immunoglobulin G (IgG) antibodies
    a. Autoantibodies to RBCs causing hemolysis
    b. Symptoms include anemia and jaundice with splenomegaly present in one-third to one-half of cases.
    c. Diagnosis by direct Coombs test
    d. Treatment with steroids
       (1) Splenectomy if steroids fail—80% success

31

SURGICAL DISEASES OF THE SPLEEN

2. Hereditary spherocytosis
   a. Abnormality in spectrin—RBC membrane protein
   b. Most common hemolytic anemia for which splenectomy is indicated
   c. Symptoms include splenomegaly, anemia, and jaundice.
   d. Diagnosis by spherocytes on peripheral blood smear and increased mean corpuscular hemoglobin concentration
   e. Treatment with splenectomy
      (1) Ideally at age 4–6 years to minimize postoperative infection
      (2) Prophylactic cholecystectomy recommended given associated symptomatic cholelithiasis in 50% of patients secondary to bilirubin stones
3. Sickle cell disease
   a. Substitution of valine for glutamic acid as the sixth amino acid of the β-globin chain creates sickle hemoglobin (HbS).
   b. Deoxygenated hemoglobin sickles and polymerizes.
   c. Symptoms include splenomegaly from splenic sequestration.
   d. Sickle cell disease often results in autosplenectomy.
   e. Treatment includes splenectomy only for acute sequestration crisis or abscesses.
4. Thalassemias
   a. They are disorders of hemoglobin synthesis and have persistent fetal hemoglobin (HbF).
   b. Symptoms include pallor, retarded body growth, and head enlargement.
   c. Treat first with transfusions and appropriate chelation therapy.
      (1) Splenectomy is indicated if excessive transfusion requirements, painful splenomegaly, or painful splenic infarction.
5. Pyruvate kinase deficiency
   a. Metabolic disorder of pyruvate kinase enzyme
   b. Results in congenital hemolytic anemia
   c. Causes altered glucose metabolism
   d. Treatment includes splenectomy for enhanced RBC survival.

C. **MYELOPROLIFERATIVE DISORDERS**
1. Chronic myelogenous leukemia
   a. Associated splenomegaly in 50% of cases
   b. Splenectomy indicated for symptomatic splenomegaly or refractory anemia
2. Polycythemia vera
   a. Treatment first with phlebotomy, aspirin, and chemotherapeutic agents
      (1) Splenectomy should be only for late-stage, symptomatic splenomegaly.
      (2) Splenectomy may improve quality of life.

D. **WHITE BLOOD CELLS DISORDERS**
1. Chronic lymphocytic leukemia
   a. There is progressive accumulation of dysfunctional lymphocytes.

b. Symptoms include weakness, fatigue, fevers, night sweats, lymphadenopathy, and frequent infections.
c. Treatment—splenectomy
   (1) May significantly improve survival in patients with hemoglobin levels less than 10 g/dL and platelet counts less than 50×10^9 per liter
   (2) May improve cytopenia and permit the administration of chemotherapy
   (3) Palliative splenectomy indicated for symptomatic splenomegaly

2. Hairy cell leukemia
   a. Rare form of leukemia—2% of cases
   b. Characterized by splenomegaly, pancytopenia, and large numbers of abnormal lymphocytes in bone marrow
   c. First line therapy: chemotherapy
   d. Splenectomy indicated for symptomatic pancytopenia or splenomegaly

3. Non-Hodgkin lymphoma
   a. Monoclonal lymphocytic proliferation; 80% B-cell type
   b. Palliative splenectomy for splenomegaly and pancytopenia

4. Hodgkin disease
   a. Four types—lymphocyte predominant (best prognosis), nodular sclerosis (most common), mixed cellularity, and lymphocyte depleted (worst prognosis)
   b. Diagnosis by Reed-Sternberg cells
   c. Staging by anatomic distribution of lymphadenopathy
   d. Previously staged by laparotomy; now mainly by imaging techniques
   e. Treatment varies with staging; if splenic involvement, chemotherapy and radiation therapy are both indicated.

E. PLATELET DISORDERS
1. Idiopathic thrombocytopenic purpura
   a. Premature removal of platelets with IgG autoantibodies from spleen
   b. Most common nontraumatic condition requiring splenectomy
   c. Symptoms include low platelet counts and petechial bleeding.
   d. Severity correlates with level of thrombocytopenia
      (1) Incidental findings: greater than 50,000 per liter
      (2) Easy ecchymosis: 30–50,000 per liter
      (3) Spontaneous petechial bleeding: 10–30,000 per liter
      (4) Increased risk for internal and intracranial bleeding: less than 10,000 per liter
   e. Diagnosis by platelet count, megathrombocytes on peripheral blood smears, and exclusion of secondary causes
   f. Adult disease—insidious onset; treat with splenectomy if medical therapy fails (prednisone and intravenous Ig). Splenectomy achieves 75%–80% cure rate with no further need for steroid therapy after surgery.

31

SURGICAL DISEASES OF THE SPLEEN

   g. Childhood course—generally self-limited disease, with 70% achieving complete remission. Manage conservatively with intermittent steroids/intravenous Ig and observation; splenectomy is rarely indicated.

2. **Thrombotic thrombocytopenic purpura**
   a. Loss of platelet inhibition results in abnormal platelet clumping/thrombosis.
   b. Deformation of vessel lumen size with resultant RBC hemolysis and splenic sequestration
   c. Symptoms include decreased platelet count, hemolytic anemia, neurologic complications, purpura, and renal dysfunction.
   d. Treat with plasma exchange, steroids, and aminosalicylic acid (ASA) (80% respond to medical therapy).
   e. Splenectomy is indicated if multiple relapses or excessive plasmapheresis.

F. OTHER SPLENIC DISORDERS

1. **Splenic abscesses**
   a. They arise from hematogenous infection, contiguous infection, hemoglobinopathies, immunosuppression, IV drug use, or trauma.
   b. Symptoms include fevers, leukocytosis, left upper quadrant pain, and splenomegaly.
   c. Diagnose by ultrasound or CT scan.
   d. Treat with broad-spectrum antibiotics and splenectomy.
      (1) Consider percutaneous drainage if there is a single abscess or if patient is unable to tolerate general anesthesia.

2. **Splenic cysts**
   a. Infectious causative agents are most commonly parasitic; the majority are *Echinococcus* species.
      (1) Treat with preoperative albendazole, splenectomy; avoid spillage of parasitic cyst contents to avoid anaphylactic shock.
   b. Noninfectious causative factor most commonly is traumatic "pseudocysts" (lack cellular lining).
      (1) Treatment: observe if asymptomatic. If symptomatic, excise if small, and unroof if larger.

3. **Felty syndrome**
   a. Immune complexes coat and sequester white blood cells (WBCs) in spleen.
   b. This has a triad of splenomegaly, rheumatoid arthritis, and neutropenia.
   c. It occurs in 3% of patients with rheumatoid arthritis; there is a female predominance.
   d. Splenectomy results in increased WBC counts in 80% of cases.

4. **Splenic artery aneurysm (>2 cm)**
   a. This is most common visceral aneurysm.
   b. There is a female predominance.
   c. It is most commonly found in the mid-to-distal artery.

    d. Rupture rate averages 3%–9%.

    e. Risk for rupture is much greater in pregnancy.

    f. Mortality rate with rupture approaches 50%.

    g. Most are diagnosed incidentally.

    h. Treatment

       (1) If symptomatic or enlarging, recommend treatment with resection or ligation.

       (2) If pregnant or of childbearing age, recommend treatment.

       (3) If greater than 2 cm and asymptomatic, consider elective resection.

       (4) If located in the distal segment, recommend splenectomy.

5. Splenic vein thrombosis

    a. It is associated with chronic pancreatitis.

    b. Gastric varices and left-sided portal hypertension are complications.

    c. If found with accompanying varices, recommended treatment is splenectomy.

IV. SURGICAL TECHNIQUES

A. OPEN SPLENECTOMY

1. Position supinely
2. Exposure
    a. Midline incision—massive splenomegaly or trauma
    b. Left subcostal incision—most elective splenectomies
3. Division of splenocolic ligament
4. Incision of lateral peritoneal attachments (splenophrenic ligament)
5. Division of short gastric arteries
6. Dissection of splenic hilum (artery, then vein)
7. Irrigation and evaluation for hemostasis

B. LAPAROSCOPIC SPLENECTOMY

1. First successful procedure performed in 1991 by Delaitre and Maignien
2. Position in right lateral decubitus at 60 degrees, 15-degree reverse Trendelenburg position
3. Dissection as with open technique, using endovascular staples, clips, or cautery
4. Removal of spleen via retrieval bag; may require morcellation of spleen to achieve removal

C. HAND-ASSISTED TECHNIQUE

1. Allows identification, retraction, and direct palpation, as well as removal of large spleens via hand port

V. POSTSPLENECTOMY CONSIDERATIONS

A. OVERWHELMING POSTSPLENECTOMY INFECTION

1. Increased susceptibility to infection by encapsulated organisms and parasites

31

SURGICAL DISEASES OF THE SPLEEN

2. Incidence rate 1%–5% over lifetime, typically within 2 years of splenectomy
3. Mortality increased in children, immunocompromised patients, and patients with hematologic conditions
4. Responsible organisms include:
   a. *Streptococcus pneumoniae* (50%–90% of cases)
   b. *Haemophilus influenzae*
   c. *Meningococcus* spp.
5. Symptoms include prodrome of fever, malaise, headache, vomiting, diarrhea, and abdominal pain.
6. Rapid progression into fulminant septic shock
7. Prevention
   a. Vaccinations
      (1) Pneumococcal, meningococcal, and *H. influenzae* vaccines
      (2) Administer vaccines 14 days prior to elective splenectomy. In nonelective splenectomy, administer 14 days after surgery
   b. Children are candidates for prophylactic antibiotics for 2 years after surgery.

B. POSTSPLENECTOMY HEMATOLOGIC CHANGES
1. Leukocytosis and thrombocytosis
2. WBC count increases on postoperative day 1 and remains increased for months.
3. Platelet count increases over several days, peaking 2–3 weeks after surgery.
4. Recommend acetylsalicylic acid for platelet count greater than 10^6 per liter.

C. HEMORRHAGE
1. Subphrenic hematoma
2. Usual source is short gastric arteries.

D. INFECTION
1. Subphrenic abscesses—increased incidence with left upper quadrant drain placement
2. Wound infection

E. PORTAL VEIN THROMBOSIS
1. Incidence of 5%–10%
2. More commonly associated with myeloproliferative disorders (up to 40%)
3. Symptoms include anorexia, abdominal pain, leukocytosis, and thrombocytosis after surgery.
4. Diagnosis by computed tomography imaging
5. Treatment with immediate anticoagulation

F. PANCREATITIS, PSEUDOCYST, FISTULA

1. Secondary to pancreatic irritation/injury during dissection of splenic hilum

RECOMMENDED READINGS

Bromberg ME. Immune thrombocytopenic purpura—the changing therapeutic landscape. *N Engl J Med*. 2006;355:1643–1645.

Ali Caditi, de Gara C. Complications of splenectomy. *Am J Med*. 2008;121:371–375.

Mebius RE, Kraal G. Structure and function of the spleen. *Nat Rev Immunol*. 2005;5:606–614.

Rajani RR, Claridge JA, Yowler CJ, et al. Improved outcome of adult blunt splenic injury: a cohort analysis. *Surgery*. 2006;140:625–632.

31

SURGICAL DISEASES OF THE SPLEEN

Bariatric Surgery

Hannah V. Lewis, MD

Thou seest I have more flesh than another man, and therefore more frailty.

—William Shakespeare

I. EPIDEMIOLOGY OF MORBID OBESITY

A. DEFINITIONS

1. Overweight—body mass index [(BMI) = weight in kg/height in m²] greater than 25–29.9
2. Obese (Class I)—BMI greater than 30–34.9
3. Severe obesity (Class II)—BMI greater than 35–39.9
4. Morbid obesity (Class III)—BMI ≥40
5. BMI for children differ
   a. Overweight: BMI greater than 85–95th percentile for age and sex
   b. Obese: BMI greater than 95th percentile for age and sex
   c. Severe obesity: BMI greater than 120% of the 95th percentile values, or BMI greater than 35—about 99th percentile.

B. CAUSES OF OBESITY

1. Genetic predisposition
2. Gestational factors
   a. Maternal diabetes mellitus (DM) during gestation
   b. Maternal smoking
3. Diet
   a. Easy access to food sources
   b. High-calorie, large-portion food choices
   c. Disinhibition—overeating
4. Lifestyle
   a. Increase in sedentary behavior
      (1) Percentage of adults participating in physical activity decreases steadily with age.
   b. Labor-saving technology
   c. Sleep deprivation—less than 7 hours a night
5. Increased caloric intake + reduced energy expenditure can equal obesity.

C. EPIDEMIOLOGY

1. Worldwide, obesity affects 1.9 billion people.
2. More than one-third of the population in the United States are obese.
3. Obesity presents a significant economic burden, accounting for 10% ($147 billion) of all direct US healthcare costs in 2008.

a. BMI greater than 30 associated with an increase of approximately $1700/year of medical spending
4. In 2013, 150,000 bariatric surgeries were performed in the United States and approximately 468,000 worldwide.

II. COMORBIDITY ASSOCIATED WITH MORBID OBESITY

A. NEOPLASIA
1. Increased risk of endometrial cancer, earlier onset of endometrial cancer, and increased risk of breast cancer in obese women
   a. May be due to higher levels of bioavailable estradiol, from increased production of estrogens in adipose tissue
2. Increased risk of colorectal cancer in both obese men and women
3. Increased risk of esophageal and gastric adenocarcinomas
   a. No association with esophageal squamous cancer

B. CARDIOVASCULAR DISEASE
1. Obesity is estimated to account for hypertension (HTN) in 26% of men and 28% of women.
   a. Risk of HTN greatest in patients with upper body and abdominal distribution of fat
2. Morbidly obese patients have a doubled risk for myocardial infarction.
3. Risk of heart failure is doubled in patients with BMI greater than 30.

C. PULMONARY DISEASE
1. Obstructive sleep apnea (OSA)
   a. A total of 63% of obese men and 22% of obese women have moderate to severe OSA.
2. Obese patients have high rates of obesity-hypoventilation syndrome.

D. ENDOCRINE DISEASE
1. Greater than 80% of type II DM cases can be attributed to obesity.
2. Obese patients are at greater risk for hypoparathyroidism.

E. GASTROINTESTINAL DISEASE
1. Morbid obesity can increase risks for the following conditions:
   a. Nonalcoholic steatohepatitis
   b. Gastroesophageal reflux disease (GERD)
   c. Cholelithiasis and choledocholithiasis
      (1) Increased production and biliary excretion of cholesterol leads to increased risk of cholesterol precipitation in gallbladder
   d. Acute pancreatitis

F. OTHER COMORBIDITIES ASSOCIATED WITH MORBID OBESITY
1. Pregnancy-related complications such as preeclampsia, early neonatal death, and meconium aspiration
2. Musculoskeletal pain in hip and knee joints
   a. Osteoarthritis increased

32

BARIATRIC SURGERY

3. Prothrombotic state caused by high intraabdominal pressures, decreased activity, and venous compression by fatty tissues
4. Altered immunologic state
5. Intertriginous dermatitis
6. Psychological complaints
   a. Depression
   b. Social isolation
   c. Decreased libido

III. MEDICAL THERAPY FOR MORBID OBESITY

1. Diet modification—low in calories, fat, and carbohydrates
2. Increased physical activity
3. Behavioral modification—avoid snacking
4. Medications
   a. Lorcaserin: appetite suppressant
      (1) Sibutramine was also an appetite suppressant; taken off the market in 2010 because of an association with increased cardiovascular events
   b. Orlistat binds to lipases in the stomach and prevents their absorption.
5. Advantages and disadvantages
   a. There is a lower cost to initiate medical therapy.
   b. Long-term results are poor: most medical weight-loss programs have a high attrition rate.
   c. Medical treatment is associated with a greater rate of rebound weight gain versus surgical treatment.

IV. TYPES OF PROCEDURES
A. MALABSORPTIVE OPERATIONS
1. Decrease the intestinal surface area used for nutrient absorption by shortening or rearranging the digestive tract.

B. RESTRICTIVE OPERATIONS
1. Reduce gastric volume and cause satiety with low food volumes.

C. COMBINED OPERATIONS ARE RESTRICTIVE AND MALABSORPTIVE.

V. PREOPERATIVE WORK-UP
A. PATIENT SELECTION CRITERIA
1. BMI ≥40
2. BMI ≥35 with associated comorbidities
3. Failure of nonsurgical weight-loss efforts
4. Well-informed, compliant, motivated patients

B. PREOPERATIVE ASSESSMENT—MULTIDISCIPLINARY APPROACH
1. Bariatric nutritional assessment
2. Psychological assessment
3. Sleep apnea study and pulmonary assessment
4. Cardiovascular assessment

C. CONTRAINDICATIONS
1. Uncontrolled/untreated psychiatric conditions
   a. Eating disorders
   b. Major depression or psychosis
2. Current drug/alcohol use
3. Poor compliance in completing preoperative work-up
4. Severe cardiac disease
5. Uncorrectable coagulopathy

VI. SURGICAL PROCEDURES FOR THE BARIATRIC PATIENT

A. LAPAROSCOPIC SLEEVE GASTRECTOMY
1. Most common bariatric procedure in the United States
2. Longitudinal greater curvature gastrectomy
3. Originally used as first step of treatment in high-risk morbidly obese, to assist in weight loss prior to duodenal switch/biliary pancreatic diversion or Roux-en-Y
4. Combines restriction with hormonal appetite suppression by removing fundus, which is where most of ghrelin is produced
5. Procedure
   a. Divide gastrocolic and gastrosplenic omentum, mobilizing stomach and rotating medially; posterior fundus is mobilized off left crus of diaphragm.
   b. Create staple line with endocutter staplers ± oversewing.
   c. Create staple line usually 2–6 cm from pylorus on the antrum, 2–4 cm from the incisura angularis, and 1–2 cm from gastroesophageal junction.
   d. Use 32–50F bougie to help with sleeve creation at the body.
6. Advantages
   a. Does not rearrange anatomy
   b. Satiety with smaller meals
   c. No dumping syndrome
7. Disadvantages
   a. Irreversible
   b. Can get dilation of the stomach if do not adhere to small meals
8. Complications
   a. Leak
      (1) Majority happen at the top of the staple line, adjacent to gastroesophageal (GE) junction. It can be related to stricture at incisura angularis or twisting leading to high pressure.
      (2) Diagnose with computed tomography (CT) scan or upper gastrointestinal (GI); treat early leak with drain placement,

32

BARIATRIC SURGERY

esophagogastroduodenoscopy (EGD), and covered stent. Treat late/chronic leak with roux limb drainage.
   b. Bleeding
      (1) Usually from gastrosplenic vessels or staple line
   c. Stricture/stenosis
      (1) Proximal—can occur after revisional surgery from gastric band to sleeve; fibrous ring remains
      (2) Middle—rare; due to malrotation/spiraling of sleeve
      (3) Distal—due to narrowing of incisura angularis from staple line
9. Contraindications
   a. Absolute: severe GERD, Barrett esophagus, cirrhosis, or severe portal HTN
   b. Relative: prohibitive anesthesia risk, noncompliance, large hiatal hernias, significant eating disorders

B. LAPAROSCOPIC ROUX-EN-Y GASTRIC BYPASS
1. Restrictive and malabsorptive
2. A 30-mL gastric pouch is created by dividing stomach, and a roux limb (~75–150 cm) is created to anastomose to the gastric pouch.
3. Requires two anastomoses
   a. Gastrojejunostomy
   b. Jejunojejunostomy
4. Excellent excess weight loss (60%–70%) and resolution of comorbidity
5. Advantages
   a. Rapid weight loss
   b. Minimal dietary restrictions
6. Disadvantages
   a. Anatomic rearrangement
   b. Increased morbidity and mortality rates (0.2%–1%) as compared with laparoscopic adjustable gastric banding
   c. Dumping syndrome associated with high carbohydrate intake
   d. Nutritional deficiencies such as vitamin B12 and iron are common.
7. Complications
   a. Leaks
      (1) Most dreaded complication
      (2) Mortality rate of 10%
      (3) Clinical characteristics—fever, tachycardia, hypotension, abdominal pain
      (4) Types
         (a) Gastric pouch leaks (49%)
         (b) Staple line leaks (9%)
         (c) Gastric remnant leaks (25%), not seen on postoperative swallow studies
         (d) Jejunojejunostomy leaks (13%)
      (5) Treatment
         (a) Percutaneous drainage

(b) Operative exploration
b. Internal hernias
   (1) More common with laparoscopic procedures than open procedures because of decreased adhesion formation
   (2) Signs of obstruction
   (3) Types
      (a) Transmesocolic (for retrocolic Roux limbs)
      (b) Mesenteric-mesocolic (Petersen hernia)
      (c) Mesenteric (at jejunojejunostomy)
   (4) Treatment: Early operative intervention for any bypass patient with obstructive symptoms can prevent intestinal strangulation and necrosis.
c. Other complications
   (1) Thrombotic events
   (2) Bleeding at the staple lines
   (3) Marginal ulceration
   (4) Gastric-gastric fistula can lead to weight regain.
   (5) Stricture formation.

C. LAPAROSCOPIC ADJUSTABLE GASTRIC BANDING
1. Silicone band lined with inflatable balloon
2. Procedure
   a. The band is connected to a subcutaneous reservoir, which controls the balloon tightness.
   b. The band is wrapped around gastric cardia, forming a 30-mL gastric pouch.
   c. Inflation of the balloon tightens the band and promotes early satiety.
3. Advantages
   a. Adjustable and reversible
   b. Least invasive bariatric surgical procedure
   c. No anatomic rearrangement
   d. Low morbidity and mortality rates
4. Disadvantages
   a. More frequent and intense follow-up with patients
   b. Slower rate of weight loss
   c. Less overall excess weight loss
5. Complications
   a. Band slippage
      (1) Anterior or posterior gastric prolapse through band
      (2) Clinically, causes pouch distention and obstructive symptoms
      (3) Treatment—deflate band, nasogastric tube drainage of pouch, operative band repositioning, or removal to prevent strangulation and necrosis
   b. Band erosion
      (1) Incidence rate of 0.2%–1.2%

(2) Diagnosis—usually endoscopy

(3) Treatment—band removal and gastric repair

D. JEJUNOILEAL BYPASS

1. Developed in the 1950s
2. Malabsorptive
3. Stomach was left intact, and the jejunum was connected to the terminal ileum.
4. Operation left a long, blind intestinal limb.
5. Excellent weight loss, but patients suffered many long-term complications, such as nutritional deficiencies, chronic diarrhea, and liver cirrhosis.
6. This procedure has been abandoned in the United States. Bacterial overgrowth in blind limb led to the doctrine of ensuring flow in all enteric limbs.

E. VERTICAL BANDED GASTROPLASTY

1. Purely restrictive operation with a stapled 30-mL pouch based off the lesser curvature
2. No anastomosis required
3. Polypropylene mesh or Silastic ring used to create gastric outlet
4. Once popular, it is now rarely performed because of weight regain and severe heartburn.
5. Laparoscopic Roux-en-Y gastric bypass has proven to have superior results to the vertical banded gastroplasty.

F. BILIOPANCREATIC DIVERSION

1. Seventy percent gastrectomy and biliopancreatic diversion with a 100-cm common alimentary channel
2. Restrictive and malabsorptive
3. Usually a two-stage procedure
4. Complex operation that yields excellent weight-loss results (70% excess body weight loss) that is sustainable more than 10 years after surgery
5. Most common variant currently performed is the duodenal switch in which the duodenum is transected proximal to the ampulla of Vater and an enteric limb is anastomosed postpylorically.

VII. RESULTS OF BARIATRIC SURGERY

A. SURGICAL THERAPY

1. Decreases mortality risk versus nonintervention or medical therapy

B. RISK REDUCTION

1. Reduction is 31.6% for death in surgical versus medical treatment for morbid obesity, according to the Swedish Obese Subjects study.

C. **LAPAROSCOPIC SLEEVE GASTRECTOMY, LAPAROSCOPIC ROUX-EN-Y GASTRIC BYPASS, AND LAPAROSCOPIC ADJUSTABLE GASTRIC BANDING**
1. Demonstrate excellent and near-complete resolution of comorbidity associated with morbid obesity, including the following conditions:
   a. Type II DM
   b. HTN
   c. GERD
   d. Sleep apnea
   e. Joint pain

E. **WEIGHT LOSS**
1. Weight loss usually reaches a maximum between 18 and 24 months after surgery.
2. Weight loss is dependent on several factors:
   a. Preoperative weight
   b. Overall patient health
   c. Procedure performed
      (1) Gastric sleeve (49%–56% excess weight loss)
      (2) Bypass surgery (55%–66% excess weight loss)
      (3) Gastric banding (40%–54% excess weight loss)
   d. Commitment to maintaining dietary guidelines
   e. Follow-up care
   f. Patient motivation

32

BARIATRIC SURGERY

RECOMMENDED READINGS

Angrisani L. Bariatric surgery worldwide 2013. *Obes Surg*. 2015;25:1822–1832.

Mechanick JL. Clinical practice guidelines for the perioperative nutritional, metabolic, and nonsurgical support of the bariatric surgery patient—2013 update: cosponsored by American Association of Clinical Endocrinologists, the Obesity Society, and American Society for Metabolic & Bariatric Surgery. *Surg Obes Relat Dis*. 2013;9:159–191.

Peterli J. Early results of the Swiss Multicentre Bypass or Sleeve Study (SM-BOSS): a prospective randomized trial comparing laparoscopic sleeve gastrectomy and Roux-en-Y gastric bypass. *Ann Surg*. 2013;258:690–694.

PART VI

Surgical Oncology

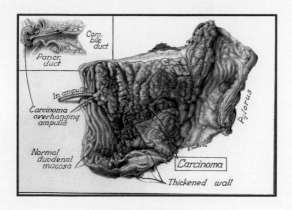

Tumor Biology, Syndromes, and Genetic Mutations

Stacey L. Doran, MD

The pathogenesis of human cancers is governed by a set of genetic and biochemical rules that apply to most and perhaps all types of human tumors.

—W.C. Hahn and R.A. Weinberg

I. SELF-SUFFICIENCY IN GROWTH SIGNALS

Mitogens are chemicals that trigger cell mitosis. In contrast with healthy cells, cancer cells have a reduced dependence on mitogens and external growth factors for replication.

A. GROWTH FACTORS
1. Tumor cells and stroma produce factors that may influence tumor growth and stimulate cell environment.
2. Transforming growth factor-beta (TGF-beta) affects angiogenesis, extracellular matrix, and production of cytokines.

B. ALTERATION OF GROWTH SIGNALING PATHWAYS
1. Growth factor receptors may be overexpressed or structurally altered.
2. Overexpression may allow cells to be stimulated by very low levels of growth factors.
3. Amplification of human epidermal growth factor receptor 2/neu (HER2/neu) is found in some forms of aggressive breast cancer.

C. SOS/RAS/RAF/MITOGEN-ACTIVATED PROTEIN KINASE PATHWAY
1. This is altered in approximately 25% of human cancers.
2. *K-ras* mutations are found in lung, pancreatic, and colon cancers.
3. The *Ras* oncogene encodes mutant protein that continuously releases mitogenic signals.

D. TUMOR GROWTH IS DEPENDENT ON MANY FACTORS
1. Angiogenesis factors, growth factors, chemokines, cytokines, hormones, enzymes, and cytolytic/cytostatic factors

II. INSENSITIVITY TO GROWTH-INHIBITORY SIGNALS

A. RETINOBLASTOMA PROTEIN
1. Retinoblastoma protein (pRB) has a central role in progression of cell through the G1 phase of the cell cycle.
2. Action may be lost through deletion or inactivation.

3. Evidence suggests that alterations leading to the loss of growth suppression by pRB exist in the majority of human cancers.

III. EVASION OF PROGRAMMED CELL DEATH

A. p53 TUMOR-SUPPRESSOR PROTEIN

1. In healthy cells, it is responsible for temporary arrest of cell growth in response to damage to allow for repair or elimination by apoptosis.
2. Action may be lost via a diverse array of mechanisms.
3. Alterations in the p53 pathway exist in the majority of human cancers.

B. EXTRINSIC APOPTOSIS INDUCTION

1. Many tumor cells upregulate programmed death-ligand 1 (PD-L1), which binds to programmed cell death protein 1 (PD-1) on T cells, thereby inactivating immune-mediated killing and permitting tumor escape.

IV. LIMITLESS REPLICATIVE POTENTIAL

1. Normal cells carry an intrinsic program that limits their ability to replicate.
   a. Independent of cell-to-cell signaling pathways
   b. Senescence reached once cells have divided a specified number of times
2. Loss of tumor suppressor proteins (p53 and pRB) leads to a crisis state.
   a. Massive cell death
   b. Karyotypic disarray
   c One in 10^7 cells achieves the ability to divide ad infinitum, termed *immortalization.*
3. Most tumor cells propagated in culture are immortalized.
4. Telomere maintenance is vital to continued replication of tumor cells.
   a. Ongoing maintenance of protective telomere sequences on the ends of chromosomes allows for immortality of cells.
   b. Reactivation of telomerase (suppressed in normal human cell types) and a telomerase-independent mechanism ("alternative lengthening of telomeres") allow for indefinite proliferation of cells.

V. SUSTAINED ANGIOGENESIS

1. Tumors cannot exceed diameters of 2 mm without acquiring a blood supply.
2. Solid tumors secrete proangiogenic factors.
   a. Vascular endothelial growth factor (VEGF)
   b. Basic and acidic fibroblast growth factor
   c. Platelet-derived growth factor
   d. anti-VEGF (Avastin)—angiogenesis inhibitor first approved for treatment of colon cancer

3. Tumors may also downregulate antiangiogenic proteins.
   a. Thrombospondin-1, which binds to CD36
   b. Interferon-β

VI. TISSUE INVASION AND METASTASIS

A. TETHERING MOLECULES ARE ALTERED
1. Cell-cell adhesion molecules
   a. E-cadherin, ubiquitously expressed on epithelial cells
      (1) Coupling of these proteins between cells leads to antigrowth signals.
      (2) Function is lost in the majority of epithelial cell tumors.
   b. Neural cell adhesion molecules (N-CAMs)
      (1) Expression is changed from a highly adhesive form to a poorly adhesive form in Wilms tumor, small cell lung cancer, and neuroblastoma.
      (2) Reduced expression is seen in invasive pancreatic and colorectal cancers.
2. Integrins link cells to extracellular matrix proteins.
   a. Successful colonization of new sites is achieved through changes in integrin α and β subunits on migrating cells.
   b. Tumor cells facilitate invasion by expressing integrins that preferentially bind degraded stromal components produced by extracellular proteases.

B. PROTEASES DEGRADE EXTRACELLULAR MATRICES
1. Protease genes are upregulated.
2. Protease inhibitors are downregulated.
3. Inactive forms of protease zymogens are converted to active forms.
4. Expression may be induced by stromal and inflammatory cells rather than the cancer cells themselves.

VII. GENETIC INSTABILITY

A. THE PREVIOUS SIX (I–VI) CHARACTERISTICS MUST BE OBTAINED THROUGH GENETIC ALTERATION
1. These alterations do not develop simultaneously because of cell's system of DNA monitoring and repair.
2. Sequential acquisition of mutations permits transition from noninvasive to locally invasive to distant metastatic tumors.
3. Somatic mutations are acquired during one's lifetime and not passed along to offspring.
4. Germline mutations are inherited and present in every cell in the body.

B. MALFUNCTION OF THE "CARETAKER" SYSTEM
1. Loss of the p53 tumor suppressor protein occurs in nearly all human cancers.

2. Inherited or acquired deficiencies in cell repair genes lead to increased DNA damage and/or inability to undergo apoptosis.

VIII. FAMILIAL CANCER SYNDROMES

A. FAMILIAL ADENOMATOUS POLYPOSIS
1. Autosomal dominant, adenomatous polyposis coli *(APC)* gene mutation
2. One percent of all colorectal cancers
3. Hundreds of colorectal polyps that progress to colorectal cancer, also upper gastrointestinal polyps, osteomas, desmoid tumors, thyroid cancer

B. HEREDITARY BREAST-OVARIAN CANCER SYNDROMES
1. Mutations in tumor suppressor genes with variable penetrance
2. A total of 5%–10% of all breast cancers
3. Breast cancer susceptibility gene 1 *(BRCA1)*—breast cancer, ovarian cancer, prostate cancer
4. Breast cancer susceptibility gene 2 *(BRCA2)*—breast cancer, male breast cancer, ovarian cancer, melanoma, prostate cancer, pancreatic cancer

C. HEREDITARY NONPOLYPOSIS COLON CANCER, LYNCH SYNDROME
1. Autosomal dominant, mutation in DNA mismatch repair genes *(hMSH2, hMLH1, hMSH6, hPMS1, hPMS2)*
2. Two percent of all colorectal cancers
3. Colorectal cancer (often right colon), endometrial cancer, ovarian cancer, gastric cancer, pancreatic cancer

D. LI-FRAUMENI SYNDROME
1. Autosomal dominant, half with p53 mutation, *hCHK2* mutation, others?
2. Increased radiation sensitivity, more likely to develop radiation-induced malignancies
3. Breast cancer, sarcomas (soft tissue and bone), brain cancers, adreno-cortical carcinoma

E. MULTIPLE ENDOCRINE NEOPLASIA
1. Multiple endocrine neoplasia type 1 (MEN1)
   a. Parathyroid hyperplasia (hyperparathyroidism), pancreatic islet cell tumors, pituitary adenomas
   b. Autosomal dominant, mutated MEN1 allele (makes menin)
2. MEN2a
   a. Parathyroid hyperplasia, pheochromocytoma, medullary thyroid cancer
   b. Mutation in *RET*
3. MEN2b
   a. Pheochromocytoma, medullary thyroid cancer, Marfan habitus
   b. Mutation in *RET*

F. **VON HIPPEL-LINDAU DISEASE**
1. Autosomal dominant mutation in tumor suppressor gene von Hippel-Lindau (VHL)
2. Renal cysts that develop into clear cell renal carcinoma, central nervous system (CNS) and retinal/CNS hemangioblastomas, pheochromocytomas

G. **COWDEN SYNDROME**
1. Mutation in *PTEN*
2. Breast, endometrial, and thyroid (follicular) cancers
3. May have macrocephaly, hamartomas, mucocutaneous lesions

H. **HEREDITARY DIFFUSE GASTRIC CANCER**
1. Mutation in *CHD1*
2. Gastric cancer, lobular breast cancer

I. **PEUTZ-JEGHERS SYNDROME**
1. Mutation in *STK11*
2. Small intestine hamartomatous polyps, mucocutaneous hyperpigmentation
3. Gastrointestinal, breast, testicular, ovarian, lung, and pancreatic cancer

IX. PHARMACOTHERAPY
A. **TUMOR GROWTH AND KINETICS**
1. Gompertzian growth
   a. Exhibit a sigmoid-shaped growth curve (Fig. 33.1)
   b. In low tumor volumes, growth is exponential. As mass increases and resources become scarce, growth plateaus.
   c. Maximum growth at 30% of maximum tumor
      (1) Nutrient and oxygen supply optimized
      (2) Point where drug efficacy may be best estimated
2. Cell cycle (Fig. 33.2)
   a. G0 phase—resting/nonproliferating
   b. G1 phase—size increase, organelle duplication
   c. S phases—DNA synthesis
   d. G2 phase—postsynthetic, final checkpoint before mitosis
   e. M phase—mitosis

B. **DRUG MECHANISMS AND THERAPEUTICS**
1. Chemotherapy mechanisms
   a. DNA damage
      (1) Alkylation
      (2) Cross-linking
      (3) Double-strand cleavage
      (4) Intercalation
      (5) Blockage of RNA synthesis

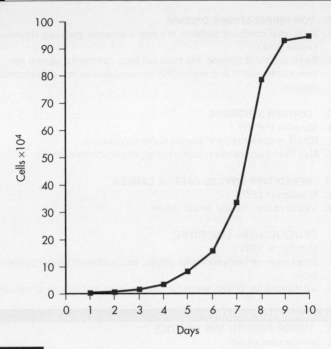

FIG. 33.1
Sigmoid-shaped curve of tumor growth.

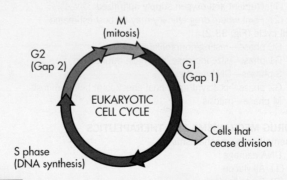

FIG. 33.2
Cell cycle of eukaryotic cell.

b. Spindle poisons arrest mitosis.
c. Antimetabolites interrupt DNA synthesis.
d. Signal transduction inhibitors
e. Oncoviral therapy involves injection of tumor-specific replicating virus to cause cancer cell destruction.
f. Gene therapy involves the transfer of wild-type genes into tumor cells.
   (1) Restore or add expression of tumor suppressor or immunostimulatory genes.
   (2) Inhibit oncogene expression.
g. Antiangiogenesis therapy
h. Immunotherapy
i. Hormonal therapy

2. Drug resistance
a. Multiple mechanisms of drug resistance may develop during cancer progression.
   (1) Increased excretion of drugs from cells. The *mdr* gene codes for membrane-bound P-glycoprotein, which serves as a channel for excretion of cellular toxins.
   (2) Decreased drug transport into cells
   (3) Reduction of drug activation
   (4) Enhanced drug metabolism
   (5) Upregulation of alternative metabolic pathways
   (6) Gene amplification to overcome drug inhibition of enzyme targets
   (7) Impairment of drug binding to target
b. Normal human cells do not develop drug resistance.
c. Drugs active as single agents may be used alone.
d. When given in combination, use drugs with different dose-limiting toxicities and different patterns of resistance.

X. CHEMOTHERAPEUTIC AGENTS: MECHANISMS, USES, AND IMPORTANT TOXICITIES

A. ALKYLATING AGENTS
1. Cyclophosphamide—may cause hemorrhagic cystitis
2. Melphalan—melanoma limb perfusion/infusion

B. ANTIMETABOLITES
1. 5-Fluorouracil (5-FU)—nucleoside analog and thymidylate synthase inhibitor; stomatitis, myelosuppression, nausea, vomiting, diarrhea
2. Methotrexate—inhibits folic acid metabolism; mucositis, myelosuppression, pulmonary fibrosis, hepatotoxicity, nephrotoxicity, diarrhea
3. Gemcitabine—nucleoside analog

C. ANTITUMOR ANTIBIOTICS
1. Bleomycin—pulmonary fibrosis
2. Doxorubicin—cardiotoxicity
3. Mitomycin C—myelosuppression

D. MITOTIC INHIBITORS
1. Etoposide (VP-16)—myelosuppression
2. Paclitaxel (Taxol)—peripheral neuropathy
3. Docetaxel (Taxotere)—myelosuppression
4. Vinblastine—myelosuppression
5. Vincristine—peripheral neuropathy

E. HORMONAL AGENTS
1. Antiestrogens (i.e., tamoxifen)—hot flashes, blood clots, increased risk for uterine cancer
2. Aromatase inhibitors (i.e., anastrozole, letrozole)—hot flashes, joint pain, osteoporosis

F. IMMUNOTHERAPY
1. Vaccine therapy
   a. Goal of stimulating tumor antigen–activated T cells
   b. Melanoma
2. Immunomodulatory pathways
   a. Immune checkpoint inhibitors enhance the ability of the immune system to recognize and kill cancer cells in vivo by preventing inhibition of T cells.
   b. Significant side effects include immune-mediated pneumonitis, colitis, nephritis, and rash.
   c. Anti-PD-1/anti-PD-L1 therapy
      (1) Nivolumab (Opdivo)— anti-PD-1; melanoma, non–small cell lung cancer, renal cell carcinoma
      (2) Pembrolizumab (Keytruda)—anti-PD-1; melanoma, non–small cell lung cancer
      (3) Atezolizumab (Tecentriq)—anti-PD-L1; urothelial carcinoma
      (4) Other PD-L1 agents such as avelumab and durvalumab under investigation but not US Food and Drug Administration (FDA)-approved
   d. Anti-cytotoxic T lymphocyte–associated protein 4 (CTLA-4)
      (1) Ipilimumab (Yervoy)—melanoma
   e. T cell adoptive therapy—tumor-infiltrating lymphocytes (TILs) or chimeric antigen receptor (CAR) T cells
3. Monoclonal antibodies
   a. Bevacizumab (Avastin)—targets VEGF-A to decrease angiogenesis; colorectal cancer; small incidence of gastrointestinal perforation
   b. Cetuximab (Erbitux)—epidermal growth factor receptor (EGFR) inhibitor; colorectal cancer, head and neck cancer
   c. Panitumumab (Vectibix)—EGFR inhibitor; colorectal cancer
   d. Trastuzumab (Herceptin)—HER2/neu epidermal growth factor inhibitor; breast cancer
   e. Growth factor receptor inhibitors
      (1) Erlotinib (Tarceva)—non–small cell lung cancer

    (2) Gefitinib (Iressa)—non–small cell lung cancer
    (3) Imatinib (Gleevec)—gastrointestinal stromal tumors
  f. B-Raf enzyme inhibitors
    (1) Targets BRAF V600E mutations, which are present in approximately 60% of melanoma
    (2) Vemurafenib (Zelboraf)—melanoma with V600E mutation
    (3) Dabrafenib (Tafinlar)—melanoma with V600E mutation

4. Cytokine therapy
  a. Interferon-α—melanoma, chronic hepatitis B and C
  b. Interleukin-2—renal cell carcinoma, metastatic melanoma

G. MISCELLANEOUS

1. Mitotane—used for adrenocortical carcinoma; causes adrenal insufficiency
2. Streptozocin—metastatic islet cell carcinomas; hypoglycemia
3. Platinums (cisplatin, carboplatin, oxaliplatin)—nephrotoxicity, neurotoxicity
4. Leucovorin—if given with methotrexate, may "rescue" the bone marrow from toxicity; if given with 5-FU has synergistic killing of cancer cells

RECOMMENDED READINGS

Feng XH, Lin X, Yu J et al. Molecular and genomic surgery. In: Brunicardi FC, Andersen DK, Billiar TR, et al. eds. *Schwartz's Principles of Surgery*. 10th ed. New York: McGraw-Hill Education; 2014:443–470.

Syngal S, Brand RE, Church JM, et al. ACG clinical guideline: genetic testing and management of hereditary gastrointestinal cancer syndromes. *Am J Gastroenterol.* 2015;110:223–262.

33

TUMOR BIOLOGY, SYNDROMES, AND GENETIC MUTATIONS

Head and Neck Malignancy

Sarah J. Atkinson, MD

Go in over your head, not just up to your neck.

—Dorothea Lange

I. EPIDEMIOLOGY

1. Worldwide, it is estimated that 300,000 people are living with oral cavity and pharynx cancer. Approximately 48,000 head and neck cancers are diagnosed in the United States annually, representing nearly 3% of cancers diagnosed in North America and 1.6% of all cancer deaths. The male-to-female ratio is almost 3:1, and the median age of onset is 62 years. The 5-year survival rate is 64% but varies greatly depending on the site of the primary.

2. The majority of these malignancies are squamous cell in origin (90%), with primary salivary gland tumors being the next most common. Squamous cell are categorized by location and are most commonly found in the oral cavity (29.5%), larynx (20.4%), hypopharynx (19.8%), oropharynx (14.7%), nose and paranasal sinuses (7%), and nasopharynx (3.2%).

3. Risk factors for head and neck squamous cell carcinoma (HNSCC) classically have been smoking and heavy alcohol exposure, which act synergistically to increase the risk of HNSCC 60–100-fold. A recent increase in human papillomavirus (HPV)–associated HNSCC is most strongly associated with tumors of the oropharynx, including tonsils and base of tongue cancers. Nearly 16,000 new cases of HPV-associated HNSCC are diagnosed each year, which now makes up 70% of oropharyngeal HNSCC. HPV-associated HNSCC have a strong male association, nearly 4:1. Fortunately, HPV-associated HNSCC of the oropharynx has a 54% better survival rate compared with HNSCC not associated with HPV. Approximately 80% of people are exposed to HPV over their lifetime, but not all exposures become clinically significant. Those who do develop malignancies typically do so 20–30 years after exposure to the virus. Some early studies have found that the HPV vaccine affords strong protection against oral HPV infections, potentially decreasing the risk of HPV-associated HNSCC.

II. WORK-UP OF A NECK MASS

1. Unknown primary: a malignant neoplasm metastatic to cervical lymph nodes without an identifiable primary tumor
   a. Vast majority will be squamous cell cancer and will present as a neck mass.

(1) Less commonly present as pain (9%), weight loss (7%), dysphagia (4%)
  b. Diagnostic algorithm (Fig. 34.1)
    (1) CT of neck
    (2) Positron emission tomography–computed tomography (PET CT) may help to identify the primary site, as well as the extent of nodal and or metastatic disease.
    (3) Fine-needle aspiration (FNA) (see diagram for FNA algorithm)
    (4) If still unable to localize, endoscopy with direct biopsies of the most common areas (base of tongue) and tonsillectomy
      (a) Panendoscopy: direct laryngoscopy, nasal endoscopy, esophagoscopy, and bronchoscopy

III. NECK DISSECTION

1. *Radical neck dissection*: removes sternocleidomastoid muscle (SCM), internal jugular (IJ) vein, and spinal accessory nerve (CN XI)
   a. This is rarely performed nowadays, because of morbidity; it is indicated only for clinically positive nodes with extracapsular extension and involvement of SCM, IJ vein, or CN XI.
   b. If bilateral is required, spare one IJ vein to avoid potential neurologic complications from venous congestion.
2. *Modified radical neck dissection:* Rationale is that lymphatics in the neck are fibroadipose tissue contained within a complex system of aponeurotic partitions that are separate from the SCM and IJ vein. There is equally effective oncologic resection with lower morbidity.
   a. Type I: spares CN XI
   b. Type II: spares IJ vein and CN XI
   c. Type III (also known as functional): spares SCM, IJ vein, and CN XI
3. *Selective neck dissection:* Rationale is that it removes nodal levels at high risk and is based on the location of the primary tumor and its known pattern of spread.
   a. En bloc resection of one or more lymph node basins
     (1) Selective neck dissections are described with respect to the lymph node levels removed. For example, a supraomohyoid neck dissection is described as a selective neck dissection (I-III).
       (a) Indication: performed in the *clinically N0 neck*
4. Lymph node groups—If you have node-positive (N+) disease, long-term survival decreases by 50%.
   a. Level i: submental and submandibular nodes
   b. Level ii: upper jugular nodes
   c. Level iii: middle jugular nodes
   d. Level iv: lower jugular and supraclavicular nodes
   e. Level v: posterior triangle nodes (postauricular, occipital, spinal accessory chain)
   f. Level vi: anterior nodes (pretracheal and paratracheal nodes, Delphian node)

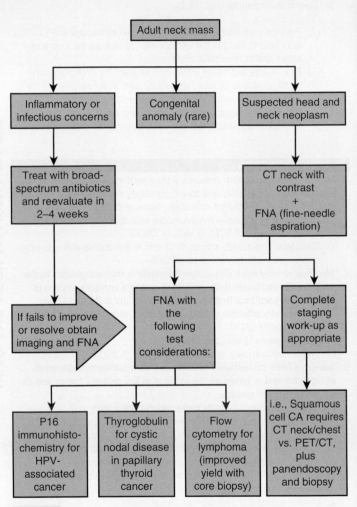

FIG. 34.1
Work-up of a neck mass. *CA,* Carcinoma; *CT,* computed tomography; *FNA,* fine-needle aspiration; *HPV,* human papillomavirus; *PET,* positron emission tomography.

IV. TREATMENT OF CANCER BY SITE

A. CARCINOMA OF THE ORAL CAVITY AND LIP

1. Physical findings suspicious for malignancy—nonhealing mucosal ulceration, violaceous mucosa, pain, bleeding, friability, leukoplakia, erythroplakia
   a. Higher rate of dysplasia and carcinoma seen with erythroplakia compared with leukoplakia
2. Tongue
   a. Exophytic—plaquelike tumor grows off tongue mucosa
   b. Infiltrative—have large submucosal extension and ulcerate late in course
   c. *Early lesions*—wide local excision, greater than 5-mm margins
      (1) Neck dissection for tumors with greater than 3-mm depth of invasion
   d. *Late lesions*—wide local excision with neck dissection adjuvant radiation and chemotherapy if indicated
   e. *Midline lesions*—bilateral neck should be treated.
3. Lip
   a. Mostly SCC
   b. *Early lesions*—local excision
   c. *Late lesions*—tumor resection with supraomohyoid neck dissection

B. OROPHARYNGEAL CARCINOMA

1. Both the incidence of oropharyngeal cancer and the proportion of HPV-related oropharyngeal cancers are rising in the United States.
2. The Centers for Disease Control and Prevention (CDC) estimates that 70% of oropharyngeal cancers are now related to HPV infections.
3. HPV-associated cancers have an improved prognosis compared with those associated with tobacco use.
   a. Tonsillar carcinoma
      (1) The tonsils are the most common site of SCC in the oropharynx.
      (2) Approximately 70% of patients present with nodal metastases.
      (3) *Early lesions*—single modality (radiation, resection)
      (4) *Advanced lesions*—multimodality therapy (resection, radiation, chemotherapy)
   b. Tongue base carcinoma
      (1) Frequently present late, 80% with nodal metastases

C. LARYNGEAL CANCER

1. Glottic cancer
   a. From laryngeal vestibule to 1 cm below vocal fold
   b. Often presents early because of persistent hoarseness
   c. Other symptoms include throat pain, referred otalgia, dysphagia, and odynophagia.
   d. Treatment
   e. *T1 lesions*—rarely present with nodal or distant metastasis because of poor lymphatic drainage

2. Single modality therapy
   a. Endoscopic excision versus primary radiation
      (1) Functional outcomes vary based on location of the tumor.
      (2) *Advanced lesions*—Treat with multimodal therapy either:
3. Concurrent chemoradiation with surgical salvage for residual or locally recurrent disease
4. Total laryngectomy with adjuvant chemotherapy and radiation
   a. Use chemotherapy for extracapsular spread, positive margins, and perineural invasion/spread.
   b. Patients with minimal laryngeal function (speech, swallow, airway) or invasion through thyroid cartilage fare better with a primary surgical modality.
   c. Supraglottic cancer
   d. General
      (1) Subsites include: suprahyoid and infrahyoid epiglottis, aryepiglottic fold, false vocal folds, arytenoids
      (2) Rich, bilateral lymphatic drainage—often presents with early neck metastases
   e. Symptoms
      (1) Throat pain, referred otalgia, dysphagia, odynophagia, and neck mass are more common than hoarseness because tumor does not involve vibrating vocal folds.
   f. Treatment
      (1) *Early lesions*—single modality treatment but must also include bilateral regional neck treatment.
5. Radiation of primary site and bilateral necks
6. Endoscopic/robotic/open supraglottic laryngectomy and concurrent selective neck dissection or neck radiation
7. N0 necks should be treated, given high rate of occult nodal metastases.
   a. *Advanced lesions*—Treat like glottic tumors with multimodal therapy.

D. **HYPOPHARYNGEAL**
1. Rare; only 5% of cancer of the aerodigestive tract, with 5-year survival rates of 35%–40%
2. Three subsites: postcricoid, pyriform sinuses, posterior pharyngeal wall
   a. Due to proximity, larynx is often involved.
3. Symptoms
   a. Most common presenting symptoms are pain, odynophagia, and dysphagia neck mass.
4. Treatment
   a. Early lesions, N0 necks
      (1) Preferred treatment modality is definitive radiation treatment of primary site and necks.
      (2) Endoscopic/open partial pharyngectomy, with ipsilateral or bilateral selective neck dissection, can be attempted.

(3) If there is vocal fold fixation or the tumor involves medial wall of pyriform (also known as T3), treat as an advanced lesion.
   b. Advanced lesion
      (1) Definitive chemoradiation with salvage laryngopharyngectomy.
      (2) Laryngopharyngectomy (and possibly partial cervical esophagectomy), bilateral neck dissections with adjuvant chemoradiation.

E. NASOPHARYNGEAL CARCINOMA
1. General
   a. Rare in the United States but common in China
   b. Associated with Epstein-Barr virus (EBV) and nickel exposure
   c. Pathology—70% are SCC.
2. Symptoms
   a. Nasal tumors present with painless neck mass, nasal obstructive symptoms, epistaxis, and chronic otitis media from eustachian tube obstruction.
   b. As tumors enlarge, adjacent cranial nerves may become involved.
3. Treatment
   a. Radiation is the mainstay of treatment.
   b. Perform surgical resection of value as salvage therapy after radiation failure.

F. SALIVARY GLAND TUMORS
1. Benign
   a. Pleomorphic adenoma or benign mixed tumor (52%)
      (1) Most commonly located in the parotid (85%) followed by minor salivary glands (10%)
      (2) Recurrence rate of 2% after treatment
      (3) Resection with wide margins for *pseudopods* extensions (cause of recurrence)
   b. Warthin tumor (papillary cystadenoma lymphomatosum) (5%)
      (1) Very slow growing
      (2) Appear almost exclusively in the tail of the parotid
      (3) Occur in men more often than women (5:1)
      (4) Associated with autoimmune diseases and smoking
      (5) Bilateral: 10%; multicentric: 10%
   c. Monomorphic adenoma (3%)
   d. Oncocytoma (oxyphilic adenoma) (1%)
   e. Godwin tumor (lymphoepithelial cysts)
   f. Hemangioma
      (1) Most common parotid tumor in kids
2. Malignant
   a. Mucoepidermoid carcinoma (12%), low grade and high grade
      (1) A total of 70% occur in parotid.
      (2) Most common type is induced by history of radiation.

b. Acinic cell tumor (6%)
 (1) Almost exclusively in parotid
 (2) Amyloid = path hallmark (apple-green birefringence with Congo red)
c. Adenocarcinoma (6%)
d. Adenoid cystic tumor (cylindroma) (4%)
 (1) Most common malignancy of the submandibular gland or minor salivary glands
 (2) A total of 50% of patients develop distant metastases.
 (3) Early perineural spread
e. Malignant mixed tumor
 (1) Growth rate is explosive.
 (2) It mostly involves parotid gland.
 (3) Prognosis is poor.
 (4) *Carcinoma ex pleomorphic adenoma* is a malignant mixed tumor that arises from a preexisting pleomorphic adenoma.
f. SCC
 (1) Lymph node metastases in 47%
g. Basal cell carcinoma
h. Lymphoma
 (1) Associated with Sjögren syndrome
i. Bilateral tumors:
 (1) Warthin
 (2) Oncocytoma
 (3) Acinic cell
j. Parotid tumors:
 (1) A total of 80% of major salivary neoplasms occur in the parotid.
3. Treatment
 a. Parotidectomy with facial nerve presentation unless the nerve is invaded, then it is sacrificed
4. Superficial versus total parotid resection
 a. Most lymph nodes are in the superficial parotid.
 (1) Spare the nerve unless it is involved.
 b. Deep lobe of parotid is addressed if the mass is in the deep lobe (positive margin) or if there is facial nerve involvement or high-grade neoplasm.
 c. With malignant tumors, radical neck dissection is performed for N+ disease, then postoperative radiation.
5. Submandibular tumors and minor salivary gland tumors
 a. These are 10% of neoplasms.
 b. Half of tumors are malignant.
 c. Adenoid cystic carcinoma is the most common malignancy (often presents with metastases).
6. Treatment: gland excision, neck dissection for N+ disease, postoperative radiation

a. Sublingual gland tumors
   (1) These are <1% of all salivary gland tumors.
   (2) Approximately 90% are malignant.

V. NECK DISSECTION INDICATIONS FOR SALIVARY GLAND MALIGNANCY

1. Obvious neck disease
2. Cancer of the submandibular gland
3. Tumor >4 cm
4. Cancer type: primary squamous cell cancer, undifferentiated cancer, high-grade mucoepidermoid, adenocarcinoma

A. RARER SITES OF CARCINOMA

1. Tumors of the paranasal sinuses
2. Mucosal melanoma

RECOMMENDED READINGS

Pasha R, Golub J. *Otolaryngology—Head and Neck Surgery: Clinical Reference Guide*. 4th ed. San Diego: Plural Publishing; 2013.

34

HEAD AND NECK MALIGNANCY

Esophageal Malignancy

Sarah J. Atkinson, MD

I. ESOPHAGEAL ANATOMY

1. The esophagus is a muscular pump bordered by two sphincters, the upper esophageal sphincter (UES) and lower esophageal sphincter (LES). Its function is to transport food and liquids in a unidirectional movement, and it possesses no endocrine, exocrine, immunologic, digestive, absorptive, or secretory functions.
2. In contrast to the rest of the gastrointestinal (GI) tract, the esophagus has no serosa, thus reducing the resistance to local spread of invasive cancer cells.

II. EPIDEMIOLOGY

1. Cancers of the esophagus are 1% of newly diagnosed malignancies in the United States.
2. The median age of diagnosis in the United States is 67 years old.
3. Most patients present with advanced disease, and their survival remains poor (5-year survival rate of 18.4%).
4. In the United States, squamous cell carcinoma is declining in incidence and adenocarcinoma is increasing in incidence.
5. In the United States, adenocarcinoma is the most common esophageal cancer (70%–75% of esophageal cancers).
   a. Incidence has increased by approximately 10% per year and is now 10 times what it was in 1976.
6. Worldwide, the incidence of squamous cell carcinoma is most common.
   a. Endemic areas—northern China, South Africa, Iran, Russia, and India.

III. HISTOLOGY AND RISK FACTORS

1. Squamous cell carcinoma typically affects the proximal and mid esophagus, whereas adenocarcinoma typically affects the lower esophagus and gastroesophageal junction.
2. Adenocarcinoma is caused by chronic gastroesophageal reflux disease (GERD).
   a. Barrett esophagus (intestinal metaplasia) is main risk factor for adenocarcinoma.
   b. Barrett develops from GERD, which can lead to low-grade dysplasia (LGD), which can develop into high-grade dysplasia (HGD) and then invasive cancer.
   c. Barrett esophagus portends a 50 times increased risk of cancer. Surveillance esophagogastroduodenoscopy (EGD) is recommended every 3–5 years after diagnosis.

d. LGD can regress with GERD treatment or can progress to HGD/cancer. Surveillance EGD is recommended every 6 months following diagnosis.

e. HGD—Treatment is recommended because 80% of patients will develop invasive cancer at 5 years. If surveillance is chosen, EGD is recommended every 3 months after diagnosis.

3. Risk factors for esophageal cancer (Table 35.1)

IV. DIAGNOSIS AND STAGING

1. Symptoms—Note that early cancers are generally asymptomatic.
   a. Dysphagia (most common and classically described as progressing from solids to liquids)
   b. Odynophagia/chest pain
   c. Weight loss
   d. Hematemesis
   e. Dyspnea, cough, hoarseness, pain, and neurologic symptoms suggest advanced disease.

2. Diagnosis
   a. Barium upper GI study
      (1) Delineate the degree of esophageal compromise.
      (2) Classic findings include polypoid tumors, strictures with mucosal irregularity, and "apple core" narrowing.
      (3) Can identify tracheoesophageal fistulas
   b. Flexible endoscopy (EGD) with biopsy is the primary method for the diagnosis of esophageal carcinoma.
      (1) This determines location, degree of obstruction, and length and extent of circumferential involvement of the tumor.
      (2) Multiple biopsies (6–8) should be performed on primary mass, as well as any additional suspicious lesions (submucosal spread or skip lesions can be present).

TABLE 35.1

EPIDEMIOLOGY OF ESOPHAGEAL MALIGNANCY

Risk Factors	Squamous Cell Carcinoma	Adenocarcinoma
First- or secondhand smoke	+++	++
Alcohol consumption	+++	−
Red meat consumption	+	+
Barrett esophagus	−	++++
Reflux symptoms	−	+++
BMI >25	−	++
Caustic injury	++++	−
Head and neck CA history	++++	−
Radiation history	+++	+++
Hot beverage consumption	+	−

−, No effect; +, suspicious effect; ++, positive effect; +++ and ++++, strong positive effect.
BMI, Body mass index; *CA,* cancer.
Data from Zhang Y. Epidemiology of esophageal cancer. *World J Gastroenterol.* 2013;19:5598–5606.

3. Staging—essential in choosing appropriate treatment plan
   a. Use computed tomography (CT) of the chest and abdomen to evaluate for metastases/disseminated disease.
      (1) If metastatic disease is present, treat nonoperatively with definitive chemoradiation therapy.
   b. Positron emission tomography (PET) evaluates for occult metastatic disease.
   c. Endoscopic ultrasonography (EUS) is used to determine depth of invasion (T stage).
      (1) Local nodal involvement (N stage) can also be evaluated by EUS.
      (2) EUS-directed needle biopsy of suspicious lymph nodes can be performed (EBUS = endobronchial ultrasound).
      (3) Tumor depth helps to predict the probability of nodal involvement, which influences decision making for treatment approach. With increasing depth (T stage), the risk of regional lymph node involvement increases.

V. TNM STAGING SYSTEM

Primary tumor (T stage)

TX—Primary tumor cannot be assessed.

T0—no evidence of primary tumor

Tis—HGD

T1a—invades lamina propria or muscularis mucosae

T1b—invades submucosa

T2—invades muscularis propria

T3—invades adventitia

T4—invades adjacent structures

T4a—resectable tumor invading pleura, pericardium, or diaphragm

T4b—unresectable tumor invading other adjacent structures, such as aorta, vertebral body, or trachea

Regional lymph nodes (N stage)

NX—Regional lymph nodes cannot be assessed.

N0—no regional lymph node metastasis

N1—metastasis in 1–2 regional lymph nodes

N2—metastasis in 3–6 regional lymph nodes

N3—metastasis in ≥7 regional lymph nodes

Distant metastasis (M stage)

MX—distant metastasis cannot be assessed.

M0—no distant metastasis

M1—distant metastasis

Histologic grade (G)

GX—grade cannot be assessed—stage grouping as G1

G1—well differentiated

G2—moderately differentiated

G3—poorly differentiated

G4—undifferentiated—stage grouping as G3 squamous (Table 35.2).

VI. TREATMENT PLANNING

1. If staging reveals a T1 (intramucosal or submucosal) or T2 (intramuscular) esophageal cancer, without evidence of lymph node involvement (i.e., local disease), treatment is resection.
2. If a full-thickness T3 lesion (associated with an 85% chance of occult nodal disease) or if lymph node involvement is revealed, regardless of tumor thickness (i.e., regional disease), treatment is with neoadjuvant therapy followed by surgical resection.

TABLE 35.2

ANATOMIC STAGE/PROGNOSTIC GROUPS

Squamous Cell Carcinoma					
Stage	T	N	M	Grade	Tumor Location
Stage 0	Tis (HGD)	N0	M0	1,X	Any
Stage IA	T1	N0	M0	1,X	Any
Stage IB	T1	N0	M0	2–3	Any
	T2–3	N0	M0	1,X	Lower, X
Stage IIA	T2–3	N0	M0	1,X	Upper, middle
	T2–3	N0	M0	2–3	Lower, X
Stage IIB	T2–3	N0	M0	2–3	Upper, middle
	T1–2	N1	M0	Any	Any
Stage IIIA	T1–2	N2	M0	Any	Any
	T3	N1	M0	Any	Any
	T4a	N0	M0	Any	Any
Stage IIIB	T3	N2	M0	Any	Any
Stage IIIC	T4a	N1–2	M0	Any	Any
	T4b	Any	M0	Any	Any
	Any	N3	M0	Any	Any
Stage IV	Any	Any	M1	Any	Any

Adenocarcinoma				
Stage	T	N	M	Grade
Stage 0	Tis (HGD)	N0	M0	1,X
Stage IA	T1	N0	M0	1–2,X
Stage IB	T1	N0	M0	3
	T2	N0	M0	1–2,X
Stage IIA	T2	N0	M0	3,X
Stage IIB	T3	N0	M0	Any
	T1–2	N1	M0	Any
Stage IIIA	T1–2	N2	M0	Any
	T3	N1	M0	Any
	T4a	N0	M0	Any
Stage IIIB	T3	N2	M0	Any
Stage IIIC	T4a	N1–2	M0	Any
	T4b	Any	M0	Any
	Any	N3	M0	Any
Stage IV	Any	Any	M1	Any

HGD, High-grade dysplasia.

35

ESOPHAGEAL MALIGNANCY

A. IMPLICATIONS FOR THERAPY

Local	Regional	Systemic
→	→	
Surgery	Chemoradiation Therapy + Surgery	Chemoradiation therapy

VII. ESOPHAGECTOMY

1. General principles
   a. Esophagus is divided proximally at or above the level of the azygous vein, and cardia of the stomach is divided distally, providing a desired 5-cm margin from the gastroesophageal junction.
   b. Mediastinal and abdominal lymphadenectomy is also performed, en bloc with the esophagus.
   c. Stomach is fashioned into a tubular conduit and anastomosed to the proximal esophagus to serve as a neoesophagus.
      (1) Stomach is most common conduit used for reconstruction. Blood supply is based on the right gastroepiploic artery.
      (2) Alternative conduits are the jejunum or colon.
   d. Truncal vagotomy is inevitable so a drainage procedure (pyloroplasty, pyloromyotomy, or Botox injection) is necessary.
   e. Feeding jejunostomy tube is placed to provide postoperative nutrition.
   f. In experienced hands, esophagectomy can be performed safely and with good quality of life.

VIII. ESOPHAGECTOMY APPROACHES

1. Transhiatal esophagectomy
   a. This is most often used for tumors involving the lower or middle third of the esophagus, but it can be considered in all patients with esophageal cancer.
   b. It is performed via upper midline abdominal incision and left cervical incision
   c. Advantages
      (1) Thoracotomy is avoided.
      (2) Intrathoracic anastomosis is avoided.
         (a) If leak occurs, it is easily managed by neck drain or by opening and packing wound.
         (b) Leak (5%–10%) is more common, but mortality associated with it is much lower than when it occurs in the chest (3%–5%).
   d. Disadvantages
      (1) Blind mediastinal dissection: controversy regarding completeness of lymph node resection

(2) Risk for hemorrhage or injury to membranous trachea

(3) Risk for recurrent anastomotic stricture

(4) Risk for recurrent laryngeal nerve injury

2. Ivor Lewis esophagectomy

a. This is performed via laparotomy incision followed by right thoracotomy.

b. It is most often used for tumors in the lower third of the esophagus.

c. The gastric conduit does not need to be as long as it does for the transhiatal esophagectomy; hence more of the proximal stomach can be resected if needed for negative margins.

d. Advantages

(1) There is better lymph node dissection (two-field lymphadenectomy/abdomen and chest) as compared with transhiatal approach, given direct visualization and sharp dissection of the periesophageal tissues en bloc with the esophagus.

(2) Leak rate is low, but if it occurs, the mortality is much higher as compared with cervical/neck leak.

(a) Anastomotic disruption leads to mediastinitis and sepsis

(b) Mortality rates of 15%–20% if leak occurs

3. Three-hole or McKeown esophagectomy

a. Right thoracotomy is followed by laparotomy and cervical incision for anastomosis.

b. Similar to transhiatal esophagectomy, it has the advantage of a cervical anastomosis (easier to treat if leaks); however, it does not avoid the risks associated with thoracotomy.

c. Similar to Ivor Lewis esophagectomy, it allows for a better lymphadenectomy.

d. Leak rate is low, but there is higher mortality if it occurs.

4. Minimally invasive esophagectomy

a. Minimally invasive Ivor Lewis esophagogastrectomy (laparoscopy and thoracoscopy)

b. Minimally invasive McKeown esophagogastrectomy (thoracoscopy, laparoscopy, and cervical incision)

c. Advantages include decreased morbidity and shorter recovery times.

IX. ENDOSCOPIC THERAPIES

1. Endoscopic mucosal resection (EMR)

a. Used to treat early-stage esophageal and esophagogastric junction (EGJ) cancers

b. Can be used as diagnostic modality or therapeutic modality in lieu of esophagectomy

c. Ideal for therapeutic EMR:

(1) Lesions less than 2 cm

(2) Well to moderately differentiated lesions

(3) Intramucosal lesions (pT1a, pT1b)

(4) No evidence of lymph node involvement

35

ESOPHAGEAL MALIGNANCY

  d. If positive margins or deeper lesion found on EMR, esophagectomy needed
    (1) Deeper lesions—higher risk of microscopic lymph node involvement, which would not be addressed by EMR alone
  e. Risks: procedural complications (perforation, stricture, bleeding) and inadequate treatment (positive margins, untreated synchronous lesions, associated nodal disease)
  f. After EMR, any associated Barrett esophagus should be treated (options: radiofrequency ablation [RFA] or cryotherapy).

2. RFA
  a. Used to treat dysplastic Barrett (i.e., Barrett with HGD) or Barrett associated with a cancer that has been treated with EMR

3. Cryoablation therapy
  a. Freezes mucosa with quick thaw to cause cell death
  b. Used to treat dysplastic Barrett (i.e., Barrett's with HGD) or Barrett associated with a cancer that has been treated with EMR
  c. Can be used to palliate cancers or to treat cancers in patients who are not candidates for other therapies.

X. CHEMOTHERAPY AND RADIOTHERAPY

1. Chemotherapy
  a. Fifty percent of patients respond.
  b. A total of 2%–5% of patients will experience complete remission.
  c. In patients with advanced disease, palliative chemotherapy does not provide any survival advantage, but it may improve quality of life in patients with metastatic or unresectable disease.

2. Radiotherapy
  a. Useful alone for palliation of obstructive symptoms.
  b. Five-year survival rate for patients treated with radiotherapy (RT) alone is 0%–10%; therefore radiotherapy alone should generally be reserved for palliation or for patients who are medically unable to receive chemotherapy.

3. Combined chemoradiation therapy
  a. Preoperative chemoradiation followed by surgery is the most common approach for patients with resectable esophageal cancer.
    (1) Proposed benefits of preoperative radiotherapy include downstaging of tumors and improving resectability and treatment of microscopic tumor extending beyond the margins of resection (locoregional control).
    (2) Chemotherapy acts systemically to eradicate micrometastatic disease (systemic control).
  b. In patients with resectable disease, preoperative chemoradiation with carboplatin and paclitaxel significantly improved overall survival and disease-free survival when compared with surgery alone.

4. CROSS trial: Patients (*n* = 366) with regional esophageal cancer were randomized to either (a) chemoradiotherapy followed by surgery or (b) surgery alone. Median overall survival was found to be significantly improved in the neoadjuvant therapy arm (58% vs. 44%).

XI. PALLIATIVE CARE

A. DYSPHAGIA AND OBSTRUCTION

1. Radiotherapy
2. Esophageal dilation and stenting
   a. Dilation may be performed using bougies, wire-guided dilators, or balloon dilators.
   b. Stents are usually placed after dilation.
      (1) Self-expanding fully covered stents placed with EGD and fluoroscopic guidance
3. Local tumor ablation
   a. Cryotherapy
   b. Intralesional injection of necrotizing agents
   c. Neodymium-doped yttrium aluminium garnet (Nd:YAG) photoablative therapy
   d. Photodynamic therapy
4. Chemotherapy

B. ESOPHAGEAL-AIRWAY FISTULA

1. This may be precipitated by radiotherapy.
2. Esophageal bypass is not well tolerated by most patients.
3. Most patients are treated with esophageal stents.

RECOMMENDED READINGS

Berry MF. Esophageal cancer: staging system and guidelines for staging and treatment, *J Thoracic Dis* 2014;6(suppl 3):S289–S297.

Cameron JL, Cameron AM. *Current Surgical Therapy.* 11th ed. Philadelphia: Elsevier Saunders; 2014.

National Comprehensive Cancer Network Guidelines for Esophageal and Esophagogastric Junction Cancers. Available at. https://www.nccn.org/professionals/physician_gls/pdf/esophageal.pdf.

35

ESOPHAGEAL MALIGNANCY

Gastric Malignancy

Gregory C. Wilson, MD

And in any case the disease generally marches to its termination with a continual increase of speed and severity, rarely receiving more than a temporary check, and ending in death about one year after it first declares itself.

—William Brinton in 1859 in Lectures on the Diseases of the Stomach. Linitis plastic is also referred to as Brinton disease, named after the English physician William Brinton.

I. ADENOCARCINOMA OF THE STOMACH

A. EPIDEMIOLOGY

1. Comprises 95% of all gastric tumors
2. Fourth most common gastrointestinal (GI) malignancy worldwide
3. Second cause of cancer mortality worldwide (behind lung cancer)
4. Approximately 25,000 cases reported in United States in 2015
5. Seventy percent of patients older than 50 (peak in seventh decade of life)
6. Male to female ratio: 2:1
7. Greatest incidence in Japan (80 times greater than in the United States)
8. Sixty-five percent of gastric cancers in the United States present at an advanced stage (T3/T4).

B. RISK FACTORS

1. Environmental factors
   a. Diet (rich in salt, smoked or poorly preserved foods, nitrates, nitrosamines)
   b. Smoking
   c. Low socioeconomic status
   d. Occupational hazards (metal, rubber, wood, asbestos)
2. Genetic factors
   a. A total of 10% of gastric cancers have an inherited/familial component (90% sporadic).
   b. Hereditary diffuse gastric cancer
      (1) Autosomal dominant, 70% penetrance
      (2) Germline mutation of *CDH-1* gene that encodes E-cadherin
   c. Additional syndromes associated with gastric adenocarcinoma: *BRCA1, BRCA2,* hereditary nonpolyposis colon cancer syndrome (HNPCC), familial adenomatous polyposis (FAP), Peutz-Jeghers syndrome, Li-Fraumeni syndrome
   d. Blood type A (relative risk, 1.2)
   e. Ethnicity—increased incidence in Asians, Native Americans, Latinos, and African Americans versus whites

3. Infectious factors
   a. *Helicobacter pylori*
      (1) Risk increased 6–8 times
      (2) Common in patients with distal cancer, not proximal cancer
   b. Epstein-Barr virus
4. **Other risk factors**
   a. Chronic atrophic gastritis (conditions associated with decreased acid production)
      (1) Hypertrophic gastropathy (Menetrier disease)—hypertrophic disease of the gastric epithelium
      (2) Pernicious anemia (3 times increased risk for development of gastric cancer)
   b. Gastric polyps
      (1) Adenomas are associated with intestinal metaplasia.
      (2) Risk of malignancy is directly increased with increased size and degree of dysplasia.
   c. Reflux gastritis after subtotal gastrectomy
      (1) Incidence of 1%–2%
      (2) Average latency of 12–30 years
      (3) Risk with Billroth II >> Billroth I reconstruction

C. PATHOLOGIC CLASSIFICATIONS
1. **Lauren classification—two subtypes: intestinal and diffuse types**
   a. Intestinal type
      (1) Most common type worldwide
      (2) More prevalent in high-risk populations (Asian and South American)
      (3) Higher association with: high salt diets, tobacco/alcohol use, chronic gastritis from *H. pylori* infection
      (4) Follow classic progression: chronic gastritis → intestinal metaplasia → dysplasia → invasive adenocarcinoma
      (5) Spread hematogenously
      (6) Distal stomach
      (7) Older patients
      (8) Based on World Health Organization (WHO) classification, these tumors can be further classified as tubular, papillary, and mucinous.
   b. Diffuse type
      (1) Arises from lamina propria, lacks organized gland formation
      (2) Loss of expression of protein epithelial cadherin *(E-cadherin)*
      (3) Common in younger patients, women, and populations with low incidence of gastric cancer (i.e., United States)
      (4) Aggressive and infiltrative growth pattern; spreads transmurally in the submucosa, classic *linitis plastica*
      (5) Lymphatic invasion and peritoneal metastasis more common
      (6) Signet ring cells are pathognomonic.

(7) Proximal stomach

(8) Not typically associated with *H. pylori*

D. CLINICAL MANIFESTATIONS

1. It often produces no specific symptoms when it is superficial and potentially curable.
2. Up to 50% of patients may have nonspecific GI complaints, such as dyspepsia.
3. Other symptoms include abdominal pain, nausea, vomiting, early satiety with bulky tumors, dysphagia, hematemesis, and melena.
   a. Patients with these symptoms are often in the late or advanced stage of disease and are incurable.
   b. Proximal tumors → dysphagia and achalasia-like symptoms
   c. Distal tumors → gastritis-like symptoms and dyspepsia
   d. Additional symptoms are related to local invasion: GI bleed, gastric perforation, colonic invasion/fistula
4. Physical examination
   a. This is unhelpful in early gastric cancer.
   b. Palpable abdominal mass, cachexia, bowel obstruction, ascites, hepatomegaly, and lower extremity edema are signs of advanced disease.
   c. Classic findings:
      (1) Blumer shelf: palpable mass on rectal examination due to peritoneal seeding of pouch of Douglas
      (2) Sister Mary Joseph nodule: peritoneal disease causing a bulging periumbilical mass
      (3) Krukenberg tumor: palpable ovarian mass on pelvic examination—drop metastasis from stomach
      (4) Virchow node: lymphatic involvement with supraclavicular lymphadenopathy
      (5) Irish node: lymphatic involvement with left axillary lymphadenopathy

E. SCREENING

1. It is cost effective only in endemic areas, such as Japan and Taiwan.
2. In the United States, endoscopic surveillance is recommended in high-risk individuals only (history of gastric polyp, FAP, HNPCC, Peutz-Jeghers syndrome).

F. DIAGNOSIS/STAGING

1. Endoscopy is the modality of choice for diagnosis.
   a. All gastric ulcers seen on endoscopy should undergo biopsy and be followed to ensure they resolve.
   b. Minimum of four biopsies is sufficient. Biopsies should be taken from the mucosa at the edge of the ulcer.
   c. Repeat biopsy may be necessary if ulcer remains despite medical therapy.
   d. Less than 3% of gastric ulcers are malignant.

2. Endoscopic ultrasound is the most useful tool for preoperative tumor and nodal staging.
   a. Evaluate depth of tumor invasion.
   b. Perform fine-needle aspiration (FNA) sampling of suspicious nodes to determine lymph node status.
3. Computed tomography (CT) scan demonstrates primary tumor extent (invasion into surrounding structures) and metastatic disease.
   a. Obtain with intravenous (IV) contrast and low-density oral contrast (water).
   b. Specific findings include peritoneal disease, liver and lung lesions, and ascites.
4. Diagnostic laparoscopy
   a. Perform in all patients with T3/4 disease and no nodal or distant disease.
   b. Examine peritoneal surface, liver, and omentum.
   c. Cytologic analysis of peritoneal washings can aid in staging.
   d. A total of 10%–15% of patients are upstaged at time of diagnostic laparoscopy.

G. **AMERICAN JOINT COMMITTEE ON CANCER TNM CLASSIFICATION**
1. T = Primary tumor
   a. **Tis**—carcinoma in situ—no invasion of lamina propria
   b. **T1a**—Tumor invades lamina propria or muscularis mucosa.
   c. **T1b**—Tumor invades submucosa.
   d. **T2**—Tumor invades muscularis propria or subserosa.
   e. **T3**—penetrates serosa
   f. **T4**—Tumor invades adjacent structures.
2. N = Regional lymph nodes involved
   a. **N0**—No regional lymph nodes involved.
   b. **N1**—metastasis in 1–2 regional lymph nodes
   c. **N2**—metastasis in 3–6 regional lymph nodes
   d. **N3a**—metastasis in 7–15 regional lymph nodes
   e. **N3b**—more than 16 regional nodes involved
3. M = Distant metastasis
   a. **M0**—no distant metastasis
   b. **M1**—distant metastasis

H. **CLASSIFICATION OF SURGICAL RESECTIONS WITH RESPECT TO FINAL PATHOLOGY**
1. R0—no residual tumor
2. R1—microscopic residual disease only
3. R2—gross residual disease

I. **SURGICAL TREATMENT**
1. Curative resection—macroscopic margin of 5–6 cm is recommended together with lymphadenectomy.

36

GASTRIC MALIGNANCY

a. Tumors in the proximal third of the stomach
   (1) Total gastrectomy with reconstruction is preferred.
   (2) Proximal subtotal gastrectomy is an alternative but not widely accepted.
   (3) Perform esophagogastrectomy for tumors of the gastroesophageal junction.
b. Tumors in the middle to distal third of the stomach
   (1) Distal subtotal gastrectomy is associated with improved quality of life over total gastrectomy and identical survival outcomes.
   (2) A 5-cm margin in the proximal stomach is needed (margin status can be confirmed with frozen biopsy).
c. Reconstruction
   (1) Billroth I: need enough stomach for tension free anastomosis (preferred reconstruction if technically feasible)
   (2) Billroth II: single anastomosis, associated with increased bile reflux, Barrett esophagus, marginal ulcers, and duodenal stump leaks
   (3) Roux-en-Y: preferred method for reconstruction when Billroth I cannot be performed
d. En bloc resection of spleen, liver, transverse colon, and/or pancreas may be required for locally advanced tumors.

2. **Lymphadenectomy**
   a. Minimum of 15 lymph nodes required for adequate staging
   b. Benefit: better staging, improved locoregional control, questionable survival benefit
   c. Nomenclature for extent of resection/lymphadenectomy
      (1) D1—omental and perigastric lymph nodes
      (2) Extended D1—omental and perigastric lymph nodes plus lymph nodes along the left gastric artery, common hepatic artery, and celiac axis
      (3) D2—extended D1 plus distal pancreatectomy and splenectomy to harvest peripancreatic and perisplenic nodes
   d. Extent of lymphadenectomy is controversial.
      (1) Japanese advocate for D2 dissection with improved survival and low mortality rate.
      (2) United States/Europe: Extended D1 dissection remains standard care. D2 lymphadenectomies are typically avoided because the potential survival benefit has not been well established and the distal pancreatectomy/splenectomy results in increased patient morbidity.

3. **Palliative surgery—for obstruction or bleeding in patients deemed unresectable for cure**
   a. Resection
      (1) Subtotal gastrectomy can improve quality of life in patients with excellent preoperative performance status.
      (2) Total gastrectomy or esophagogastrectomy is less likely to improve quality of life given the high associated morbidity and poor prognosis in these patients.

b. GI bypass—for patients who can tolerate a laparotomy and are not candidates for gastric resection

4. Endoscopic mucosal resection for early gastric cancer—limited to experienced centers
   a. Incidence of lymph node metastasis in early gastric cancer is less than 10%.
   b. Close endoscopic follow-up is necessary.
   c. If submucosal invasion is seen on permanent sectioning, gastrectomy with lymphadenectomy is required.
   d. Indications are nonulcerated tumors, ulcerated tumors less than 3 cm, any tumor smaller than 3 cm, and less than 0.5-mm invasion into submucosa.
   e. Contraindications: diffuse tumor, deep submucosal invasion (>0.5 mm)

J. NEOADJUVANT/ADJUVANT THERAPY

1. Perioperative chemotherapy (Medical Research Council Adjuvant Gastric Infusional Chemotherapy [MAGIC] trial)
   a. Three cycles of preoperative chemotherapy
   b. Surgery followed by three additional cycles of chemotherapy
   c. MAGIC regimen = epirubicin, cisplatin, and infused fluorouracil
   d. Five-year survival rate of 36% versus 23% (surgery alone)

2. Adjuvant chemoradiation therapy (Intergroup trial INTO116)
   a. Postoperative 5-fluorouracil and leucovorin and 45-Gy radiation
   b. Overall 5-year survival 43% versus 28% in surgery alone

3. Adjuvant chemotherapy (Capecitabine and Oxaliplatin Adjuvant Study in Stomach Cancer [CLASSIC] study)
   a. Six months of postoperative chemotherapy (capecitabine and oxaliplatin)
   b. Improved 5-year survival and recurrence rates over surgery alone

K. PROGNOSIS (5-YEAR SURVIVAL)

1. Overall 5-year survival rate varies based on geographic location: 90% in Japan to 30% in United States
2. Patients after R0 resection: 35%–60%
3. Patients with T1 cancer: 90%
4. Patients with T3 or greater tumors: less than 50%
5. Patients with nodal involvement: less than 30%

II. GASTRIC LYMPHOMA

A. GENERAL CONSIDERATIONS

1. Second most common malignancy of the stomach after adenocarcinoma
2. Two percent of all non-Hodgkin lymphoma, most common extranodal lymphoma
3. Strongly associated with *H. pylori*

36

GASTRIC MALIGNANCY

4. Average age at presentation: 60 years
5. Five-year survival rate of 80% for stage I and II tumors

B. CLINICAL PRESENTATION
1. It is distinguishable from gastric adenocarcinoma at presentation.
2. A total of 42% present as emergencies (bleeding, perforation, obstruction).

C. PATHOLOGY
1. B-cell non-Hodgkin lymphoma is most common, with histiocytic subtype

D. DIAGNOSIS
1. Endoscopy with biopsy and brush cytology—80% accuracy
2. Staging—chest radiograph, chest and abdominal CT, bone marrow biopsy, biopsy of enlarged lymph nodes, routine laboratory tests, lactate dehydrogenase

E. TREATMENT
1. Chemotherapy regimen (doxorubicin and cyclophosphamide) produces complete response in 80% of all gastric lymphomas.
2. Use radiation therapy and surgery if there is an incomplete response to chemotherapy or recurrence.
3. Perform bone marrow transplant for aggressive disease.
4. Mucosal-associated lymphoid tissue (MALT) lymphoma can often be eradicated by *H. pylori* treatment alone.
   a. If this treatment fails, radiation or chemotherapy is usually sufficient to eradicate the tumor.

III. GASTROINTESTINAL STROMAL TUMORS

A. GENERAL CONSIDERATIONS
1. Comprise less than 1% of all GI malignancies
2. Previously described as leiomyoma, leiomyoblastoma, and epithelioid leiomyosarcoma
3. Stomach: most common site of gastrointestinal stromal tumors (GISTs)—52% of cases

B. OTHER CHARACTERISTICS
1. A total of 95% of GISTs express CD117 (c-kit).
2. They appear to arise from the interstitial cell of Cajal that variably expresses CD117 (94%) and histologic features of smooth muscle and neural tissue.
3. Mutation of c-kit proto-oncogene results in ligand-independent activation of the Kit receptor tyrosine kinase and unopposed cell cycle.
4. Tumor develops submucosally.
5. It presents as bulky mass with central necrosis.

C. DIAGNOSIS
1. Upper GI—smooth-lined filling defect with sharp borders
2. Endoscopy—endophytic lesion on gastric wall. Overlying mucosa usually intact; ulceration/bleeding can occur
3. Endoscopic ultrasound—hypoechoic mass contiguous with muscularis propria

D. PATHOLOGIC LESIONS
1. They are heterogeneous, ranging from well-differentiated tumors (myoid, neural, or ganglionic) to incomplete or mixed differentiation.
2. Hematogenous spread is common; liver is frequently involved.

E. TREATMENT
1. R0 resection is treatment of choice.
2. Indications for adjuvant imatinib (Gleevec) therapy include ruptured GIST, tumor size greater than 10 cm, mitotic rate greater than 10/50 high-power field (HPF), tumor size greater than 5 cm, and greater than 5 mitoses/HPF.
3. Patients with unresectable or metastatic disease are given imatinib mesylate (Gleevec), an oral tyrosine kinase inhibitor that targets c-kit, and then reevaluated for potential resection if they respond to this treatment.
4. Neoadjuvant therapy should be considered in patients with tumors with extensive organ involvement, duodenal GIST, rectal GIST, or gastroesophageal junction GIST.
5. Patients who do not respond to Gleevec can be given sunitinib (Sutent).

36

GASTRIC MALIGNANCY

RECOMMENDED READINGS
Bang YJ, et al. Adjuvant capecitabine and oxaliplatin for gastric cancer after D2 gastrectomy (CLASSIC): a phase 3 open-label, randomised controlled trial. *Lancet*. 2012;379:315–321.

Cunningham D, et al. Perioperative chemotherapy versus surgery alone for resectable gastroesophageal cancer. *N Engl J Med*. 2006;355:11–20.

Small Bowel Malignancy

Brent T. Xia, MD

I. EPIDEMIOLOGY

A. INCIDENCE

1. Although the small intestine comprises 90% of the surface area of the gastrointestinal (GI) tract, less than 3% of primary GI neoplasms occur in this region. Theories for this discrepancy include:
   a. The dilute and liquid contents of the small bowel cause less mucosal irritation.
   b. The rapid transit of intestinal contents provides for shorter exposure to carcinogens.
   c. The lower bacterial load results in less conversion of bile acids into carcinogens by anaerobic organisms.
   d. Carcinogens in food, such as benzpyrene, is degraded to less toxic metabolites by enzyme benzpyrene hydroxylase, which is abundant in the small bowel.
   e. Increased concentration of lymphoid tissue and production of immunoglobulin A (IgA) may have a protective effect.
2. The majority of tumors are discovered incidentally. Improvements in endoscopy and radiologic techniques have led to an increase in detection rates. Symptoms are often from obstruction, bleeding, intussusception, or metastatic disease.
3. Incidence increases with:
   a. Male sex
   b. Middle age or older
   c. Consumption of red meat
   d. Ingestion of smoked or cured foods
   e. Prior diagnosis of colon adenocarcinoma
4. The incidence/detection of carcinoid tumors has increased fourfold in the past 3 decades and is largely responsible for the overall increased incidence of small bowel malignancies.

B. TUMOR CHARACTERISTICS

Carcinoid tumors (44%) are the most common small bowel cancers, followed closely by adenocarcinomas (33%). Lymphomas and sarcomas comprise 8% and 17% of small bowel cancers, respectively (Table 37.1).

1. Carcinoid tumors
   a. Most common location is the ileum
   b. They are well-differentiated tumors.
   c. They appear as firm intramucosal or submucosal nodules.
   d. Approximately half of carcinoids greater than 2 cm metastasize to the liver.

TABLE 37.1

SMALL BOWEL NEOPLASM CHARACTERISTICS

Tumor Type	Incidence (%)	Most Common Site	Genetic Risk Factors
Carcinoid/ neuroendocrine	44	Ileum	MEN1
Adenocarcinoma	33	Duodenum	FAP PJS JPS Cowden syndrome Lynch syndrome/ HNPCC
Sarcoma	17	Evenly distributed throughout small intestine	Familial GIST syndrome
Lymphoma	8	Ileum	Autoimmune disorders with chronic immunodeficiency states

CD, Crohn's disease; *FAP*, familial adenomatous polyposis; *GIST*, gastrointestinal stromal tumor; *HNPCC*, hereditary nonpolyposis colorectal cancer; *JPS*, juvenile polyposis syndrome; *MEN1*, multiple endocrine neoplasia type 1; *PJS*, Peutz-Jeghers syndrome.

2. Adenocarcinoma
   a. Most common location is the duodenum
   b. Risk is elevated in patients with a history of colorectal cancer (see Section I.C).
3. Primary small bowel lymphoma
   a. Immunoproliferative small intestinal disease (IPSID) (a variant of mucosa-associated lymphoid tissue [MALT])
   b. Enteropathy-associated T-cell lymphoma (EATL), associated with gluten-sensitive enteropathy
4. Sarcoma
   a. Evenly distributed throughout the small bowel
   b. Most common type: gastrointestinal stromal tumor (GIST)
      (1) Derived from interstitial cell of Cajal
      (2) Positive c-kit (receptor tyrosine kinase) expression, a protooncogene leading to uninhibited cell growth
      (3) Small intestine: second most common site of this tumor
5. Metastatic lesions
   a. Tumors that tend to spread to the peritoneal cavity are ovarian, colon, and gastric cancers.
   b. Small intestine is the most common site of GI metastases in advanced-stage melanoma.

C. GENETIC PREDISPOSITION AND PATHOGENESIS
1. Sporadic tumors
   a. Majority of adenocarcinomas arise from adenomas.
   b. Carcinogenesis pathway is similar to that of colon cancer, with high incidence of tumor-suppressor genes p53 and KRAS mutations.

2. High-risk inherited syndromes for small bowel adenocarcinoma (see Table 37.1)
   a. Familial adenomatous polyposis (FAP)
      (1) Autosomal dominant mutation of adenomatous polyposis coli (APC) tumor suppressor gene
      (2) A total of 50%–90% chance of developing duodenal adenomas, with 1 in 20 progressing to malignancy
      (3) Elevated risk of developing desmoid tumors in the small bowel or its mesentery
   b. Peutz-Jeghers syndrome (PJS)
      (1) Autosomal dominant mutation of *STK11* tumor suppressor gene
      (2) Manifests with the development of hamartomas throughout the GI tract, which also increase the risk of intussusception
      (3) Elevated risk of small and large bowel adenocarcinomas
      (4) Similar manifestations in juvenile polyposis syndrome (JPS) and Cowden syndrome
   c. Hereditary nonpolyposis colorectal cancer (HNPCC)/Lynch syndrome
      (1) Mutation in DNA mismatch repair genes
      (2) Four percent lifetime risk of small bowel adenocarcinoma
      (3) Responsible for 5%–10% of small bowel adenocarcinomas
      (4) Increased risk of colorectal cancer and endometrial cancer
   d. Multiple endocrine neoplasia type I (MEN1): neuroendocrine tumors of duodenum.
3. **Diseases causing chronic inflammation of the small bowel**
   a. Crohn's disease (CD)
      (1) CD patients have a higher risk (20–30-fold) of small bowel adenocarcinoma than do patients without CD.
      (2) Risk increases with duration of disease and extent of small bowel involvement.
      (3) It commonly presents as a small bowel stricture.
   b. Celiac disease
      (1) Eight percent prevalence of small intestinal adenocarcinoma, with a relative risk of 10 compared with general population.
4. Immunodeficiency/suppression: increased risk of small bowel lymphoma—for example, in congenital and acquired immunodeficiency states, such as with use of chronic immunosuppressive drugs and celiac disease

II. DIAGNOSIS

1. Clinical presentation
   a. Patients may be asymptomatic or present with nonspecific symptoms, most commonly abdominal pain, followed by nausea/vomiting.
      (1) Given vague symptoms, the majority of patients are diagnosed with advanced stage III–IV disease.
   b. Carcinoid syndrome includes symptoms that occur with serotonin and other active compounds secreted by carcinoid tumors, typically in the setting of hepatic metastases.

   (1) Skin flushing
   (2) Wheezing
   (3) Diarrhea
   (4) Palpitations, tricuspid insufficiency
   (5) Peripheral edema

2. Imaging modalities
  a. Computed tomography (CT) scan
    (1) Eighty percent sensitivity, increases with use of enterography
    (2) Allows for evaluation of distant spread and regional lymph node involvement
  b. Positron emission tomography (PET) scan
    (1) It is useful for workup of adenocarcinomas and sarcomas.
    (2) No study has demonstrated superiority to CT scan with intravenous contrast.
    (3) It is not accurate for carcinoid tumors, which tend to have low uptake of radiotracer ^{18}F-deoxyglucose.
  c. Somatostatin receptor scintigraphy: 88% sensitivity and 97% specificity for detecting small bowel carcinoid tumors

3. Procedural modalities
  a. Endoscopy
    (1) This allows tissue biopsy.
    (2) Best for lesions of the duodenum—Push techniques allow visualization further down jejunum or into ileum from colonoscopy.
    (3) Diagnostic efficacy decreases for lesions past the proximal jejunum.
  b. Capsule endoscopy
    (1) Less invasive than push endoscopy
    (2) A total of 87% yield for detecting lesions
    (3) Superior to push endoscopy for lesions past the proximal jejunum and in instances of obscure GI bleeds
  c. Double-balloon endoscopy
    (1) "Push-pull" or "double-bubble" enteroscopy
    (2) Alternatively inflating and deflating two balloons, thus pleating the small intestine over the endoscope. Allows for access beyond that of conventional push endoscopy
    (3) Complementary to capsule endoscopy, allows for tissue sampling

4. Laboratory tests
  a. Serum carcinoembryonic antigen (CEA)
    (1) Often elevated in small bowel adenocarcinomas; however, lacks sensitivity/specificity
  b. Urine 5-hydroxyindoleacetic acid (5-HIAA)
    (1) A breakdown product of serotonin, secreted by carcinoid/neuroendocrine tumors
    (2) Variable sensitivity but highly specific if elevated for neuroendocrine tumors

c. Serum chromogranin-A (Cg-A)
(1) A glycoprotein that is secreted by neuroendocrine cells.
(2) It may also be elevated in patients with liver disease, renal insufficiency, or inflammatory bowel disease.
(3) Falsely elevated levels are also seen in patients who take proton pump inhibitors.

III. STAGING

A. ADENOCARCINOMA
Tumor Node Metastasis (TNM) system of the American Joint Committee on Cancer (AJCC)/ International Union Against Cancer (UICC)

B. LYMPHOMA
Lugano Classification (adapted from Ann Arbor staging system for Hodgkin lymphoma)

C. SARCOMA AND CARCINOID TUMORS
Adapted from the TNM system of the AJCC/UICC

IV. MANAGEMENT

A. SURGERY
1. Localized tumors: wide segmental resection with mesentery (for regional lymph nodes)
2. Tumors of D1 and D2: pancreaticoduodenectomy
3. Tumors of D3 and D4: no survival benefit observed in retrospective studies between segmental resection versus pancreaticoduodenectomy, as long as R0 resection can be obtained
   a. Exception: Patients with FAP should undergo a pancreaticoduodenectomy given predilection for multiple and sessile polyps in the periampullary region.
4. Tumors of the distal ileum: resection of distal ileum and right colectomy with shared mesenteric draining lymph nodes

B. CHEMOTHERAPY
1. Adjuvant therapy indications
   a. Lymph node positive
      (1) Extrapolated from data on node-positive colon cancer (MOSAIC trial: FOLFOX—fluorouracil, oxaliplatin, leucovorin).
   b. Small bowel GISTs
      (1) Oral tyrosine kinase inhibitors (TKIs) such as imatinib significantly improved disease recurrence rates.
      (2) Adjuvant imatinib is indicated for resected GIST ≥3 cm or other high-risk features such as rupture or elevated mitotic rate.
2. Chemotherapy for advanced disease
   a. Adenocarcinomas: based on guidelines established for metastatic colorectal cancer

b. GISTS: Majority of patients with metastatic burden treated with oral TKIs demonstrated response or disease stability.

c. Neuroendocrine tumors: See Chapter 52.

d. Lymphoma: dependent on histologic subtype

RECOMMENDED READINGS

Aparicio T, Zaanan A, Svrcek M, et al. Small bowel adenocarcinoma: epidemiology, risk factors, diagnosis and treatment. *Dig Liver Dis*. 2014;46:97–104.

Bilimoria KY, Bentrem DJ, Wayne JD, et al. Small bowel cancer in the United States: changes in epidemiology, treatment, and survival over the last 20 years. *Ann Surg*. 2009;249:63–71.

Cusack JC, Overman MJ. Epidemiology, clinical features, and types of small bowel neoplasms. In: Post TW, ed. UpToDate. Waltham, MA: Wolters Kluwer. Available at http://www.uptodate.com/contents/epidemiology-clinical-features-and-types-of-small-bowel-neoplasms. Accessed July 11, 2016.

Ecker BL, McMillan MT, Datta J, et al. Efficacy of adjuvant chemotherapy for small bowel adenocarcinoma: a propensity score-matched analysis. *Cancer*. 2016;122:693–701.

37

SMALL BOWEL MALIGNANCY

Malignant Colorectal and Perianal Disease

Joshua Kuethe, MD

Colon cancer screening is probably one of the most underused ways that exist to save a person's life from cancer.

—Michael Thun, MD

I. COLORECTAL CANCER: EPIDEMIOLOGY

A. **EACH YEAR IN THE UNITED STATES, 135,000 CASES OF COLORECTAL CANCER WILL BE DIAGNOSED.**

1. Colon cancer: 95,000
2. Rectal cancer: 40,000

B. **ALMOST 50,000 PEOPLE DIE OF COLORECTAL CANCER ANNUALLY IN THE UNITED STATES.**

1. Mortality is steadily decreasing since 1990.
2. Still the third most common cause of cancer death in the United States

II. RISK FACTORS

1. Personal history of colorectal cancer or polyps
2. Age—increase in incidence after age 50
3. Family history—up to 20% of patients have family history of colorectal cancers; genetic syndromes account for less than 5% of colorectal cancers.
   a. Hereditary nonpolyposis syndromes (e.g., hereditary nonpolyposis colorectal cancer [HNPCC])
   b. Hereditary polyposis syndromes (e.g., familial adenomatous polyposis [FAP], *MYH*)
4. Environmental and dietary factors
   a. Low-fiber, high-fat diet increases risk for colorectal cancer.
   b. High-fiber, calcium, selenium, vitamins A, C, and E, carotenoids, and plant phenols appear to be protective.
   c. Cigarette smoking is associated with increased risk, especially more than 35 years of smoking.
5. Inflammatory bowel disease—after 10 years, the risk for cancer in left-sided colitis or pancolitis is 1%–2% per year. The risk appears to be similar between ulcerative colitis and Crohn proctocolitis.

III. SIGNS AND SYMPTOMS

1. The majority of patients are asymptomatic at presentation.
2. Colon cancer signs and symptoms

a. Anemia—microcytic; chronic, intermittent occult blood loss in the stool
b. Systemic complaints—anorexia, fatigue, weight loss, or dull, persistent abdominal pain; abdominal mass with more advanced tumors
c. Change in bowel habits—obstipation, alternating constipation and diarrhea, small-caliber "pencil" stools
d. Obstructive symptoms—less common but more prominent on the left because of growth pattern of tumor, small caliber of bowel, and solid stool

3. Rectal cancer
   a. Blood streaking in stools, tenesmus
   b. This finding must not be attributed to hemorrhoids without further investigation.
   c. Obstruction is less common but is a poor prognostic sign when present.

IV. SCREENING GUIDELINES FOR COLORECTAL CANCER

A. AVERAGE-RISK PATIENT, STARTING AT AGE 50–75 YEARS—ANY OF THE FOLLOWING SCREENING MODALITIES ARE ACCEPTED:

1. Colonoscopy every 10 years (preferred method)
2. Annual fecal occult blood test and flexible sigmoidoscopy every 5 years
3. Air contrast barium enema every 5 years
4. Yearly fecal occult blood test
5. Computed tomography (CT) colonography or fecal DNA—promising screening tools for colorectal cancer, but there are insufficient data to conclude screening interval or follow-up at present

B. INFLAMMATORY BOWEL DISEASE—INITIAL COLONOSCOPY AT DIAGNOSIS

1. Colonoscopy 8 years after diagnosis for pancolitis
2. Colonoscopy 12–15 years after diagnosis of left-sided colitis
3. Colonoscopy every 1–2 years after that

C. FAMILIAL ADENOMATOUS POLYPOSIS

1. Colonoscopy yearly starting at 10–12 years of age
2. Yearly flexible sigmoidoscopy to look for evidence of the polyposis

D. HEREDITARY NONPOLYPOSIS COLORECTAL CANCER

1. Colonoscopy at 20–25 years of age
2. Repeat colonoscopy every 1–2 years after initial

E. FAMILY HISTORY

1. Screening colonoscopy at 40 years of age or 10 years before the age of youngest affected relative
2. Repeat colonoscopy every 5 years after initial

V. POLYPS

1. Characterized by histology, presence of dysplasia or cancer, and anatomy (polypoid or sessile)
2. Broadly classified as follows:
   a. Nonadenomatous: Hyperplastic and hamartomatous polyps have no malignant potential.
   b. Adenomatous: Adenomas, tubular adenomas, tubulovillous, and villous adenomas are mostly premalignant, although 1%–2% of all polyps will harbor an invasive cancer.
3. Predictors of invasive carcinoma within a polyp
   a. Size
      (1) 1–2 cm—2%–9%
      (2) Larger than 2 cm—20%–50%
   b. Villous or tubulovillous histology
   c. Left-sided location
   d. Age greater than 60 years
4. Haggitt classification of malignant nonsessile polyps:
   a. Level 0—carcinoma in situ
   b. Level 1—invasion into submucosa but limited to the head of the polyp
   c. Level 2—invasion into the neck of the polyp
   d. Level 3—carcinoma invading stalk
   e. Level 4—invasion into submucosa below the stalk, or sessile polyps
5. Management of polyps
   a. Polypectomy using endoscopic forceps or a snare is appropriate for all polyps found during colonoscopy.
   b. For adenomatous polyps not amenable to endoscopic treatment (usually because of size or sessile anatomy), biopsies should be obtained and a formal colectomy should be performed if the patient is medically fit for surgery.
6. Management of malignant polyps removed endoscopically
   a. Haggitt levels 1, 2, and 3 have less than 1% chance of nodal metastases, and no further therapy is required, except in cases of lymphovascular invasion, poor differentiation, or cancer being present less than 2 mm to resection margin.
   b. Haggitt level 4 has 12%–25% risk for nodal metastases and requires colectomy.
   c. Most sessile polyps harboring a malignancy are managed with colectomy.

VI. PATHOGENESIS

A. LOSS OF HETEROZYGOSITY PATHWAY—80% OF CASES

1. *APC* (adenomatous polyposis coli) tumor suppressor gene: first studied in familial adenomatous polyposis. Inactivation/mutation is present in 80% of sporadic colorectal cancers.

2. *K-ras*—proto-oncogene; mutation leads to uncontrolled cell division
3. *DCC* (deleted in colorectal carcinoma)—tumor suppressor gene. This mutation is present in more than 70% of colorectal cancers.
4. *p53*—gene crucial for initiation of apoptosis. Mutations are present in 75% of colorectal cancers.

B. REPLICATION ERROR REPAIR PATHWAY—20% OF CASES
1. Mismatch repair genes include *hMSH2, hMLH1, hPMS1, hPMS2, hMSH6/GTPB.*
2. Mutations result in microsatellite instability—variable lengths of short-base-pair segments repeated several times
3. Tumors of replication error repair pathway tend to be right-sided and have overall better prognosis.

C. ADENOMATOUS POLYPOSIS SYNDROMES
1. Familial polyposis—adenomatous polyposis of the colon with a 100% risk for malignancy; may also occur in the stomach and duodenum, including increased risk for ampullary adenocarcinoma; autosomal dominant inheritance. Associated with *APC* mutation
2. *MYH*-associated polyposis—similar to an attenuated FAP; fewer polyps; 43%–100% risk of malignancy; increased risk of upper gastrointestinal (GI) polyps; autosomal recessive inheritance. Associated with *MYH* gene mutation on chromosome 1
3. Gardner syndrome—subtype of FAP, colorectal polyposis associated with extracolonic soft tissue tumors, and osteomas; also has a 100% incidence rate of malignant degeneration
4. Turcot syndrome—polyposis of the colon associated with central nervous system tumors; autosomal recessive inheritance
5. Cronkhite-Canada syndrome—GI polyposis with alopecia, nail dystrophy, hyperpigmentation; minimal malignant potential; no inheritance pattern

D. NONADENOMATOUS POLYPOSIS SYNDROMES
1. Peutz-Jeghers syndrome—hamartomatous polyps of the entire GI tract with mucocutaneous deposition of melanin in lips, oral cavity, and digits; hamartomas do not have malignant potential, but increased rate of GI tract cancers are a common comorbidity; autosomal dominant inheritance
2. Juvenile polyposis syndrome—hamartomatous polyps found in the colon and rectum but can be diffuse; hamartomas do not have malignant potential but increase risk for colorectal cancer; autosomal dominant inheritance

E. NONPOLYPOSIS SYNDROMES
1. Hereditary nonpolyposis syndrome (Lynch syndromes)—replication error repair pathway and the most common inheritable colorectal cancer syndrome account for 2%–7% of all colorectal cancers.

a. Lynch syndrome—colorectal cancer, endometrial and ovarian cancer, transitional cell cancer of the ureter and renal pelvis, gastric cancer, pancreatic cancer
b. Amsterdam II criteria—assists in the identification of patients who may have Lynch syndrome
   (1) Three or more relatives with an associated cancer (colorectal cancer, or cancer of the endometrium, small intestine, ureter, or renal pelvis)
   (2) Two or more successive generations affected
   (3) One or more relatives diagnosed before the age of 50 years
   (4) One should be a first-degree relative of the other two.

VII. PREOPERATIVE EVALUATION

A. COMPLETE HISTORY
With emphasis on personal and family history of malignancies or polyps

B. COLONOSCOPY
With complete visualization of entire colon to cecum
1. Synchronous cancers are present in 2%–5% of patients.
2. If unable to perform complete colonoscopy before surgery because of obstruction, a complete colonoscopy should be performed 3–6 months after surgery.

C. RECTAL CANCER
1. Endorectal ultrasound is used to determine tumor invasion and to detect enlarged lymph nodes.
2. Pelvic magnetic resonance imaging (MRI) is the preferred method of tumor staging because it can predict surgical resection margins.

D. CARCINOEMBRYONIC ANTIGEN
1. Increased level is an independent prognostic factor of decreased disease-free survival and increased risk for metastases.

E. CHEST, ABDOMINAL, AND PELVIC COMPUTED TOMOGRAPHY SCAN
1. Evaluates for metastatic disease
2. Determines local tumor extension
3. Can detect regional lymphadenopathy
4. Useful in operative planning if synchronous resection of metastases is considered
5. Positron emission tomography (PET) scan—not routinely used

F. COLORECTAL CANCER STAGING—AMERICAN JOINT COMMITTEE ON CANCER STAGING SYSTEM
1. Primary tumor (T):

a. Tis: The cancer is in the earliest stage (in situ). It is only in the mucosa and has not grown beyond the muscularis mucosa (thin inner muscle layer).

b. T1: The tumor has grown through the muscularis mucosa and extends into the submucosa.

c. T2: The tumor has grown through the submucosa and extends into the muscularis propria.

d. T3: The tumor has grown through the muscularis propria and into the outermost layers of the colon or rectum but not through them. It has not reached any nearby organs or tissues.

e. T4a: The cancer has grown through the serosa (also known as the visceral peritoneum), the outermost lining of the intestines.

f. T4b: The cancer has grown through the wall of the colon or rectum and is attached to or invades into nearby tissues or organs.

2. Regional lymph nodes (N):

a. Nx: No description of lymph node involvement is possible because of incomplete information.

b. N0: No cancer is found in nearby lymph nodes.

c. N1: Cancer cells are found in or near one to three nearby lymph nodes.

d. N1a: Cancer cells are found in one nearby lymph node.

e. N1b: Cancer cells are found in two to three nearby lymph nodes.

f. N1c: Small deposits of cancer cells are found in areas of fat near lymph nodes but not in the lymph nodes themselves.

g. N2: Cancer cells are found in four or more nearby lymph nodes.

h. N2a: Cancer cells are found in four to six nearby lymph nodes.

i. N2b: Cancer cells are found in seven or more nearby lymph nodes.

3. Distant metastasis (M):

a. M0: No distant spread is seen.

b. M1a: The cancer has spread to one distant organ or set of distant lymph nodes.

c. M1b: The cancer has spread to more than one distant organ or set of distant lymph nodes, or it has spread to distant parts of the peritoneum (the lining of the abdominal cavity).

4. Staging: based on American Joint Committee on Cancer (AJCC) 7th edition; 5-year disease-specific survival

Stage 1:	Any T1–2, N0, M0	92%
Stage 2A:	T3, N0, M0	86%
Stage 2B:	T4a, N0, M0	79%
Stage 2C:	T4b, N0, M0	65%
Stage 3A:	T1–2, N1–2a, M0	89%
Stage 3B:	T1–4b, N1b–2a, M0	69%
Stage 3C:	T3–4b, N1–2b, M0	53%
Stage 4A:	Any T, Any N, M1a	11%
Stage 4B:	Any T, Any N, M1b	11%

VIII. TREATMENT OF COLON CANCER

A. GENERAL PRINCIPLES

1. An adequate cancer operation requires resection of tumor-containing bowel with margins of 2–5 cm and resection of the mesentery at the origin of the arterial supply, including the primary lymphatic drainage of the tumor.
2. At least 12 lymph nodes are required for adequate staging.
3. Only 70% of colorectal cancer patients can undergo resection for cure at presentation.
4. Synchronous colon cancers can be addressed by segmental resections or a total colectomy.

B. SURGICAL THERAPY FOR RESECTABLE MASSES

1. A nonobstructing, nonmetastatic colon cancer is treated with one-stage R0 resection with en bloc resection of the mesentery and lymph node basins, depending on the location of the tumor (Fig. 38.1).
2. If the mass is obstructing and nonmetastatic, most surgeons would proceed with R0 resection and diversion.
3. Clinical T4b masses (invasion of adjacent organs) should undergo neoadjuvant chemotherapy to improve resection margins.
4. Tumors that are unresectable or in patients who are medically inoperable should undergo systemic chemotherapy (see later).
   a. Tumors of the cecum and ascending colon are generally treated by resection of the distal ileum to the mid-transverse colon, including the ileocolic, right colic, and right branch of the middle colic vessels with accompanying mesentery.
   b. Tumors of the left transverse colon and splenic flexure require resection of the transverse and proximal descending colon. The middle and left colic arteries are removed.
   c. Tumors in the descending and sigmoid colon require removal from the splenic flexure to the rectosigmoid. The inferior mesenteric artery is ligated.

C. CHEMOTHERAPEUTIC REGIMENS

1. Adjuvant therapy for stage 3
   a. FOLFOX (fluorouracil [5FU], leucovorin, oxaliplatin) alone or
   b. CapeOx (capecitabine, oxaliplatin) alone or
   c. 5FU and leucovorin, if oxaliplatin cannot be tolerated
2. Adjuvant therapy for stage 4
   a. FOLFOX or
   b. FOLFIRI + Avastin or cetuximab[a]

D. STAGE-SPECIFIC THERAPY

1. Stage I: resection alone
2. Stage II: "low risk" (T1–3, N0), resection alone

---

[a] For patients who have wild-type (WT) *KRAS, NRAS, or BRAF*. Patients with mutations are unlikely to respond to panitumumab or cetuximab.

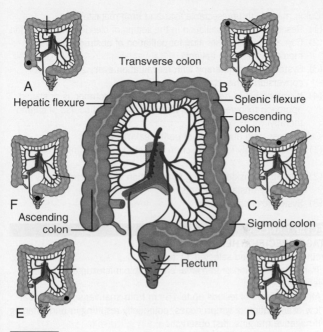

FIG. 38.1

Anatomic resection commonly used for cancer at different sites within the large bowel. (A) Right hemicolectomy. (B) Extended right hemicolectomy. (C) Transverse colectomy. (D) Left hemicolectomy. (E) Sigmoid colectomy. (F) Abdominal perineal resection. Black circles signify the location of the cancer.

3. Stage II: "high risk" (T3 with clinical obstruction or perforation at presentation, fewer than 12 nodes in surgical specimen, poorly differentiated or lymphovascular invasion), should undergo resection and be considered for adjuvant chemotherapy
4. Stage III: resection followed by systemic chemotherapy
5. Stage IV:
   a. Colon mass with resectable, isolated liver or lung metastases
      (1) Synchronous or staged resection, followed by systemic chemotherapy
      (2) Versus colon resection + local therapy with ablation or stereotactic body radiation therapy (SBRT) is also an option, followed by chemotherapy
      (3) Versus neoadjuvant chemotherapy for 3 months followed by synchronous or staged resection and observation of shortened course of adjuvant chemotherapy
      (4) Versus colectomy, followed by 2–3 months of adjuvant chemotherapy, then resection of metastatic disease

MALIGNANT COLORECTAL AND PERIANAL DISEASE

38

b. Colon mass with unresectable liver and lung metastases
   (1) Resection only for palliation in the setting of bleeding or obstruction
   (2) Can also consider stenting for palliation of obstructing mass in medically unstable patients
   (3) Systemic chemotherapy with reevaluation every 2 months for conversion to resectable
   (4) If conversion to resectable, proceed with synchronous or staged approach followed by observation or shortened course of chemotherapy
c. Colon mass with abdominal or peritoneal metastasis
   (1) Resection only for palliation in the setting of bleeding or obstruction
   (2) Can also consider stenting for palliation of obstructing mass in medically unstable patients
   (3) Systemic chemotherapy

IX. RECTAL CANCER

A. STAGE-SPECIFIC THERAPY

1. Carcinoma in situ and selected T1 lesions:
   a. Transanal resection or transanal endoscopic microsurgery (TEM) technique
   b. Allows excision of lesions up to 15 cm from anal verge; does not allow examination of lymph nodes, potentially resulting in understaging
   c. If negative margins, just observation
   d. If high-risk features on pathology (positive margins, lymphovascular invasion, or poorly differentiated), will require resection by transabdominal approach
2. T2–3, any T with +N1–2
   a. Neoadjuvant chemoradiation (5-FU + radiation therapy [RT])
   b. Neoadjuvant therapy may significantly downstage tumors:
      (1) Followed by resection (total mesorectal excision)
      (2) Followed by adjuvant therapy
      (3) Potential for sphincter preservation
3. **Distant metastatic disease treated with palliative procedure and approached similar to colon cancer**

B. OPERATIVE APPROACH

1. Transanal resection
   a. <30% circumference of bowel
   b. <3 cm in size
   c. Margin clear (>3 mm)
   d. Mobile, nonfixed
   e. Within 8 cm of anal verge
   f. T1 (low-risk subtype) only
   g. Endoscopically removed polyp with cancer or indeterminate pathology
   h. No lymphovascular invasion or perineural invasion

2. Transabdominal resection with total mesorectal excision
   a. Plane between the mesorectum and presacral fascia
   b. Decreases local recurrence and blood loss
   c. Minimizes injury to pelvic nerves
   d. Extend 4–5 cm below distal edge of tumors for an adequate meso-rectal excision.
   e. In distal rectal cancers (i.e., <5 cm from anal verge), a negative margin of 1–2 cm may be acceptable.
   f. Full rectal mobilization allows for a negative distal margin and adequate mesorectal excision.
   g. Lymph node dissection
   h. Removal of clinically suspicious nodes
   i. Low anterior resection (LAR) or abdominoperineal resection (APR)
   j. Tumors in the upper mid and upper third of the rectum are treated by a LAR.
   k. Tumors in the lower third of the rectum (2–5 cm) may be amenable to a LAR with coloanal anastomosis.
   l. APR (Miles procedure) with a permanent end-sigmoid colostomy is offered to those patients who are not candidates for LAR.
      (1) Direct adherence of the tumor to adjacent structures may result from inflammation rather than from tumor extension. A cure in the presence of local invasion may still be possible with en bloc resection of the involved structures, or if local invasion is more extensive, by total pelvic exenteration.

C. CHEMOTHERAPEUTIC REGIMENS
1. Neoadjuvant chemoradiation, followed by resection 6–8 weeks
   a. 5FU + RT (45–50 Gy in 25–28 fractions)
   b. Capecitabine + RT
2. Adjuvant therapy
   a. 5FU, leucovorin (if oxaliplatin cannot be tolerated)
   b. FOLFOX (5FU, leucovorin, oxaliplatin)
   c. CapeOx (capecitabine, oxaliplatin)

X. POSTOPERATIVE FOLLOW-UP

Approximately 80% of recurrences occur within 2 years of resection, most often in the form of hepatic metastases or local recurrence.

A. DIAGNOSIS AND TREATMENT
1. Careful history, physical examination, and carcinoembryonic antigen (CEA) screening identify more than 90% of recurrent disease.
2. Follow-up protocol
   a. Routine physical examination, complete blood cell count, liver function tests—every 3 months for 2 years, then every 6 months for 2 years, then annually

38

MALIGNANT COLORECTAL AND PERIANAL DISEASE

b. CEA—every 3 months for 2 years, then every 6 months for 2 years, then annually

c. Colonoscopy—1 year, then 3 years, then 5 years

d. Barium enema—performed if complete visualization is not achieved by colonoscopy

3. **CEA is most helpful if initially increased and returns to normal after resection.**

4. **An increase in CEA (>5 ng/mL) requires repeat level to confirm the result, followed by prompt investigation.**

a. CT scan of the chest, abdomen, and pelvis

b. Colonoscopy

c. PET scan

(1) When conventional imaging fails to identify the site of presumed recurrence, PET scan can be used as an adjunct.

(2) In cases when resectable disease is found on standard imaging, PET scan can be used to rule out additional sites of disease.

(3) If all imaging, including PET scan, is negative, follow up with repeat PET scan in 3–6 months.

(4) If PET scan detects disease, determination of resectability can be made based on imaging alone.

d. Laparotomy is reserved for patients found to have resectable disease.

B. TREATMENT OF LOCAL RECURRENT DISEASE

1. Should attempt a cure by resection in selected patients or to palliate symptoms whenever possible

2. Debulking procedures (tumor resections with gross disease left behind) are not indicated.

3. Recurrence after LAR usually requires an APR.

4. Pelvic recurrences after APR are usually unresectable, but occasionally pelvic exenteration is possible.

XI. ANAL CANCER

1. Epidemiology

a. Approximately 7000 cases of anal cancer will be diagnosed each year in the United States.

2. In the United States, 800 people die of anal cancer annually.

3. Malignancies of the anal canal are relatively uncommon and represent only 2%–3% of all anorectal carcinomas. However, the incidence appears to be increasing.

2. Risk factors

3. Signs and symptoms

4. Screening

5. Anatomy and characterization

XII. TUMORS OF THE ANAL CANAL

1. Human papillomavirus (HPV)
   a. Present in 84% of anal cancers
   b. Estimated that 90% of anal cancers are from HPV
2. Multiple sexual partners/receptive anal intercourse
   a. Likely related to HPV exposure
   b. Seventeen-fold increase in anal cancer
3. Smoking
4. Immunosuppression (solid organ transplant or human immunodeficiency virus [HIV])

XIII. SIGNS AND SYMPTOMS

1. Rectal pain/pressure
2. Bleeding
3. Palpable or visible mass
4. Itching
5. Change in bowel habits
6. Discharge

XIV. SCREENING

There is no consensus recommended screening regimen for anal cancer. Small series have demonstrated benefit from annual Papanicolaou (Pap) smear in high-risk individuals, but no definitive recommendations have been established.

XV. ANATOMY AND CHARACTERIZATION

A. ANAL TUMORS ARE CLASSIFIED INTO TWO GROUPS.

1. Anal canal tumors and anal margin tumors
2. Based on location within the canal/verge
3. Derived from biologic behavior of the tumors and difference in lymphatic drainage in these two areas
4. Most tumors spread by direct extension and lymphatic drainage. Hematologic spread is less common.

B. ANATOMY

1. The superior border anal canal, separating it from the rectum, has been defined as the palpable upper border of the anal sphincter and puborectalis muscles of the anorectal ring.
2. The inferior border starts at the anal verge, the lowermost edge of the sphincter muscles, corresponding to the introitus of the anal orifice.
3. It is approximately 3–5 cm in length.

XVI. TUMORS OF THE ANAL CANAL

A. ANAL INTRAEPITHELIAL NEOPLASIA

1. Squamous carcinoma in situ
2. Precursor to invasive squamous cell carcinoma (SCC)

38

MALIGNANT COLORECTAL AND PERIANAL DISEASE

3. Associated with infection of human papillomavirus types 16 and 18
4. High-risk, immunosuppressed patients should have Pap smears every 3–6 months.
5. Abnormal Pap smear should be followed by high-resolution anoscopy, biopsy, and ablation.
6. Treatment—resection or ablation

B. SQUAMOUS CELL CARCINOMAS (BASALOID, CLOACOGENIC, OR TRANSITIONAL CARCINOMAS)

1. Although each has different histologic features, they exhibit similar biologic behavior and are thus grouped together.
2. These are typically seen in patients 50–70 years of age, more frequently in women.
3. Two cell types exist: squamous cell (keratinizing) and transitional cell (nonkeratinizing).
4. Approximately 40%–50% of patients have pelvic lymph node involvement at diagnosis, whereas 15%–36% have inguinal nodal involvement and 10% have distant metastasis.
5. Excellent prognosis when discovered before nodal involvement and invasion to adjacent structures; 80% of tumors are cured by chemotherapy/radiation therapy alone (the Nigro protocol).

C. DIAGNOSIS

1. Digital rectal examination (DRE)
2. Inguinal lymph node evaluation
   a. Biopsy or fine-needle aspiration (FNA) if suspicious nodes
3. Chest x-ray or chest CT
4. Anoscopy
5. Abdominal/pelvic CT or MRI
6. Consider HIV testing + CD4 level if indicated
7. Gynecologic examination for women, including screening for cervical cancer

D. STAGING

1. Tumor
   a. Tis (carcinoma in situ): In situ means that the cancer is in the earliest stage and has not grown beyond the lining of rectum.
   b. T1: The tumor is 2 cm or less.
   c. T2: The tumor is between 2 and 5 cm.
   d. T3: The tumor is greater than 5 cm.
   e. T4: A tumor of any size invades nearby organs, such as the vagina, urethra, and bladder.
2. Regional lymph nodes (N)
   a. NX: Regional lymph nodes cannot be assessed.
   b. N0: The cancer has not spread into the lymph nodes.
   c. N1: The cancer has spread to perirectal lymph nodes.
   d. N2: The cancer has spread to unilateral internal iliac and/or inguinal lymph nodes.

    e. N3: The cancer has spread to perirectal and inguinal and/or bilateral internal iliac and/or inguinal lymph nodes.

3. Distant metastasis (M)
    a. M0: The cancer has not spread to distant organs.
    b. M1: The cancer has spread to distant organs.

4. Stage I: T1, N0, M0
5. Stage II: T2–3, N0, M0
6. Stage IIIA: T1–3, N1, M0 or T4, N0, M0
7. Stage IIIB: T4, N1, M0 or any T, N2–3, M0
8. Stage IV: any T, any N, M1

E. TREATMENT
1. Any T, N0, or N+, proceed with Nigro protocol
2. Mitomycin C, 5-FU, and RT with 45 Gy
3. Metastatic, proceed with systemic cisplatin-based chemotherapy
4. Patients with locoregional recurrence or progression after primary treatment should undergo APR.
5. Patients with evidence of regional recurrence with positive inguinal lymph nodes can undergo lymph node dissection ± radiation and chemotherapy.

F. ADENOCARCINOMA OF THE ANAL CANAL
Patients with adenocarcinoma of the anal canal are managed in the same manner as patients diagnosed with rectal cancer. Refer to the guidelines in the previous section on Rectal Cancer.

XVII. TUMORS OF THE ANAL MARGIN

A. SQUAMOUS CELL CARCINOMA
1. Represent 25%–30% of all squamous cell carcinoma (SCC) of the anus
2. Typically well or moderately well differentiated
3. Better prognosis than anal canal SCC
4. Typically occur in individuals greater than 60 years old

B. DIAGNOSIS AND STAGING
1. DRE
2. Inguinal lymph node evaluation
    a. Biopsy or FNA if suspicious nodes
3. Chest x-ray or chest CT
4. Anoscopy
5. Abdominal/pelvic CT or MRI
6. Consider HIV testing + CD4 level if indicated
7. Gynecologic examination for women, including screening for cervical cancer

C. TREATMENT
1. T1, N0, well differentiated—proceed with local excision

38

MALIGNANT COLORECTAL AND PERIANAL DISEASE

a. If adequate margins, observe
b. If inadequate, repeat resection versus RT and 5FU-based chemotherapy
2. Any T, N0, or N+ proceed with Nigro protocol
3. Metastatic proceed with systemic cisplatin-based chemotherapy
4. Patients with locoregional recurrence or progression after primary treatment should undergo APR.
5. Patients with evidence of regional recurrence with positive inguinal lymph nodes can undergo lymph node dissection ± radiation and chemotherapy.

XVIII. MALIGNANT MELANOMA OF THE ANAL MARGIN/CANAL

1. This is 0.5%–1% of malignant anal tumors.
2. Anal canal is the third most common site after skin and eyes.
3. This most typically occurs adjacent to the dentate line.
4. Rectal bleeding is the most frequent complaint.
5. Most are not highly pigmented, and diagnosis is difficult.
6. Tumor is aggressive and often widely metastatic.

A. DIAGNOSIS AND STAGING

1. Same as work-up and staging of cutaneous malignant melanoma
2. Refer to the section on Malignant Melanoma.

B. TREATMENT

1. APR is indicated in selected patients, although some small studies have advocated for wide local excision in select patients.
2. If metastatic, patients should undergo systemic chemotherapy in the same manner as cutaneous metastatic melanoma.

RECOMMENDED READINGS

National Comprehensive Cancer Network (NCCN) Practice Guidelines for Anal Cancer. Available at http://www.tri-kobe.org/nccn/guideline/colorectal/english/anal.pdf.
National Comprehensive Cancer Network (NCCN) Practice Guidelines for Colon Cancer. Available at https://www.nccn.org/patients/guidelines/colon/files/assets/common/downloads/files/colon.pdf.
National Comprehensive Cancer Network (NCCN) Practice Guidelines for Rectal Cancer. Available https://www.tri-kobe.org/nccn/guideline/colorectal/english/rectal.pdf.

Malignant Pancreas Disease

Gregory C. Wilson, MD

Tumor biology is King; selection of cases is Queen, and the technical details of surgical procedures are princes and princesses of the realm who frequently try to overthrow the powerful forces of the King and Queen, usually to no long-term avail.

—Adapted from Blake Cady, MD presidential address of the 77th meeting of the New England Surgical Society

I. PANCREATIC ADENOCARCINOMA

A. EPIDEMIOLOGY

1. Fourth most common cause of adult cancer mortality in the United States (8th leading cause worldwide)
2. Approximately 50,000 new cases/year nationally with high expected mortality
3. Slight male sex predominance; 1.3:1 male/female ratio
4. Dramatically increases after age 45; peaks in seventh and eighth decades of life
5. Higher incidence in Western and industrialized world
6. Incidence rates are highest in native inhabitants of New Zealand and Hawaii and in Black Americans
7. Overall lifetime risk for developing pancreatic cancer is 0.5% by age of 70

B. CAUSATIVE FACTORS

1. Cigarette smoking (2–3× increased risk)—increases with duration and amount; risk is reduced with smoking cessation. May account for up to 25% of all cases
2. Genetic Predisposition and Familial Pancreatic Cancer—account for ~10% of pancreatic cancers
   a. *BRCA1*—3× increased risk
   b. *BRCA2*—3–10× increased risk
      (1) PALB2 mutations—PALB2 localizes with *BRCA2* and has similar effect of *BRCA2* mutations.
   c. Lynch syndrome—mismatch repair gene mutations
   d. PRSS1 mutations—chronic pancreatitis, 50% of patients will develop pancreatic cancer by age 70
   e. Peutz-Jeghers
   f. Ataxia-telangiectasia
   g. Li-Fraumeni syndrome p53 mutation
   h. Familial pancreatic cancer: defined as patients with two or more first-degree relatives with pancreatic cancer, unknown genetic predisposition,

4–10-fold increased risk for development of pancreatic cancer, which increases directly proportional to the number of affected family members
3. Chronic pancreatitis—extent of risk is controversial but may be up to 15-fold increase.
4. Others factors are less clear.
   a. Diabetes mellitus
   b. Caffeine
   c. Alcohol
   d. Obesity
   e. ABO blood group: A, AB, and B blood types may have increased risk.
   f. *Helicobacter pylori* infection

C. PATHOLOGY

1. Ninety-five percent of pancreatic neoplasms originate from exocrine cells (remainder are of endocrine origin).
2. Pancreatic adenocarcinoma subtypes/variants include ductal adenocarcinoma (90% of cases), giant cell carcinoma—(4%), adenosquamous carcinoma—(3%), mucinous carcinoma—(2%), mucinous cystadenocarcinoma—(1%), acinar cell carcinoma—(1%)
3. Most common rumor location: head (60%), body (10%), tail (5%)
4. Ninety-five percent of pancreatic adenocarcinomas have KRAS mutations
5. Precursor lesions
   a. Pancreatic intraepithelial neoplasia (PANIn) is a pancreatic ductal lesion that does not penetrate the basement membrane but demonstrates neoplastic growth and genetic mutations. Considered a precursor lesion to adenocarcinoma
   b. Graded from 1 to 3 based on number of mitoses, necrosis, nuclear atypia, and papillary component
   c. PANIn grade 3 lesions are found in over half of individuals with invasive pancreatic cancer.
   d. Presence of PANIn lesions at resection margin does not affect survival/recurrence.
   e. Multi-hit phenomenon from PANIn to carcinoma follows a particular sequence of genetic alterations: KRAS → CDKN2A → p53 and SMAD4.

D. PRESENTATION

1. Most common presentation symptoms/signs: pain, weight loss, and jaundice
   a. Pain—usually poorly localized and of low intensity; increases in intensity and is in lower back in advanced disease, invading celiac and superior mesenteric neural plexuses
   b. Weight loss—90% of cases at presentation; because of a combination of malnutrition from malabsorption and anorexia
   c. Painless jaundice—occurs in tumors of the pancreatic head or uncinate process. Associated with dark urine and acholic stool

  d. Additional signs/symptoms include:
    (1) New-onset diabetes—a concern in patients younger than 40 years
    (2) Gastric outlet obstruction
    (3) Courvoisier sign (palpable, nontender gallbladder on examination)
    (4) Abdominal mass
    (5) Ascites
    (6) Trousseau syndrome (migratory, superficial thrombophlebitis)

E. DIAGNOSTIC EVALUATION/STAGING
1. Imaging modalities
    a. Computed tomography (CT) scan (pancreas protocol) of abdomen. Typically the mass is first identified with another CT imaging modality.
      (1) Provides information regarding the tumor, extension, lymph node involvement, and vascular invasion
      (2) Needs to be triple-phase (arterial, attenuation, portal venous)
      (3) Greater than 80% accuracy in predicting resectability
      (4) Double duct sign: dilated pancreatic and bile ducts
      (5) Additional findings: pancreatic duct dilation, abrupt caliber change of pancreatic duct, pancreatic atrophy
      Note: These findings are not conclusive but should rather lead to additional imaging modalities.
    b. MRI/MRCP—useful in patients allergic to CT contrast dye
    c. Positron emission tomography (PET) scan—no definitive role in staging and is currently not recommended, however may improve identification of subclinical metastatic disease
    d. CT scan of the chest can evaluate for lung metastases.
2. Endoscopic modalities
    a. Endoscopic retrograde cholangiopancreatography (ERCP)
      (1) Useful when CT is equivocal because rarely have a normal pancreatogram with pancreatic cancer
      (2) Stent can be used to palliate when surgery is not an option immediately or if needed to resolve symptoms or sepsis prior to surgery.
      Pearl: *A greater wound infection rate exists for patients with a stent placed before surgery.*
      (3) Consider magnetic resonance cholangiopancreatography if ERCP not technically possible.
      (4) Brushings can be obtained if strictures are present.
    b. Endoscopic ultrasound (EUS)
      (1) Provides information regarding vascular involvement (tumor-vessel interface) and assess for lymphadenopathy
      (2) Can be combined with fine-needle aspiration (tissue diagnosis is needed for neoadjuvant or palliative therapy)
        (a) Suspected lymphadenopathy can also be sampled to help guide treatment plans.
      (3) Pancreatic adenocarcinoma = hypoechoic mass with irregular contour

39

MALIGNANT PANCREAS DISEASE

3. **Tumor markers**
   a. Serum carbohydrate or cancer-associated antigen 19-9 (CA 19-9)
      (1) Altered serum protein that is selectively produced by malignant cells (but can also be expressed in benign dx)
      (2) Cut-off level of 37 U/mL results in sensitivity of 77% and specificity of 87% for malignancy.
      (3) CA 19-9 levels greater than 100 U/mL associated with unresectability
      (4) Normal or reduced CA 19-9 levels after resection associated with improved survival
      (5) Postoperative surveillance: increased levels associated with metastatic or recurrent disease

4. **Diagnostic laparoscopy**
   a. A total of 10%–25% of patients are found to be unresectable at time of laparotomy.
   b. Current indications—pancreatic head tumors greater than 3 cm, tumors located in the body or tail, any suspicious CT findings, patients with CA 19-9 levels greater than 100 U/mL
   c. Usefulness of peritoneal washings has not been demonstrated and would not preclude resection.

5. **Clinical staging**
   a. TNM classification
      1. Primary tumor (T):
         (a) **Tx**—Primary tumor cannot be assessed.
         (b) **T0**—no evidence of primary tumor
         (c) **T1**—tumor limited to pancreas and ≤2 cm in diameter
         (d) **T2**—tumor limited to pancreas and >2 cm in diameter
         (e) **T3**—tumor extends beyond pancreas; celiac axis and superior mesenteric artery not involved
         (f) **T4**—Tumor involves celiac axis or superior mesenteric artery.
      2. Regional lymph nodes (N):
         (a) **Nx**—Regional lymph nodes cannot be assessed.
         (b) **N0**—regional lymph nodes not involved
         (c) **N1**—regional lymph nodes involved
      3. Distant metastasis (M):
         (a) **M0**—no evidence of distant metastasis
         (b) **M1**—distant metastasis present
   b. Staging system:
      (1) **Stage IA**—T1, N0, M0
      (2) **Stage IB**—T2, N0, M0
      (3) **Stage IIA**—T3, N0, M0
      (4) **Stage IIB**—T1–3, N1, M0
      (5) **Stage III**—T4, any N, M0
      (6) **Stage IV**—any T, any N, M1

F. SURGICAL THERAPY/RESECTABILITY

1. Typically only 15%–20% of patients are surgical candidates at the time of diagnosis.
2. Surgical resection offers the only potential cure but median survival after surgery alone remains 11–20 months.
3. Resectability determined by extent of local tumor growth, tumor-vessel interface, and presence of metastatic disease
   a. Resectable disease
      (1) No arterial involvement
      (2) Less than 180-degree involvement superior mesenteric vein (SMV) or portal vein (PV), patent SMV-PV confluence
      (3) No evidence of metastatic disease
      Treatment: proceed with surgical resection. Upfront surgery versus neoadjuvant therapy in this patient population remains controversial with merits to both sides of the argument.
   b. Locally advanced, borderline resectable disease
      (1) Arterial involvement less than 180 degrees, short segment involvement of hepatic artery
      (2) Greater than 180-degree involvement of SMV/PV, short segment occlusion.
      (3) No evidence of metastatic disease
      Treatment: neoadjuvant therapy followed by surgical resection
   c. Locally advanced, unresectable disease
      (1) Greater than 180-degree involvement of superior mesenteric artery or celiac axis
      (2) Involvement of SMV/PV not amenable to reconstruction
      (3) Involvement of inferior vena cava or aorta
      Treatment: initial chemotherapy followed by restaging
   d. Metastatic disease
4. In addition to tumor morphology, patient functional status, comorbidities, and ability to tolerate a major operation play an important role in treatment plan.
5. Operative procedures
      Initial step of any definitive procedure is a thorough intraabdominal metastatic evaluation, which includes examining the liver, peritoneum, paraaortic lymph nodes, and mesentery.
   a. Pancreaticoduodenectomy (i.e., Whipple procedure)—pancreatic head disease, also used to resect periampullary tumors
   b. Distal pancreatectomy—consider for pancreatic body and tail disease.
   c. Total pancreatectomy—consider if anastomosis not possible or unable to get negative margins.
   d. Central pancreatectomy (Appleby procedure)—resection of body tumor with resection of celiac axis

39

MALIGNANT PANCREAS DISEASE

G. NEOADJUVANT THERAPY

1. Potential benefits of neoadjuvant therapy
   a. With surgery alone approach survival remains poor. Neoadjuvant therapy ensures patients complete their multimodal treatment regimen.
   b. Test the biology of the disease. The morbidity and mortality of a major resection can be avoided in those patients that would have likely progressed regardless. Also ensures adequate response of the tumor to the therapeutic regimen
   c. Improved R0 resection rates (most common positive resection margin is the uncinate/retroperitoneal margin along the SMA)
   d. Micrometastases are presumed at the time of diagnosis and can only be effectively treated with chemotherapy.
   e. Potential to downstage tumors that are initially locally advanced and unresectable
2. Remains an area of active research
3. Need tissue diagnosis prior to induction; also need to consider biliary stenting
4. Recommended regimen: FOLFIRINOX (fluorouracil, leucovorin, irinotecan, and oxaliplatin) followed by chemoradiation therapy

H. ADJUVANT THERAPY

1. Pancreatic cancer is considered a systemic disease at diagnosis; therefore all patients with disease ≥T1N0 should undergo adjuvant therapy.
2. Gemcitabine is the previous standard of care for adjuvant chemotherapy. ESPAC 4 study demonstrated superiority of gemcitabine plus capecitabine, which is now the standard of care.
3. Multiple randomized control led trials demonstrate improved survival over surgery alone.
4. Controversy remains about the role of chemoradiation in the adjuvant setting: American institutions continue to favor the use of chemoradiation while European centers do not.

I. SURVEILLANCE

1. Recommended routine surveillance after treatment includes follow-up every 3–4 months for 2 years with clinical evaluation, liver function tests, CA 19-9 level, and CT. After 2 years, routine surveillance can be spaced out to every 6 months.
2. The practice of routine surveillance after treatment for pancreatic cancer remains controversial and varies by center given the poor prognosis of recurrent or metastatic disease.

J. SURVIVAL

1. Median survival after resection is 11–20 months.
2. Five-year survival after resection is 25% for node negative disease and 10% for patients with nodal disease.
3. 80% of patients have disease recurrence within 2 years after resection.

4. Stage specific survival: (based on recent National Cancer Database (NCDB) data)
   a. Stage IA: median survival = 24 months, 5-year survival = 31%
   b. Stage IB: median survival = 21 months, 5-year survival = 27%
   c. Stage IIA: median survival = 15 months, 5-year survival = 15%
   d. Stage IIB: median survival = 13 months, 5-year survival = 8%
   e. Stage III: median survival = 10.6 months, 5-year survival = 7%
   f. Stage IV: median survival = 4.5 months, 5-year survival = 3%

II. PREMALIGNANT CYSTIC NEOPLASMS OF THE PANCREAS

A. MUCINOUS CYSTIC NEOPLASMS (MCNs)

1. Dysplastic lesions with malignant potential; mucin-producing tumors from the epithelium of the pancreatic duct; often detected by endoscopic aspiration of mucin
2. Predominantly found in women and almost always located in body or tail of the pancreas
3. Ovarian-type stroma—pathognomonic finding
4. CT finding of cystic lesion of the pancreas should spurn additional endoscopic evaluation.
5. Endoscopy with EUS
   a. Cyst fluid aspiration
      (1) Cytology—aspiration of cyst wall may reveal atypical or malignant cells.
      (2) Mucin staining
      (3) Amylase level: determines connection to pancreatic duct (if elevated). MCNs should have low amylase levels whereas high amylase levels would suggest connection to pancreatic duct and would be more indicative of intraductal papillary mucinous neoplasms (IPMN).
      (4) Carcinoembryonic antigen (CEA)—level greater than 200 ng/mL distinguishes mucinous neoplasm from nonmucinous lesions. No correlation with carcinoma
6. Treatment: surgical resection, most commonly subtotal distal pancreatectomy
7. Approximately 50% of resected MCNs contain either high-grade dysplasia or invasive carcinoma.
8. Survival for MCN with invasive carcinoma is similar to pancreatic adenocarcinoma.

B. INTRADUCTAL PAPILLARY MUCINOUS NEOPLASMS

1. Papillary cystic lesions of pancreas
2. Produce mucin and are in direct communication with the pancreatic ductal system
3. Classically categorized based on their relationship with the pancreatic ducts
   a. Main duct IPMN (MD-IPMN): higher malignant potential with approximately 50% harboring high-grade dysplasia or invasive carcinoma
   b. Branch duct IPMN (BD-IPMN)

39

MALIGNANT PANCREAS DISEASE

4. Indications for surgical resection

a. Based on the 2012 International or Fukuoka Consensus Guidelines
   (1) All MD-IPMNs should be resected.
   (2) BD-IPMNs with any of the following high-risk stigmata should be resected.
      (a) Obstructive jaundice with cystic lesion in the head of the pancreas
      (b) Enhancing solid component in the cyst
      (c) Pancreatic main duct ≥10 mm
   (3) BD-IPMNs with any of the following worrisome features should be considered for resection versus close surveillance (management of these lesions remains an area of active research and ongoing debate)
      (a) Cyst ≥3 cm
      (b) Thickened/enhancing cyst wall
      (c) Main duct size 5–9 mm
      (d) Nonenhancing cyst wall nodule
      (e) Abrupt caliber change of pancreatic duct with distal gland atrophy
      (f) Regional lymphadenopathy
      (g) Pancreatitis
   (4) BD-IPMNs *without* high-risk stigmata or worrisome features should undergo close surveillance.
   (5) Pathologic classification for IPMN-associated invasive adenocarcinoma
      (a) Colloid: increased mucin production, less aggressive and may have more indolent course
      (b) Tubular: more aggressive and behaves similar to pancreatic ductal adenocarcinoma

RECOMMENDED READINGS

Neoptolemos JP, Stocken DD, Friess H, et al. A randomized trial of chemoradiotherapy and chemotherapy after resection of pancreatic cancer. *N Engl J Med*. 2004;350: 1200–1210.

Oettle H, Post S, Neuhaus P, et al. Adjuvant chemotherapy with gemcitabine vs observation in patients undergoing curative-intent resection of pancreatic cancer. *JAMA*. 2007;297:267–277.

Royal RE. The multimodality treatment of patients with pancreatic cancer. *Cancer*. 2004;16:1–16.

Tempero MA, Behrman S, Ben-Josef E, et al. Pancreatic adenocarcinoma. *J Natl Compr Canc Netw*. 2005;3:598–625.

Diseases of the Breast

Stacey L. Doran, MD

The results of operations for cancer, whether of the breast or elsewhere, would be much better than they now are if they could always be taken during the early development of the disease.

—Thomas Bryant

I. ANATOMY AND PHYSIOLOGY

A. ANATOMY BASICS

1. Modified sweat glands of ectodermal origin. Develop along the bilateral mammary ridges, where accessory breasts (polymastia) or nipples (polythelia) may be found, if intrauterine reabsorption is incomplete
2. Enveloped by superficial and deep layers of fascia on the anterior chest wall
3. Consist of 15–20 lobules drained by lactiferous ducts that coalesce at the nipple
4. Fibrous septa (Cooper ligaments) extend from the deep pectoral fascia to the dermis to provide structural support.
5. Boundaries
   Base of the breast = extends from the second to the sixth rib
   Medial border = lateral margin of sternum
   Lateral border = midaxillary line. Axillary tail of Spence pierces deep fascia and enters axilla.

B. LYMPHATIC DRAINAGE

1. Lymph node involvement is the most important prognostic factor for survival.
2. Any part of the breast can drain to any set of nodes.
3. Axillary nodes—receive 75%–95% of drainage from ipsilateral breast. Axillary nodes secondarily drain to supraclavicular and jugular nodes.
4. Levels of axillary nodes—All nodes are below the axillary vein.
   Level I—lateral to pectoralis minor; includes anterior/external mammary, posterior/subscapular, and lateral/axillary vein groups
   Level II—deep to pectoralis minor muscle; includes central and inter-pectoral nodal groups
   Level III—medial to pectoralis minor and extending up to apex of axilla; includes central nodal groups
5. Internal mammary nodes receive up to 20% of drainage.
6. Interpectoral (Rotter) nodes lie between pectoralis major and pectoralis minor muscles.
7. Abdominal and paravertebral nodes receive less than 5% of drainage.

C. NERVES

1. Intercostobrachial nerve—crosses the axilla from the chest wall to supply cutaneous sensation to upper medial arm. Injury results in anesthesia of upper medial arm.
2. Long thoracic nerve (of Bell)—courses with the lateral thoracic artery along the medial border of axilla to innervate serratus anterior muscle. Injury results in a "winged" scapular deformity.
3. Thoracodorsal nerve—courses along lateral border of axilla to innervate the latissimus dorsi muscle. Loss weakens arm adduction, golf swing, and pull-ups.
4. Lateral pectoral nerve—innervates only the pectoralis major muscle. It exits medial to the medial pectoral nerve (is named lateral because it arises from the lateral cord of the brachial plexus, whereas medial pectoral nerve arises from the medial cord)
5. Medial pectoral nerve—innervates both the pectoralis minor and major muscles. It emerges lateral to the lateral pectoral nerve.
6. Lateral cutaneous branches of intercostal nerves are responsible for cutaneous sensation of the breast.

D. BLOOD SUPPLY

1. Internal thoracic artery, intercostal arteries, thoracoacromial artery, and lateral thoracic artery
2. Batson plexus—valveless venous drainage that allows metastasis to the spine

E. PHYSIOLOGY

1. Phases of breast development depend on pituitary and ovarian hormones.
   a. Estrogen—promotes ductal development, fat deposition, growth of glandular tissue
   b. Progesterone—in conjunction with estrogen, promotes lobular-alveolar development, maturation of glandular tissue
   c. Prolactin (from the anterior pituitary)—milk production
   d. Oxytocin (from the posterior pituitary)—milk ejection
2. Menstruation: Cyclic hormones levels lead to cyclic increase in density of breasts and may cause associated breast pain (mastodynia).
3. Menopause: Decline in hormone levels leads to involution of breast tissue, atrophy of lobules, loss of stroma, and replacement with fatty tissue (less dense breasts easier to interpret on mammography).

II. HISTORY

A. AGE

1. Fibrocystic changes increase with age after puberty and until menopause.
2. Fibroadenoma is most common breast lesion in women younger than 30 years.
3. Risk for breast cancer increases with increasing age—rare (<1%) in patients younger than 30 years of age; average age is 62 years.

TABLE 40.1	
CHARACTERISTICS OF NIPPLE DISCHARGE	
Physiologic	Pathologic
Bilateral	Unilateral
Clear/milky	Bloody
Multiple ducts/quadrants	Single duct/quadrant
Not spontaneous	Spontaneous
Negative for occult blood	Positive for occult blood
No mass	Palpable mass

B. MASS

1. Determine when and how it was first noted, tender versus nontender, change in size with time/in relation to the menstrual cycle, and fixed versus mobile.

C. NIPPLE DISCHARGE (TABLE 40.1)

1. Bloody—benign intraductal papilloma most common. Discharge cytology has poor specificity for determining cancer, so papilloma must be excised to rule out invasive papillary cancer.
2. Milky (galactorrhea)—pregnancy, lactation, pituitary adenoma, acromegaly, hypothyroidism, excessive daily nipple stimulation, stress, drugs (oral contraceptives, antihypertensives, certain psychotropic drugs). Evaluation should include urine or serum pregnancy tests and prolactin levels.
3. Serous—normal menses, oral contraceptives, fibrocystic change, early pregnancy
4. Yellow/green—fibrocystic change, galactocele
5. Purulent—breast abscess

D. BREAST PAIN (MASTODYNIA)

1. Determine pain quality, relation to menses, duration, and location. Rule out musculoskeletal, radicular (pinched nerve) origins.
2. Rarely a symptom of breast cancer. Pain can be cyclic or continuous and associated with menstrual irregularity, premenstruation, exogenous ovarian hormones during or after menopause, or fibrocystic change.
3. Discontinue caffeine and nicotine.
4. Treat with evening primrose oil or nonsteroidal antiinflammatory drugs. Diet may be low in unsaturated fatty acids (UFAs), so increase dietary intake of foods higher in UFAs. If symptoms are debilitating, danazol (Danocrine) may be used for a maximum of 4–6 months.

E. GYNECOLOGIC HISTORY

1. Woman's age at the birth of first child, age of menarche, age at menopause, use of oral contraceptives, and use of hormone replacement therapy (see Breast Cancer section)

40

DISEASES OF THE BREAST

F. MEDICAL HISTORY

1. History of benign breast disease (e.g., fibrocystic change), breast cancer, radiation therapy to the breast or axilla, and recent trauma

G. SURGICAL HISTORY

1. History of breast biopsy, lumpectomy, mastectomy, axillary node dissection, hysterectomy, oophorectomy, or adrenalectomy

H. FAMILY HISTORY

1. History of any breast disease, especially in immediate family (i.e., parents, siblings, children). Also include history of other cancers, especially breast, ovarian, and prostate cancer.

I. CONSTITUTIONAL SYMPTOMS

1. Anorexia, weight loss, dyspnea, cough, chest pain, hemoptysis, headache, central nervous system (CNS) symptoms, abdominal pain, nausea, and bone pain

III. PHYSICAL EXAMINATION

A. INSPECTION

1. Examine the patient seated with arms at the side, seated with arms raised over the head, seated with hands on the hips, and supine.
2. Note breast size, shape, contour, and symmetry; skin coloration, dimpling, edema, erythema, peau d'orange, and excoriation; and nipple inversion, retraction, symmetry, or discharge.

B. PALPATION

1. With the patient in the sitting position, palpate the cervical region and supraclavicular fossae. Then support the patient's arm and palpate each axilla. Note node size, character, and mobility.
2. With the patient in the supine position, palpate the breasts both with the arms stretched above the head and with the arms at the sides. Identify any masses, noting location, size, shape, consistency, tenderness, overlying skin changes, and mobility. Use the flat portion of your fingers for the examination. Carcinoma is typically firm, nontender, poorly circumscribed, and asymmetric with contralateral side.
3. Palpate the areola for subareolar masses. Look for nipple discharge, and try to isolate to palpated lobule.

C. SCREENING

1. There is much controversy in screening recommendations, with the American Cancer Society (ACS), National Comprehensive Cancer Network (NCCN), and United States Preventative Services Task Force (USPSTF), differing on points such as at what age to start screening, frequency of screening, what age to stop screening if at all, and the use of self-breast examinations.

2. The most recent ACS guidelines for women at average risk recommend:
   a. Annual clinical breast examination beginning age 18 and mammogram annually beginning at age 40
   b. Self-examinations are optional (the USPSTF recommends against).
   c. Continue mammography while in good health and life expectancy is at least 5 years.
3. For high-risk women, defined as a greater than 20% lifetime risk of breast cancer by risk-prediction models:
   a. Annual breast magnetic resonance imaging (MRI) and mammogram
   b. Clinical breast examination every 6 months
   c. Screening should begin 5–10 years before the age at which the youngest relative was diagnosed or at age 25 in *BRCA* mutation carriers.

IV. RADIOGRAPHIC STUDIES

A. MAMMOGRAPHY
1. Sensitivity and specificity vary with breast density, approximately 90% for both

B. MAMMOGRAPHIC FINDINGS SUGGESTIVE OF MALIGNANCY
1. Irregular margins
2. Stellate or spiculated mass
3. Architectural distortion, fibrosis, and asymmetrical thickening
4. Pleomorphic microcalcifications with a linear, branched, or rodlike pattern, especially when focal or clustered (≥3 calcifications)
5. Increased vascularity
6. Altered subareolar duct pattern
7. Unclear borders of a mass
8. Breast imaging reporting and data system (BIRADS) classification

C. ULTRASONOGRAPHY
1. Useful for distinguishing between cystic and solid masses
2. Can visualize lesions larger than 0.5 cm in diameter
3. Helpful in evaluating dense breast tissue
4. May resolve questionable mammographic findings, both by appearance of lesions and in conjunction with biopsy

D. MAGNETIC RESONANCE IMAGING
1. Recommended for screening in women with greater than 20% lifetime risk of cancer but not currently recommended for standard screening
2. May be useful as follow-up imaging in women with findings of unknown significance on mammography/ultrasonography and for preoperative planning for known breast cancers

E. DIGITAL BREAST TOMOSYNTHESIS
1. Advanced mammography that takes multiple images of the breast at different angles to construct 0.5-mm slices
2. May be useful in dense breasts or to visualize the relationship between multiple abnormalities

V. EVALUATION OF BREAST MASS

A. NIPPLE DISCHARGE
1. Evaluation
   a. History and physical examination
   b. Ultrasound
   c. Mammogram
   d. Occult blood
   e. Galactogram
2. Worrisome characteristics—spontaneous, recurrent, unilateral, involving a single duct
3. Treatment—excision of intraductal lesion or duct found on ultrasound/ductogram to rule out malignancy

B. PALPABLE LESIONS
1. Cystic—well demarcated, mobile, firm, and fluctuates with menstrual cycle; ultrasound to further characterize
   a. Simple cysts on ultrasound that are asymptomatic may be treated with reassurance.
   b. Symptomatic cysts or with atypical imaging findings should be treated with fine-needle aspiration (FNA).
      (1) No further work-up or cytology is required if fluid is nonbloody (serous) and mass disappears.
      (2) If bloody fluid, residual mass after aspiration, septations, or cyst recurs more than twice, place clip at time of aspiration and proceed to excisional biopsy. Send fluid for cytology.
2. Solid
   a. If there is any elevated concern for malignancy, proceed immediately to diagnostic mammography and biopsy (only 20% reveal malignancy).
   b. For benign-appearing lesions (e.g., fibroadenoma), may use "triple-diagnosis strategy"—serial clinical breast examinations, mammography, and FNA. Monitor the mass for at least 1 year in 3- to 6-month intervals. If all modalities indicate that mass is benign, then there is 95% confidence of being benign, but this DOES NOT RULE OUT CANCER.

C. FINE-NEEDLE ASPIRATION BIOPSY
1. Accuracy rates approach 90%–94%.
2. Nondiagnostic cytology (no epithelial cells present in aspirate) requires excisional biopsy.

3. Diagnostic cytology—discuss cancer treatment options if cancer cells present. This cannot discern between invasive and noninvasive.
4. If inconsistent with mammogram, perform excisional biopsy.

D. CORE NEEDLE BIOPSY (PERCUTANEOUS)
1. Used for palpable masses, nonpalpable masses, or calcifications
2. Can be used in conjunction with image guidance, such as mammogram or ultrasound, for nonpalpable masses
3. Papilloma: 10% sampling error rate
4. Atypia: 25% chance of missing adjacent cancer

E. EXCISIONAL BIOPSY
1. This is a definitive method for tissue diagnosis.
2. Nonpalpable lesion—image-guided core biopsy or excision with wire localization. If core shows papilloma or atypical cells, then must excise to rule out adjacent cancer. Perform postbiopsy mammogram in 3–6 months to confirm removal of the lesion.
3. Biopsy incisions—plan incision with regard to natural skin tension lines: curvilinear incisions in the upper hemisphere of the breast, radial incisions in the lower hemisphere of the breast, and circumareolar incisions for masses just beneath the areola. Incision should be made so that subsequent mastectomy can incorporate biopsy site. All breast biopsies should be performed with the assumption that the lesion is malignant.
4. The entire mass with a surrounding >2-mm rim of normal tissue should be excised. The specimen should be processed for hormone receptor analysis, human epidermal growth factor receptor 2 (HER2)/neu/erbB-2, and fluorescence in situ hybridization (FISH) in specimens with equivocal HER2 staining.

VI. BENIGN BREAST DISEASE
A. GALACTORRHEA
1. Differential diagnosis includes elevated prolactin, oral contraceptives, tricyclic antidepressants, phenothiazines, metoclopramide, α-methyldopa, and reserpine.
2. It can be induced by frequent nipple stimulation.
3. It is often associated with amenorrhea, if pituitary adenoma.

B. FIBROCYSTIC CHANGES
1. Wide spectrum of clinical and histologic findings, including cyst formation, breast nodularity, stromal proliferation, and epithelial hyperplasia. May represent an exaggerated response of normal breast stroma and epithelium to circulating and locally produced hormones and growth factors
2. Three categories—nonproliferative lesions, proliferative lesions, and atypia

40

DISEASES OF THE BREAST

3. Incidence greatest around age 30–40 years but may persist into eighth decade of life
4. Usually presents as breast pain, swelling, and tenderness associated with focal areas of nodularity, induration, or gross cysts. Frequently bilateral. Varies with menstrual cycle
5. Slightly increased risk of breast cancer
6. Treatment
   a. (Rule out) Evaluate for carcinoma by core needle biopsy or excisional biopsy of any discrete mass. Any sampling biopsy should be interpreted in light of examination and imaging. Any discordance requires excisional biopsy.
   b. Repeat breast examinations at different times in menstrual cycle.
   c. Perform baseline mammogram for patients aged 35–39 years and annual mammogram for patients older than 40 years to identify any new or changing lesions.
   d. Patient should avoid xanthine-containing products (coffee, tea, chocolate, cola drinks) and nicotine.
   e. Danazol, a weak estrogen with androgen qualities, may be prescribed for severe mastodynia. It must be continued for 2–3 months to see a potential effect. Administer for maximum of 4–6 months. Recurrence rate is 50% within 1 year of discontinuing drug.
   f. Tamoxifen, which binds to estrogen receptors, has been used for severe symptoms, although it is not US Food and Drug Administration (FDA)–approved for this indication. Adverse effects include hot flashes, thrombosis, cataracts, and increased risk for uterine cancer.

C. FIBROADENOMA

1. Most common breast lesion in women younger than 30 years
2. Round, well-circumscribed, rubbery, mobile, nontender mass. Usually solitary but may be multiple and bilateral
3. Hormonally dependent; may increase in size with normal menses, pregnancy, lactation, and use of oral contraceptives
4. Ultrasound and biopsy to confirm diagnosis
5. Treatment—small lesions may be observed. Excisional biopsy if lesion is greater than 2 cm, rapid increase in size (to rule out phyllodes tumor), or patient complains of significant pain/anxiety

D. PHYLLODES TUMOR AND CYSTOSARCOMA PHYLLODES

1. Malignant versus benign: differentiated by the number of mitoses per high-power field
2. May occur at any age, but mean patient age is 30–40 years
3. Smooth, rounded, well-circumscribed, painless, mobile mass. Overlying skin may be red, warm, shiny, and have venous engorgement. Median size of 4–5 cm. Characterized by rapid growth
4. Contains both mesenchymal and stromal components. Approximately 90% are benign.
5. Spreads hematogenously

6. High rate (15%) of local recurrence after simple excision or enucleation
7. Treatment—wide local excision (WLE) with a negative margin. Lymph node sampling not required

E. INTRADUCTAL PAPILLOMA

1. Benign, solitary polypoid lesion involving epithelium-lined major subareolar ducts
2. May present as bloody nipple or clear discharge in premenopausal women
3. Major differential diagnosis: intraductal papilloma versus invasive papillary carcinoma
4. Treatment—excision of involved duct or papilloma site after localization by physical examination, ultrasound, or ductogram
5. Diffuse papillomatosis—involves multiple ducts of both breasts. Minimal increased risk for breast cancer

F. FAT NECROSIS

1. May be ecchymotic, tender, firm, ill-defined mass, often accompanied by skin or nipple retraction. Almost impossible to differentiate from carcinoma by physical examination or mammography. Usually located in superficial breast tissue, averaging only 2 cm in diameter. More common in overweight women or those with pendulous breasts
2. History of antecedent trauma may or may not be elicited. Can also be caused by surgery, infection, duct ectasia, and aseptic saponification
3. Treatment: if a clear history of trauma, observation; otherwise, excision to rule out malignancy

G. PLASMA CELL MASTITIS AND PERIDUCTAL MASTITIS

1. There is subacute inflammation of ductal system characterized by dilated mammary ducts (ectasia) with inspissated secretions, marked periductal inflammation, and infiltration of plasma cells causing yellowish white viscous nipple discharge.
2. Occurs at or after menopause. History of difficult nursing may be elicited.
3. Presenting symptoms include noncyclical, focal breast pain associated with nipple retraction or discharge, and subareolar masses.
4. Usually presents with minimal radiographic findings, maybe enhanced echogenicity with ultrasound. Excisional biopsy is indicated to rule out carcinoma.

H. GALACTOCELE

1. Occurs after cessation of lactation secondary to an obstructed lactiferous duct
2. Round, well-circumscribed, mobile, tender subareolar mass with milky yellow or greenish yellow nipple discharge
3. Treatment—needle aspiration; excision indicated if cyst cannot be aspirated or cyst becomes infected

40

DISEASES OF THE BREAST

I. MASTITIS AND BREAST ABSCESS

1. Common in lactating women after the third week. Patient may develop generalized cellulitis of breast tissue or abscess.
2. This presents with fevers and with a hard, painful, erythematous breast.
3. Progression from mastitis to abscess formation occurs in 5%–10% of cases.
4. Most common causative organisms are skin flora, such as *Staphylococcus aureus* and *S. epidermidis,* but are usually multimicrobial if abscessed.
5. Treatment
   a. Culture breast milk; begin broad-spectrum antibiotics (dicloxacillin or amoxicillin and clavulanate potassium [Augmentin] for 2 weeks; add metronidazole [Flagyl] if abscess). Patient should continue breast-feeding/pumping.
   b. Incise and drain if fluctuant and not improved with appropriate antibiotic therapy.
   c. Recurrent infection is best treated by excision of diseased subareolar ducts.
   d. If woman is lactating, encourage pumping or continued breastfeeding to fully empty the breast.
6. Differential diagnosis must include inflammatory carcinoma. When incision and drainage is performed, send biopsies of abscess cavity in all patients.

J. MONDOR DISEASE

1. Superficial thrombophlebitis of the thoracoepigastric vein. Usually secondary to trauma or surgery
2. Presents as a tender, palpable, subcutaneous area or linear skin dimpling
3. Finding of palpable cord along the inframammary fold is diagnostic. Vein is deep to breast.
4. Treatment—nonsteroidal antiinflammatory drugs for pain. Resolves spontaneously. Mammogram if patient is older than 35 years

K. GYNECOMASTIA

1. Physiologic
   a. Benign proliferation of male breast glandular tissue. In an adult, defined as >2 cm in diameter
   b. Newborns—caused by exposure to maternal estrogens
   c. Pubertal (ages 13–17 years)—may be bilateral or unilateral; greatest prevalence in adolescence beginning at 10–12 years of age with complete involution by age 16 or 17. Treat with reassurance.
   d. Senescent (age >50 years)—caused by male "menopause" with relative estrogen increase; frequently unilateral; breast tissue is enlarged, firm, and tender; usually regresses spontaneously within 6–12 months

2. Drug induced—associated with use of estrogens, digoxin, thiazides, phenothiazines, phenytoin, theophylline, cimetidine, antihypertensives (reserpine, spironolactone, methyldopa), diazepam, tricyclics, antineoplastic drugs, marijuana, anti–human immunodeficiency virus medication. Treatment is discontinuation of offending drug or surgery. It can recur after surgery if etiology is not identified and eliminated.
3. Pathologic—associated with cirrhosis, renal failure, malnutrition, hyperthyroidism, adrenal dysfunction, testicular tumors, hermaphrodism, hypogonadism (e.g., Klinefelter syndrome)
4. Any dominant or suspicious mass should undergo biopsy to rule out carcinoma, especially in the senescent male individual.
5. Resect if it is causing social problems or is disfiguring.

L.   POLAND SYNDROME
1. Hypoplasia of chest wall and shoulder, absence of breast, and absence of pectoralis major muscle

VII. BREAST CANCER
A.   EPIDEMIOLOGY
1. Most common nonskin cancer in US women—12% of women in the United States (1/8 or 230,000 US women each year) will experience development of breast cancer during their lifetime, and 3.5% (40,000 US women each year) will die of the disease; it constitutes 30% of cancers diagnosed in women.
2. It is a disease of developed nations.
3. Incidence increases with increasing age.
4. It is leading cause of death in US women 40–55 years of age.
5. Age-adjusted incidence appears to be increasing, whereas age-adjusted death rate appears to be decreasing.
6. Screening decreases mortality rate by 25% because of diagnosis at an earlier age.
7. Incidence in men is rising more rapidly than in women.

B.   RISK FACTORS
1. Sex—female-to-male ratio for breast cancer is 100:1 to 150:1.
2. Age—risk increases with increasing age.
3. Family history of breast cancer—overall risk depends on number of first-degree relatives with breast cancer, their ages at diagnosis, and whether the disease was unilateral or bilateral.
4. Genetic mutations account for 10% of all breast cancers.
   a. High-risk genetic mutations, with up to a 50% chance of a second malignancy in 5 years: BRCA1 gene—chromosome 17q, associated with ovarian, prostate, and colon cancer; breast cancer at earlier age (40–50 years); BRCA2 gene—chromosome 13, associated with male breast cancer, bladder cancer, and pancreatic cancer; breast cancer at older age (>50 years)

b. Multiple other genetic mutations of intermediate risk, with a 20%–50% risk of a second malignancy in ten years: tp53 (Li-Fraumeni syndrome), PTEN (Cowden syndrome), ATM (ataxia-telangiectasia syndrome), PALB2, CDH1, BARD1, BRIP1, MRE11A, MUTYH, NBN, NF1, RAD50, RAD51C, RAD51D

5. Atypical ductal or lobular hyperplasia identified on breast biopsy
6. Noninvasive carcinoma (ductal carcinoma in situ [DCIS] and lobular carcinoma in situ [LCIS])
7. Cumulative duration of menstruation, early menarche (<12 years of age) or late menopause (>55 years of age). Risk is increased for women who menstruate for more than 30 years.
8. Nulliparity or age older than 30 years at first delivery
9. Exogenous combined hormone replacement use. Current use of oral contraceptives. Risk declines to baseline within months after discontinuation.
10. Exposure to low-dose ionizing radiation
11. Alcohol consumption, especially before 30 years of age

C. CLINICAL PRESENTATION

1. Nonpalpable, suspicious lesion on mammogram requires needle localization biopsy or stereotactic FNA biopsy for diagnosis.
2. Palpable mass—typically nontender, firm, irregular, relatively immobile, most commonly located in upper outer quadrant of breast. It may be multifocal, multicentric, or bilateral.
3. Skin changes include skin dimpling (due to tension of Cooper ligaments), nipple retraction or inversion, erythema, warmth, edema, peau d'orange (dermal lymphatic invasion), ulceration, eczema or excoriation of superficial epidermis of nipple (as in Paget disease), and en cuirasse (leatherlike) changes.
4. Nipple discharge—bloody; it most commonly is caused by intraductal papilloma, but invasive papillary carcinoma must be ruled out
5. Metastatic spread—spreads lymphatically to bone, lungs, brain, liver; it may present with anorexia, weight loss, cachexia, dyspnea, cough, hemoptysis, bony pain (especially vertebral), pathologic fractures, headache, motor/sensory loss

D. TNM CLASSIFICATION

1. Primary tumor (T)
   a. **TX:** Primary tumor cannot be assessed.
   b. **T0:** no evidence of primary tumor
   c. **Tis:** Tis (ductal) or Tis (lobular)—DCIS or LCIS. Tis (Paget)—Paget disease of nipple without tumor.
   d. **T1:** tumor ≤2 cm. T1mi ≤1 mm. T1a >1 mm but ≤5 mm. T1b >5 mm but ≤10 mm. T1c >10 mm but ≤20 mm
   e. **T2:** tumor >2 cm but ≤5 cm
   f. **T3:** tumor >5 cm

g. **T4:** tumor of any size invading adjacent or distant structures. T4a—extending to chest wall. T4b—ulceration and/or ipsilateral satellite nodules that do not meet the criteria for inflammatory carcinoma. T4c—both T4a and T4b. T4d—inflammatory carcinoma

2. Lymph nodes (N):
   a. **NX:** Lymph nodes cannot be assessed.
   b. **N0:** no regional lymph node metastases
   c. **N1:** metastases to movable ipsilateral level I or II axillary lymph nodes
   d. **N2a:** metastases to fixed or matted ipsilateral level I or II axillary lymph nodes
   e. **N2b:** clinically apparent metastases to ipsilateral internal mammary nodes without clinically apparent axillary node involvement
   f. **N3a:** metastases to ipsilateral infraclavicular (level III) lymph nodes
   g. **N3b:** clinically apparent metastases to ipsilateral internal mammary nodes with clinically apparent axillary node involvement
   h. **N3c:** metastases to ipsilateral supraclavicular lymph nodes

3. Distant metastases (M):
   a. **MX:** Metastases cannot be assessed.
   b. **M0:** no distant metastasis
   c. **M1:** distant metastasis—includes cervical or contralateral internal mammary lymph nodes

E. STAGING
1. Stage 0—Tis N0 M0
2. Stage IA—T1 N0 M0
3. Stage IB—T0–1 N1mi M0
4. Stage IIA—T0 N1 M0, T1 N1 M0, T2 N0 M0
5. Stage IIB—T2 N1 M0, T3 N0 M0
6. Stage IIIA—T0 N2, M0, T1–3 N2 M0 + T3 N1 M0
7. Stage IIIB—T4 N0–2 M0
8. Stage IIIC—any T N3 M0
9. Stage IV—any T any N M1

F. PATHOLOGIC LESIONS
1. Growth patterns
   a. Broadly divided into epithelial tumors arising from cells lining ducts or lobules (most common) versus nonepithelial tumors arising from supporting stroma (i.e., angiosarcoma, malignant cystosarcoma phyllodes, primary stromal sarcomas; less common)
   b. May be noninvasive (absence of invasion through the basement membrane) or invasive
   c. May be multifocal (disease within same breast quadrant as dominant lesion), multicentric (disease in distant quadrant within the same breast), or bilateral (disease in both breasts)

TABLE 40.2		
COMMON HISTOLOGIC TYPES OF IN SITU BREAST CANCER		
Characteristics	DCIS	LCIS
Age	Postmenopausal	Premenopausal
Mass	Rare	None
Mammogram	Microcalcifications	None
Risk	Associated invasive ductal cancer	Associated invasive ductal or lobular cancer
	Ipsilateral breast	Either breast
Nodes	Rare	None
Treatment	Lumpectomy ± radiation or simple mastectomy	Observation vs. prophylactic bilateral simple mastectomy
	No ALND	No ALND

ALND, Axillary lymph node dissection; *DCIS,* ductal carcinoma in situ; *LCIS,* lobular carcinoma in situ.

2. **Common histologic types of breast cancer**
   a. Noninvasive (Table 40.2)
      (1) DCIS—malignant epithelial cells completely contained within breast ducts; does not invade the basement membrane
         (a) More common than LCIS
         (b) Solid, cribriform, papillary, micropapillary, and comedo subtypes; comedo subtype poorest prognosis—most likely to recur
         (c) Average age at diagnosis: 50s
         (d) Greater than 90% of DCIS lesions are nonpalpable and are found as clustered microcalcifications on screening mammography. Prevalence has increased as screening mammography has improved.
         (e) Tends to be multicentric (35%)
         (f) Occult invasive carcinoma found on final pathology in 10%–25% of cases
         (g) Standard surgical treatment is breast-conserving therapy followed by radiation versus simple mastectomy. Hormonal therapy should be considered in estrogen receptor–positive DCIS. Ten-year survival is excellent at over 95%.
      (2) LCIS—traditionally considered a marker for malignancy and not a premalignant condition. Also called lobular neoplasia, along with atypical lobular hyperplasia
         (a) Risk for subsequent invasive carcinoma (usually ductal) is increased 7–18 times in both the ipsilateral and the contralateral breast. Lifetime risk of developing invasive breast cancer is 30%–40%.
         (b) Mean age of diagnosis is 44–46 years, with 80%–90% of cases in premenopausal women.
         (c) It does not form a palpable mass and is not visible on mammogram. It is usually discovered incidentally on biopsy for another abnormality; it is identified in up to 4% of biopsy specimens obtained for benign disease.

(d) Tends to be multicentric (50% of cases). LCIS is identified in the contralateral breast in 30% of cases.

b. Invasive

(1) Infiltrating ductal carcinoma

(a) This is most common breast malignancy (80%).

(b) Originates from ductal epithelium and infiltrates supporting stroma. Less common forms include medullary carcinoma, colloid carcinoma, tubular carcinoma, and papillary carcinoma.

(c) Most commonly presents as a palpable mass or mammographic abnormality

(2) Invasive lobular carcinoma

(a) This accounts for 5%—10% of all invasive breast malignancies.

(b) It originates from lobular epithelium and infiltrates supporting stroma.

(c) Prognosis is similar to invasive ductal carcinoma.

(d) Presents as a palpable mass or mammographic abnormality. Does not form microcalcifications. Within patient's lifetime, 30%–40% can occur bilaterally.

(3) Paget disease of the nipple

(a) This accounts for 1%–3% of all breast malignancies.

(b) Usually associated with intraductal carcinoma (DCIS) or invasive carcinoma just beneath the nipple (95%). Histologically, there are malignant cells along the basement membrane through the milk ducts to the nipple and areola.

(c) It presents initially as thickened erythema and mild eczematous changes that become erosions and ulcerations.

(d) Diagnose by scrape cytology, shave biopsy, punch biopsy, or nipple excision.

(e) Treat with mastectomy or, if limited to retroareolar area, excision of nipple-areolar complex.

(4) Inflammatory breast carcinoma

(a) Accounts for 1%–4% of all breast malignancies

(b) Characterized by peau d'orange of the skin secondary to dermal lymphatic invasion. Presents as diffuse induration, erythema, warmth, edema

(c) More common among African-American women and has a median age of diagnosis of 54 years

(d) Commonly presents with axillary metastases (60%–85%) and distant metastases (17%–36%)

(e) Most rapid and lethal malignancy; usually poorly differentiated

(f) Treatment—Start with chemotherapy, follow with a modified radical mastectomy (MRM), then chest wall/axillary radiation. Combined-modality therapy: 30%–40% 10-year survival rate

   c. Staging is more important than histology in determining prognosis.

   d. Other prognostic indicators include nuclear and histologic grade, presence or absence of estrogen and progesterone receptors, HER2/neu DNA content, and proliferative fraction (S-phase).

G. SURGICAL TREATMENT OPTIONS

1. WLE, lumpectomy, and partial mastectomy—breast-conserving therapy
   a. Two major objectives are:
      (1) Complete excision of tumor with tumor-free margins
      (2) Good cosmetic result
   b. Usually accompanied by sentinel lymph node biopsy and/or axillary node dissection and radiation therapy to the whole breast
   c. Has been shown to have equivalent survival outcomes to mastectomy when combined with appropriate adjuvant treatment
   d. Contraindications to breast-conserving therapy
      (1) Absolute
         (a) Two or more primary tumors in separate quadrants (multi-centricity)
         (b) Diffuse malignancy with microcalcifications
         (c) History of breast irradiation
         (d) Scleroderma
         (e) Persistent positive surgical margins
      (2) Relative
         (a) Collagen vascular disease other than scleroderma
         (b) Pregnancy
         (c) Tumors larger than 4 cm in diameter
         (d) Multiple tumors in the same quadrant
         (e) Large breast size
2. Subcutaneous mastectomy—removes breast tissue only, sparing nipple-areolar complex, skin, and nodes. Experimental cancer operation, but may be considered for prophylactic surgeries
3. Simple mastectomy with skin-sparing—mastectomy (removal of breast tissue) with sacrifice of the nipple-areolar complex. Allows for retention of the skin envelope for reconstruction purposes, with cancers not close to skin or chest wall
4. Simple mastectomy (total mastectomy)—often performed for DCIS or LCIS. Removes breast tissue, nipple-areolar complex, and skin without axillary node dissection
5. MRM—removes breast tissue, nipple-areolar complex, skin, pectoralis fascia, and axillary lymph nodes in continuity. Spares pectoralis major muscle.
6. Radical mastectomy (Halsted)—removes breast tissue, nipple-areolar complex, skin, pectoralis major and minor muscles, and axillary lymph nodes in continuity. Leaves bare chest wall with significant cosmetic and functional deformity. Was historically preferred until clinical trials

showed that there is no significant difference between MRM and radical mastectomy for disease-free survival, distant disease-free survival, or overall survival. Now used only when tumor significantly invades muscle

7. Sentinel lymph node biopsy
   a. Technetium sulfur colloid radionuclide tracer is injected around areola 2–16 hours before surgery ± isosulfan blue (Lymphazurin) injected periareolar at time of surgery.
   b. Collect the hottest node and all nodes that have emitted counts greater than 10% of the hottest node.
   c. Isosulfan blue (Lymphazurin) dye may cause type I hypersensitivity reaction or skin necrosis (1%–3%).
   d. If the sentinel node(s) is negative, then a formal axillary lymph node dissection (ALND) is not required.
   e. If no radionuclide or blue dye is found within the axillary nodes, then a formal ALND is required.
   f. If clinically positive nodes are present, a formal ALND may be performed, or if radiation of the axilla is included, it may replace the ALND if little disease is found in 1–2 nodes.
   g. It is contraindicated during pregnancy, multicentric disease, previous axillary surgery, and neoadjuvant therapy.

8. ALND
   a. Collect all level I and II nodes.
   b. Boundaries of axilla are lateral border latissimus dorsi muscle (posterior), axillary vein (superior), lateral border pectoralis major (anterior), inframammary fold (inferior), lateral pectoralis minor muscle (superficial), and depth of thoracodorsal and long thoracic nerves (deep).
   c. Complications
      (1) Axillary vein thrombosis—sudden, early postoperative swelling; rare
      (2) Lymphedema—slow swelling of upper extremity or breast/chest over 18 months
      (3) Lymphangiosarcoma (Stewart-Treves syndrome)—dark purple bruiselike discoloration on arm 10–20 years after ALND + radiotherapy
      (4) Intercostal brachiocutaneous nerve—most commonly injured nerve, paresthesia of lateral chest wall and inner arm

H. SURGICAL TREATMENT BY STAGE

1. Stage 0
   a. DCIS—total ipsilateral mastectomy versus WLE with 2-mm to 3-mm margin plus radiation therapy. Mastectomy if multicentric, large multifocal, comedo type, larger than 2.5 cm, or unable to obtain clear margins. No ALND
   b. LCIS—prophylactic treatment: bilateral total mastectomy versus tamoxifen coupled with surveillance. No ALND

c. Clinically occult invasive carcinoma—MRM versus WLE with radiation therapy

d. Paget disease—total mastectomy versus MRM. Approximately 95% coupled with invasive disease within the breast

2. **Stages I and II—represent 85% of breast cancers**

a. Current treatment recommendations are MRM versus WLE with axillary assessment (sentinel lymph node biopsies and/or axillary node dissection) plus radiation therapy.

b. Clinical trials have shown WLE with axillary assessment plus radiation therapy to be equivalent to MRM in terms of disease-free survival, distant disease-free survival, and overall survival.

c. Adjuvant chemotherapy is indicated for node-positive patients and high-risk, node-negative patients. Preoperative chemotherapy may have a role in converting tumors to make breast conservation surgery possible.

d. Factors associated with high risk for recurrence include the following:

   (1) Age younger than 35 years
   (2) Tumor size larger than 2 cm
   (3) Poor histologic (scirrhous) and nuclear grade (II, III)
   (4) Absence of estrogen and progesterone receptors
   (5) Aneuploid DNA content
   (6) High-proliferative fraction (S-phase)
   (7) Overexpression of epidermal growth factor receptor II
   (8) Presence of cathepsin D
   (9) Amplification of HER2/neu (c-erbB2) oncogene
   (10) Lymphatic or vascular invasion
   (11) p53 or Ki67 mutations
   (12) Extensive DCIS component (>25% of tumor)

e. Five-year survival rates for stage I and II breast cancers are 95% and 85%, respectively.

3. **Stages III and IV**

a. Multimodality therapy including surgery, radiation therapy, and systemic therapy is usually used.

b. Surgical therapy must be individualized based on extent of tumor and technical ease of resection.

c. Preoperative chemotherapy followed by MRM and chest wall local radiation therapy is the mainstay of treatment for inflammatory breast carcinoma.

d. Five-year survival rates for stage III and IV breast cancers are 45% and 15%, respectively.

I. RADIOTHERAPY TO CHEST AND BREAST

1. **Lumpectomy**

a. May qualify for a partial breast radiotherapy technique if older than 50 years, no lymphovascular invasion, singular lesion

b. Whole breast radiotherapy if multiple lesions, younger than 50 years, lymphovascular invasion

2. **Greater than three positive lymph nodes**

3. Skin or chest wall involvement
4. Positive margins
5. Tumor larger than 5 cm
6. Inflammatory cancer
7. Fixed axillary or internal mammary nodes

J. CHEMOTHERAPY AND HORMONAL THERAPY

1. Surgery and radiation therapy are used to achieve locoregional control, whereas chemotherapy and hormonal therapy are used to achieve systemic control.
2. Adjuvant therapy
   a. Decision to offer systemic therapy because of the risk for metastatic disease is based on tumor size, involvement of regional lymph nodes, tumor biology (estrogen receptor, progesterone receptor and HER2 receptor status). Chemotherapy may also be offered to those with (the extent and rate of progression of) metastatic disease, relative to their prognostic factors, degree and progression of symptoms, and the patient's ability to tolerate therapy without significant toxicity. Oncotype DX is a multiple gene panel that correlates to risk of recurrence and responsivity (and thus improved survival) to chemotherapy, used only for those invasive tumors that express estrogen receptor.
   b. Chemotherapy should be considered for patients with hormone receptor–negative tumors, tumors with HER2 overexpression, aggressive metastatic disease, and the ability to tolerate adverse effects of cytotoxic drugs.
   c. Hormonal therapy should be considered for patients with hormone receptor–positive tumors and relatively indolent metastatic disease. Tamoxifen is the treatment of choice for premenopausal patients and should be used for at least 5 years. Aromatase inhibitors are the drugs of choice for postmenopausal women unless they have significant osteoporosis (in which case, use tamoxifen).
3. Neoadjuvant therapy is the administration of hormonal or chemotherapy before surgical management. It is usually offered to those with a large tumor, who may desire a lumpectomy if not immediately a candidate (enables lumpectomy in approximately 30% post chemotherapy), those with lymph node involvement, or those with HER2 overexpression within the tumor.
4. Cytotoxic chemotherapy
   a. Combination chemotherapy is more effective than single-agent chemotherapy.
   b. It is associated with greater toxicity than hormonal therapy and may be poorly tolerated by older or debilitated patients.
   c. Premenopausal patients tend to have better response to cytotoxic chemotherapy, whereas postmenopausal patients tend to have better response to hormonal therapy.
   d. Genomic profiling (such as with Oncotype DX) may be used for

risk stratification in women with estrogen receptor–positive breast cancers when determining if they are likely to benefit from adjuvant chemotherapy. The profile will score a patient as low, intermediate, or high risk. This test should only be performed in women who are candidates to receive chemotherapy (i.e., no comorbid health conditions) and who have not already qualified to need chemotherapy (i.e., inflammatory breast cancer).

  e. Options
    (1) CMF—cyclophosphamide, methotrexate, 5-fluorouracil
    (2) Anthracycline (e.g., doxorubicin, epirubicin) + a taxane (e.g., Taxol, Taxotere)
    (3) Docetaxel and cyclophosphamide

5. Hormonal therapy
  a. Indications
    (1) Adjuvant therapy for hormone receptor patients
    (2) Palliative therapy for relatively indolent metastatic disease in patients with hormone receptor–positive tumors
  b. Tamoxifen versus aromatase inhibitors (anastrozole, letrozole)
    (1) Tamoxifen is a competitive estrogen antagonist that is effective in premenopausal women. It is as effective as oophorectomy.
    (2) Aromatase inhibitors block estradiol formation. It is effective in postmenopausal women.
    (3) Prophylactic tamoxifen reduces breast cancer risk by approximately 50%–60%.
    (4) Side effects include blood clots, endometrial cancer, ovarian cysts, and accelerated cataract growth.
  c. Alternatives to tamoxifen
    (1) Aromatase inhibitors
    (2) Estrogen receptor downregulators (fulvestrant)
    (3) Oophorectomy—only indication is in the treatment of metastatic breast cancer in premenopausal, hormone receptor–positive patients. However, tamoxifen has been shown to be equally effective.
  d. Immunotherapies
    (1) Trastuzumab (Herceptin)—synthetic monoclonal antibody to HER2. Used only with HER2 overexpression in tumor
    (2) Pertuzumab (Perjeta)—synthetic antibody to HER2 molecule, with a different idiotype than trastuzumab. Acts synergistically with trastuzumab. Only studied in neoadjuvant setting
  e. Treatment scheme is presented in Table 40.3.

K. BREAST CANCER AND PREGNANCY
1. Diagnosis is more difficult and frequently delayed because of breast engorgement, tenderness, and increased nodularity and density.
2. Suspicious masses detected during pregnancy should undergo FNA or core biopsy.

TABLE 40.3
INDICATIONS FOR SYSTEMIC THERAPY

Nodes	Menopausal Status	Estrogen Receptor Status	Therapy
Positive	Premenopausal	Positive	Oncotype DX testing to determine if high risk; if high risk, then Chemotherapy; Tamoxifen after radiation
	—	Negative	Chemotherapy
	Postmenopausal	Positive	Oncotype DX testing to determine if high risk; if high risk, then Chemotherapy; Aromatase inhibitor after radiation
	—	Negative	Chemotherapy
Negative	Premenopausal	Positive	Oncotype DX testing to determine if high risk; if high risk, then Chemotherapy; Tamoxifen after radiation
	—	Low risk (tumor <1 cm)	Tamoxifen
	—	High risk	Chemotherapy + tamoxifen
	—	Negative	Chemotherapy
	—	Low risk (tumor <0.5 cm)	None
	—	High risk	Chemotherapy
	Postmenopausal	Positive	Oncotype DX testing to determine if high risk; if high risk, then Chemotherapy; Tamoxifen after radiation
	—	Low risk (tumor <2 cm)	Aromatase inhibitor vs. tamoxifen
	—	High risk (tumor ≥2 cm)	Aromatase inhibitor vs. tamoxifen + chemotherapy
	—	Negative	
	—	Low risk	Likely chemotherapy, followed by radiation, if indicated
	—	High risk	Chemotherapy

40

DISEASES OF THE BREAST

3. If malignancy is identified, subsequent treatment decisions are influenced by specific trimester of pregnancy. The goal of treatment is the cure of breast cancer without injury to the fetus.
   a. Radiation is contraindicated during pregnancy.
   b. Studies have demonstrated that termination of pregnancy, in hopes of decreasing hormonal tumor stimulation, has no added benefit.
   c. For cancer detected during first and second trimesters, MRM is the treatment of choice. However, immediate breast reconstruction should not be performed because a symmetrical result is impossible until the postpartum appearance of the contralateral breast is known.
   d. In the second and third trimesters, preoperative adjuvant chemotherapy can be given followed by breast conservation, with radiation therapy deferred until after delivery. Studies have shown no increased risk of fetal malformation for chemotherapy administered during the second and third trimesters. An increased incidence of spontaneous abortion and congenital malformation is associated with chemotherapy given during the first trimester.
   e. For cancer detected during the third trimester, WLE and axillary node dissection may be safely performed, with radiation therapy delayed until after delivery.

L. MALE BREAST CANCER
1. Incidence rate is 1% of all breast cancers.
2. Increased risk may be associated with hyperestrogenic states—Klinefelter syndrome, liver disease, and exogenous estrogen use (metastatic prostate cancer, transvestites). Low-dose radiation is also implicated. Forty percent of men with breast cancer have the *BRCA2* mutation.
3. Mean age at diagnosis is 60–65 years.
4. Because of scant breast tissue in men, the skin and pectoralis major muscle is more often involved than in women. Delay in diagnosis may result in more advanced stage at presentation and worse prognosis.
5. Infiltrating ductal carcinoma is most common histologic type of breast cancer in men.
6. Node-negative disease—prognosis similar to that in women. Node-positive disease has a significantly worse prognosis than in women.
7. Treatment depends on stage and local extent of tumor.
   a. DCIS—perform simple mastectomy and rarely lumpectomy with radiotherapy.
   b. Invasive carcinoma—total mastectomy with axillary assessment. If underlying pectoralis major muscle is involved, then radical mastectomy is recommended.
   c. Postoperative radiation therapy improves local control but does not affect survival.
   d. Node-positive or high-risk, node-negative patients—adjuvant chemotherapy or hormonal therapy. Greater than 80% of male breast cancers are hormone receptor positive; therefore tamoxifen may play an important role.

M. BREAST RECONSTRUCTION AFTER MASTECTOMY—DELAYED OR IMMEDIATE

1. No evidence to suggest that breast reconstruction after mastectomy compromises efficacy of adjuvant chemotherapy, increases incidence of local recurrence, or delays diagnosis of recurrence on chest wall
2. Significantly improves patient's concept of body image
3. With early cancers, may be performed immediately. If advanced, delay until after radiation therapy is completed.
4. Types of reconstructive procedures
    a. Prosthetic breast implant—filled with silicone or saline, inserted between the pectoral muscles (subpectorally) after expansion
    b. Myocutaneous flap reconstruction—more complicated procedure but better long-term cosmetic results
        (1) Transverse rectus abdominis flap—based on superior mesenteric artery and vein; entire contralateral rectus abdominis muscle is transposed with transverse ellipse of skin and subcutaneous tissue from lower abdomen
        (2) Latissimus dorsi flap is based on thoracodorsal artery and vein.
        (3) Free rectus abdominis flap—Thoracodorsal or anterior serratus vessels are anastomosed to internal mammary or axillary vessels to maintain blood supply to the flap.
        (4) Greater omentum pedicle flap is covered with a skin graft.
        (5) Gluteus maximus free flap
    c. Deep inferior epigastric perforator flap—free-flap based on individual vessels from the rectus, through the anterior fascia. The flap spares the muscle. Patient must have sufficient vessels and flow. Certain prior abdominal surgeries may preclude its use.
    d. Nipple-areolar reconstruction may be performed after prosthetic breast implant or myocutaneous flap reconstruction after the reconstructed breast attains its final shape and position, typically in 6–12 weeks.
    e. Nipple-areolar complex-sparing incisions typically require the tumor tissue involvement to be away from the base of the nipple.
5. Complications of breast reconstruction
    a. Infection
    b. Tissue loss and skin flap necrosis, especially because of vascular compromise. More common in smokers
    c. Poor cosmetic result
    d. Slippage of prosthetic implant or capsular contraction
    e. Fat necrosis

40

DISEASES OF THE BREAST

RECOMMENDED READINGS

Oeffinger KC, Fontham ETH, et al. Breast cancer screening for women at average risk: 2015 guideline update from the American Cancer Society. *JAMA*. 2015;314:1599–1614.

Sabel M. Anatomy and physiology of the breast. In: *Essentials of Breast Surgery.* Philadelphia: Mosby Elsevier; 2009:1–18.

Siu AL; U.S. Preventive Services Task Force. Screening for breast cancer: U.S. Preventive Services Task Force Recommendation Statement. *Ann Intern Med*. 2016;164:279–296.

Malignant Skin Lesions

Meghan C. Daly, MD

Challenges are what make life interesting and overcoming them is what makes life meaningful.

—Joshua J. Marine

I. BASAL CELL CARCINOMA

A. GENERAL
1. Most common skin malignancy
2. Originates from epidermis: basal epithelial cells and hair follicles
3. Clinical presentation
   a. Waxy or cream-colored
   b. Classically described with pearly, rolled borders
   c. Central ulceration common; slow, indolent growth
   d. 70% occur on face
   e. Local destruction; rarely metastatic disease
4. Types
   a. Nodular—classic type
   b. Superficial—slow growing, scaly, pink plaque
   c. Sclerosing/morpheaform—rarest form (5%–10%), resembles scar, most aggressive
5. Risk factors
   a. Ultraviolet light, radiation therapy (XRT), immunosuppression, arsenic
   b. Genetic predisposition: basal-nevus syndrome (PTCH-1), xeroderma pigmentosa (XP), other rare conditions

B. DIAGNOSIS
1. Punch biopsy
2. Excisional biopsy for smaller lesions

C. TREATMENT
1. Surgical excision with 3–5-mm margins ideal
2. Electrodissection and curettage/photodynamic therapy (PDT)/laser ablation for smaller lesions/premalignant lesions
3. Mohs micrographic surgery
   a. For cosmetically sensitive areas, high-risk or recurrent lesions
   b. Serial excision of tumor with immediate evaluation of frozen sections until normal tissue margins obtained
4. Radiation therapy
5. Topical treatment with 5-fluorouracil (5FU)/imiquimod cream for multiple lesions, low-risk superficial lesions
6. Systemic treatment for rare metastasis or locally advanced disease not amenable to surgery or radiation: Smoothened (SMO) inhibitors

II. SQUAMOUS CELL CARCINOMA
A. GENERAL
1. Second-most common skin malignancy
2. Squamous cell carcinoma greater than 2 cm or if poorly differentiated has an increased likelihood of metastasis compared with basal cell carcinoma of similar size
3. Associated with ultraviolet exposure, chronic scars, and irradiated skin, immunosuppression, genetic disorders (e.g., XP)
4. Precursor is actinic keratosis majority of time
5. Clinical presentation
   a. Arises in sun-exposed areas (i.e., face, extremities)
   b. Erythematous, scaly plaque, ulcerated mass or nodule
6. Bowen disease
   a. Squamous cell carcinoma in situ
   b. Five percent develop into invasive squamous cell carcinoma
7. Marjolin ulcer—squamous cell carcinoma arising in old burn scar
8. Erythroplasia of Queyrat—in situ squamous cell carcinoma of penis

B. DIAGNOSIS
1. Punch biopsy
2. Excisional biopsy

C. TREATMENT
1. Surgical excision with 5–10-mm margins
2. Alternative treatments include XRT
3. Other less common treatments: electrodesiccation and curettage for small low-risk lesions, topical 5FU, PDT
4. Regional lymph node dissection for clinically positive nodes
5. Can consider sentinel node biopsy for high-risk primary lesions and clinically negative nodes
6. Systemic cytotoxic chemotherapy for distant metastatic disease (uncommon)

III. MALIGNANT MELANOMA
A. GENERAL
1. Originates from neural crest cells (melanocytes) in basal layer epidermis
2. Risk factors
   a. Previous melanoma
   b. Large number of dysplastic nevi
   c. Ultraviolet exposure, previous XRT, tanning beds
   d. Fair complexion, light-colored eyes
   e. Family history (10% of melanomas familial), genetic syndrome (e.g., CDK2NA, CDK4, XP, BRCA2, others)
   f. Immunosuppression
   g. Age

41

MALIGNANT SKIN LESIONS

B. CLINICAL PRESENTATION
1. A—asymmetry
2. B—border irregularity
3. C—color variation
4. D—diameter greater than 6 mm
5. E—evolution

C. TYPES OF MELANOMA
1. Superficial spreading: most common
   a. Long radial growth phase before vertical growth
2. Nodular: most aggressive
   a. Predominately vertical growth phase
   b. Bluish black with smooth borders, can be amelanotic
3. Lentigo maligna: least aggressive
   a. Minimal invasion
   b. Targets face/neck/dorsum of hands, older population
   c. Best prognosis given thin depth
4. Acral lentiginous
   a. Palms/soles/subungual region
   b. Predominant subtype in dark-skinned individuals
   c. "Hutchinson sign"—pigmented proximal/lateral nail folds
   d. Very aggressive but least common type.

D. PROGNOSTIC FACTORS
1. Depth of invasion is most important prognostic factor.
2. Presence of ulceration increases aggressiveness.
   a. Ulceration shown to correlate with increased angiogenesis
3. Vertical growth phase and mitotic rate are inversely related to prognosis.
4. Anatomic location—extremities more favorable than trunk/face/scalp

E. STAGING
1. Clark level of staging—based on anatomic depth
   a. Level I—superficial to basement membrane (in situ)
   b. Level II—papillary dermis through basement membrane
   c. Level III—papillary and reticular dermis junction
   d. Level IV—reticular dermis
   e. Level V—subcutaneous fat
2. Breslow level of staging—based on vertical thickness
   a. More important than Clark level for prognosis
   b. Less than 1 mm—thin
   c. 1–4 mm—intermediate
   d. Greater than 4 mm—thick
3. TNM staging system—most current staging system, developed by American Joint Committee on Cancer
   a. Primary tumor thickness (T)

Each T stage is subgrouped into "a" and "b" denoting the absence or presence of ulceration, respectively. T1 lesions can be designated T1b if they have ≥1 mitosis/mm^2:

    (1) T1: less than 1.0 mm

    (2) T2: 1.01–2.0 mm

    (3) T3: 2.01–4.0 mm

    (4) T4: greater than 4.01 mm

b. Nodal status (N)

    (1) N1: metastasis in one regional node

        (a) N1a—micrometastasis

        (b) N1b—macrometastasis

    (2) N2: metastasis in two–three regional nodes

        (a) N2a—micrometastasis

        (b) N2b—macrometastasis

        (c) N2c—negative nodes with in-transit or satellite metastasis

    (3) N3: metastasis 4+ nodes, matted nodes, or in-transit metastasis with positive nodes

c. Metastases (M)

    (1) M0: no evidence of metastatic disease

    (2) M1a: distant skin, subcutaneous, or nodal disease with normal lactate dehydrogenase (LDH) level

    (3) M1b: lung metastasis with normal LDH

    (4) M1c: all other distant metastases or any distant site with elevated LDH

d. Stages

    (1) Stage 1a: T1a, N0, M0

    (2) Stage 1b: T1b, N0, M0

        (a) T2a, N0, M0

    (3) Stage IIa: T2b, N0, M0

        (a) T3a, N0, M0

    (4) Stage IIb: T3b, N0, M0

        (a) T4a, N0, M0

    (5) Stage IIc: T4b, N0, M0

    (6) Stage III: any T, N1–3, M0

    (7) Stage IV: any T, any N, M1

F. DIAGNOSIS

1. Excisional biopsy
2. Punch biopsy
3. Shave biopsy although common, not recommended if too superficially performed as may transect tumor and not measure thickness of lesion accurately

G. TREATMENT

1. Wide local excision of remaining lesion and biopsy scar
   a. Lesions with 1-mm depth or less: 1-cm margins recommended

b. Lesions 1–2 mm in thickness: 1–2-cm margins recommended

c. Lesions with greater than 2-mm depth: 2-cm margins recommended

d. Must excise to the level of underlying fascia, smaller margins considered for cosmetic and functional issues

2. Lymph node evaluation

a. Regional lymph nodes most common site of metastatic disease

b. All palpable lymphadenopathy requires therapeutic nodal dissection.

c. Sentinel lymph node dissection

(1) Appropriate for clinically node-negative disease in lesions ≥1 mm and selected patients in some centers with lesions ≤1 mm (>0.75 mm, ulceration or ≥1 mitosis per mm^2)

(2) Techniques: Radiolabeled (technitium-99m) sulfa colloid, albumin or tilmanocept, is injected intradermally around the lesion, lymphoscintigraphy is usually performed and using a gamma probe intraoperatively, the sentinel lymph nodes are identified and removed; 1% isosulfan blue dye, patent blue dye V, or methylene blue is also often injected around the target lesion, highlighting the appropriate sentinel lymph node allowing for easier identification

d. If a positive sentinel node is identified, a completion node dissection is usually recommended; however, a clinical trial testing the survival benefit of additional surgery is currently maturing.

3. **Clinically positive nodes without distant disease usually mandate a therapeutic nodal dissection.**

4. Adjuvant therapy for stage III disease

a. Interferon-α2b in standard or PEG formulations, ipilimumab (CTLA-4 inhibitor), clinical trials

(1) Can prolong disease-free survival but overall survival benefits are controversial or unproven

5. Metastatic disease

a. BRAF/MEK inhibitors combinations: BRAF (vemurafenib, dabrafenib), MEK (trametinib, cobimetinib), others in development.
Only indicated in approximately 50% of melanoma patients with the BRAF V600 activating mutation

b. IL-2

c. Ipilimumab

d. PD-1 inhibitors

e. Cytotoxic chemotherapy

f. Clinical trials

6. **Other treatments in selected patients**

a. Surgical resection of metastatic disease can be therapeutic or palliative.

b. Radiation therapy as adjunct treatment for nodal basins at high risk for recurrence, brain metastases, or selected settings

c. Isolated limb perfusion (ILP) or isolated limb infusion (ILI) with melphalan for extremity locally advanced disease/in transit disease

d. Intralesional therapies (talimogene laherparepvec [T-VEC], Bacillus Calmette-Guérin [BCG], others)

IV. MERKEL CELL CARCINOMA

A. GENERAL

1. Rare
2. Aggressive with high propensity for local recurrence and regional lymph node metastases
3. Risk factors include: fair-skin, immunosuppression, B-cell malignancies
4. Clinically present as rapidly growing, painless, firm, red to purple nodule/indurated plaque commonly in head and neck region
5. Have neuron-specific enolase (NSE), cytokeratin, and neurofilament protein

B. TREATMENT

1. Wide local excision
2. Sentinel lymph node biopsy
3. Adjuvant radiation

RECOMMENDED READINGS

Larkin J, Ascierto PA, Dreno B, et al. Combined vemurafenib and cobimetinib in BRAF-mutated melanoma. *N Engl J Med*. 2014;371:1867–1876.

Long GV, Stroyakovskiy D, Gogas H, et al. Combined BRAF and MEK inhibition versus BRAF inhibition alone in melanoma. *N Engl J Med*. 2014;371:1877–1888.

Shaih AH, Yeh I, Kovalyshyn I, et al. The genetic evolution of melanoma from precursor lesions. *N Engl J Med*. 2015;373:1926–1936.

Sosman JA, Kim KB, Schuchter L, et al. Survival in BRAF V600-mutant advanced melanoma treated with vemurafenib. *N Engl J Med*. 2012;366:707–714.

41

MALIGNANT SKIN LESIONS

PART VII

Hepatobiliary Surgery

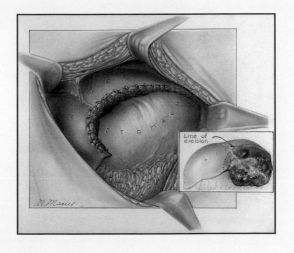

Benign Gallbladder and Biliary Tree

Carey L. Watson, MD

*The gallbladder should be removed not because it contains
stones, but because it forms them.*

—Carl Langenbuch

I. ANATOMY

A. GALLBLADDER

1. Pear-shaped sac lying in gallbladder fossa on inferior surface of liver with 30–50-mL capacity, greater than 300-mL capacity when obstructed
2. Divided into four anatomic portions: fundus, corpus, infundibulum, and neck
3. Demarcates anatomic division between left and right hepatic lobes (Cantlie line runs between gallbladder and inferior vena cava [IVC] and divides liver in two lobes)
4. Supplied by the cystic artery
   a. Originates from the right hepatic artery in 90%; can arise from left hepatic, common hepatic, gastroduodenal, or superior mesenteric arteries
   b. Courses superiorly and posteriorly to the cystic duct until it reaches the peritoneal surface of the gallbladder and divides
5. Venous drainage
   a. Rarely a cystic vein drains to right portal vein.
   b. Primarily through small veins, these drain directly into liver
6. Cystic duct
   a. Connects the gallbladder to the common duct system
   b. Sits just anterior to the right hepatic artery
   c. Valves of Heister—mucosal folds at the gallbladder/cystic duct junction
   d. Highly variable in length and anatomic course
7. Calot triangle
   a. Common hepatic duct, liver, cystic duct define the boundaries (modern definition)
   b. Cystic artery, right hepatic artery, and the cystic duct lymph node (Calot node) lie within this triangle.

B. BILE DUCTS

1. Left and right hepatic ducts join to form a common hepatic duct.
   a. Left is longer than right and is at increased risk for dilatation from distal obstruction.
   b. They are joined by the cystic duct to form the common bile duct (CBD).

2. CBD is approximately 8–11.5 cm in length and 2–10 mm in diameter.
3. There are three portions to the CBD: suprapancreatic, intrapancreatic, and intraduodenal.
4. CBD empties into the duodenum in one of two patterns:
   a. Unites with the pancreatic duct outside the duodenum and enters the duodenum as a single duct (75%)
   b. Exits into the duodenum via a separate orifice (25%)
5. Blood supply of CBD is from gastroduodenal artery and right hepatic artery.

C. ANOMALIES
Awareness of the highly variable nature of the gallbladder and associated structures is critical in the approach to the patient undergoing gallbladder or biliary surgery.
1. Gallbladder—duplication, intrahepatic, left-sided, or bilobed
2. Cystic duct—short or absent, long with alternative course, double cystic duct, accessory cystic duct, ducts of Luschka (drain directly from liver into gallbladder and may require clipping to prevent postoperative biloma)
3. Cystic artery and hepatic arteries—double cystic artery, accessory left hepatic artery, replaced right hepatic artery

II. CHOLELITHIASIS
A. INCIDENCE
1. Found in 12% of general population
2. Majority (80%) are asymptomatic.
3. Predisposing conditions
   a. Sex distribution—twice as common in women
   b. Age—found in 20% of adults older than 40 years and 30% of adults older than 50
   c. Medical—obesity, pregnancy, rapid weight loss, total parenteral nutrition, diabetes, pancreatitis, chronic hemolytic states, malabsorption, Crohn disease, spinal cord injuries, increased triglycerides, decreased high-density lipoprotein
   d. Drugs—exogenous estrogens, clofibrate, octreotide, ceftriaxone
   e. Ethnic factors—Pima Indians, other Native Americans, Scandinavians, persons living in Chile

B. CAUSATIVE FACTORS
Three principal defects contribute to gallstone formation.
1. Cholesterol supersaturation—most critical to stone formation
   a. Three major constituents in bile:
      (1) Bile salts—primary: cholic and chenodeoxycholic acids; secondary: deoxycholic and lithocholic
      (2) Phospholipids—90% lecithin
      (3) Cholesterol—Bile containing excess cholesterol relative to bile salts and lecithin is predisposed to gallstone formation.

2. Accelerated nucleation
   a. Mucin and bilirubin are pronucleators associated with increased stone formation.
3. Gallbladder hypomotility/stasis

C. TYPES OF GALLSTONES
1. Mixed (75%)
   a. Most common, relatively small in size, usually multiple
   b. Predominantly cholesterol (at least 50% of content)
2. Pure cholesterol (10%)
   a. Often solitary with large, round configuration
   b. Usually not calcified
3. Pigment (15%)
   a. Result from bilirubin precipitation
   b. More common in women and Asian individuals
   c. Black pigment—associated with cirrhosis and chronic hemolytic states
   d. Brown pigment—usually associated with biliary infection and more common in biliary tree than in gallbladder
   e. Approximately 50% are radiopaque.

D. TREATMENT OF ASYMPTOMATIC CHOLELITHIASIS
1. Prophylactic cholecystectomy is not indicated in most patients (only approximately 20% become symptomatic).
2. Certain subgroups may benefit from prophylactic cholecystectomy.
   a. American Indians with gallstones who have a greater rate of gallbladder cancer
   b. Heart and lung transplant patients because the morbidity of acute cholecystitis is severe in this subgroup (kidney transplant candidates do not appear to benefit)
   c. Diabetes is *no longer* considered an indication for prophylactic cholecystectomy.
   d. Gastric bypass with prophylactic cholecystectomy is controversial; it does not appear to improve outcome.

III. SYMPTOMATIC CHOLELITHIASIS

A. BILIARY COLIC
Defined as pain arising from the gallbladder without established inflammation or infection
1. Pathology—results from intermittent obstruction of the cystic duct by stone
2. Natural history
   a. Rate of recurrence is between 50% and 70% after first episode.
   b. Risk for development of biliary complications is 1%–2% per year.
3. Clinical manifestations
   a. Severe pain, often visceral in nature, involving right upper quadrant (RUQ) or midepigastrium
   b. May radiate to back or below right scapula

   c. Often follows a fatty meal

   d. Pain lasts between 1 and 6 hours (if >6 hours, think cholecystitis).

   e. Steady pain, not undulating like that of renal colic

   f. Can be associated with nausea and vomiting

4. **Physical examination—usually normal, only mild-to-moderate tenderness during an attack or mild residual tenderness lasting for a few days after an attack; usually negative Murphy sign**

5. Diagnosis

   a. Reference laboratory values

   b. Ultrasound is 95% sensitive and 90% specific for diagnosis of cholelithiasis and is diagnostic procedure of choice.

   c. Plain radiography detects only 10%–15% of cholesterol stones (50% of pigment stones).

6. Complications

   a. Prolonged obstruction can lead to acute cholecystitis.

   b. Stones may pass into the CBD, resulting in choledocholithiasis, cholangitis, or pancreatitis.

7. **Treatment: patients with biliary colic and documented gallstones generally treated with an elective laparoscopic cholecystectomy (lap chole)**

B. ACUTE CALCULOUS CHOLECYSTITIS

Defined as pain arising from inflammation of the gallbladder wall

1. Pathology

   a. Impacted stone in the cystic duct results in prolonged obstruction.

   b. Stasis of bile damages gallbladder mucosa, resulting in the release of enzymes and inflammatory mediators.

   c. Histology ranges from mild acute inflammation to edema to necrosis and perforation of the gallbladder wall.

   d. Forty percent of bile cultures are positive for bacteria in this setting.

     (1) Usually single-organism growth

     (2) Most likely organisms include *Escherichia coli, Klebsiella, Enterococcus, Enterobacter.*

2. Natural history

   a. Seventy-five percent of cases report previous attack of biliary pain.

   b. If untreated, 80% resolve within 7–10 days.

   c. Complications develop in approximately 17%.

3. Clinical manifestations

   a. As inflammation progresses, visceral pain gives way to parietal pain localized to RUQ.

   b. Duration of pain is beyond 6 hours.

   c. Nausea and vomiting are more common than in biliary colic.

4. Physical examination

   a. Fevers are common.

   b. Murphy sign—During palpation of the RUQ and deep inspiration, the inflamed gallbladder comes in contact with the examiner's hand, resulting in pain and inspiratory arrest (patient stops breathing momentarily).

   c. The gallbladder is palpable in one-third of the patients.

5. Diagnosis
   a. Laboratory tests—Leukocytosis is common; there are increases in alkaline phosphatase and serum aminotransferase, and serum bilirubin level between 2 and 4 mg/dL can also occur.
   b. Ultrasound is useful in diagnosing acute cholecystitis and is diagnostic procedure of choice.
      (1) Sonographic Murphy sign in the presence of stones predicts acute cholecystitis 90% of the time.
      (2) Gallbladder wall is thickened and there is pericholecystic fluid in up to 50% of patients with acute cholecystitis.
      (3) Ultrasound shows echoic shadowing from stones.
   c. Computed tomography (CT) scan is useful in diagnosing complications of acute cholecystitis (empyema, perforation, or emphysematous cholecystitis).
   d. Cholescintigraphy (i.e., hepatobiliary iminodiacetic acid [HIDA] scan)
      (1) Intravenously administer gamma-emitting technetium 99m (^{99m}Tc)-labeled hydroxyl iminodiacetic acid, which is rapidly taken up by the liver and secreted into bile.
      (2) Nonfilling of the gallbladder within 4 hours with preserved excretion into the CBD and small bowel indicates an obstructed cystic duct.
      (3) Accuracy in diagnosing acute cholecystitis is 95%, which is superior to ultrasound.
6. Complications
   a. If left untreated and the cystic duct remains obstructed, the gallbladder can fill with a clear mucoid fluid—*hydrops of the gallbladder*.
      (1) This can lead to ischemia/necrosis/perforation of gallbladder wall.
   b. Results are gangrenous cholecystitis 7% of the time, gallbladder empyema (6%), perforation (3%), and emphysematous cholecystitis (<1%).
7. Treatment
   a. Intravenous hydration and correction of electrolyte imbalance may be necessary.
   b. Antibiotics
      (1) They are not necessary in mild acute cholecystitis.
      (2) Coverage for gram-negative organisms can be initiated if severe or complicated cholecystitis is suspected (first-generation or second-generation cephalosporin is first choice).
      (3) Patients who have more severe complications or are toxic in appearance should be given broad-spectrum antibiotics, including anaerobic coverage.
   c. Cholecystectomy is the definitive treatment for acute cholecystitis and its complications.
      (1) This can usually be performed laparoscopically.
      (2) Cholecystectomy within 72 hours of symptom onset is optimal, but Cochrane review suggests no difference in outcomes if inter-

val cholecystectomy is delayed and performed 6–12 weeks after initial cool-down period.

(3) Patients who are immunosuppressed (steroid use, diabetes) should have immediate cholecystectomy.

(4) Delayed cholecystectomy (initial conservative management with intravenous fluids and antibiotics followed by cholecystectomy on an elective basis) is justified in some patients who are at high surgical risk.

(5) In patients who are not stable enough to undergo anesthesia, ultrasound or CT-guided percutaneous cholecystostomy with external drainage can be performed to decompress the gallbladder; this is followed by delayed cholecystectomy when the patient is more stable.

d. Intraoperative cholangiogram (IOC) can be helpful to define ductal anatomy when dissection is difficult due to inflammation or biliary tract variation.

IV. CHOLEDOCHOLITHIASIS

Choledocholithiasis is the occurrence of stones in the bile ducts.

A. CAUSATIVE FACTORS AND NATURAL HISTORY

1. Up to 15% of patients with gallstones have CBD stones.
2. Primary CBD stones (rare)
   a. Brown pigment stones often form as a result of bacterial action on phospholipids and bile and form de novo in the duct usually as a result of obstruction.
   b. Those with a history of biliary sphincterotomy are at greater risk.
3. Secondary CBD stones (more common)
   a. Cholesterol stones and black pigment stones form in the gallbladder and pass into the CBD.
4. CBD stones may remain asymptomatic for years and pass silently into the duodenum.
5. Laboratory values can be normal; however, increases in serum bilirubin, alkaline phosphatase, or amylase are often seen.

B. TREATMENT

Complications of CBD stones, such as acute pancreatitis or cholangitis, can be life threatening; therefore all stones, even if asymptomatic, require removal. For gallstone pancreatitis, removal of gallbladder during same admission, within 48 hours of admission, results in shorter hospital stay with no difference in technical difficulty of case and no apparent increase in complications despite pain level and lab values.

1. If choledocholithiasis is identified before cholecystectomy, there are two alternatives:
   a. Lap chole with IOC and either transcystic duct or direct CBD exploration results in fewer procedures and a shorter overall stay. The majority of CBD can be removed at the same setting as the lap chole.

b. Endoscopic retrograde cholangiography (ERC) with endoscopic papillotomy to clear the CBD before cholecystectomy is also acceptable.
   (1) Exceptions—suspicion of neoplasm, worsening pancreatitis, severe cholangitis, unfit for surgery
2. **When choledocholithiasis is identified on cholangiogram during cholecystectomy, there are three alternatives:**
   a. Laparoscopic transcystic duct or direct CBD exploration (success depends on experience of surgeon)
      (1) Initial attempt—transcystic approach via a cholangiography catheter. Glucagon may be given to relax the sphincter of Oddi and then saline irrigation to flush the stone from the CBD. If this fails, a balloon catheter may be passed into the duct, inflated, and pulled back to withdraw the stone. For proximal stones, it is possible to "milk" the stone back through the duct and have it exit the incision in the cystic duct. If this approach fails, the next attempt can be made with a wire basket catheter passed under fluoroscopy to catch the stones and extract them from the duct.
      (2) Last attempt—If the cystic duct is well dilated, a choledochoscope may be passed into the biliary tree, and under direct visualization the stones may be caught via a wire basket or pushed into the duodenum.
      (3) If stone extraction fails by all of the methods previously mentioned, open choledochotomy is required (T-tube or antegrade stent necessary).
   b. Convert to open procedure and perform CBD exploration.
      (1) Initial attempt—transcystic approach (as previous)
      (2) If fails, choledochotomy required (T-tube or antegrade stent is necessary)
   c. Complete cholecystectomy and ERC with endoscopic sphincterotomy to clear stones
      (1) Sphincterotomy is technically successful in 90% of patients.
      (2) Complete clearance of CBD stones is possible in only 70%–80% of patients.
      (3) In such cases, a second attempt at stone clearance may be necessary.
3. **Retained CBD stones**
   a. If T-tube is in place, cholangiogram can be performed 4–6 weeks after surgery, or earlier if obstructive symptoms occur, to evaluate for retained stones.
   b. If retained stones persist, they can be removed percutaneously using basket through a mature T-tube tract (4 weeks) under fluoroscopic control (>90% success rate). If no stones are retained, T-tube may be removed.
   c. Perform ERC with sphincterotomy or transduodenal "basket" removal of stones for unstable patients, malfunctioning T-tubes, or unsuccessful percutaneous extraction.
   d. Percutaneous transhepatic approach
   e. Reoperation

42

BENIGN GALLBLADDER AND BILIARY TREE

V. CHOLANGITIS

A. CAUSATIVE FACTORS AND PATHOPHYSIOLOGY

1. Eighty-five percent of cases are caused by impacted stone in the bile ducts, resulting in stasis of bile in the presence of bacteria.
2. Pus under pressure in the bile ducts leads to rapid bacteremia and sepsis.
3. Other causes include neoplasm, strictures, parasitic infections, and congenital abnormalities.
4. Most common organisms include *E. coli, Klebsiella, Pseudomonas,* enterococci, and *Proteus.*
   a. Anaerobic organisms (*Bacteroides* and *Clostridium)* in 15% of cases

B. CLINICAL FEATURES AND DIAGNOSIS

1. *Charcot triad* is fever (95%), RUQ pain (90%), and jaundice (80%).
   a. Full triad present in only 70% of cases
2. *Reynolds pentad* is Charcot triad plus altered mental status and hypotension.
   a. This occurs in severe suppurative cholangitis.
   b. Older patients may present solely with delirium or an altered mental status.
3. Intrahepatic abscess can present as a late complication.
4. Laboratory and radiographic evaluation
   a. Leukocytosis is common—A normal white blood cell count can be accompanied by a severe left shift.
   b. Bilirubin level is increased to more than 2 mg/dL in 80% of cases, although it can initially be normal.
   c. Serum alkaline phosphatase concentration is usually increased.
   d. RUQ ultrasound shows CBD dilatation in 75% of cases.
   e. Abdominal CT is useful in diagnosing such complications as abscess and pancreatitis.

C. TREATMENT

1. If suspected, blood cultures should be taken and antibiotics started as indicated for the severity of infection.
2. Aggressive resuscitation with intensive care unit admission is often necessary.
3. The patient's condition should improve within 6–12 hours of starting antibiotics, with defervescence, white blood cell count decline, and relief of discomfort occurring within 2–3 days.
4. If the patient's condition declines within 6–12 hours, immediate CBD decompression must be undertaken.
   a. ERC with endoscopic decompression, sphincterotomy, and stent placement is the treatment of choice (mortality rate of 5%–6%).
   b. Percutaneous transhepatic biliary drainage can also be used with reasonable success if ERC is unsuccessful or unavailable (mortality rate of 9%–16%).
   c. Emergency laparotomy with open CBD exploration is associated with high mortality rates (up to 50% mortality rate).

VI. ACALCULOUS CHOLECYSTITIS

A. EPIDEMIOLOGY AND PATHOGENESIS

1. Most cases occur in the setting of prolonged fasting, immobility, and hemodynamic instability.
   a. With prolonged fasting, the gallbladder is not stimulated by cholecystokinin to empty and bile stagnates in the lumen.
   b. Dehydration can lead to formation of extremely viscous bile, which may obstruct or irritate the gallbladder.
   c. Bacteremia may result in the seeding of the stagnant bile.
   d. Septic shock with resultant mucosal hypoperfusion can result in ischemia of the gallbladder wall.
2. Less commonly, it may occur in children, patients with vascular disease or systemic vasculitis, bone marrow transplant recipients, immunocompromised patients, and patients receiving cytotoxic drugs via the hepatic artery.

B. NATURAL HISTORY

1. Patients are often in the intensive care unit with multiple medical problems, resulting in a difficult and often delayed diagnosis.
2. By the time diagnosis is made, gangrene, perforation, empyema, bacterial superinfection, or cholangitis has occurred in 50% of patients.
3. Mortality rate is reported to be as high as 50%.

C. CLINICAL MANIFESTATION AND DIAGNOSIS

1. A high degree of suspicion is required.
2. RUQ tenderness is helpful but is absent in three-fourths of patients initially.
3. Fevers and hyperamylasemia are often the only signs.
4. Ultrasound
   a. Bedside availability is a major advantage in this setting.
   b. Thickened gallbladder wall (>4 mm) and pericholecystic fluid in the absence of hypoalbuminemia and ascites can be detected.
   c. Sonographic Murphy sign is reliable when the patient is cooperative.
   d. Sensitivity ranges between 62% and 90%; specificity is greater than 90%.
5. CT scan
   a. Gallbladder wall thickening, pericholecystic fluid, subserosal edema, intramural gas, and sloughed gallbladder mucosa can be detected.
   b. This often detects gallbladder disease in patients with a normal ultrasound.
   c. Patient must be stable enough to travel to the CT scanner.

D. TREATMENT

1. Cholecystectomy, laparoscopic or open, is the definitive treatment; however, patients are often too unstable.
2. Percutaneous cholecystostomy under radiographic guidance can be performed, followed by definitive cholecystectomy when the patient is stable.

BENIGN GALLBLADDER AND BILIARY TREE

42

VII. OTHER DISORDERS OF THE GALLBLADDER

A. GALLSTONE DISEASE IN PREGNANCY

1. Lap chole can be undertaken with minimal fetal and maternal morbidity.
2. Indications include severe biliary colic, acute cholecystitis, gallstone pancreatitis, and when the underlying disease poses a threat to the pregnancy.
3. Surgery traditionally is considered to be safest during the second trimester; however, several series demonstrate that lap chole is safe at all stages of pregnancy.

B. BILIARY DYSKINESIA

1. Delayed gallbladder emptying in the absence of stones or sludge is predictive of pain relief after cholecystectomy.
2. Low gallbladder ejection fraction also predicts outcome.
   a. Ejection fraction less than 35% is considered abnormal.
   b. Cholecystectomy improves symptoms 67%–90% of the time.
3. Both delayed emptying and gallbladder ejection fraction can be detected with HIDA scan.

C. BILIARY SLUDGE

1. Generally a complication of biliary stasis
2. Pathogenesis, natural history, and treatment—similar to gallstones
3. Commonly found in patients in the intensive care unit
4. Less chance of recurrence after single episode of colic

D. MIRIZZI SYNDROME

1. Stone impacted in the gallbladder neck or cystic duct compresses the common hepatic duct, resulting in bile duct obstruction and jaundice.
2. This is found in 1% of patients undergoing cholecystectomy.
3. It presents as recurrent bouts of abdominal pain, fever, and jaundice.
4. Ultrasound shows stones in a contracted gallbladder with moderate dilatation of the hepatic bile ducts.
5. Type I—compression of hepatic duct by large stone
   a. Subsequent inflammation can result in a stricture of the hepatic duct.
6. Type II—cholecystocholedochal fistula from stone erosion into the hepatic duct
7. Treatment
   a. Mirizzi syndrome type I—cholecystectomy with or without CBD exploration. If severe inflammation is present, perform partial cholecystectomy with postoperative endoscopic sphincterotomy to ensure clearance of CBD stones.
   b. Mirizzi syndrome type II—Perform partial cholecystectomy and cholecystocholedochoduodenostomy.

E. GALLSTONE ILEUS

Bowel obstruction resulting from impaction of gallstone in the intestinal lumen

1. Cause of obstruction in less than 1% of patients younger than 70 years; 5% in patients older than 70
2. Results from erosion of a large gallstone (>2.5 cm) into the intestinal lumen via a *cholecystenteric fistula*
   a. Most commonly into the duodenum but also can erode into the colon or stomach
3. Classic symptoms and signs of bowel obstruction (cramping abdominal pain, vomiting, abdominal distention, small bowel dilatation on radiograph)
4. Described as a *tumbling ileus*—as the stone passes through the length of the gut, symptoms wax and wane, intermittently obstructing the bowel lumen.
5. Complete obstruction generally occurs in the terminal ileum where the bowel lumen is the narrowest.
6. Pneumobilia is present on radiograph in 50% of patients.
7. *Bouveret syndrome*—gallstone impaction in pylorus or duodenum resulting in symptoms of gastric outlet obstruction
8. Ultrasound can confirm presence of gallstones and, on occasion, identify the fistula.
9. Treatment involves laparotomy with removal of the stone via a small enterotomy proximal to the point of obstruction.
   a. Resection is only necessary if perforation or ischemia
   b. The cholecystenteric fistula is left alone because many close spontaneously, and recurrence rate is only 5%.

F. EMPHYSEMATOUS CHOLECYSTITIS

1. Infection of the gallbladder wall with gas-forming bacteria, usually anaerobes
2. More common in individuals with diabetes and can rapidly progress to gangrene and perforation
3. Prompt cholecystectomy is imperative.

G. CALCIFIED "PORCELAIN" GALLBLADDER

1. Intramural calcification of the gallbladder wall
2. Seen on CT or abdominal radiograph
3. Gallbladder carcinoma in 20%
4. Prophylactic treatment with open or lap chole

VIII. MEDICAL TREATMENTS

A. ORAL DISSOLUTION THERAPY

1. Chenodeoxycholic acid is effective in reducing the ratio of cholesterol to bile salt.
2. Use for small (<10 mm), noncalcified cholesterol stones in patients with a functioning gallbladder.
3. Therapy takes 6–12 months.
4. Five-year recurrence rate is approximately 50%.

42

BENIGN GALLBLADDER AND BILIARY TREE

B. EXTRACORPOREAL SHOCK WAVE LITHOTRIPSY

1. This uses high-energy sound waves to physically fragment gallstones into pieces small enough to be passed into the duodenum.
2. Outcomes and overall effectiveness are no better than dissolution therapy alone.

IX. LAPAROSCOPIC CHOLECYSTECTOMY

Laparoscopic cholecystectomy is a safe and well-tolerated procedure with reduced perioperative morbidity and improved cost effectiveness when compared with the open approach.

A. SETUP

1. Antibiotics—Use first-generation cephalosporin or clindamycin. They may be unnecessary in uncomplicated biliary colic or cholecystitis.
2. Place patient on fluoroscopy-compatible table for possible IOC.

B. TECHNIQUE (FIGS. 42.1 AND 42.2)

1. Four trocars are traditionally placed (see Fig. 42.1).
   a. Veress or Hassan technique via infraumbilical or supraumbilical 11-mm port. Use an angled (30-degree) laparoscope for best visualization.
2. Assistant, standing on the right, elevates the gallbladder toward the ipsilateral diaphragm and retracts the infundibulum of the gallbladder toward the right hip.
3. Surgeon, standing on the left, dissects the cystic artery and duct from the gallbladder wall.
4. Dissection of the peritoneum over Calot triangle reveals the "critical view" (see Fig. 42.2D) where the cystic duct and artery can be seen at their junction with the gallbladder.
   a. This view is crucial to avoid inadvertently mistaking the CBD for the cystic duct or the right hepatic artery for the cystic artery.
5. Metallic clips are placed across the cystic duct at the gallbladder origin, and a small incision is made in the cystic duct for cholangiogram catheter placement.
   a. Cholangiography is performed to confirm ductal anatomy (difficult dissection, abnormal appearance of structures) or to exclude choledocholithiasis (increased liver function tests, history of pancreatitis or jaundice).
   b. If available, laparoscopic biliary ultrasound is also an effective modality for visualizing the biliary tree.
6. The cystic duct and artery are secured with metal clips and divided.
7. Gallbladder is dissected off the liver bed with cautery and removed in an EndoCatch bag via the periumbilical port.

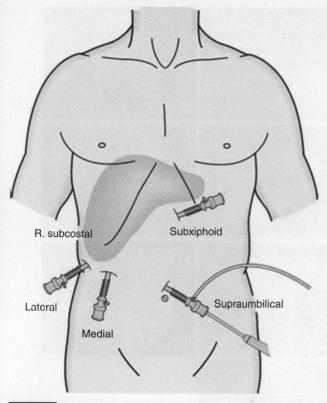

FIG. 42.1

Trocar placement for laparoscopic cholecystectomy. The laparoscope is placed through a 10-mm port just above the umbilicus. Additional ports are placed in the epigastrium and subcostal in the midclavicular and near the anterior axillary lines. (Reproduced from Cameron J. *Atlas of Surgery.* Vol. 2. Philadelphia: BC Decker; 1994.)

C. POSTOPERATIVE CARE

1. Patients can generally go home the day of surgery on a regular diet and mild oral analgesics.
2. Full physical activity can be resumed within 1 week.

D. COMPLICATIONS

1. Overall morbidity rate is 7%.
2. Operative mortality rate is 0.12%.
3. Bile duct injury occurs in 0.35% of cases.

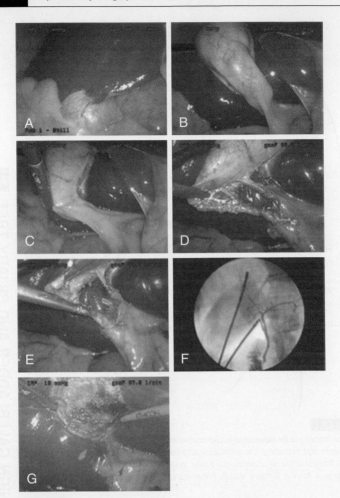

Laparoscopic cholecystectomy. (A) Gallbladder in situ. (B) Cephalad retraction of the fundus toward the right shoulder exposes the infundibulum of the gallbladder. (C) Retraction of the infundibulum toward the right lower quadrant opens up the hepatocystic triangle. The hepatocystic triangle is the area bordered by the cystic duct, gallbladder edge, and liver edge. (D) Division of the peritoneum overlying the anterior and posterior aspects of the hepatocystic triangle exposes "the critical view." (E) Cholangiogram catheter in the cystic duct. (F) Normal cholangiogram. (G) Gallbladder removed from the gallbladder fossa with electrocautery. (Reproduced with permission from Feldman M. *Sleisenger & Fordtran's Gastrointestinal and Liver Disease,* 8th ed. Philadelphia: Elsevier; 2006.)

RECOMMENDED READINGS

Aboulian A, Chan T, Yaghoubian A, et al. Early cholecystectomy safely decreases hospital stay in patients with mild gallstone pancreatitis. *Ann Surg.* 2010;251:615–619.

Gurusamy KS, Davidson C, Gluud C, Davidson BR. Early versus delayed laparoscopic cholecystectomy for people with acute cholecystitis. *Cochrane Database Syst Rev.* 2013;6:CD005440.

Hunter JG. Avoidance of bile duct injury during laparoscopic cholecystectomy. *Am J Surg.* 1991;162:71–76.

Malignant Gallbladder and Biliary Tree

Carey L. Watson, MD

Jaundice is a disease that your friends diagnose.
—William Osler

I. GALLBLADDER CANCER

A. GENERAL CONSIDERATIONS

1. In the United States, 1.2 cases per 100,000 people annually; world-wide, sixth most common gastrointestinal tumor and represents more than 80% of biliary tumors
2. Found in 0.1%–0.5% of all cholecystectomy specimens
3. Associated with gallstones in more than 90% of cases
4. Increased incidence in certain ethnic groups—Alaskan, Native Americans
5. Other factors—porcelain gallbladder, cholecystenteric fistulas, anomalous pancreaticobiliary junction, inflammatory bowel disease, Mirizzi syndrome
6. Male/female ratio of 1:2
7. Adenocarcinoma—most common cell type; 82% of cases
8. Grave prognosis, with 5-year survival rates of less than 5% in untreated patients and median overall survival less than 6 months; 50% of patients with lymph node disease at time of diagnosis

B. PRESENTATION

1. It is usually found incidentally at the time of elective cholecystectomy or advanced disease stage.
   a. Loss of clear dissection planes in the gallbladder bed or near the hilum is common.
2. Symptoms include right upper quadrant pain, jaundice, and symptoms secondary to metastasis.
3. Carcinoembryonic antigen (CEA) or cancer-associated antigen (CA) 19-9 may be increased.

C. TREATMENT

1. If carcinoma is suspected before surgery, perform open cholecystectomy with hepaticoduodenal lymphadenectomy; goal is R0 resection.
2. Carcinoma in situ and T1 tumors (invades lamina propria or muscle layer)
   a. Cholecystectomy alone is adequate therapy—survival rate approaches 100%.

3. T2 lesions (invades perimuscular connective tissue but not beyond serosa or into liver)
   a. Incidence rate of lymph node metastasis is 43%.
   b. Extended cholecystectomy with resection of gallbladder and portal lymph nodes
   c. Wedge resection of gallbladder bed (segments IVb and V) is also performed at some centers but remains controversial.
4. Locally advanced tumors, T3 (perforates serosa/invades liver and/or invades one other adjacent organ) or T4 (invades hepatic artery, portal vein, or multiple extrahepatic organs)
   a. Associated with long-term 5-year survival rates less than 5%
   b. Often present with lymph node or peritoneal metastasis and are therefore unresectable
   c. Some studies report improved 5-year survival rates as high as 21%–44% in patients who underwent radical resection with tumor-free margins.
5. Adjuvant chemoradiation therapy has been recently shown to be associated with improved survival in stages 1–3 disease independent of node status when reviewing data from the National Cancer Database.

II. BILE DUCT CANCER (CHOLANGIOCARCINOMA)

A. GENERAL CONSIDERATIONS
1. Rare cancer. Accounts for only 2%–3% of malignancies
2. Divided into intrahepatic or extrahepatic cholangiocarcinoma
3. Known risk factors for cholangiocarcinoma (causes of chronic inflammation of bile ducts: primary sclerosing cholangitis, choledochal cysts, chronic Salmonella typhi infection, and parasitic infections [liver flukes]).
4. CEA and CA 19-9 levels may be elevated and can be useful for postoperative surveillance.

B. INTRAHEPATIC CHOLANGIOCARCINOMA
1. This is the second most common liver cancer after hepatocellular carcinoma (HCC). It originates from intrahepatic bile ducts.
2. In most patients, the tumor is discovered incidentally.
3. Most patients do not have underlying liver disease.
4. On computed tomography (CT), it usually appears as a large hypovascular tumor with central necrosis. It is important to identify before surgery the extent of the portal vein or hepatic artery involvement. Magnetic resonance imaging (MRI) is often most helpful for anatomy and is superior when distinguishing between other hepatic lesions.
5. Biopsy is usually not helpful in immunohistochemistry (IHC). Pathology is rarely definitive. Rule out metastatic disease to liver because biopsy will usually show adenocarcinoma.
6. Resection with negative margins remains the only viable therapy. Chemotherapy or radiotherapy has not been shown to improve survival.

The presence of metastasis or regional lymph nodes outside the hepatoduodenal ligament is a contraindication to resection.

7. If patient has unresectable disease, consider palliative options, such as radiofrequency ablation (RFA), chemoembolization, or radiation.

C. EXTRAHEPATIC CHOLANGIOCARCINOMA

1. A total of 60%–70% arise in perihilar region (Klatskin tumors), 20%–25% arise in distal bile duct (periampullary), and less than 10% are multifocal.

2. Reported 5-year survival is a dismal 10%–20%.

3. Distal cholangiocarcinoma requires pancreaticoduodenectomy; perihilar cholangiocarcinoma requires resection of involved ducts with Roux-en-Y hepaticojejunostomy for both right and left ducts. If bile duct margins are positive, the surgeon must be prepared to do a hepatectomy. Preoperative planning is extremely important and can be complex.

4. Recent review of data from the National Cancer Database suggests that adjuvant chemoradiation after surgical resection in high-risk extrahepatic cholangiocarcinoma (with positive lymph nodes or positive margins) is associated with improved survival.

5. Unresectable disease treatment options:
   a. Palliative therapy: Goal is to relieve biliary obstruction with biliary drainage (stenting or percutaneous liver drains).
   b. Photodynamic therapy

RECOMMENDED READINGS

Hoehn RS, Wima K, et al. Adjuvant chemotherapy and radiation therapy is associated with improved survival for patients with extrahepatic cholangiocarcinoma. *Ann Surg Oncol.* 2015;22(suppl 3):S1133–S1139.

Hoehn RS, Wima K, et al. Adjuvant therapy for gallbladder cancer: an analysis of the National Cancer Data base. *J Gastroint Surg.* 2015;19:1794–1801.

Benign Liver Disease, Cirrhosis, and Portal Hypertension

Alex Chang, MD

> *The cruise director is the ship's liver . . . everything you can think of filters through you at some point.*
> —Willie Aames

Cirrhosis is the end-stage of chronic liver disease characterized by degeneration of the normal hepatic architecture and replacement with fibrosis. Clinically these patients present with loss of hepatocellular function, including coagulopathy, encephalopathy, and jaundice. The hepatocellular fibrosis causes increased resistance to transhepatic flow, leading to portal hypertension, ascites, varices, and a number of physiologic syndromes.

44

I. PATHOPHYSIOLOGY

1. Acute and chronic liver injury leads to generation of cytokines interleukin-1, interleukin-6, tumor necrosis factor (TNF)-α, transforming growth factor β-1, and epidermal growth factor.
2. Progressive destruction of hepatocytes, bile ducts, and vascular endothelial cells results in cellular proliferation, regeneration, and fibrous scar formation.
3. Activation of hepatic stellate cells (Ito cells) leads to proliferation, vitamin A depletion, fibrosis, contraction, and obliteration of the perisinusoidal space of Disse.

II. MORPHOLOGY

Fibrous septa seen in cirrhosis due to the accumulation of extracellular matrix divides hepatic regenerative nodules.

1. Micronodular—smaller than 3 mm, uniform nodules involving virtually every hepatic lobule indicative of early disease
2. Macronodular—nodules of varying sizes greater than 3 mm with irregular hepatocytes
3. Mixed—micronodular and macronodular present in equal proportions

III. ETIOLOGY

The etiology of cirrhosis in the United States is shown in Table 44.1.

1. *Alcohol* abuse is responsible for up to 30% of cases of cirrhosis in the United States. Characteristically, micronodular cirrhosis is seen in alcoholics. Metabolism of alcohol into acetaldehyde by alcohol dehydrogenase is responsible for the majority of cellular and biochemical damage.

TABLE 44.1

MOST COMMON CAUSES OF CIRRHOSIS IN THE UNITED STATES

Hepatitis C	33%
Alcohol	28%
NAFLD/cryptogenic	18%
Hepatitis B	15%
Miscellaneous	5%
Autoimmune	
Primary biliary cirrhosis	
Primary sclerosing cholangitis	
Metabolic liver disease	
Budd-Chiari syndrome	
Right heart failure	

NAFLD, Nonalcoholic fatty liver disease.

2. *Hepatitis B virus* (HBV)—chronic infection with HBV develops in less than 5% of acute HBV infections. Cirrhosis develops in 10%–20% of chronic HBV infections.

3. *Hepatitis C virus* (HCV)—75%–85% of infections become chronic, with a high rate of chronic hepatitis and 10%–15% incidence of cirrhosis. Treatment depends on virus genotype with success rates greater than 90% in genotype 1 with ledipasvir and sofosbuvir. Interferon- and ribavirin-based therapy are still used in genotype 3 HCV.

4. *Hepatitis D virus* (HDV)—an RNA virus, requires HBV to be pathologic. Superinfection with HBV and HDV has 80% incidence of cirrhosis.

5. *Nonalcoholic fatty liver disease* (NAFLD)—nonalcoholic steatohepatitis (NASH) develops in the background of insulin resistance, lipotoxicity, oxidative stress. Most cases of cryptogenic cirrhosis are thought to be due to end-stage NASH.

6. *Cholestasis*—Chronic obstruction of bile outflow from the liver due to intrahepatic or extrahepatic obstruction results in proliferation of the bile ducts, fibrosis, and biliary cirrhosis due to toxicity to hepatocytes.
   a. Intrahepatic cholestasis—primary biliary cirrhosis (associated with antimitochondrial antibodies), primary sclerosing cholangitis, lymphoma, amyloidosis, Alagille syndrome, and cystic fibrosis
   b. Extrahepatic cholestasis—choledocholithiasis, pancreatic cancer, cholangiocarcinoma, pancreatic and choledochal cystic disease, acquired immunodeficiency syndrome, bile duct strictures, biliary atresia

7. *Autoimmune hepatitis*—due to anomalous human leukocyte antigen (HLA) class II antigen on the surface of hepatocytes. It can be due to acute infection or genetic predisposition.

8. *Inheritable factors* implicated in cirrhosis include hemolytic anemia, cystic fibrosis, glycogen storage disease, α1-antitrypsin deficiency, hemochromatosis, and Wilson disease.

9. *Toxins*—Chemical exposure to carbon tetrachloride, beryllium, and vinyl chloride has been associated with cirrhosis.

TABLE 44.2

STIGMATA OF HEPATOCELLULAR FAILURE AND PORTAL HYPERTENSION

Stigmata of Hepatocellular Failure	Signs of Portal Hypertension
Jaundice	Ascites
Dark urine	Caput medusae
Muscle wasting	Splenomegaly
Purpura	"Venous hum" over right upper quadrant
Encephalopathy	Gastroesophageal varices
Spider angiomata	
Asterixis	
Gynecomastia	
Testicular atrophy	
Palmar erythema	
Loss of body hair	
Dupuytren contractures	

10. *Other* less common causes of cirrhosis include schistosomiasis, chronic parenteral nutrition, venoocclusive disease (right heart failure, constrictive pericarditis, Budd-Chiari syndrome).

IV. DIAGNOSIS

1. Clinical history
   a. Often consistent with common causes of cirrhosis, progressive unintentional weight gain or weight loss and fatigue. Patients with new coagulation abnormality, thrombocytopenia should be screened
2. Physical examination
   a. Frequently shows stigmata of hepatocellular failure or portal hypertension shown in Table 44.2
3. Laboratory evaluation
   a. Bilirubin
      (1) Direct hyperbilirubinemia is due to excess conjugated bilirubin caused by overproduction or underexcretion.
      (2) Indirect hyperbilirubinemia is an excess of unconjugated bilirubin primarily caused by enzymatic deficiency in conjugating bilirubin.
      (3) Clinical jaundice is apparent when total bilirubin level is greater than 2 mg/dL.
      (4) Conjugated bilirubin is water soluble and excreted by the kidney.
   b. Serum enzymes
      (1) Alkaline phosphatase
         (a) It is produced in bone, placenta, and liver.
         (b) It is excreted in bile.
         (c) Increased alkaline phosphatase can signal obstruction of bile ducts (in the absence of bone disease and pregnancy).
      (2) Transaminases—may be normal in long-standing disease, despite acute exacerbation
         (a) Aspartate aminotransferase (serum glutamic-oxaloacetic transaminase)

BENIGN LIVER DISEASE, CIRRHOSIS

44

(b) Alanine aminotransferase (serum glutamic-pyruvic transaminase)

(c) Alanine aminotransferase greater than aspartate aminotransferase in viral hepatitis

(d) Aspartate aminotransferase greater than alanine aminotransferase in alcoholic hepatitis

c. Serum proteins (measure synthetic function)

(1) Albumin—low level when hepatic function is impaired

(a) Coagulation factors

(i) Prothrombin time reflects adequate fibrinogen, prothrombin, and coagulation factor (V, VII, IX, X) production.

(ii) Prothrombin time is prolonged when fat absorption, and subsequent vitamin K absorption, is impaired (i.e., biliary obstruction, malnutrition, and hepatocellular insufficiency).

(iii) Thrombocytopenia, a common finding, is reflective of hypersplenism and portal hypertension.

4. Radiologic procedures

a. Ultrasound—may be 90% sensitive in diagnosing cirrhosis when the findings of multiple nodular irregularities along the ventral surface of the liver are demonstrated. Hepatic ductal anatomy may also be visualized.

b. Computed tomography/magnetic resonance imaging can assess size, ascites, and presence of varices.

c. Angiography—can directly measure hepatic artery pressures and define portal vein flow during the venous phase. Computed tomographic angiography can be useful in determining portal and systemic vessel patency, as well as hepatobiliary pathology.

d. Hepatic vein cannulation, see section VI

5. Percutaneous liver biopsy

a. Permits histologic diagnosis of fibrosis

b. Contraindications—coagulopathy, thrombocytopenia, cholangitis, tense ascites

c. Complications—bile leak or peritonitis, pneumothorax, bleeding, pain

6. Paracentesis

a. Relieves dyspnea and anorexia caused by increased intraabdominal pressure

b. Cytologic examination of ascitic fluid—can distinguish cause (cancer vs. cirrhosis) and diagnose spontaneous bacterial peritonitis

c. Complications—infection, bleeding, perforation of viscus

V. CLASSIFICATION

1. Child score

a. The Child-Turcotte-Pugh score was initially developed to determine risk of mortality in cirrhotics undergoing portal decompressive surgery and has been extrapolated to assess liver function and prognosticate risk with all surgical procedures.

  b. Cumulative score from Table 44.3 determines the Child classification and is correlated to risk of mortality after major surgery.

    (1) Child A = 5–7 points (2% mortality risk)

    (2) Child B = 8–10 points (10% mortality risk)

    (3) Child C ≥11 points (>50% mortality risk)

2. Model for End-Stage Liver Disease (MELD)

  a. The MELD scoring system was initially developed to predict 3-month mortality after transjugular intrahepatic portosystemic shunt procedure and is now used to prioritize organ allocations in the United States and Europe.

  b. The original model uses patient's serum bilirubin, creatinine, and international normalized ratio (INR) for prothrombin time.

  c. The MELD scoring system was updated in 2016 to the MELD-Na depending on the patient's serum sodium concentration, shown in Table 44.4.

  d. Patients undergoing hemodialysis twice weekly are given a creatinine value of 4.0, and patients with a serum bilirubin below 0.8 are given a bilirubin of 1.0 to ensure the sodium-MELD score remains a positive number.

VI. CONSEQUENCES OF CIRRHOSIS

It is important to understand that the liver is the "metabolic clearinghouse" and regulates almost every aspect of metabolism to appreciate the impact

TABLE 44.3
CHILD-TURCOTTE-PUGH MODIFIED CLASSIFICATION OF CIRRHOSIS

Characteristics	1 Point	2 Points	3 Points
Ascites	None	Controlled	Uncontrolled
Bilirubin (mg/dL)	<2.0	2.0–2.5	>3.0
Encephalopathy	None	Minimal	Refractory
Prothrombin time (s)	1–4	4–6	>6
Albumin (g/dL)	>3.5	3.0–3.5	<3.0

TABLE 44.4
MODEL FOR END-STAGE LIVER DISEASE

MELD Score

MELD score = $10 \times [(0.957 \times \ln (creatinine)) + (0.378 \times \ln (bilirubin)) + (1.12 \times \ln (INR))] + 6.43$

Sodium-MELD For Patients With Na Range 125–140 mmol/L

MELD-Na = $\text{MELD} - sodium \text{ (mmol/L)} - [0.025 \times \text{MELD} \times (140 - sodium \text{ (mmol/L)})] + 140$

INR, International normalized ratio; *MELD,* Model for End-Stage Liver Disease.

of cirrhosis. Although cirrhosis implies nothing about the state of hepatic function, a cirrhotic liver is metabolically dysfunctional. Alterations in liver function and physiologic changes due to increased hepatic venous resistance characterize the patient with cirrhosis.

1. **Portal hypertension**
   a. Pathophysiology
      (1) Obstruction to portal venous flow due to increased resistance through hepatic sinusoids
      (2) Hepatic vasoconstriction due to endothelin, norepinephrine, angiotensin, and depletion of nitric oxide and prostaglandins
      (3) Splanchnic vasodilation—multifactorial due to neurogenic, humoral, and local mediators
      (4) Systemic hyperdynamic circulation due to decreased systemic vascular resistance exacerbates splanchnic hyperemia
      (5) Hepatic venous pressure gradient (HVPG), defined as the difference between portal vein pressure and vena cava pressure, greater than 10 is diagnostic of portal hypertension regardless of clinical signs.
   b. Classification of portal hypertension by level of venous obstruction
      (1) Prehepatic (presinusoidal)—portal vein, superior mesenteric vein, splenic vein thrombosis, primary biliary cirrhosis, schistosomiasis, congenital hepatic fibrosis, and external compression
      (2) Intrahepatic (sinusoidal)—alcoholic, steatohepatitis, Wilson disease, posthepatitis cirrhosis, hemochromatosis
      (3) Posthepatic (postsinusoidal)—Budd-Chiari syndrome, vena caval web, right heart failure, and constrictive pericarditis
      (4) In the absence of obstruction, portal hypertension can occur with high flow states (i.e., arteriovenous fistula, massive splenomegaly).
   c. Diagnosis
      (1) Portal venography—obtained by venous phase imaging during mesenteric arteriography
         (a) Defines size and location of dilated veins and provides qualitative estimate of hepatic portal perfusion
         (b) Hepatopetal flow (away from liver) versus hepatofugal flow (toward liver)
      (2) Hepatic vein cannulation
         (a) Contrast injection can visualize portal vein if hepatopetal flow present
         (b) Used to determine adequacy of portal perfusion
      (3) Measurement of portal pressure
         (a) Direct—measured during operation or portal venography
         (b) Indirect—wedged hepatic vein pressure; compare with inferior vena caval pressure. HVPG can help to predict the risk of variceal bleeding or response to therapy aimed at reducing portal pressure.

2. Varices
   a. Depending on the severity of cirrhosis, 20%–70% of patients with cirrhosis have varices.
   b. Thirty percent of varices result in associated acute gastrointestinal bleeding.
   c. Mortality rate is 20%–50% for the initial bleeding episode.
   d. Of those who survive, 30% experience rebleeding within 6 weeks, and up to 70% rebleed within 1 year.
   e. Portal pressure is most commonly relieved through several venous routes.
      (1) Esophagogastric varices (esophageal venous plexus, coronary vein, splenophrenic, short gastric veins)
      (2) Abdominal wall (umbilical vein)
      (3) Hemorrhoidal (inferior mesenteric vein, veins of Retzius)
      (4) Diaphragm (diaphragmatic veins of Sappey and splenophrenic veins)
   f. Primary prophylaxis
      (1) Endoscopic screening should begin at the time of cirrhosis diagnosis and continue every 2–3 years. Once detected, small varices should be screened annually for progression.
      (2) Nonselective beta-blockers (NSBBs) are recommended for an HVPG 20% lower than baseline or less than 12 mm Hg.
      (3) Use H_2 blockers or proton pump inhibitor (PPI) therapy to neutralize stomach pH.
      (4) Perform endoscopic variceal ligation (EVL) for the presence of medium or large varices.
   g. Acute variceal bleeding
      (1) Bleeding is rare unless wedged hepatic venous pressure (WHVP) is greater than 12 mm Hg.
   h. Initial management is aimed at airway protection, nasogastric lavage, and early blood product resuscitation goal hemoglobin of 7–8 mg/dL.
   i. Balloon tamponade (Sengstaken-Blakemore, Minnesota tubes)
      (1) Gastric balloon is inflated with 200 mL of air and traction is pulled against the gastroesophageal junction.
      (2) Esophageal balloon may be inflated to 40 mm Hg if bleeding persists.
      (3) Initial control must be promptly followed by additional maneuvers because rebleeding occurs in 40%–70% and complications occur with prolonged use.
   j. Pharmacologic treatment
      (1) Administer octreotide 250 mcg intravenous (IV) bolus, followed by continuous infusion of 25–50 mcg/h for 5 days.
      (2) Administer vasopressin 20 units IV bolus followed by 0.2–0.4 units/min.
      (3) Pharmacologic control can be achieved in 50%–75% of patients.
   k. Antibiotic prophylaxis should be initiated at admission with oral quinolones in most patients and IV ceftriaxone in advanced cirrhosis or with history of quinolone-resistant bacteria.

44

BENIGN LIVER DISEASE, CIRRHOSIS

l. Early endoscopic therapy is recommended in all cases.
  (1) EVL is recommended in most cases, with endoscopic injection sclerotherapy reserved for technically difficult cases.
  (2) Injection with tissue adhesive (*N*-butyl-cyanoacrylate) is recommended for bleeding isolated gastric varices and type 2 gastroesophageal varices that extend beyond the cardia.
  (3) Complications include chest pain, esophageal perforation, ulceration, and bacteremia.

m. Transjugular intrahepatic portosystemic shunt (TIPS)
  (1) Preferred mode of portal decompression. Contraindications are listed in Table 44.5.
  (2) Ultrasound confirmation of patency of portal vein
  (3) Cannulation of hepatic vein via right internal jugular (usually right hepatic vein)
  (4) Passage of needle from hepatic vein into portal vein branch through the liver parenchyma
  (5) Seldinger technique used to pass guidewire from hepatic vein into portal vein branch, and subsequent dilation of needle tract and stent placement creating hepatic vein–portal vein fistula
  (6) Ninety percent success rate at controlling acute variceal hemorrhage; reported 10% rebleeding incidence rate
  (7) Complications include hepatic encephalopathy (25%) and accelerated liver failure (5%).

n. Surgical decompression
  (1) Total portosystemic shunt procedures involve decompression of the hypertensive portal circulation into the low-pressure systemic venous system.
    (a) Deprives the liver of important hepatotrophic growth factors and routes cerebral toxins directly into the systemic circulation
    (b) Principal complication is the development of accelerated hepatic failure and hepatic encephalopathy.
  (2) Nonselective shunts eliminate portal venous flow; they are most effective at controlling bleeding but are followed by a high rate of encephalopathy and hepatic failure.
    (a) Portacaval end-to-side shunt (Eck fistula) and side-to-side portacaval shunts are the gold standard by which other shunts are evaluated.

TABLE 44.5

CONTRAINDICATIONS TO TIPS PROCEDURE

Absolute Contraindications	Relative Contraindications
Congestive heart failure	Single hepatic cyst or central hepatoma
Severe pulmonary hypertension	Hepatic or portal vein thrombosis
Multiple hepatic cysts	Severe coagulopathy
Active infections or sepsis	Severe thrombocytopenia
Unrelieved biliary obstruction	

        (b) H-graft interposition shunts—mesocaval, portacaval, and
             mesorenal
             (i) Function depends on shunt diameter.
             (ii) Higher rates of thrombosis
        (c) Central splenorenal shunt (Linton shunt)
             (i) Includes splenectomy with anastomosis of portal side of
                 splenic vein to the left renal vein
             (ii) Physiologically and hemodynamically similar to a side-
                  to-side portacaval shunt
    (3) Selective shunts preserve portal venous flow while decompress-
        ing esophagogastric flow.
        (a) Distal splenorenal (Warren-Zeppa) shunt
             (i) Prototypical selective shunt used in United States.
                 Splenic vein ligated near hilum and end-to-side
                 anastomosis to left renal vein. Spleen remains in situ,
                 and the coronary vein is ligated.
             (ii) Varices are decompressed via the short gastric veins.
                  It decompresses the varices while maintaining portal
                  perfusion in 90% of patients.
             (iii) Operative mortality (7%–10%) and long-term survival
                   are similar to nonselective shunts in patients with
                   alcoholic cirrhosis. Survival seems to be improved in
                   patients with nonalcoholic cirrhosis.
             (iv) Possibly lower incidence of late hepatic failure and
                  encephalopathy compared with nonselective shunts.
             (v) Long-term survival (60% 5-year survival rate) after
                 distal splenorenal shunt is similar to that of endoscopic
                 sclerotherapy. Rate of rebleeding is greater in sclero-
                 therapy, whereas shunting may lead to progression of
                 liver dysfunction.
             (vi) Splenic vein must be greater than 7 mm in diameter,
                  and ascites must be absent or medically controlled.
    o. Esophageal devascularization (Sugiura procedure)
    p. Liver transplantation
       (1) Definitive treatment for portal hypertension and its complications
       (2) Avoid portacaval shunt in patients awaiting transplant—use
           banding, sclerotherapy, TIPS, or selective shunting when possible
           to preserve portal anatomy for transplant purposes.
3. **Ascites**
   a. Due to increased hydrostatic pressure, decreased intravascular
      oncotic pressure, and lymphatic outflow obstruction
   b. Secondary hyperaldosteronism
      (1) Caused by increased secretion and/or decreased inactivation of
          aldosterone by the impaired liver
      (2) Results in increased total body water and sodium caused by
          augmented sodium resorption in the distal tubule

BENIGN LIVER DISEASE, CIRRHOSIS

44

    c. Increased antidiuretic hormone secretion
      (1) Caused by relative hypovolemia, as detected by the carotid body and the central nervous system
      (2) Results in decreased free water clearance
    d. Initial management consists of low sodium diet (<2 g daily) and spironolactone 100 mg/day titrated up to 400 mg/day.
      (1) Loop diuretics may be added if spironolactone is ineffective alone; amiloride is an alternative agent if significant gynecomastia develops secondary to spironolactone.
    e. High-volume paracentesis
      (1) Relieves symptoms related to ascites including dyspnea and anorexia
      (2) Offers temporary relief because ascites always recurs unless liver dysfunction and portal hypertension are addressed
      (3) May require simultaneous albumin infusions to minimize the effects of volume shifts
      (4) Often used as a bridge to transplantation
    f. Surgical treatment of ascites
      (1) Peritoneovenous shunt is the treatment of choice if medical therapy fails.
      (2) It allows for drainage of peritoneal fluid directly into the superior vena cava.
      (3) LeVeen shunt is a one-way valve that opens when intraabdominal pressure exceeds 3 cm H_2O.
      (4) Denver shunt incorporates manual subcutaneous pump to prevent clogging.
      (5) Close monitoring for disseminated intravascular coagulation (DIC) is necessary after shunt placement; if DIC and coagulopathy cannot be corrected, shunt ligation is indicated.
      (6) Other complications include sepsis, congestive heart failure, hypokalemia, air embolism, vena cava thrombosis, and shunt malfunction.

4. Encephalopathy
    a. Characterized by altered consciousness, asterixis (flapping tremor elicited by wrist extension), rigidity, hyperreflexia, and electroencephalographic changes
    b. Seen in both acute and chronic hepatic dysfunction
    c. Due to abnormal circulation and metabolism of portal blood factors including ammonia, mercaptans, aromatic amino acids, and others
    d. NH_3 (easily absorbed and delivered to the liver via the portal circulation) is readily converted to NH_4, which is poorly absorbed, because of the change in colonic pH.
    e. Is often precipitated by gastrointestinal hemorrhage, portosystemic shunting procedures, spontaneous bacterial peritonitis (SBP) and other infection, excess protein in diet, constipation, narcotics, or sedatives.

f. Treatment includes neomycin 500 mg orally every 6 hours to alter intestinal flora production of ammonia, and lactulose 15–30 mL orally every 12 hours to mobilize organic acids in the colon.
g. Maintaining nutritional status in liver failure patients requires as much as 1.1 g protein/kg per day to maintain nitrogen balance.
h. HepatAmine (American McGaw) is a total parenteral formulation high in branched chain amino acids and low in aromatic amino acids; useful in patients at risk for hepatic encephalopathy

VII. HEPATIC SYNDROMES

1. Hepatorenal syndrome (HRS) results as oliguria, increased blood urea nitrogen and creatinine secondary to liver dysfunction; associated with poor prognosis
    a. Type 1 HRS—rapid onset; treatment includes relief of ascites, improvement in volume status, and improved renal perfusion
    b. Type 2 HRS—progressive onset; associated with liver dysfunction, portal hypertension with splanchnic vasodilation and renal vasoconstriction; characterized by a failure of kidneys to secrete sufficient sodium despite diuretic therapy
    c. Urine sodium excretion—typically less than 10 mEq/L
2. Pulmonary syndromes
    a. Hepatopulmonary syndrome (HPS)
        (1) Associated with widened alveolar arterial oxygen gradient greater than 20 mm Hg and intrapulmonary vasodilation
        (2) Insidious onset dyspnea especially while standing, digital clubbing, and cyanosis
        (3) Intrapulmonary nitric oxide regulation is implicated in HPS.
        (4) Supportive care with supplemental oxygen as a bridge to transplantation
        (5) Transplantation is curative in 80% of HPS.
    b. Portopulmonary hypertension (PPH)
        (1) It is associated with mild hypoxemia, pulmonary vasoconstriction, and right heart failure.
        (2) Treatment with IV prostacyclins may bridge patients to transplantation.

RECOMMENDED READINGS

Bosch J, Abraldes JG, Groszmann R. Current management of portal hypertension. *J Hepatol*. 2003;38:S54–S68.

de Franchis R. Revising consensus in portal hypertension: report of the Baveno V consensus workshop on methodology of diagnosis and therapy in portal hypertension. *J Hepatol*. 2010;53:762–768.

Garcia-Isao G, Bosch J. Management of varices and variceal hemorrhage in cirrhosis. *N Engl J Med*. 2010;362:823–832.

44

BENIGN LIVER DISEASE, CIRRHOSIS

Liver Tumors

Alex Chang, MD

Growth for the sake of growth is the ideology of the cancer cell.

—Edward Abby

Hepatic masses are commonly encountered because of increased frequency of advanced cross-sectional imaging. They range from benign to malignant, with and without underlying liver disease, and their management requires knowledge of the pathology, radiologic appearance, and clinical behavior of each lesion.

1. Solid liver lesions

   Important considerations when working up solid liver lesions are to differentiate between malignant and benign disease and, if benign (which is far more common), whether the patient needs any further follow-up or treatment.

   a. Benign lesions

      (1) Hemangioma—congenital tumor consisting of disorganized vasculature and fibrous tissue most commonly identified in the fourth to sixth decade, with a female to male ratio of at least 2:1

         (a) This is the most common benign tumor; prevalence rate is 7%–20% in ultrasound and autopsy series.

         (b) They are well-circumscribed, compressible lesions; 80% are less than 4 cm, although they may be much larger.

         (c) Majority are asymptomatic; rapid growth may cause compression of neighboring organs or pain due to stretching of Glisson capsule.

         (d) There is peripheral to central filling in contrast-enhanced computed tomography (CT) scanning.

         (e) Magnetic resonance imaging (MRI) is most sensitive and specific with the tumor enhancement on T2-weighted images. Cessation of hormonal contraception in female patients with asymptomatic hepatic hemangioma may be recommended.

         (f) Biopsy is contraindicated because of risk of bleeding.

         (g) It may be observed; resection or enucleation is indicated in symptomatic patients.

         (h) Transcatheter intraarterial embolization followed by surgical excision is the preferred approach to acute hemorrhage (rare) when resources are available.

         (i) Kasabach-Merritt syndrome is characterized by rare massive cavernous hemangioma associated with diffuse intravascular coagulopathy requiring urgent embolization or resection.

      (2) Focal nodular hyperplasia (FNH)

         (a) Second most common benign liver lesion

         (b) Incidence of 4%–8%, with a strong predilection for females

45

(c) Firm, hyperplastic, light-colored mass without a true capsule usually in the subcapsular parenchyma

(d) Disorganized hepatocytes and bile ductules with fibrous septa and areas of necrosis

(e) Radiographically seen as isoattenuated circumscribed mass with a central stellate hypoattenuated scar on unenhanced CT; arterial phase enhancement with small feeding vessels seen with delayed enhancement of the central scar

(f) Lacks malignant potential

(g) Surgical resection reserved for rare symptomatic cases or those that cannot be radiographically distinguished from hepatic adenoma (HA) or fibrolamellar carcinoma

(3) HA

(a) Rare lesion consisting of benign hepatocytes laden with glycogen and lipids

(b) Annual incidence approximately 1 in 1,000,000; 500-fold increased risk with longtime use of contraceptives; female to male ratio up to 11:1

(c) Usually solitary lesions 4–8 cm in size, although up to 30% may present with multiple lesions

(d) Well-defined lesions with isointense or hyperintense density on T1-weighted and T2-weighted imaging and arterial phase enhancement on contrast-enhanced MRI

(e) May be difficult to differentiate between FNH on cross-sectional imaging; technetium 99m sulfur colloid scan may be useful in these cases because adenomas are absent of Kupffer cells required for radiotracer uptake

(f) Low risk of rupture or malignant degeneration

(g) Surgical resection indicated in most cases, given diagnostic uncertainty and risk of malignancy

(h) Small lesions (<4 cm) may regress with cessation of oral contraceptives. Annual follow-up is required to confirm tumor response.

(i) Behavior of HAs during pregnancy is unpredictable, and resection before pregnancy is recommended.

b. Malignant lesions

(1) Metastatic disease

(a) Metastatic lesions are the most common malignant lesions in the liver. They most commonly originate from colorectal, lung, pancreas, breast, carcinoid, neuroendocrine, and urogenital cancers.

(b) In the course of disease, 50% of colorectal cancers will develop hepatic metastases.

(c) CT, positron emission tomography, and tumor marker carcinoembryonic antigen (CEA) are helpful in the diagnosis of metastatic disease.

45

LIVER TUMORS

    (d) It most commonly appears as hypoattenuated mass on portal phase with ringlike peripheral enhancement in arterial phase contrast-enhanced CT.

    (e) Hypervascular metastases are renal cell carcinoma, carcinoid tumors, adrenal tumors, thyroid carcinoma, pancreatic islet cell tumors, and neuroendocrine tumors.

    (f) Resection of select synchronous and metachronous colorectal metastases to the liver provides survival benefit in large series.

    (g) Resection for questionably resectable lesions should be reconsidered after systemic chemotherapy and restaging.

    (h) Portal vein embolization can be used in patients with inadequate hepatic reserve to tolerate resection.

    (i) Radiofrequency ablation (RFA) should be considered for patients unfit for surgery.

    (j) Oligometastases may require a combined approach with resection and RFA or systemic chemotherapy before resection to achieve an R0 resection.

(2) Primary hepatocellular carcinoma (HCC)

    (a) Incidence is up to six cases per 100,000 people in the United States, with a male to female ratio of 3:1.

    (b) Most common risk factor is cirrhosis of any etiology, most frequently chronic hepatitis C virus infection with 3%–7% increased annual risk of HCC.

    (c) Patients may present with anorexia, weight loss, lethargy, nausea, right upper quadrant pain, and symptoms related to cirrhosis, such as ascites, jaundice, and encephalopathy.

    (d) α-Fetoprotein (AFP) level is increased in approximately 75% of HCCs, but it is nonspecific and related to size.

    (e) AFP >200 ng/mL together with an imaging study showing a hypervascular mass is considered diagnostic of HCC.

    (f) Screening with hepatic ultrasound and AFP determination is recommended in high-risk patients.

    (g) Cross-sectional imaging appearance of HCC may vary. Typical characteristics include arterial enhancement with early washout.

    (h) Percutaneous biopsy of a suspicious lesion should be performed with caution because of the risk for needle seeding (approximately 2%).

    (i) Treatment options include resection, liver transplantation, ethanol or FRA, or chemoembolization. Treatment consensus is commonly based on the Barcelona Clinic Liver Cancer staging system, which stratifies patients based on degree of liver disease and stage of tumor burden.

    (j) Child A and early B patients are offered resection, and late B and C patients are best treated by transplantation.

(k) Liver transplantation has been historically reserved for patients within the Milan criteria, defined as a single tumor less than 5 cm or up to three tumors with none being greater than 3 cm and absence of macrovascular invasion.

(l) Locoregional therapy for HCC, including RFA, transarterial chemoembolization (TACE), microwave ablation, percutaneous ethanol injection, cryotherapy, and transarterial yttrium 90 microsphere therapy, is increasing in popularity; however, results have yet to be validated in large series.

(m) Fibrolamellar carcinoma is a variant of HCC more frequent in young women. It is not associated with underlying liver disease, and AFP is usually normal. Complete surgical resection is the treatment of choice.

(3) Intrahepatic cholangiocarcinoma (CCA)

(a) This is second most common primary hepatic malignancy.

(b) It is derived from progenitor cells giving rise to intrahepatic bile ducts.

(c) Cirrhosis is the only known risk factor, although most cases are not associated with underlying liver disease.

(d) Poor prognosis compared with HCC because of common asymptomatic presentation with advanced disease.

(e) Biopsy is necessary to differentiate CCA because lesions appear hypointense on contrast-enhanced studies.

(f) Surgical resection is the only effective therapy, with 5-year survival ranging from 25%–31% after an R0 resection with no vascular invasion. Lymph node positivity portends a poor prognosis.

2. **Cystic liver lesions**

Cystic lesions of the liver are common, and the vast majority of cystic lesions are benign.

a. Benign lesions

(1) Simple hepatic cyst

(a) Congenital lesion with no malignant potential

(b) Rarely becomes symptomatic

(c) Large dominant cysts occasionally become symptomatic and require surgical resection or marsupialization.

(d) Polycystic liver disease (PCLD) is an autosomal dominant disease with variable penetrance ranging from asymptomatic cysts to disabling cystic hepatomegaly; treatment with liver transplantation is reserved for refractory symptoms or liver dysfunction.

(2) Hepatic cystadenoma

(a) Hepatic cystadenomas arise from the biliary epithelium.

(b) It accounts for 5% of all cystic liver lesions.

(c) It usually is a single, large tumor presenting with abdominal pain or discomfort because of the size of the lesion.

45

LIVER TUMORS

    (d) Ultrasonography shows a fluid-filled cyst with irregular margins, septations, and mural nodules.

    (e) Treatment with surgical resection is indicated if symptomatic or when indistinguishable from cystadenocarcinoma.

(3) Mesenchymal hamartoma

    (a) It is an uncommon benign lesion composed of bile ducts and immature mesenchymal cells.

    (b) It may appear multiseptated and be indistinguishable from biliary cystadenoma.

    (c) Most occur in childhood and progressively increase in size, although spontaneous regression is possible. Malignant transformation is rare.

    (d) Treatment is surgical resection.

(4) Infectious cystic lesions

    (a) Pyogenic liver abscess

       (i) It results from bacterial infection of the liver parenchyma.

      (ii) Most common cause is ascending cholangitis, followed by pyelophlebitis (complicated appendicitis, diverticulitis, pancreatitis, inflammatory bowel disease), trauma, or causes of abdominal sepsis.

     (iii) A total of 20%–45% occur with no clear causative factor.

     (iv) Most common organisms are aerobic gram-negative (*Escherichia coli*, *Klebsiella* spp., *Enterococcus* spp.), *Streptococcus* spp., *Staphylococcus aureus*, and anaerobes (*Bacteroides* spp., *Clostridia*). Fungal abscesses are common in immunocompromised patients.

      (v) Blood cultures are negative in up to half of patients.

     (vi) Patients present with acute to subacute symptoms, including fever, right upper quadrant pain, and hepatomegaly.

    (vii) Characteristic contrast CT appearance is that of a round or irregularly shaped hypoattenuating mass with a peripheral capsule that shows enhancement.

   (viii) Treatment includes broad-spectrum antibiotics followed by percutaneous drainage and treatment of the underlying cause, if identified.

    (ix) Surgical drainage is reserved for those who fail percutaneous drainage or have multiloculated abscesses unamenable to percutaneous drainage.

     (x) Mortality rates are 2%–6% in most cases but can be as high as 30%–43% if patient presents with ruptured hepatic abscess.

    (b) Amebic abscess

       (i) Caused by *Entamoeba histolytica,* which travels to the liver from the intestines via the portal blood

(ii) Patients often have recent travel history to tropical areas.

(iii) Occurs in up to ⅓ of patients with amebic colitis

(iv) Presents with acute onset right upper quadrant pain, fever, anorexia, and acute colitis

(v) Appears as solitary, round, hypoattenuating mass with an enhancing ring on CT, most commonly in the right lobe

(vi) Diagnosis confirmed by serum indirect hemagglutination assay

(vii) Treatment with metronidazole (750 mg 3 times a day for 5–10 days); effective in 95% of cases

(c) Echinococcal cysts

(i) Hydatid disease is caused by the dog tapeworm *Echinococcus granulosus*, with sheep being the usual intermediate host.

(ii) Ingestion of contaminated foods allows for ova to travel to the portal circulation, to the liver (50%–77%), and subsequently lungs (10%–40%), brain, and bones.

(iii) Cysts consist of a germinal and laminar layer that are surrounded by a fibrous capsule, which becomes calcified in 50% of cases. It may present as a palpable hepatic mass.

(iv) Hepatocytes undergo liquefactive necrosis resulting in a pus-filled cavity appearing as "anchovy paste."

(v) Classic ultrasonographic or CT findings are a thick, often calcified, cyst wall and with internal daughter cysts.

(vi) Diagnosis is made by enzyme-linked immunosorbent assay or indirect hemagglutination tests. Eosinophilia is present in 40% of cases.

(vii) Medical therapy with albendazole has a low success rate (<30%), and definitive therapy requires complete surgical excision of living parasites, including removal of the active cyst lining or liver resection.

(viii) The operative field must be protected from spillage, and the remaining cavity after aspiration may be injected with ethyl alcohol or 20% sterile saline to kill remaining parasite. This should be avoided if biliary involvement is suspected.

(ix) Rupture or surgical spillage of cyst contents into the peritoneal cavity may cause anaphylaxis and development of multiple intraabdominal cysts.

(x) Percutaneous techniques (puncture, aspiration, injection, and reaspiration [PAIR]) may be attempted in poor surgical candidates.

b. Malignant lesions
   (1) Cystadenocarcinoma
       (a) Biliary cystadenocarcinoma accounts for a minority of cystic hepatic lesions.
       (b) It typically presents in middle-aged women and can vary greatly in size from 1.5 to 30 cm.
       (c) It can occur from malignant degeneration of cystadenoma or de novo.
   (2) Cystic HCC
       (a) Results from central necrosis, systemic, or local treatment of HCC
   (3) Cystic metastases
       (a) Mucinous adenocarcinomas from colorectal or ovarian origin may present with metastases to the liver.
       (b) Treatment follows similar guidelines as solid metastatic disease.

RECOMMENDED READINGS

Blumgart LH, ed. *Surgery of the Liver and Biliary Tract*. 5th ed. Philadelphia: Saunders; 2012.
Cameron JL, ed. *Current Surgical Therapy*. 11th ed. Philadelphia: Saunders; 2013.
Lee JKT, Sagel SS, Stanley RJ, Heiken JP, eds. *Computed Body Tomography With MRI Correlation*. 4th ed. Lippincott Williams & Wilkins; 2006.

PART VIII

Transplant Surgery

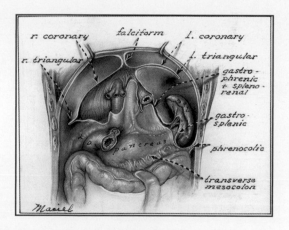

Renal Transplantation

Alexander Cortez, MD

Post-operatively the transplanted kidney functioned immediately with a dramatic improvement in the patient's renal and cardiopulmonary status. This spectacular success was a clear demonstration that organ transplantation could be life-saving.

—Joseph Murray, MD

I. GENERAL CONSIDERATIONS

A. HISTORY AND EPIDEMIOLOGY

1. First kidney transplant performed between identical twins by Joseph Murray in 1954
2. Early transplantation halted by lack of adequate immunosuppression
   a. Initially attempted total body irradiation and mercaptopurine (6-MP), which had significant toxicity
   b. Steroids and azathioprine initiated in 1960s opened the door to further efforts due to more acceptable maintenance regimens.

B. IMMUNOLOGY OF RENAL TRANSPLANTATION

1. ABO antigens: required for organ transplantation; ABO antigens behave as strong antigens and incompatibility may lead to irreversible hyperacute rejection
2. Human leukocyte antigen (HLA) matching
   a. Class I antigens (A, B, C) are located on all nucleated cell membranes.
   b. Class II antigens (DP, DQ, DR) are located on immune, dendritic, and endothelial cell membranes.
   c. In transplant, the most important major histocompatibility genes are HLA-A, HLA-B, and HLA-DR.
3. Panel-reactive antibody
   a. Patient's serum is incubated with B and T cells from a panel of donors selected to represent HLA antigens commonly found in the local population.
   b. Results are expressed as the percentage of panel cells that are killed by the serum.
   c. Result of 60% panel-reactive antibodies suggests that 60% of donors will be unacceptable for the patient because there are circulating antibodies that react with one or more of the donor's HLA antigens.

C. IMMUNOSUPPRESSION

1. Corticosteroids—work via cytoplasmic binding of DNA that prevents production of cytokines, resulting in lymphocyte depletion, impaired immune activation, and broad antiinflammatory effects

2. Calcineurin inhibitors (cyclosporine and tacrolimus [Prograf])—inhibit interleukin-2 (IL-2) production
3. Antimetabolites
   a. Mycophenolate mofetil (CellCept)—inosine monophosphate dehydrogenase (IMPDH) inhibitor that disrupts de novo synthesis of purines in lymphocytes
   b. Azathioprine—purine analog that interferes with DNA and RNA synthesis
4. Mechanistic target of rapamycin (mTOR) inhibitors (sirolimus and everolimus)—inhibits lymphocyte response to IL-2
5. Monoclonal and polyclonal antibodies
   a. Antithymocyte globulin (thymoglobulin)—rabbit-derived antibodies against human T and B cells
   b. Muromonab-CD3 (OKT3)—anti-CD3 on T cells
   c. Belatacept—binds to cytotoxic T lymphocyte–associated protein 4 (CTLA-4) on T cells to halt costimulation and subsequent T-cell activation
   d. Rituximab—anti-CD20 on B cells; used for antibody-mediated rejection
   e. Basiliximab and daclizumab—anti-CD25 of IL-2 receptor on T cells

II. EVALUATION OF CANDIDATES FOR TRANSPLANTATION

A. INDICATIONS
1. For end-stage renal disease, transplantation offers best long-term outcomes among renal replacement options.
2. Patient life expectancy is longer than expected graft life (i.e., avoid patients dying before graft fails).

B. ABSOLUTE CONTRAINDICATIONS—ULTIMATELY THESE ARE CENTER SPECIFIC
1. Active, untreated malignancy (except nonmelanocytic skin cancer and incidental renal cell carcinoma)
2. Active infection
3. Uncontrolled cardiopulmonary disease
4. Acute viral hepatitis

C. RELATIVE CONTRAINDICATIONS
1. Ongoing substance abuse issues
2. Poorly controlled psychiatric illness
3. History of noncompliance
4. Untreated human immunodeficiency virus (HIV) (no longer an absolute contraindication as a result of highly active antiretroviral therapy [HAART] treatment outcomes)
5. Renal diseases with high recurrence rates

D. PATIENT EVALUATION
1. Patients with glomerular filtration rate (GFR) ≤30 (chronic kidney disease [CKD] stage 4) should be referred to a nephrologist for transplant evaluation.

2. Detailed history and physical examination with special emphasis on:
   a. Underlying renal disease
   b. Estimated urine output and dialysis needs
   c. Medical history, namely cardiovascular
   d. Screening for previously mentioned contraindications
3. Once GFR is less than 20, transplantation should be pursued.

E. INDICATION FOR PRETRANSPLANT NATIVE NEPHRECTOMY
1. Chronic renal parenchymal infection
2. Infected stones or reflux
3. Heavy proteinuria
4. Intractable hypertension
5. Polycystic kidney disease that is massive, recurrently infected, or bleeding
6. Suspicion of adenocarcinoma

III. KIDNEY DONATION

A. LIVING DONOR KIDNEY TRANSPLANTATION
1. Increases number of available organs for transplantation
2. Risks of donation
   a. Mortality rate after donor nephrectomy is estimated at 0.03%.
   b. Reoperation rate and readmission rates are less than 1% each.
   c. Incidence of other postoperative complications approximates 3%.
3. Exclusion criteria for living kidney donation—ultimately these are center specific.
   a. Inadequately treated psychiatric disease or active substance abuse
   b. Evidence of renal disease
   c. Abnormal renal anatomy
   d. Recurrent or bilateral nephrolithiasis
   e. Obesity, diabetes, hypertension, or significant cardiopulmonary disease
   f. Active infection or malignancy
   g. Hereditary hypercoagulable disorder

B. CLASSICALLY DEFINED DONOR CATEGORIES
1. Standard criteria donor (SCD)
2. Extended criteria donor (ECD)
   a. Donors older than 60 years
   b. Donors aged 50–59 years with two additional risk factors, including hypertension (HTN), death from cerebrovascular accident (CVA), or increased serum creatinine (Cr) greater than 1.5 mg/dL
   c. ECD kidneys have 70% increased risk of failure within 2 years when compared with SCD kidneys.
3. Donor after cardiac death (DCD)
   a. Health care team determines that recovery is unlikely and maintains donor life on ventilator.
   b. Ventilator is disconnected in operating room and if heart stops beating within designated time frame, procurement proceeds.

46

RENAL TRANSPLANTATION

4. Kidney Donor Profile Index (KDPI)—newer scoring system that incorporates a variety of donor factors into a single number that summarizes the likelihood of graft failure after deceased donor kidney transplantation
   a. Lower scores are associated with longer estimated function, and higher scores are associated with shorter estimated function.
   b. Factors include age, weight, height, race, cause of death, history of diabetes mellitus (DM) and HTN, hepatitis C virus (HCV) status, baseline Cr, and DCD status.

IV. SPECIFIC OPERATIVE CONSIDERATIONS

A. LIVING DONOR NEPHRECTOMY

1. Left kidney is preferred because of longer renal vein.
2. Laparoscopic ± hand-assist nephrectomy is preferred technique at most centers.
3. Colon is reflected medially, and the liver or spleen is retracted away from the kidney.
4. Renal artery and vein are carefully identified and divided with a vascular stapler (clips avoided given concern for falling off and postoperative hemorrhage).
5. Ureter is ligated distally, and kidney is brought out through hand port or Pfannenstiel.
6. Kidney is flushed with preservation solution, placed on ice, and transported.

B. TRANSPLANT PROCEDURE

1. Kidney is placed in pelvic cavity (heterotopic) because of less surgical burden and easier access for evaluation after transplant (i.e., biopsy).
2. Right iliac fossa favored for transplant site because vessels are more superficial.
3. Oblique incision cranial to inguinal ligament—muscles are spared and linea semilunaris divided so that peritoneum can be retracted medially to expose the iliac vessels.
4. Donor vessels are generally anastomosed to recipient external iliac vessels in end-to-side fashion.
5. Ureteral anastomosis should include a 1-cm submucosal tunnel to prevent reflux using tension-free, watertight sutures.

V. POSTOPERATIVE CONSIDERATIONS

A. POSTOPERATIVE CARE

1. Monitoring of hourly urine output is important to determine early degree of graft function.
2. Avoid volume depletion caused by posttransplant diuresis by providing fluid replacements.
3. Central venous pressure (CVP) monitoring is a useful guide to intravascular volume status.

4. Closely monitor electrolyte abnormalities.
5. Foley catheter is left in place for 2–5 days after surgery, depending on recipient bladder size and function.

B. ASSESSMENT OF GRAFT FUNCTION
1. Urine output: Decreased urine output may indicate hypovolemia, urinary obstruction, ureteral compromise, vascular compromise, acute tubular necrosis, or rejection.
   a. Less reliable if native kidney made urine prior to transplant
2. Creatinine: Decrease in Cr indicates graft function even if patient made urine preoperatively.
3. Ultrasound demonstrates patency of artery and vein and detects fluid collection and hydronephrosis.
   a. Renal ultrasound is first step following finding of postoperative laboratory abnormality.
4. Renal biopsy may yield definitive pathologic diagnosis in cases of dysfunction.

C. COMPLICATIONS
1. Wound infection (1%–10%)
2. Delayed graft functioning (DGF): defined as a dialysis requirement within the first week after transplantation
3. Bleeding: more commonly related to anticoagulation or coagulopathy than technical error
   a. May present as decreased urine output as a hematoma develops and causes graft compression
   b. Hemorrhage and shock: less common in kidney transplants
4. Graft thrombosis (<1%)
   a. Most devastating complication because usually results in graft loss
   b. Occurs within first week after transplant
   c. Presents as sudden cessation in urine output and a rapid increase in creatinine
   d. Risk factors include hypercoagulopathy, peripheral vascular disease (PVD), procurement damage or intimal damage, or vessel kinking.
   e. Diagnosed by Doppler ultrasound
5. Lymphocele (1%–18%)
   a. Many are asymptomatic; may present with mass effect or lymph fistula
   b. Diagnosed by ultrasound
   c. Definitively treated by creating an intraperitoneal window
      (1) Percutaneous drainage may contain fluid leak, as well as differentiate lymphocele (elevated triglyceride) from urinoma (elevated Cr)
6. Renal artery stenosis (1%–23%)
   a. Usually occurs 3 months to 2 years after transplantation
   b. Presents with refractory hypertension or unexplained increase in creatinine

46

RENAL TRANSPLANTATION

    c. Diagnosed by Doppler ultrasound or angiography

    d. Percutaneous transluminal balloon angioplasty offers the safest mode of treatment.

7. **Ureteral stricture (2%–15%)**

    a. This is most common urinary complication, usually the result of obstruction (hematoma, kinking, edema, etc.).

    b. Late-onset obstruction is related to fibrosis from ischemia or BK viremia.

    c. It manifests as oliguria, increased creatinine, and potentially sepsis.

    d. Management includes percutaneous nephrostomy, percutaneous dilation and stenting, and surgical revision.

8. **Urine leak (3%–10%)**

    a. Related to ureteral ischemia and anastomotic tension

    b. Usually occurs in the first month after transplant

    c. Presents with pain, graft swelling, fever, sepsis, and urine fistula

    d. Treatment of percutaneous nephrostomy and stenting or operative revision

9. **Malignancy**

    a. Immunosuppression predisposes to the development of malignancy.

    b. Incidence of nonskin malignancies in renal transplant recipients is up to $3.5\times$ greater than that of age-matched control subjects.

    c. Posttransplant lymphoproliferative disorder (PTLD) and Kaposi sarcoma tend to occur early after transplant; other tumors tend to occur later.

VI. OUTCOMES

A. SURVIVAL BENEFIT OF RENAL TRANSPLANTATION

1. Kidney transplantation offers improved quality of life and increased cost effectiveness compared with dialysis.

2. Survival benefit of transplantation versus remaining on the waiting list (Fig. 46.1)

    a. In the early period after transplant, the risk of death is greater for transplant recipients than for waitlisted patients.

    b. Within a short period, the risk of death and chances of survival equalize, and thereafter transplantation has a persistent survival benefit.

3. The longer a patient receives dialysis, the greater the risk for posttransplant morbidity, mortality, and graft loss.

B. SURVIVAL

1. Graft versus patient survival (Fig. 46.2)

2. Kidney graft survival at 1, 5, and 10 years, respectively:

    a. Living donor: 96%, 81%, 58%

    b. SCD: 92%, 70%, 44%

    c. ECD: 85%, 55%, 26%

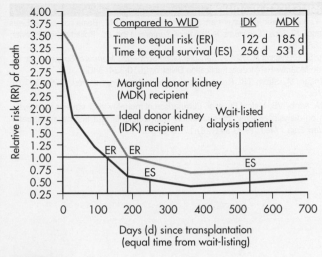

FIG. 46.1

Relative risk of death after kidney transplant compared with remaining on waiting list.

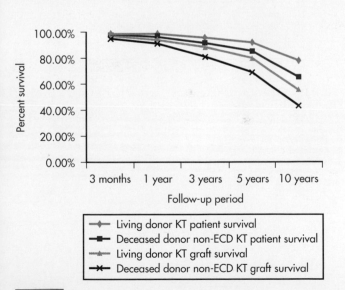

FIG. 46.2

Survival after kidney transplant (KT). *ECD,* Extended criteria donor.

RECOMMENDED READINGS

Becker Y. Kidney and pancreas transplant. In: Townsend CM, Beauchamp RD, Evers BM, Mattox KL, eds. *Sabiston's Textbook of Surgery*. 19th ed. Philadelphia: Elsevier; 2012:666–681.

Schwartz SI, Brunicardi FC. *Kidney Transplantation Schwartz's Manual of Surgery*. 10th ed. New York: McGraw-Hill Medical Publication Division; 2010:334–340.

Suthanthiran M, Strom TB. Renal transplantation. *New Engl J Med*. 1994;331(6): 365–376.

Wolfe RA, Ashby VB, Milford EL, et al. Comparison of mortality in all patients on dialysis, patients on dialysis awaiting transplantation, and recipients of a first cadaveric transplant. *New Engl J Med*. 1999;341(23):1725–1730.

Liver Transplantation

Peter L. Jernigan, MD

Liver, brain and heart, these sovereign thrones.

–William Shakespeare

I. GENERAL CONSIDERATIONS

A. HISTORY

1. 1967—Starzl performed the first successful liver transplant.
2. 1983—Venovenous bypass was introduced for use during anhepatic phase; cyclosporine was approved for transplant immunosuppression.
3. 1984—Broelsch and associates introduced the reduced-size liver transplantation.
4. 1989—first successful living related transplant
5. 1998—first successful living donor transplant to adult recipient
6. Approximately 7000 liver transplants are currently performed yearly in the United States.

B. INDICATIONS AND LISTING PROCESS FOR TRANSPLANTATION

1. Acute liver failure and complications of cirrhosis (ascites, spontaneous bacterial peritonitis, encephalopathy, variceal hemorrhage, synthetic dysfunction, portal hypertension, hepatocellular carcinoma [HCC])
2. Metabolic disease with systemic manifestations (α1-antitrypsin deficiency, familial amyloidosis, glycogen storage disease, hemochromatosis, Wilson disease, primary oxaluria)
3. Systemic complications of chronic liver disease (hepatopulmonary syndrome, hepatorenal syndrome, portopulmonary hypertension)
4. Organs distributed by United Network for Organ Sharing (UNOS) based on patient's Model for End-stage Liver Disease (MELD) score
   a. Scoring system from 6 to 40 that estimates 3-month survival (90% survival for MELD = 6, 7% for MELD = 40) without liver transplant
   b. Based on creatinine, sodium, bilirubin, and international normalized ratio
   c. Exception points for HCC start at 28 after 6-month observation on waiting list to assess tumor biology (maximum 36)
5. UNOS previously used Child-Turcotte-Pugh score (total bilirubin, serum albumin, prothrombin time, ascites, encephalopathy) for liver allocation but replaced it with MELD score in 2006.

C. SPECIFIC INDICATIONS

1. Viral hepatitis
   a. Type A, B, and C (HAV, HBV, HCV, respectively) may all be associated with fulminant hepatic failure, but this is most common with HAV and uncommon overall.

b. HCV most commonly causes cirrhosis and chronic liver failure—most common indication for liver transplant in the United States

c. Positive HBV or HCV titers at time of transplant are associated with high risk for recurrence. Antiviral therapy with sustained viral response is associated with similar 5-year survival after transplant as nonviral cirrhosis.

2. Acute fulminant hepatic failure—secondary to drug toxicity, hepatitis, metabolic disease, pregnancy, Budd-Chiari syndrome, mushroom intoxication, and others. Acetaminophen toxicity is the most common cause.

3. Biliary disease—primary biliary cirrhosis, primary sclerosing cholangitis, extrahepatic biliary atresia (most common causative factor in children)

4. HCC
   a. Multifocal disease is common in cirrhotic liver. Criteria for transplant vary by center, but Milan criteria are commonly used: 1 nodule ≤5 cm or ≤3 nodules of 3 cm or less.
   b. Unresectable HCC in a noncirrhotic liver may be indication for transplant, even outside Milan criteria.
   c. Treatment for HCC may include neoadjuvant therapy or other procedures to downstage disease before transplantation.

D. CONTRAINDICATIONS

1. Absolute
   a. Patient cannot undergo surgery or is unlikely to survive surgery (i.e., severe cardiovascular or pulmonary disease)
   b. Active sepsis or untreated infection—transplant in human immunodeficiency virus (HIV)–positive patients is uncommon but performed at certain centers in select patients.
   c. Life expectancy after transplant is too short to justify risks of operation (i.e., extrahepatic malignancy or organ dysfunction)
   d. Active alcohol or substance abuse
   e. Surgery impossible for technical reasons (morbid obesity, multiple venous thrombi)
   f. Patient refusal of operation

2. Relative
   a. Advanced age—varies by center, functional status is generally more important
   b. Cholangiocarcinoma—may be considered in select cases but risk of recurrence is high
   c. Previous malignancy
   d. Chronic or refractory infections
   e. Poor social support

E. ORGAN SELECTION

1. In general, standard criteria apply, including a hemodynamically stable donor with no evidence of sepsis or non–central nervous system

primary malignancy, and ABO compatibility. Human leukocyte antigen (HLA) matching is not necessary.

2. Cadaveric whole organ
   a. Standard criteria donor (SCD)—brain dead donor, less than 80 years old, harvested and stored in cold preservation fluid less than 12 hours
   b. Factors associated with increased risk of graft failure—advanced donor age, HCV or HBV positive, cold ischemia time greater than 12 hours, steatotic liver, use of vasoactive medications
   c. Donation after cardiac death (DCD)—organ harvested after life support is withdrawn and the heart stops beating

3. Cadaveric reduced-size grafts and split-liver grafts
   a. Full right, full left, or left lateral lobe graft
   b. Cadaveric reduced-size grafts may be used to prevent large-for-size mismatch and hypoperfusion; these are less common now with use of split-liver grafts.
   c. Split-liver transplantation, together with living donor liver transplantation (LDLT) (next section), has increased the pool of pediatric-sized livers.
   d. Optimal selection of donor and recipient is key to successful transplant.

4. LDLT
   a. Originally there were only left or left lateral lobe grafts for pediatric recipients, but this has expanded to full right or left lobe grafts and adult recipients.
   b. This remains a limited source of liver grafts in the United States.
   c. Overall patient survival is comparable to deceased donor grafts, but LDLT is associated with increased complications and higher rates of retransplantation.
   d. Graft-to-recipient weight ratio of less than 0.8% is associated with increased risk of small-for-size syndrome and graft failure.
   e. There is increased risk of biliary and vascular complications with reduced-size, split-liver, and living donor grafts, but this has improved with increasing experience with techniques.

II. SPECIFIC OPERATIVE CONSIDERATIONS

A. TRADITIONAL OPERATIVE TECHNIQUE

1. Bilateral subcostal incision with midline extension to xiphoid process
2. Mobilization of the native liver; isolation of the suprahepatic and infrahepatic venae cavae; skeletonization of the hilar structures—portal vein, bile duct, and hepatic artery
3. Establishment of venous-venous bypass to decompress the splanchnic venous system; selectively used with intestinal edema, hypotension after test clamping of the vena cava, extensive portal hypertension bleeding, and difficult hepatectomy; cannulas (percutaneous or cut-down) from the portal and femoral veins drain blood into the axillary vein
4. Recipient hepatectomy
5. Vascular anastomoses—suprahepatic vena cava, infrahepatic vena cava, hepatic artery, and portal vein

47

LIVER TRANSPLANTATION

6. Biliary anastomosis—end-to-end bile duct anastomosis or choledocho-jejunostomy
7. Abdominal fascial closure with nonabsorbable sutures

B. PIGGYBACK TECHNIQUE

1. Recipient hepatectomy altered to leave the recipient retrohepatic vena cava intact
2. Hilar dissection performed as in traditional technique
3. Recipient liver remains attached to vena cava only by hepatic veins.
4. Recipient hepatectomy
5. Vascular anastomosis—donor suprahepatic vena cava to recipient inferior vena cava in end-to-side fashion, donor infrahepatic vena cava ligated, hepatic artery, and portal vein
6. Remainder of procedure done as in traditional technique

C. LIVING DONOR HEPATECTOMY

1. Techniques vary significantly depending on type of graft, institution, and patient anatomy.
2. Open or laparoscopic approaches are routinely used.
3. Meticulous preoperative evaluation is necessary to ensure adequate graft for recipient (especially for adult recipients) and sufficient remnant liver for donor (especially for right hepatectomy).

III. POSTOPERATIVE CONSIDERATIONS

A. POSTOPERATIVE CARE

1. Hemodynamic monitoring and resuscitation with the aid of pulmonary artery catheter
2. Correction of coagulopathy with blood products
3. Ventilatory support often for 24–48 hours after transplantation
4. Electrolyte management—correction of glucose, calcium, potassium, magnesium, and phosphate is particularly important.
5. Infection surveillance and prophylaxis—trimethoprim/sulfamethoxazole, fluconazole, and ganciclovir prophylaxis

B. IMMUNOSUPPRESSION (PROTOCOLS VARY BY INSTITUTION)

1. Induction suppression
   a. Corticosteroids—methylprednisolone (most common), prednisone, or prednisolone. First line of treatment for acute cellular rejection
   b. T cell–depleting monoclonal antibodies—muromonab-CD3 (OKT3), alemtuzumab (Campath-1H)
   c. T cell–depleting polyclonal antibody—ATG (Thymoglobulin)
   d. Interleukin-2 receptor subunit a (IL-2Ra) monoclonal antibody—daclizumab (Zenapax), basiliximab (Simulect)
2. Maintenance suppression
   a. Calcineurin inhibitors—tacrolimus (Prograf, FK506) is preferred, also cyclosporine (Neoral, Sandimmune, Gengraf); all are nephrotoxic

b. Antimetabolites—mycophenolate mofetil (CellCept, Myfortic), azathioprine (Imuran)

c. Mechanistic target of rapamycin (mTOR) inhibitors—sirolimus (Rapamune), everolimus (Afinitor)

C. ASSESSMENT OF GRAFT FUNCTION

1. Routine laboratory tests: Transaminase levels, alkaline phosphatase, factor V function (best predictor of early graft function), serum bilirubin, and coagulation parameters are nonspecific but are usually used to follow trends in graft function.

2. Liver biopsy: This is most specific for differentiating rejection from recurrent hepatitis, steatosis, ischemia, or other causes of graft dysfunction.

D. COMPLICATIONS

1. Primary nonfunction—has become a relatively rare cause of graft dysfunction since the introduction of storage solutions, such as University of Wisconsin (UW) solution. Manifested by failure to regain hepatic function in the early postoperative period (first 24–48 hours). Urgent retransplantation is usually indicated.

2. Rejection—occurs at some time in 60% of liver transplant patients; diagnosis made by biopsy of graft
   a. Acute cellular rejection—initially treated with high-dose corticosteroids; 80%–90% are steroid responsive
   b. Chronic ductopenic rejection (vanishing bile duct syndrome)—typically greater than 2 months after transplant; requires retransplant

3. Donor-to-recipient size mismatch
   a. Small-for-size syndrome—associated with graft dysfunction in the absence of rejection or vascular insufficiency; graft-to-recipient weight ratio less than 0.8% is predictive; requires retransplantation
   b. Large-for-size mismatch—typically seen in pediatric recipients with hypoperfusion and dysfunction of the graft; may lead to ischemia/necrosis and retransplantation; graft-to-recipient weight ratio greater than 4% increases risk

4. Hepatic artery thrombosis
   a. May occur intraoperatively because of intimal dissection—repair with donor iliac allograft, saphenous vein autograft, or synthetic graft.
   b. Postoperatively, diagnosis is made by angiogram, after screening with ultrasound/Doppler examination.
   c. Most common arterial complication—increased risk with pediatric transplant or split grafts

5. Portal vein thrombosis
   a. Early postoperative—usually due to technical errors and managed with reoperation, thrombectomy, systemic anticoagulation
   b. Late postoperative—due to intimal hyperplasia; difficult to manage and may require selective shunting

47

LIVER TRANSPLANTATION

6. Vena caval obstruction—rare, usually can be managed nonoperatively
7. Biliary complications—manifested by fever and increasing bilirubin and alkaline phosphatase levels; frequently secondary to hepatic artery insufficiency; diagnosed by cholangiogram
   a. Biliary leak—typically can be managed with stenting and/or drainage; may require conversion to hepaticojejunostomy if associated with necrosis; associated with lifelong risk of biliary stricture
   b. Biliary stricture—anastomotic stricture usually due to technical errors or edema, nonanastomotic stricture usually due to arterial insufficiency; must always rule out hepatic artery thrombosis/stenosis; often managed endoscopically but may require surgical revision or conversion to hepaticojejunostomy
8. Renal dysfunction—may be secondary to hypotension/hypovolemia; increased risk with calcineurin inhibitors
9. Infection and immunosuppressive drug complications
   a. Bacterial infection most common in first postoperative month; viral and fungal infections may occur at any time; preoperative screening and postoperative prophylaxis are important
   b. Posttransplantation lymphoproliferative disorder (PTLD)—associated with Epstein-Barr virus and cytomegalovirus; polyclonal PTLD usually resolves with decreased immunosuppression and antivirals; monoclonal PTLD is more difficult and may require chemotherapy, radiation, or resection
10. Recurrence of native disease (viral hepatitis, malignancy, some metabolic disorders)
11. Hypertension and hyperlipidemia are common after transplant and should be managed closely

E. **RESULTS (ORGAN PROCUREMENT AND TRANSPLANTATION NETWORK/SCIENTIFIC REGISTRY OF TRANSPLANT RECIPIENTS 2014 ANNUAL REPORT)**
1. Patient survival and graft survival vary significantly based on indication for transplant.
   a. Malignancy associated with lowest 5-year graft survival; cholestatic disease with highest
2. Graft survival rates (liver transplants performed in 2009)
   a. Deceased donor, adult recipient: 86% and 71% at 1 and 5 years, respectively
   b. Living donor, adult recipient: 85% and 77% at 1 and 5 years, respectively
   c. Deceased donor, pediatric recipient: 86% and 79% at 1 and 5 years, respectively
   d. Living donor, pediatric recipient: 89% and 86% at 1 and 5 years, respectively

RECOMMENDED READINGS

deLemos AS, Vagefi PA. Expanding the donor pool in liver transplantation: extended criteria donors. *Clin Liver Dis*. 2013;2:156–159.

Martin P, DiMartini A, Feng S, et al. Evaluation for liver transplantation in adults: 2013 practice guideline by the American Association for the Study of Liver Diseases and the American Society of Transplantation. *Hepatology*. 2014;59:1144–1165.

Moini M, Schilsky ML, Tichy EM. Review on immunosuppression in liver transplantation. *World J Hepatol*. 2015;7:1355–1368.

OPTN/SRTR 2014. Annual Data Report: Liver. *Am J Transplant*. 2016;16:69–98.

Pancreas Transplantation

Alexander Cortez, MD

The pancreas is by far the most complex organ in the body.

—Patrick Soon-Shiong, MD

I. GENERAL CONSIDERATIONS

A. HISTORY AND EPIDEMIOLOGY

1. First pancreas transplant was performed in 1966 at the University of Minnesota.
2. More than 25,000 US and 10,000 worldwide pancreas transplants have taken place since the original operation.
3. Type 2 diabetes mellitus (DM) is associated with an increased risk of blindness (25×), kidney disease (17×), gangrene (20×), heart disease (2×), and stroke (2×) compared with patients without DM.

B. INDICATIONS FOR PANCREAS TRANSPLANTATION

1. Insulin-dependent (type 1) diabetics who show C-peptide deficiency, although some insulin-independent (type 2) diabetics may be considered
2. "Brittle diabetics": patients who are insulin dependent and suffer from wide fluctuations in glucose levels
   a. Urgency increases with "hypoglycemic unawareness," in which hypoglycemic episodes are not recognized by the patient.
3. Patients with end-stage or impending renal disease secondary to diabetes

C. TYPES OF PANCREAS TRANSPLANTS

1. Simultaneous pancreas and kidney (SPK) transplant—80% of pancreas transplants
   a. Patients with concurrent DM and end-stage renal disease (ESRD)
   b. Provides a dialysis-free and insulin-independent life
   c. Advantage—insulin control protects longevity of renal allograft.
   d. Lowest incidence of pancreas graft thrombosis (5%) and immunologic graft loss (2%)
2. Pancreas after kidney (PAK) transplant—15% of pancreas transplants
   a. Patients with prior renal transplant and difficult-to-control diabetes
   b. Limits damage of poorly controlled diabetes on renal allograft
   c. Higher rates of graft thrombosis (8%) and immunologic graft loss (5.5%) than with SPK
3. Pancreas transplant alone (PTA)—5% of pancreas transplants
   a. Nonuremic, labile diabetics with hypoglycemic unawareness
   b. Consider when risk of secondary complications from DM outweighs the risk of surgery and immunosuppression

c. Similarly, higher rates of graft thrombosis (7%) and immunologic graft loss (6.6%) than with SPK

D. ORGAN SELECTION

Almost all are performed from cadaveric donors. In addition to standard criteria for donor selection, specific contraindications to pancreas donor eligibility at most centers include:

1. Presence of DM or first-degree relative with DM
2. Chronic pancreatitis
3. Pancreatic damage secondary to trauma
4. History of alcohol abuse

II. SPECIFIC OPERATIVE CONSIDERATIONS

A. TRANSPLANT ANATOMY

1. Recipient bed is prepared in the right iliac fossa.
2. Venous drainage may be systemic or portal.
   a. Systemic: donor portal vein to recipient iliac or inferior vena cava (IVC) (most common)
   b. Portal: donor portal vein to recipient superior mesenteric vein (SMV)
3. Arterial anastomosis is performed using a donor common iliac "Y-graft."
   a. Donor external iliac of Y-graft to donor superior mesenteric artery (SMA)
   b. Donor internal iliac of Y-graft to donor splenic artery
   c. Donor common iliac of Y-graft to recipient common iliac artery

B. MANAGEMENT OF EXOCRINE SECRETIONS

1. Enteric drainage: donor duodenum (harvested en bloc with pancreas) anastomosed to recipient small bowel
   a. More physiologic method of drainage
   b. More common in the United States
2. Bladder drainage: donor duodenum anastomosed to bladder
   a. Risk of contamination with enteric content is decreased.
   b. There is the ability to monitor urinary amylase for rejection (exocrine rejection precedes endocrine rejection).
   c. Disadvantages include metabolic acidosis, urinary tract infection, dysuria, and cystitis.

III. POSTOPERATIVE CONSIDERATIONS

A. POSTOPERATIVE CARE

1. Vascular thrombosis is the most common cause of early graft loss.
   a. Therefore patients are typically anticoagulated perioperatively with aspirin, systemic heparinization, or low-molecular-weight heparin.
2. Graft function can be monitored by amylase levels and glucose homeostasis.
   a. It is specific but not sensitive, because 90% of the pancreas may be lost before glucose homeostasis is impaired.

b. Exogenous insulin use is avoided in the perioperative setting to ensure that serum glucose levels reflect pancreas function.

3. Duplex ultrasound or radionuclide perfusion scans are used to evaluate allograft blood flow.

4. Ultimately there is no reliable technique for diagnosis of rejection.
   a. Rejection may be monitored by following creatinine levels with SPK.
      (1) Increases in creatinine precede decrease in pancreatic exocrine function in 90% of cases.
   b. Biopsy of allograft can provide histologic diagnosis.

5. Immunosuppressive regimens vary, but most centers use induction with antilymphocyte globulin or muromonab-CD3 (OKT3) and maintenance with cyclosporine or tacrolimus (FK506), prednisone, azathioprine, and/or mycophenolate mofetil.
   a. Rejection accounts for up to 32% of graft loss in the first year.

B. COMPLICATIONS

1. **Graft pancreatitis (up to 35%)**
   a. Secondary to preservation injury and ischemia
   b. Suggested by hyperamylasemia and local graft pain
   c. May require drainage of peripancreatic collections or operative debridement of necrotic pancreas

2. **Graft thrombosis (5%–15%)**
   a. Most common cause of sudden early graft loss
      (1) May present as a sudden increase in insulin requirement or as a sharp drop in urinary amylase levels
   b. Presents with swollen and tender allograft
   c. Thought to occur because the pancreas is a low-flow organ; venous thrombosis is more common than arterial thrombosis
   d. Diagnosis typically based on Doppler ultrasound and treatment usually requires graft pancreatectomy

3. **Anastomotic leak (2%–10%)**
   a. Presents with fever, abdominal pain, nausea, vomiting, and tachycardia
   b. Rare with bladder drainage
   c. Best mode of diagnosis: computed tomography with oral contrast

4. **Bleeding (6%–8%)**
   a. Immediate bleeding usually occurs from the pancreatic parenchyma.
   b. Delayed bleeding typically occurs from the enteric anastomosis and presents as a gastrointestinal (GI) bleed.
   c. It is usually related to use of anticoagulation in perioperative period.

5. **Rejection—average nearly 30% within the first year**

C. OUTCOMES

1. Patient survival among all three categories of pancreas transplants is greater than 95% at 1 year and 90% at 3 years.
   a. SPK graft (pancreas) function rates are 80%, 68%, and 45% at 5, 10, and 20 years, respectively.

b. PAK graft function rates are 62%, 46%, and 16% at 5, 10, and 20 years, respectively.
c. PTA graft function rates are 59%, 39%, and 12% at 5, 10, and 20 years, respectively.
2. Pancreas graft half-life (50% function) is 14, 7, and 7 years for SPK, PAK, and PTA, respectively.
3. Insulin independence at 1 year is 81%, 71%, and 62% for SPK, PAK, and PTA, respectively.
4. Data support potential reversal of diabetic neuropathy and decreased recurrence of nephropathy in SPK.

IV. ISLET CELL TRANSPLANTATION

A. BACKGROUND
1. PTA is rarely performed for diabetics with labile disease but who do not experience hypoglycemic unawareness given high risk of perioperative morbidity and need for immunosuppression.
2. By isolating insulin-producing beta cells from islets of Langerhans, the risk of transplantation may be avoided.
3. Advantages to islet cell transplantation over exogenous insulin include:
   a. Restoring beta-cell secretory capacity
   b. Improving glucose counterregulation
   c. Improved glucose homoeostasis, which restores hypoglycemia awareness

B. INDICATIONS
1. Allotransplantation in patients with type 1 diabetes with hypoglycemic unawareness or inability to tolerate major transplant operation
2. Autotransplantation after pancreatectomy for carcinoma or refractory pancreatitis

C. TECHNIQUE
1. Pancreatic tissue obtained from pancreatectomy or cadaveric source is enzymatically digested.
   a. Usually requires two cadaveric pancreas grafts to harvest approximately 1 million islets or 300,000+ islet cell equivalents in autotransplant
2. Islet cells are extracted and purified via gradient separation.
3. Microencapsulation is used to decrease immunogenicity in allotransplant.
4. Islet cells are infused into hepatic parenchyma via injection into the portal vein or liver directly.

D. OUTCOMES
1. Since 1990, approximately 1500 transplants have occurred.
2. Islet cell transplantation outcomes have significantly improved since 2000, with the introduction of the Edmonton immunosuppression protocol.

48

PANCREAS TRANSPLANTATION

3. However, multiple challenges must be overcome before islet cell transplantation becomes routinely successful.
   a. Creation of an ideal microencapsulation vehicle that may facilitate xenotransplantation efforts is paramount.
   b. There is no routine way to detect rejection until hyperglycemia ensues.
4. Insulin independence at 1 year is up to 70% but less than 35% at 3 years.
   a. Despite not being insulin independent, many patients are freed from hypoglycemic events, with more easily controlled diabetes.

V. PANCREAS VERSUS ISLET CELL TRANSPLANTATION

1. These should not be viewed as mutually exclusive but rather complementary therapeutic interventions.
2. Pancreas transplantation typically results in higher likelihood of insulin independence than does islet cell transplantation.
3. Islet cell transplantation is not associated with same surgical risk as pancreas transplant and is therefore a suitable option for patients with multiple medical comorbidities.

RECOMMENDED READINGS

Becker Y. Kidney and pancreas transplant. In: Townsend CM, Beauchamp RD, Evers BM, Mattox KL, eds. *Sabiston's Textbook of Surgery*. 19th ed. Philadelphia: Elsevier; 2012:666–681.

Gruessner RWG, Gruessner AC. The current state of pancreas transplantation. *Nat Rev Endocrinol*. 2013;9(9):555–562.

Redfield RR, Scalea JR, Odorico JS. Simultaneous pancreas and kidney transplantation. *Curr Opin Organ Transplant*. 2015;20(1):94–102.

Schwartz SI, Brunicardi FC. Pancreas transplantation. In: Brunicardi FC, Andersen DK, Billiar TR, Dunn DL, Hunter JG, Pollock RE, eds. *Schwartz's Manual of Surgery*. 10th ed. New York: McGraw-Hill Medical Pub Division; 2010:340–345.

PART IX

Endocrine Surgery

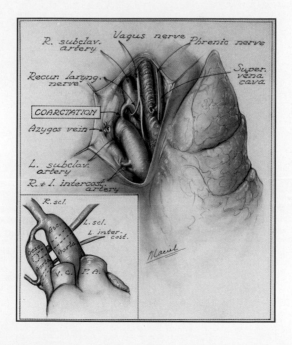

Endocrine Surgery

Thyroid

Emily Midura, MD

The extirpation of the thyroid gland for goiter typifies, perhaps better than any other operation, the supreme triumph of the surgeon's art.

—William Halsted

I. EMBRYOLOGY

A. THYROID DEVELOPMENT

1. At 3 weeks' gestation, this is the first endocrine organ to develop.
2. It originates as an outgrowth of the pharyngeal endoderm at the base of the tongue (foramen cecum).
3. Epithelialized endoderm migrates down the middle of the neck anterior to the hyoid bone and larynx.
4. The thyroglossal duct is the tubular tract that forms along the migratory path and obliterates at 8 weeks' gestation.

B. DEVELOPMENTAL ANOMALIES

1. Aberrant and ectopic thyroid tissue can form anywhere along the migratory tract.
2. Thyroglossal duct cyst can form if the migratory tract fails to obliterate. Presents clinically as a midline mobile mass (1–2 cm), and 80% occur near the hyoid bone. Treatment is with Sistrunk operation (cyst and middle hyoid bone resection), and 1% contains malignant cells.
3. Lingual thyroid occurs if thyroid tissue fails to descend to the neck during development and may be only functioning thyroid tissue. Medical or surgical intervention required only if obstructive symptoms
4. Pyramidal lobe results from the failure of the distal end of the thyroglossal duct to obliterate.

II. ANATOMY

A. OVERVIEW

1. Weighs approximately 15–30 g in adults
2. Right and left lobes are connected by isthmus in midline; 50% of patients have pyramidal lobe.
3. Pretracheal layer of the deep cervical fascia forms outer capsule. Suspensory ligaments of Berry form posterior connections.

B. ARTERIAL SUPPLY

1. Superior thyroid artery—first branch of the external carotid, divides into anterior and posterior branches
2. Inferior thyroid artery—branch of the thyrocervical trunk

3. Thyroid IMA artery—small, single artery that replaces the inferior arteries in 10% of people, can branch off aorta, innominate, or carotid

C. VENOUS DRAINAGE
1. Superior and middle thyroid veins—drain to the internal jugular vein
2. Inferior thyroid veins—drain to the brachiocephalic vein

D. NERVES
1. Recurrent laryngeal nerves (RLNs) are branches of the vagus and innervate the intrinsic muscles of the larynx except the cricothyroid; 70% are located in the tracheoesophageal groove and are identified near the inferior thyroid arteries. Injury to unilateral nerve causes hoarseness; bilateral can cause airway obstruction necessitating urgent tracheostomy.
2. Superior laryngeal nerves are also branches off the vagus, innervate the cricothyroid muscle, and can be found near the superior thyroid artery.

E. LYMPHATICS
1. Extensive lymphatic drainage to all levels of lymph nodes in the neck (levels I–VI) and anterior mediastinum (level VII)

F. HISTOLOGY
1. Lobules contain thyroid follicles lined with cuboidal epithelium that secrete colloid when stimulated by thyroid-stimulating hormone (TSH).
2. C cells or parafollicular cells are neuroendocrine cells located in the upper thyroid poles in the interfollicular stroma that secrete calcitonin.

III. PHYSIOLOGY

A. IODINE METABOLISM
1. Iodine is converted to iodide and absorbed in the stomach and jejunum.
2. Thyroid follicular cells store 90% of the body's iodine; the remainder is renally excreted.

B. THYROID HORMONE SYNTHESIS
1. Iodide trapping in the thyrocyte occurs via active transport.
2. Thyroid peroxidase (TPO) catalyzes organification and coupling reactions.
3. Organification: Iodide is oxidized and converted to iodine, and iodination of tyrosine residues on thyroglobulin (Tg) creates monoiodotyrosine (MIT) and diiodotyrosine (DIT).
4. Coupling of iodotyrosines results in formation of iodothyronines, triiodothyronine (T3) (MIT + DIT) and thyroxine (T4) (DIT + DIT).

C. THYROID HORMONE FUNCTION
1. Circulating thyroid hormones enter cells through diffusion and bind nuclear proteins.

2. They impact almost every system in the body and increase metabolic rate, cardiac function, intestinal motility, respiratory drive, and glucose metabolism.

D. THYROID HORMONE REGULATION
1. Controlled by the hypothalamus-anterior pituitary-thyroid axis.
2. Thyrotropin-releasing hormone (TRH) released by the hypothalamus stimulates the anterior pituitary to release TSH.
3. TSH increases iodine trapping, thyroid hormone synthesis and release, peripheral conversion of T4–T3, and thyroid cell proliferation.
4. Negative feedback loop with T3 inhibits the release of TRH, and both free T3 and T4 inhibit the release of TSH.

E. CALCITONIN
1. Regulates calcium homeostasis
2. Released by parafollicular C cells in response to high calcium levels
3. Inhibits osteoclasts (bone resorption), stimulates osteoblasts (bone formation), and inhibits renal absorption of calcium to decrease circulating calcium levels

IV. WORK-UP OF THYROID DISEASE
A. CLINICAL PRESENTATION
1. Hyperthyroidism: excessive thyroid hormone, presents with weight loss, heat intolerance, sweating, tremors, hyperreflexia, diarrhea, palpitations, tachycardia
2. Hypothyroidism: insufficient thyroid hormone, presents with weight gain, lethargy, cold intolerance, hyporeflexia, constipation, bradycardia, coarse/dry skin, slow mentation, irregular menses
3. Nontoxic goiter: enlarged thyroid gland without evidence of thyroid dysfunction or physiologic derangement
4. Thyroid nodule: usually asymptomatic and identified on physical examination or incidentally on imaging

B. LABORATORY DATA
1. Thyroid function panel usually consists of TSH, free T3, and free T4.
2. TSH levels reflect ability of anterior pituitary to detect free T4; this is a common screening test and is diagnostic of hypothyroidism versus hyperthyroidism.
3. T3/T4: Free levels are usually used to confirm hyper/hypothyroidism diagnosis; total levels may reflect changes in Tg levels.
4. Thyroid antibodies: Anti-Tg and anti-TPO usually indicate autoimmune thyroiditis but can be associated with Graves disease, multinodular goiter, and neoplasms.
5. Tg: elevated with neoplastic disease and gland destruction. Levels are used to monitor for recurrence after neoplastic resection.

49

THYROID

C. IMAGING

1. Radionuclide imaging: Radioactive iodine is used to determine gland shape/size and functional activity.[123]I ($T_{1/2}$ = 12–14 hours) is used to diagnose lingual thyroids and goiters, whereas [131]I ($T_{1/2}$ = 8–10 days) is used to image malignant disease. Areas with less radioactivity than the surrounding gland are "cold," and those with increased activity are "hot." Technetium scanning and fluorodeoxyglucose–positron emission tomography (FDG-PET) scans can be used to evaluate nodal disease.
2. Ultrasound: evaluation of nodules and goiters to determine solid versus cystic, size, multicentricity as well as cervical lymphadenopathy
3. CT/MRI: used for large goiters or invasive tumors not amenable to ultrasound to determine relation to airway and vascular structures

D. BIOPSY

1. Fine-needle aspiration (FNA) biopsy is used to differentiate between benign and malignant nodules; results include benign, malignant, nondiagnostic, or suspicious. Nondiagnostic FNAs can be repeated and can also be sent for Gram stain and culture in infectious presentations.
2. Surgical biopsy is used when FNA is suspicious or nondiagnostic with other concerning imaging findings; it consists of thyroid lobectomy or total thyroidectomy, depending on pathologic findings.

V. HYPERTHYROIDISM

A. DIFFUSE TOXIC GOITER—GRAVES DISEASE

1. Clinical presentation: age 30–40 years, female predominance (6:1), associated with exophthalmos, pretibial myxedema, goiter, and symptoms of hyperparathyroidism
2. Pathophysiology: autoimmune disorder caused by TSH-receptor (TSH-R) antibodies, histology reveals diffuse lymphocytic invasion
3. Diagnosis: low TSH, high free and total T3/T4, circulating TSH-R antibodies increased iodine uptake, and enlarged gland on radionuclide scan
4. Treatment: medical, radioiodine, and surgery
   a. Medical: first line therapy with thionamides (propylthiouracil [PTU] and methimazole), which inhibit TPO and take several weeks until baseline hormone levels are depleted; should treat for at least 6 months; high-dose iodine also used in combination with thionamides to inhibit T3/T4 release and treat thyroid storm and severe thyrotoxicosis; when discontinued thyrotoxicosis can worsen
   b. Radioiodine ablative therapy (RAI): [131]I used as ablative therapy; only 50% of patients are euthyroid after 6 months; high risk of hypothyroidism; 10% have worsening exophthalmos
   c. Surgery: bilateral subtotal thyroidectomy leaves 4–6 g thyroid tissue; used in poor candidates for medical or RAI therapies (young, pregnant, significant orbitopathy, large goiters, or with suspicious thyroid mass), risks include RLN injury (1%) and hypothyroidism (1%); preoperative treatment with antithyroid medications required

to achieve euthyroid state and high-dose iodine therapy given 7–10 days preoperative decreases size and vascularity of gland

B. TOXIC ADENOMA

1. Clinical presentation: age 30–40 years, single slow growing, smooth, firm neck mass
2. Pathophysiology: TSH-R gene mutation leads to development of an autonomously functioning follicular adenoma; hyperthyroidism develops when size greater than 3 cm; rarely malignant
3. Diagnosis: increased iodine uptake or "hot" nodule on radionuclide scan; lab tests can vary
4. Treatment: small nodules are managed with antithyroid medications and RAI; surgical management with lobectomy if large nodules or in younger patients; need to be euthyroid preoperatively but do not need iodine treatment because adenomas are not hypervascular

C. TOXIC MULTINODULAR GOITER—PLUMMER DISEASE

1. Clinical presentation: older than 50 years, with long history of goiter; usually presents with atrial fibrillation, tachycardia, congestive heart failure, or airway obstruction, along with hyperthyroidism symptoms
2. Pathophysiology: nonfunctioning multinodular goiter becomes autonomous; can be precipitated by iodine containing drugs
3. Diagnosis: low TSH, high free and total T3/T4, and ultrasound with multiple thyroid nodules
4. Treatment: RAI or surgical resection with subtotal thyroidectomy

D. THYROID STORM

1. Clinical presentation: present with fever, central nervous system (CNS) depression, and cardiac dysfunction in the setting of hyperthyroidism
2. Pathophysiology: usually precipitated by trauma, infection, or surgery; amiodarone administration also a trigger
3. Treatment: supportive care, iodine, PTU, steroids, and beta-blockade to decrease peripheral T4 conversion to T3 and hyperthyroid symptoms

VI. HYPOTHYROIDISM

A. CHRONIC LYMPHOCYTIC THYROIDITIS—HASHIMOTO THYROIDITIS

1. Clinical presentation: age 30–50 years; female predominance (1:10–20); present with enlarged, firm, lobulated thyroid gland; only 20% with hypothyroid symptoms
2. Pathophysiology: autoimmune disease with anti-Tg, TPO, and TSH-R antibodies, as well as cytotoxic T-cell infiltration, which results in thyroid cell apoptosis and destruction, rarely develops thyroid lymphoma
3. Diagnosis: elevated TSH, decreased T3/T4, thyroid autoantibodies
4. Treatment: thyroid hormone replacement, surgical resection for suspicious lesions, or symptomatic gland enlargement

49

THYROID

VII. THYROIDITIS AND NONTOXIC GOITERS

A. ACUTE SUPPURATIVE THYROIDITIS

1. Clinical presentation: more common in children; often preceded by upper respiratory infection (URI) or otitis media; presents with severe neck pain radiating to jaw/ear with fevers, chills, odynophagia, dysphonia; if untreated can result in sepsis, tracheal/esophageal rupture, sympathetic trunk paralysis
2. Pathophysiology: can result from hematogenous/lymphatic spread; direct spread from thyroglossal duct cyst, persistent pyriform sinus, penetrating trauma, or immune suppression; 70% streptococcus or anaerobes
3. Diagnosis: FNA with Gram stain, cytology, and culture; computed tomography (CT) to determine extent of infection
4. Treatment: intravenous (IV) antibiotics, drainage of abscess, complete resection of pyriform sinus tract if involved

B. SUBACUTE THYROIDITIS

1. Clinical presentation: painful versus painless disease
   a. Painful presents in 30–40-year-old females with neck pain and enlarged, tender firm thyroid gland; may be preceded by URI; patients start with hyperthyroid symptoms, followed by euthyroid, hypothyroid, and finally return to euthyroid state
   b. Painless presents 6 weeks postpartum in women 30–60 years of age
2. Pathophysiology: usually self-limited; painful thyroiditis likely viral/postviral immune response; associated with HLA-B23 genotype and painless autoimmune and seen postpartum
3. Diagnosis: TSH, T3/T4, elevated erythrocyte sedimentation rate (ESR) in painful thyroiditis, radionuclide uptake minimal due to destruction of thyroid tissue
4. Treatment: nonsteroidal antiinflammatory drugs (NSAIDs), steroids in severe cases, beta-blockade or levothyroxine if symptomatic, thyroidectomy in refractory disease

C. RIEDELS THYROIDITIS (INVASIVE FIBROUS THYROIDITIS)

1. Clinical presentation: presents in women 30–60 years old as painless anterior neck mass with progression to compressive symptoms; late in disease can have hypothyroidism and hypoparathyroidism; gland is enlarged, "woody," firm, and adherent to surrounding tissues
2. Pathophysiology: autoimmune; replacement of all thyroid parenchyma with fibrous tissue
3. Diagnosis: open thyroid biopsy with isthmus wedge resection; FNA is often nondiagnostic
4. Treatment: excision of thyroid isthmus decompresses the trachea; further resection not recommended due to risk of injuring surrounding structure; levothyroxine replacement as needed; steroids and tamoxifen for refractory cases

D. NONTOXIC GOITER

1. Clinical presentation: any enlargement of the thyroid gland; endemic goiters seen in areas of iodine deficiency, usually asymptomatic but as they grow can develop compressive symptoms; gland is soft and enlarged on examination
2. Pathophysiology: iodine deficiency or inherited enzyme deficiency causes inadequate thyroid hormone synthesis, TSH stimulation, and subsequent gland hyperplasia.
3. Diagnosis: TSH, T3/T4, FNA if dominant nodule or painful/enlarging nodule; CT to evaluate compressive symptoms
4. Treatment: iodine administration for deficiency; levothyroxine to suppress TSH if symptomatic; subtotal thyroidectomy if compressive symptoms

VIII. THYROID NODULES

A. CLINICAL PRESENTATION

1. Age less than 20 years or greater than 70 years, family history, previous neck radiation
2. Solitary nodule, dominant nodules in multinodular gland or large goiter, nonpalpable nodule greater than 8 mm, especially those that are firm, fixed and nontender with associated cervical lymphadenopathy

B. CLINICAL EVALUATION

1. Low TSH suggests toxic nodule; obtain radionuclide scan and treat with ablation or surgery. "Hot" nodules are rarely malignant.
2. Normal TSH requires FNA to rule out malignancy.
3. FNA results: 70% benign (colloid nodule, thyroiditis), 15% nondiagnostic, 10% suspicious/indeterminate, 5% malignant

C. MANAGEMENT BASED ON FINE-NEEDLE ASPIRATION RESULTS

1. Benign: follow clinically; if it grows, requires repeat FNA
2. Nondiagnostic: repeat FNA; if it remains nondiagnostic, observe if low risk, surgical excision if high risk
3. Suspicious: surgical excision because FNA cannot differentiate follicular and Hürthle cell adenomas from carcinomas and 20% will be malignant
4. Malignant: proceed with surgery.

D. CYSTIC NODULES

1. Evaluation: FNA and cytology of both fluid and solid components; if cytology is nondiagnostic and does not recur, no further work-up indicated; if it does recur, repeat FNA
2. Treatment: surgery required if malignant or suspicious cells on FNA, recurrence of cyst after two aspirations, nondiagnostic solid component to cyst

49

THYROID

E. INCIDENTALOMA

1. Evaluation: nonpalpable nodules found incidentally on head and neck imaging, FNA should be performed if greater than 15 mm in size; any size nodule with features concerning for malignancy or nodules found in patients at high risk for thyroid cancer

IX. THYROID NEOPLASMS

A. EPIDEMIOLOGY

1. A total of 15,000 new cases annually, 1.5% of all cancers in the United States
2. Classification: well differentiated (papillary, follicular, and Hürthle cell), undifferentiated (anaplastic), medullary, and lymphoma
3. Prognostic factors: age, size, extrathyroidal invasion, metastasis; of note, lymph node metastasis is NOT an important prognostic indicator

B. PAPILLARY THYROID CARCINOMA

1. Clinical presentation: 80% of all thyroid cancers; asymptomatic neck mass at age 20–40 years, with female predominance (2:1); previous neck irradiation
2. Diagnosis: FNA demonstrates fibrosis and calcifications (psammoma bodies) with Orphan Annie eye nucleic features; can have cystic component
3. Treatment: surgical excision, extent based on size and staging; see Table 49.1 for risk factors and Table 49.2 for staging

---

TABLE 49.1

RISK GROUPS FOR WELL-DIFFERENTIATED THYROID CANCER

High Risk	Low Risk
Age ≥45 years	Age <45 years
Extrathyroidal invasion	Tumor confined to the thyroid
Major invasion of the tumor capsule (follicular)	No distant metastasis
Distant metastasis	Tumor size <4 cm
Tumor size >4 cm	Well-differentiated or moderately differentiated tumor
High grade (tall-cell variants, poorly differentiated)	

TABLE 49.2

THYROID CANCER STAGING

	Papillary or Follicular			
Stage	Age <45 Years	Age ≥45 Years	Medullary	Anaplastic
I	M0 (any T, N)	T1	T1	—
II	M1	T2, T3	T2, T3, T4	—
III	—	T4 or N1	N1	—
IV	—	M1	M1	Any

M0, No metastasis; *M1*, metastasis present; *N0*, no nodal involvement; *N1*, nodal involvement; *T1*, tumor ≤1 cm; *T2*, tumor >1 cm but ≤4 cm; *T3*, tumor >4 cm; *T4*, extrathyroidal invasion.

a. Less than 1 cm or minimal papillary thyroid carcinoma (PTC) without local invasion or metastasis undergo lobectomy and isthmectomy
b. Low risk: lobectomy or total thyroidectomy
c. High risk: total thyroidectomy
d. Modified radical neck dissection (MRND) only performed when palpable lymph nodes in high-risk patients to decrease local recurrence; does not alter survival in patients less than 45 years

C. FOLLICULAR THYROID CARCINOMA

1. Clinical presentation: 10% thyroid cancers, presents at age 40–50 years with female predominance (2:1); more common in iodine deficiency; usually present with a single nodule
2. Diagnosis: FNA can diagnose cell type but cannot differentiate malignant disease; need structural information to diagnose carcinoma; lesions have tumor capsule and spread hematogenously; minimally invasive disease has intact tumor capsule; widely invasive disease has capsular and vascular invasion
3. Treatment: thyroid lobectomy to determine if benign adenoma or carcinoma, which is adequate treatment for minimally invasive disease; if find widely invasive disease, require completion thyroidectomy; MRND only indicated with clinically palpable nodes

D. HÜRTHLE CELL CARCINOMA

1. Clinical presentation: 3% of thyroid cancers; variant of follicular thyroid carcinoma (FTC) and presents at age 40–50 years with 2:1 female predominance; more aggressive than FTC with almost a third with multifocal disease, lymph node involvement, and/or distant metastasis
2. Diagnosis: FNA to diagnose cell type; surgical excision to differentiate adenoma and carcinoma
3. Treatment: requires total thyroidectomy and central node dissection (paratracheal and pretracheal lymph nodes) with radical neck dissection on side with palpable lymph nodes

E. MEDULLARY THYROID CANCER

1. Clinical presentation: neuroendocrine tumor that arises from parafollicular C cells; 5% thyroid cancers, 20% are hereditary (familial medullary thyroid cancer [MTC] and multiple endocrine neoplasia [MEN] II), which are more often bilateral; patients present with firm neck mass that may be painful; secretes calcitonin and carcinoembryonic antigen (CEA) and can secrete hormones that cause cushingoid features (adrenocorticotropic hormone [ACTH]) and watery diarrhea (vasoactive intestinal peptide)
2. Diagnosis: FNA with amyloid deposits and modified calcitonin molecules
3. Treatment: total thyroidectomy and central neck dissection because disease is often bilateral and multifocal, and local lymph node involvement

49

THYROID

is common; if tumor is greater than 1 cm or there is clinically apparent lymph node involvement, ipsilateral MRND is required; if bilateral tumor or lymph node involvement, bilateral MRND is performed

4. Hereditary disease: autosomal dominant with almost complete penetrance; germline mutation in RET proto-oncogene tyrosine kinase; can diagnose with genetic testing, and patients with RET mutations require prophylactic total thyroidectomy and central neck dissection only if nodule identified; calcitonin is elevated or there is lymph node disease; patients with MEN need treatment of pheochromocytoma before thyroid resection

   a. MEN2a: MTC in 100%, pheochromocytoma in 50%, parathyroid neoplasm in 10%–35%, total thyroidectomy at age 5

   b. MEN2b: MTC in 100%, pheochromocytoma in 50%, neuromas (mucosal, gastrointestinal) in almost 100%, total thyroidectomy at age of diagnosis as very aggressive disease

   c. Familial MTC: total thyroidectomy at age 5

F. ANAPLASTIC THYROID CANCER

1. Clinical presentation: 1% of thyroid cancer; presents at age 50–70 years; 10% with preexisting goiter; 20% with previous well-differentiated tumor; present with rapidly enlarging neck mass and dysphonia, dyspnea, and dysphagia from highly aggressive and invasive tumors

2. Diagnosis: FNA; surgical biopsy if equivocal results

3. Treatment: poor prognosis, multimodal therapy with surgical resection, chemotherapy, and radiation

G. THYROID LYMPHOMA

1. Clinical presentation: 1% of thyroid cancer; majority are B-cell type; increased incidence with Hashimoto thyroiditis; presents as painless neck mass with compressive/obstructive symptoms

2. Diagnosis: FNA; surgical biopsy if equivocal results

3. Treatment: chemoradiation, surgical resection if compressive/obstructive symptoms

H. ADJUVANT THERAPY

1. Differentiated thyroid cancer (PTC, FTC, and Hürthle cell): Tg levels and radionuclide scans to detect recurrence; increased Tg and iodide uptake signify recurrence after total thyroidectomy; difficult to monitor for recurrence after partial thyroid resection

   a. I^{131} ablative therapy: used after total thyroidectomy in high-risk patients to destroy remaining thyroid tissue

   b. Levothyroxine: titrate to TSH less than 0.01 mU/L to prevent TSH stimulation of tumor cell growth

2. Radiation therapy: controversial, may improve local control in high-risk patients or in those with grossly positive margins

3. Chemotherapy: can be considered in anaplastic disease as adjuvant therapy; no role in differentiated disease

RECOMMENDED READINGS

Baskin HJ, Cobin RH, Duick DS, et al. American Association of Clinical Endocrinologists medical guidelines for clinical practice for the evaluation and treatment of hyperthyroidism and hypothyroidism. *Endocr Pract.* 2002;8:457–469.

Bliss RD, Gauger PG, Delbridge LW. Surgeon's approach to the thyroid gland: surgical anatomy and the importance of technique. *World J Surg.* 2000;24:891–897.

Brunicardi FC, Andersen DK, Billiar TR, et al., eds. Thyroid, parathyroid and adrenal. In: *Schwartz's Principles of Surgery.* New York: McGraw-Hill; 2014.

Cabanillas ME, Dadu R, Hu MI, et al. Thyroid gland malignancies. *Hematol Oncol Clin North Am.* 2015;29:1123–1143.

Gough J, Scott-Coombes D, Fausto Palazzo F. Thyroid incidentaloma: an evidence-based assessment of management strategy. *World J Surg.* 2008;32:1264–1268.

National Comprehensive Cancer Network (NCCN). *NCCN Clinical Practice Guidelines in Oncology. Thyroid Carcinoma Version 1.2016*; 2016. Available at https://www.nccn.org/professionals/physician_gls/f_guidelines.asp.

Padur AA, Kumar N, Guru A, et al. Safety and effectiveness of total thyroidectomy and its comparison with subtotal thyroidectomy and other thyroid surgeries: a systematic review. *J Thyroid Res.* 2016;2016:7594615.

49

THYROID

Parathyroid

Ashley Walther, MD

The greatest challenge in parathyroid localization is to localize a good parathyroid surgeon.

—John L. Doppman

I. PARATHYROID EMBRYOLOGY AND ANATOMY

A. EMBRYOLOGY

1. Superior parathyroid glands—derived from fourth branchial pouch (same as thyroid)
   a. Most common location: posterior aspect of upper and middle thyroid lobes at level of cricoid cartilage (80%)
   b. Alternative locations: tracheoesophageal groove, paraesophageal or retroesophageal, middle or posterior mediastinum, intrathyroidal, carotid sheath
2. Inferior parathyroid glands—derived from third branchial pouch (same as thymus)
   a. Most common location: within 1 cm of intersection of inferior thyroid artery and recurrent laryngeal nerve
   b. Alternative locations: in the thymus, mediastinal, intrathyroidal, thyrothymic ligament, submandibular; variable due to long descent pathway

B. ANATOMY

1. Most patients have four glands; 13% have more than four; 3% have fewer than 4.
2. Golden yellow to light brown color
3. Measure up to 7 mm
4. Weigh 40–50 mg each
5. Superior—dorsal to recurrent laryngeal nerve
6. Inferior glands—ventral to recurrent laryngeal nerve
7. Main blood supply: branches of inferior thyroid artery, branch of superior thyroid artery may supply upper glands; drain via ipsilateral thyroid veins
8. Histology: composed of chief cells (which produce parathyroid hormone [PTH]) and oxyphil cells

C. PHYSIOLOGY

1. Total serum calcium level: 8.5–10.5 mg/dL
2. PTH acts to increase calcium at:
   a. Bone—stimulates osteoclasts, releasing calcium and phosphate
   b. Kidney—absorption in proximal convoluted tubule, limits excretion in distal convoluted tubule

   c. Intestine—enhanced 1-hydroxylation of 25-hydroxyvitamin D, indirectly increases absorption

II. PRIMARY HYPERPARATHYROIDISM

A. GENERAL
1. Increased PTH production from abnormal parathyroid glands leads to increased enteral absorption, increased hydroxylation of vitamin D, and decreased renal clearance.
2. Incidence: 0.1%–0.3%; more common in women
3. Single gland or parathyroid adenoma (80%); multiple adenomas or hyperplasia (15%–20%); parathyroid carcinoma (1%)

B. CAUSATIVE FACTORS
1. Unknown; ionizing radiation, familial predisposition, declining renal function
2. Inherited disorders (autosomal dominant): multiple endocrine neoplasia 1 and 2a, family hyperparathyroidism

C. PRESENTATION
1. Most have minimal symptoms or asymptomatic and are found incidentally on lab studies
2. Symptomatic hypercalcemia more common in parathyroid carcinoma versus benign conditions
3. Symptoms: "Stones, bones, groans, and psychic overtones"
   a. Stones—nephrolithiasis in 20%–25%; nephrocalcinosis—less than 5%
      (1) Chronic hypercalcemia impairs concentration, leading to polyuria, polydipsia, and nocturia.
   b. Bone disease (15%)—osteopenia, osteoporosis, and osteitis fibrosa
      (1) Reduction in bone mineral density common; bone pain and tenderness, with pathologic fractures being rare
   c. Abdominal groans (20%)—peptic ulcer disease, cholelithiasis, pancreatitis
   d. Psychic overtones (50%)—fatigue and muscle weakness, depression, anxiety, irritability, lack of concentration, and insomnia

D. DIAGNOSIS
1. Physical examination—rarely palpable; if palpable neck mass, suspect parathyroid cancer or thyroid anomaly
2. Laboratory studies
   a. Elevated serum calcium in setting of elevated PTH level
   b. Decreased serum phosphate
   c. Elevated chloride:phosphate ratio (>33)
3. Work-up for other causes of hypercalcemia, including malignancy, adrenal insufficiency, pheochromocytoma, vitamin D toxicity, granulomatous disease, immobility, drug induced (thiazide diuretics, lithium, antacids leading to milk-alkali syndrome), familial hypocalciuric hypercalcemia

E. MANAGEMENT

1. **Medical treatment**
   a. Hypercalcemic crisis
      (1) Symptoms: anorexia, nausea, emesis, polyuria, polydipsia, abdominal pain, lethargy, bone pain, muscle weakness
      (2) Treatment: normal saline resuscitation, furosemide drip (10–20 mg/h) once isovolemic
      (3) Hemodialysis to reduce levels quickly
   b. Medications
      (1) Selective estrogen receptor modifiers and bisphosphonates: lower serum calcium and increase bone mineral density
      (2) Calcimimetics: lower serum calcium and PTH
      (3) No long-term outcome data. Parathyroidectomy more cost-effective than medical management or strict follow-up
2. **Surgical treatment**
   a. Indications for parathyroidectomy
      (1) Serum calcium greater than 1 mg/dL above upper limits of normal
      (2) Life-threatening hypercalcemic episode
      (3) Creatinine clearance reduced to less than 60 mL/min
      (4) 24-hour urinary calcium excretion: not indicated (some physicians still regard >400 mg as indication for surgery)
      (5) T score less than −2.5 at any site and/or previous fracture fragility
      (6) Age less than 50 years
      (7) Long-term medical surveillance not desired or possible
   b. Preoperative localization tests—technetium 99m (99mTc)-labeled sestamibi most widely used; sensitivity 80%–90% for detecting adenomas
      (1) Allow for minimally invasive unilateral or focused exploration
      (2) Mandatory for reoperative exploration
      (3) Complemented by ultrasound; identify intrathyroidal glands
      (4) Multiphase computed tomography (CT)
   c. Surgical resection
      (1) Adenoma—resection is curative.
      (2) Hyperplasia—3½- or 4-gland removal with reimplantation of ½ gland in forearm or sternocleidomastoid muscle
      (3) Carcinoma—bilateral neck exploration, en bloc excision of tumor and ipsilateral thyroid lobe
      (4) Modified radical neck dissection in presence of abnormal nodes
      (5) Ectopic location (15%–20%)
         (a) Carotid sheath: 5%–19%
         (b) Paraesophageal: 28%–33%
         (c) Intrathyroidal: 5%–10%
         (d) Intrathymic: 12%–24%

(e) Anterior mediastinum: 17%–20%

(f) High cervical position: 1%

d. Intraoperative PTH: compare preoperative PTH level with level taken 10 minutes after removal of gland

(1) If PTH falls by ≥50% and is normal or near normal, high likelihood of successful resection

e. Indication for sternotomy

(1) Not recommended at initial operation unless Ca^{2+} >13 mg/dL

(2) Use if localization studies detect anterior mediastinal or intrathymic tumors.

f. Postoperative care

(1) Risk of recurrent laryngeal nerve injury (1%)

(2) Hypocalcemia and "hungry bone syndrome"

(a) Most common if bone disease present

(b) Mild: treat with oral calcium supplementation (2–4 g of elemental calcium per day).

(c) Severe, symptomatic: treat with intravenous (IV) calcium.

(d) Vitamin D supplementation for refractory hypocalcemia

III. SECONDARY HYPERPARATHYROIDISM

A. CAUSATIVE FACTORS

1. Most common: chronic renal failure

2. Hypocalcemia from malabsorption or inadequate calcium or vitamin D intake

B. SYMPTOMS

1. Psychiatric disorders, bone pain, pruritus, headache, muscle weakness, weight loss, fatigue, renal osteodystrophy, soft tissue calcification

C. TREATMENT

1. Medical

a. Low-phosphate diet, phosphate binders, adequate intake of calcium, and vitamin D

b. Calcimimetics

2. Surgical

a. Indications: symptoms, calcium greater than 11 mg/dL with increased PTH; used only when medical therapy is unsuccessful

b. Dialysis the day before surgery

c. Bilateral neck exploration, subtotal or total parathyroidectomy with autotransplantation and upper thymectomy

d. Postoperative management of hungry bone syndrome

IV. TERTIARY HYPERPARATHYROIDISM

A. CAUSATIVE FACTOR

1. Persistent hyperparathyroidism after renal transplantation

2. Parathyroid gland hyperplasia with autonomous PTH production

50

PARATHYROID

B. SYMPTOMS
1. Pathologic fractures, bone pain, renal stones, peptic ulcer disease, pancreatitis, and mental status changes

C. TREATMENT
1. Surgical treatment for symptomatic disease or autonomous PTH greater than 1 year after transplant
2. Subtotal or total parathyroidectomy with autotransplantation and upper thymectomy

V. PARATHYROID CARCINOMA
1. Rare, accounts for less than 1% of all hyperparathyroidism
2. Younger, more symptomatic
   a. Higher elevation of calcium, PTH, and alkaline phosphatase levels
   b. Palpable gland (>50%)
3. Treatment
   a. Radical resection of involved gland, ipsilateral thyroid lobe, and regional lymph nodes
   b. If recurs, attempt to resect to avoid uncontrolled hypercalcemia
   c. Prognosis is poor, depends on complete initial resection

RECOMMENDED READINGS

Bilezikian JP, Brandi ML, Eastell R, et al. Guidelines for the management of asymptomatic primary hyperparathyroidism: summary statement from the Fourth International Workshop. *J Clin Endocrinol Metab*. 2014;99(10):3561–3569.

Judson BL, Shaha AR. Nuclear imaging and minimally invasive surgery in the management of hyperparathyroidism. *J Nucl Med*. 2008;49(11):1813–1818.

Mariani G, Gulec SA, Rubello D, et al. Preoperative localization and radioguided parathyroid surgery. *J Nucl Med*. 2003;44(9):1443–1458.

Phitayakorn R, McHenry CR. Incidence and location of ectopic abnormal parathyroid glands. *Am J Surg*. 2006;191(3):418–423.

Shen W, Duren M, Morita E, et al. Reoperation for persistent or recurrent primary hyperparathyroidism. *Arch Surg*. 1996;131(8):861–867.

Adrenal Gland

Emily Midura, MD

*War will never cease until babies begin to come into the world
with larger cerebrums and smaller adrenal glands.*

—H.L. Mencken

I. EMBRYOLOGY AND ANATOMY

A. GENERAL
1. Paired, retroperitoneal glands superior and medial to kidney
2. Weight 4–5 g; yellow in color because of high lipid content

B. ARTERIAL SUPPLY
1. Superior adrenal artery—branch of inferior phrenic artery
2. Middle adrenal artery—branch of aorta
3. Inferior adrenal artery—branch of renal artery

C. VENOUS DRAINAGE
1. Single major adrenal vein, 5%–10% of patients with accessory venous drainage
2. Right adrenal vein—short, drains directly into inferior vena cava (IVC)
3. Left adrenal vein—longer, empties into left renal vein

D. CORTEX
1. Embryology: It is derived from mesodermal tissue on adrenogenital ridge at the fifth week of gestation near gonads and can have ectopic tissue near sex organs.
2. Outer portion of gland consists of three zones:
   a. Zona glomerulosa—outer layer, produces mineralocorticoid aldosterone (salt)
   b. Zona fasciculata—middle layer, produces glucocorticoid cortisol (sugar)
   c. Zona reticularis—inner layer, produces androgens (sex)

E. MEDULLA
1. Embryology: It is derived from ectodermal tissue arising from the neural crest and can have ectopic tissue in paraaortic/paravertebral locations; organ of Zuckerkandl at aortic bifurcation is a collection of neural crest cells similar to the adrenal medulla.
2. Inner portion of gland contains chromaffin cells, which produce catecholamine hormones epinephrine and norepinephrine.

II. ZONA GLOMERULOSA—MINERALOCORTICOIDS

A. PHYSIOLOGY

1. Aldosterone secretion is regulated by renin-angiotensin system.
   a. Juxtaglomerular cells in kidney stimulate renin release with decreased renal blood flow, decreased plasma Na^+, and increased sympathetic tone.
   b. Renin induces conversion of angiotensinogen to angiotensin I.
   c. Angiotensin I is cleaved by angiotensin-converting enzyme (ACE) in lungs to angiotensin II.
   d. Angiotensin II is a potent vasoconstrictor and increases aldosterone synthesis/release.
   e. Aldosterone acts on distal convoluted tubule to increase Na^+ reabsorption and H^+/K^+ excretion.

B. PRIMARY ALDOSTERONISM/CONN SYNDROME

1. Presentation: presents at 30–50 years of age with hypertension not controlled with multimodal therapy, hypokalemia, muscle weakness and fatigue, polydipsia, polyuria, and headaches
2. Pathophysiology: 70% single functional adrenal adenoma, 30% bilateral adrenal hyperplasia (BAH), differential includes renal artery stenosis, cirrhosis, congestive heart failure (CHF), and adrenocortical carcinoma
3. Laboratory evaluation: hypernatremia, hypokalemia, and metabolic alkalosis; elevated aldosterone and low renin activity (ratio >1:30); failure to suppress aldosterone with sodium loading
4. Imaging: computed tomography (CT) or magnetic resonance imaging (MRI) (less sensitive) with intravenous (IV) contrast to identify adenoma
5. Selective venous catheterization: used with bilateral gland enlargement and when there is inability to identify an adenoma on imaging; cannulate bilateral adrenal veins and measure aldosterone and cortisol levels after adrenocorticotropic hormone (ACTH) stimulation; greater than fourfold difference in measurements is diagnostic
6. Scintigraphy: nuclear medicine scan; ^{131}I-6-iodomethyl noriodocholesterol (NP-95) is taken up in the adrenal cortex, and adenomas appear as "hot" nodules, whereas BAH has bilateral increased uptake
7. Treatment: surgical excision after preoperative potassium supplementation and control of hypertension with spironolactone (aldosterone antagonist), amiloride (K^+ sparing diuretic), calcium channel blocker, and ACE-inhibitor; patients may require mineralocorticoid replacement; monitor closely for adrenal insufficiency in immediate postoperative period

III. ZONA FASICULATA—GLUCOCORTICOIDS

A. PHYSIOLOGY

1. Cortisol release regulated by hypothalamic-pituitary-adrenal axis
   a. Hypothalamus secretes corticotropin-releasing hormone (CRH).
   b. CRH induces the anterior pituitary to secrete ACTH (derived from proopiomelanocortin hormone [POMC]).

   c. ACTH stimulates secretion of glucocorticoids, mineralocorticoids, and androgens.

   d. ACTH secretion is stimulated by stress, pain, hypoxia, hypothermia, trauma, and hypoglycemia; basal levels at peak in morning and at nadir in late afternoon.

   e. Cortisol binds to receptors in cytosol of target cells to stimulate gene transcription.

   f. Axis is controlled by a negative feedback loop.

B. CUSHING SYNDROME

1. Presentation: patients present with hirsutism, characteristic fat deposition (moon facies, buffalo hump, central obesity), diabetes, hypertension, amenorrhea, and abdominal striae; female predominance (1:8)
2. Pathophysiology: hypercortisolism; can be ACTH independent or dependent
   a. ACTH independent usually secondary to exogenous steroid use, adrenal adenoma/carcinoma, or BAH
   b. ACTH dependent: 70% are Cushing disease (pituitary adenoma) that causes BAH; can also have ectopic ACTH hypersecretion from carcinoid, bronchial tumors, primary adrenal neoplasm, or ectopic CRH production
3. Laboratory evaluation: elevated 24-hour urine cortisol, low-dose dexamethasone suppression test (cortisol production will not be suppressed in autonomous adrenal gland), high-dose dexamethasone suppression test (ectopic ACTH-producing tumor if cortisol not suppressed >50%)
4. Bilateral petrosal venous sampling: measure ACTH in petrosal sinus; an elevated central to peripheral ACTH gradient is diagnostic of a pituitary source.
5. Imaging: CT or MRI (less sensitive) with IV contrast to identify adenoma; MRI of head to evaluate for pituitary lesion
6. Treatment: adrenalectomy for adrenal adenoma; bilateral adrenalectomy for BAH; pituitary adenomas treated with transsphenoidal excision or radiation with bilateral adrenalectomy to avoid hypopituitarism; treatment of underlying extraadrenal tumor; medical treatment for nonsurgical candidates includes ketoconazole, metyrapone, and aminoglutethimide

IV. ZONA RETICULARIS—ANDROGENS

A. PHYSIOLOGY

1. ACTH stimulates production of androgens (dihydroepiandrosterone [DHEA], androstenedione, testosterone, and estrogen) from 17-hydroxypregnenolone; during development adrenal androgens promote male genitalia formation.

B. ANDROGEN-BASED TUMORS

1. Virilizing tumors
   a. Present in children with early growth spurts, premature development of facial and pubic hair, acne, and enlarged genitals

51

ADRENAL GLAND

b. Present in females with hirsutism, amenorrhea, infertility, masculine features
c. Can be hard to diagnose in males
d. Diagnosed with elevated plasma or urine DHEA/17-ketosteroids

2. Feminizing tumors
   a. Males present at 30–50 years of age with gynecomastia, impotence, and testicular atrophy.
   b. Women present with irregular menses and uterine bleeding.
   c. Female children present with breast enlargement and early menarche.
   d. Elevated urine 17-ketosteroids and estrogens are diagnostic.

3. Treatment: tumors treated with adrenalectomy; metastatic disease controlled with adrenolytic medications (mitotane, aminoglutethimide, and ketoconazole)

V. ADRENOCORTICAL CANCER

1. Presentation: rare; bimodal age distribution in childhood and 30–40 years of age; 50% have nonfunctioning tumors; if functioning tumors, present with Cushing syndrome and virilizing factors

2. Diagnosis: renal panel to rule out hypokalemia; low-dose dexamethasone test, 24-hour urine cortisol, 17-ketosteroids, and catecholamines
   a. CT/MRI demonstrate large, heterogeneous mass with irregular margins (>6 cm predicts malignancy) and possible hemorrhage, surrounding lymphadenopathy, or liver metastasis.
   b. Staging CT chest and pelvis for staging for metastatic lesions

3. Treatment: en bloc resection with lymph nodes and adjacent structures if invasion present; mitotane used as adjuvant agent for invasive disease, metastatic disease, or unresectable tumors; other chemotherapeutic agents with inconsistent response (etoposide, cisplatin, doxorubicin, paclitaxel); bony metastasis treated with radiation
   a. Resection margins are best predictor of survival: 30%–50% survival at 5 years with complete resection; less than 1 year for incomplete

4. Metastatic disease to the adrenals includes lung cancer (small cell carcinoma), renal cell carcinoma, melanoma, gastric adenocarcinoma, hepatocellular adenocarcinoma, esophageal adenocarcinoma, and breast cancer.

VI. ADRENAL MEDULLA

A. PHYSIOLOGY

1. It produces and releases catecholamine hormones—epinephrine, norepinephrine, and dopamine.
2. Metabolism in liver and kidneys forms metabolites metanephrines, normetanephrines, and vanillylmandelic acid.

B. **PHEOCHROMOCYTOMA—CATECHOLAMINE-SECRETING TUMOR**
1. Presentation: presents at 30–40 years of age, with palpitations, headache, diaphoresis, anxiety, tremulousness, flushing, chest pain, nausea, and vomiting
   a. Located in adrenals or along sympathetic ganglia, including organ of Zuckerkandl, neck, mediastinum, abdomen, and pelvis
   b. Follows "rule of 10s"—10% bilateral, familial, malignant, extraadrenal, and present in children
   c. Associated with multiple endocrine neoplasia (MEN) IIa and IIb, von Hippel-Lindau disease, Sturge-Weber syndrome; hereditary tumors tend to be multiple and bilateral
2. Pathophysiology: Adrenal tumors secrete epinephrine; extraadrenal sites secrete norepinephrine because they lack phenylethanolamine-*N*-methyltransferase (converts norepinephrine to epinephrine).
3. Diagnosis: measure 24-hour urine catecholamines, metanephrines, vanillylmandelic acid, plasma metanephrines; CT abdomen and pelvis without contrast; MRI or metaiodobenzylguanidine (MIBG) scan
4. Treatment: adrenalectomy after preoperative volume resuscitation; alpha blockade with phenoxybenzamine (1–3 weeks before surgery) and subsequent beta blockade to prevent perioperative hypertensive crisis and congestive heart failure
   a. Perioperative monitoring with arterial line; central line for access
   b. Postoperative hypotension common because of loss of adrenergic stimulation
   c. Malignant tumors diagnosed by local invasion; may metastasize to bone, liver, regional lymph nodes, lung, and peritoneum; treated with en bloc resection, metastasectomy, and adjuvant chemotherapy

VII. INCIDENTALOMA

A. **EPIDEMIOLOGY**
1. Adrenal lesion found during routine imaging; excludes tumors discovered for evaluation of hormone hypersecretion or staging of known cancers
2. Incidence 0.4%–4%
3. Differential includes:
   a. Benign functioning lesion—aldosteronoma, cortisol- or sex steroid–producing adenoma, pheochromocytoma
   b. Malignant functioning lesion—adrenocortical cancer, malignant pheochromocytoma
   c. Benign nonfunctioning lesion—cortical adenoma, myelolipoma, cyst, ganglioneuroma, hemorrhage
   d. Malignant nonfunctioning lesion—metastasis

B. **CLINICAL EVALUATION**
1. Asymptomatic patients with cysts, hemorrhage, myelolipoma, or diffuse metastatic disease need no further work-up.
2. Identify surgical candidates—functioning tumors, malignant tumors

51

ADRENAL GLAND

a. Perform low-dose dexamethasone suppression test or 24-hour urine cortisol to rule out subclinical Cushing syndrome.

b. Perform 24-hour urine collection for catecholamines, metanephrines, and vanillylmandelic acid to rule out pheochromocytoma.

c. Measure serum electrolytes, plasma aldosterone, and renin to rule out aldosteronoma.

d. Imaging: Lesions greater than 6 cm have 35% risk for malignancy; hyperattenuation, inhomogeneous, irregular borders, local invasion, and adjacent adenopathy all suggest malignancy.

e. Fine-needle aspiration (FNA) is useful in patients with known malignancy and a solitary adrenal mass. *Note: Must rule out pheochromocytoma before biopsy.*

C. MANAGEMENT

1. Perform surgical resection for functioning tumors or malignancy.
2. Lesions less than 4 cm are followed with yearly CT scan.
3. Nonfunctional lesions of 4–6 cm can be managed conservatively or operatively depending on patient risk factors.

VIII. ADRENAL INSUFFICIENCY

A. PATHOPHYSIOLOGY AND CLINICAL PRESENTATION

1. Primary (adrenal source) or secondary (ACTH deficiency)
2. It can be caused by autoimmune disease, infections, metastatic deposits, hemorrhage (Waterhouse-Friderichsen syndrome from fulminant meningococcemia), trauma, severe stress, or exogenous steroid discontinuation.
3. Patients often present with symptoms that mimic sepsis—fever, nausea, vomiting, lethargy, abdominal pain, hypotension—after recent steroid withdrawal or significant clinical stress.

B. DIAGNOSIS

1. Laboratory evaluation: hyponatremia, hypokalemia, hypoglycemia, eosinophilia, and low cortisol levels
2. ACTH stimulation test

C. TREATMENT

1. Volume resuscitation, steroid replacement, and correction of underlying cause
   a. Administer IV hydrocortisone.
   b. Fludrocortisone (mineralocorticoid) may also be required.

IX. ADRENAL SURGERY

A. ADRENLAECTOMY

1. Right adrenalectomy: requires mobilization of the right hepatic lobe to enter the retroperitoneum; minimal transverse colon mobilization; dissection of the gland starts with an inferomedial approach with ligation of feeding arteries and identification of the right adrenal vein draining into the IVC

2. Left adrenalectomy: requires mobilization of the inferior pole of the spleen, tail of the pancreas, and left colon to expose the retroperitoneum; the adrenal vein is identified first and divided, followed by division of arterial branches in a superolateral to medial approach

B. OPEN ADRENALECTOMY

1. Indications: known malignancy, large tumor, local invasion, need for metastasectomy
2. Operative approaches: anterior transabdominal, thoracoabdominal, posterior retroperitoneal
   a. Anterior approach: patient in reverse Trendelenburg; ipsilateral or bilateral subcostal incisions
   b. Thoracoabdominal: used for large, locally invasive tumors; patient positioned with ipsilateral flank raised and arm extended above the head; incision is in the 10th–11th intercostal space in the posterior axillary line and extended to abdominal midline
   c. Posterior approach: used in smaller tumors in patients with previous abdominal operations; largely replaced by laparoscopic approach; patients lie prone and flexed at the waist; incision from midline of the 10th rib to the posterior iliac crest; retroperitoneum is entered through the lumbodorsal fascia, exposing Gerota fascia, which is entered and the kidney mobilized to expose the adrenal gland; the adrenal vein is identified and divided, and the gland is mobilized lateral to medial, dividing all feeding arterial branches

C. LAPAROSCOPIC ADRENALECTOMY

1. Indications: small (<6 cm), benign tumors
2. Approach: anterior and posterior retroperitoneal approaches
   a. Anterior: patient in lateral decubitus with affected side up; dissection similar to open anterior abdominal approach
   b. Posterior retroperitoneal: used in patients with previous abdominal operations and bilateral adrenalectomies because patient does not require repositioning to expose the contralateral gland; patient positioned in prone jackknife; dissection is similar to the open retroperitoneal approach

51

ADRENAL GLAND

RECOMMENDED READINGS

Brunicardi FC, Andersen DK, Billiar TR, et al., eds. Thyroid, parathyroid and adrenal. In: *Schwartz's Principles of Surgery*. New York: McGraw-Hill; 2014.

Carroll TB, Findling JW. The diagnosis of Cushing's syndrome. *Rev Endocr Metab Disord*. 2010;11:147–153.

Husebye ES, Allolio B, Arlt W, et al. Consensus statement on the diagnosis, treatment and follow-up of patients with primary adrenal insufficiency. *J Intern Med*. 2014;275:104–115.

Iacobone M, Citton M, Viel G, Rossi GP, Nitti D. Approach to the surgical management of primary aldosteronism. *Gland Surg*. 2015;4:69–81.

Libe R. Adrenocortical carcinoma (ACC): diagnosis, prognosis, and treatment. *Front Cell Dev Biol*. 2015;3:45.

National Comprehensive Cancer Network (NCCN). *NCCN Clinical Practice Guidelines in Oncology. Neuroendocrine Tumors Version 2.* 2016. Available at https://www.nccn.org/professionals/physician_gls/f_guidelines.asp.

Okoh AK, Berber E. Laparoscopic and robotic adrenal surgery: transperitoneal approach. *Gland Surg.* 2015;4:435–441.

Shen WT, Sturgeon C, Duh QY. From incidentaloma to adrenocortical carcinoma: the surgical management of adrenal tumors. *J Surg Oncol.* 2005;89:186–192.

Terzolo M, Bovio S, Pia A, Reimondo G, Angeli A. Management of adrenal incidentaloma. *Best Pract Res Clin Endocrinol Metab.* 2009;23:233–243.

Neuroendocrine Tumors

Teresa C. Rice, MD

When Robert Zollinger, MD, told his parents about his plans to be a surgeon, his father gave him one piece of advice: "If you're going to be a doctor, be a good one."

Walter Zollinger

I. NEUROENDOCRINE TUMORS

A. DEMOGRAPHICS

1. Incidence is rising, likely because of increased detection; the majority are found in the gastrointestinal (GI) tract and pancreas.
2. Peak incidence is in sixth to seventh decade of life.

B. CLASSIFICATION (MULTIPLE SYSTEMS AND EVOLVING TERMINOLOGY)

1. Histologic: well differentiated (previously known as carcinoid tumors) versus poorly differentiated (G3) (previously known as neuroendocrine carcinomas)
2. Well-differentiated neuroendocrine tumors (NETs) can be further subgrouped into low (G1) and intermediate grade (G2) by mitotic rate (<2 mitoses/10 high-power field [hpf] vs. 2–20 mitoses/10 hpf) or Ki67 labeling index (<3% vs. 3%–20%).

C. LOCATION

1. Majority originate from enterochromaffin cells in GI tract.
2. Other locations include bronchopulmonary tract, larynx, pancreas (islet cell tumors), biliary tract, thymus, ovary, kidney, and skin.

D. PRESENTATION

1. This varies depending on physical characteristics, origin, and if hormones are produced.
2. Ninety percent of patients are hormonally asymptomatic; hormonal products must obtain direct access to the systemic circulation (hepatic metastases, significant retroperitoneal disease, primary tumor not draining to portal venous circulation) to be active and not cleared by liver.
3. Mass of tumor can cause intussusception or obstruction (e.g., small bowel obstruction [SBO], jaundice, appendicitis, pancreatitis).
4. Hormone secretion can cause carcinoid symptoms, such as:
   a. Flushing—bradykinin, hydroxytryptophan, prostaglandins
   b. Diarrhea—serotonin
   c. Cramping—serotonin
   d. Endocardial fibrosis—serotonin
   e. Pellagra—depletion of niacin stores due to serotonin

f. Bronchospasm—bradykinin, histamine, prostaglandins
g. Telangiectasia—vasoactive intestinal peptides, serotonin, prostaglandins, bradykinin
h. Glucose intolerance—serotonin
i. Arthropathy—serotonin
j. Hypotension—serotonin

5. Symptoms can be induced by consumption of ethanol, chocolate, or blue cheese and by exertion and surgery.
6. Metastatic potential is related to grade, location, and size.
7. Urinary 5-hydroxyindoleacetic acid, serum chromogranin A, and substance P are most commonly measured.

E. STAGING AND LOCALIZATION

1. Chest computed tomography (CT) scan—bronchial NET
2. Endoscopy/endoscopic ultrasound (EUS)—ability to biopsy gastric, duodenal, distal small ileal NETs, colorectal carcinoids, and pancreas
3. Multiphasic CT scan and/or CT enterography—liver metastases, retroperitoneal masses, and carcinomatosis
4. Nuclear medicine scans (pentetreotide indium-111, gallium Ga-68 Dotatate positron emission tomography [PET] scan, and MIBG [metaiodobenzylguanidine I123])
5. Angiography/selective venous sampling—may be useful in difficult cases

F. MANAGEMENT

1. Appendiceal
   a. Less than 1 cm, low grade without mesoappendix invasion and negative margin—appendectomy
   b. One to 2 cm—controversial because risk of metastases is rare, particularly if smaller than 1.5 cm
   c. Greater than 2 cm or other higher risk factors for lymphatic metastases in good-risk patient—right hemicolectomy
2. Small bowel (more likely to metastasize)
   a. Multicentric in 20%–40%—must examine all of small bowel and colon
   b. Resection of involved small bowel and mesentery; can consider cholecystectomy if somatostatin analogs are likely to be used in future
3. Rectal
   a. Less than 1 cm, T1, low grade—endoscopic/transanal excision
   b. One to 2 cm, low grade controversial
   c. Greater than 2 cm, T2 or other higher-risk factors, low anterior resection (LAR) or abdominoperineal resection (APR) to resect and clear draining nodes
4. Gastric
   a. Type 1 associated with chronic atrophic gastritis and achlorhydria: endoscopic resection of small tumors and surveillance, antrectomy for progression to reduce gastrin secretion or more radical resection for more advanced disease

    b. Type 2 associated with gastrinoma: treat primary

    c. Type 3 sporadic NET not in association with chronic atrophic gastritis: partial or total gastrectomy and regional node resection

5. **Metastatic disease**
   a. Observation in asymptomatic patients with very slow progression
   b. Systemic therapy
      (1) Somatostatin analogs, both for symptoms and for tumor growth
      (2) Molecular therapies targeting mechanistic target of rapamycin (mTOR), thymidine kinase (TK), or vascular endothelial growth factor (VEGF), such as everolimus, sunitinib, bevacizumab
      (3) Interferon-α
      (4) Radiolabeled somatostatin analogs
      (5) Cytotoxic chemotherapy, particularly for high-grade or rapidly growing cancers
   c. Surgical intervention
      (1) Obstruction, perforation, bleeding, or other tumor-related symptoms
      (2) Potentially resectable disease
      (3) Severe carcinoid symptoms for which sufficient debulking anticipated with low morbidity
   d. Regional intraarterial therapy
   e. Radiofrequency or stereotactic body radiation therapy (SBRT) ablative therapies

II. GASTRINOMA

A. DEMOGRAPHICS

1. This is found in 0.1% of individuals with duodenal ulcers and 2% of individuals with ulcers refractory to medical therapy.
2. Twenty-five percent of gastrinomas are associated with multiple endocrine neoplasia syndrome type 1 (MEN1).
3. Gender distribution is 60% male, 40% female.
4. Mean onset of symptoms is before sixth decade of life.

B. LOCATION

1. Eighty-five percent of gastrinomas are located in the gastrinoma triangle, more commonly in duodenum than in pancreas itself (Fig. 52.1).
2. Ectopic locations include splenic hilum, gastric wall, mesentery, and liver.

C. PRESENTATION

1. Symptoms are secondary to hypergastrinemia; increased gastrin leads to acid hypersecretion by parietal cells and peptic ulceration.
2. Abdominal pain and diarrhea are most common symptoms.
   a. It may be caused by ulcers that 90% of individuals have endoscopically confirmed in the upper GI tract.

52

NEUROENDOCRINE TUMORS

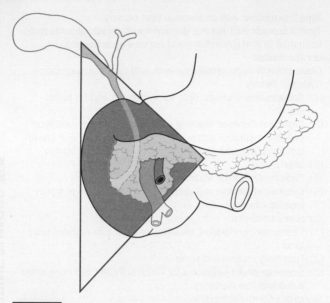

FIG. 52.1

The gastrinoma triangle. Boundaries are the junction of the cystic duct and common bile duct, the second and third portion of the duodenum, and the neck and body of the pancreas.

b. Ulcers may also lead to bleeding (30%–50%) and perforation (5%–10%).
c. Diarrhea presents as only symptom in 20% of cases. It is caused by acid hypersecretion, injury to small bowel mucosa, malnutrition caused by inactivated enzymes, and increased motility.
3. Gastroesophageal reflux

D. DIAGNOSIS

1. Serum gastrin level
   a. Increased in 90% of patients (reference range, 100–200 pg/mL)
   b. Fasting serum gastrin level greater than 1000 pg/mL in presence of gastric acid diagnostic
   c. For serum gastrin levels 200–1000 pg/mL, secretin stimulation testing can distinguish gastrinomas from G-cell hyperplasia
2. Localization
   a. Endoscopy/EUS, multiphasic CT, or magnetic resonance imaging (MRI)
   b. Somatostatin receptor scintigraphy or Ga-68 Dotatate PET/CT
      (1) Most gastrinomas have somatostatin receptors.

(2) False-negative rate for small duodenal wall gastrinomas is high.

 c. Angiography with selective arterial secretin stimulation and venous sampling

 d. Intraoperative

E. MANAGEMENT

1. Medical therapy

 a. Initially control acid hypersecretion with high-dose proton pump inhibitor.

 b. Octreotide may be added to decrease gastrin secretion.

 c. Evaluate for MEN1.

2. Exploration

 a. For sporadic disease, exploration is indicated.

  (1) Initial assessment for metastatic disease

  (2) Mobilization of pancreas with intraoperative ultrasound

  (3) Transduodenal illumination/duodenotomy with palpation if fail to find tumor

  (4) Enucleation for small tumors less than 2 cm; resection for larger tumors

  (5) Resections without localization not indicated

  (6) Regional node resection

 b. For MEN1, surgery is controversial because most believe that surgery will fail to resolve hypergastrinemia as it is often multifocal. Some reserve this for tumors greater than 2 cm and resistance to medical therapies. Surgery should include duodenotomy and may include distal pancreatectomy.

3. Metastatic disease—as with other metastatic NETs discussed previously

III. INSULINOMA

A. DEMOGRAPHICS

1. Most common islet cell tumor
2. Slight female gender predominance
3. Age of presentation from fifth to sixth decade of life
4. Ninety percent sporadic; 10% associated with MEN1 syndrome

B. PRESENTATION

1. Whipple triad

 a. Fasting hypoglycemia

 b. Blood glucose level of less than 50 mg/dL at fasting

 c. Resolution of symptoms with glucose administration

2. Common symptoms—visual disturbances, altered consciousness, weakness, seizures, diaphoresis, tremors, and tachycardia

C. DIAGNOSIS

1. Biochemical tests

 a. Seventy-two-hour supervised fast

(1) Measure serum glucose and insulin levels every 4 hours.
(2) When glucose level is less than 60 mL/dL, measure levels every hour.
(3) Diagnosis is confirmed with symptoms of hypoglycemia, serum insulin level greater than 6 μU/mL, and insulin:glucose ratio greater than 0.3.

b. Elevated C peptide levels (will not be elevated with surreptitious administration of insulin), no circulating oral hypoglycemic medications, no anti-insulin antibodies

c. Equivocal cases: Consider C peptide suppression test and tolbutamide test but more common to proceed with imaging tests to identify mass

2. Localization
   a. Usually small (<2 cm) and single (90%)
   b. Metastatic disease at diagnosis in 10% of patients
   c. Multiphasic CT scan and/or MRI—detects majority of primary tumors and evaluates for metastatic disease
   d. EUS
   e. Visceral angiography, selective arterial calcium stimulation, and portal vein/hepatic vein sampling
   f. Somatostatin analog scintigraphy not as useful as insulinomas—often lack appropriate receptors

D. MANAGEMENT

1. Exploration
   a. Enucleation for small lesions away from the pancreatic duct
   b. Distal pancreatectomy for body and tail near the duct, and pancreaticoduodenectomy for lesions in the head that are large
   c. For MEN1, local excision of head lesions and distal pancreatectomy
   d. Pancreatic biopsy if no tumor is found to evaluate for beta-cell hyperplasia and adult nesidioblastosis

2. Metastatic disease
   a. Resection
      (1) Both to prolong survival and for palliation
      (2) Debulking—may improve control of symptoms
   b. Medical therapy
      (1) Diazoxide—inhibits release of insulin
      (2) Somatostatin analogs
      (3) Other NET systemic therapies
   c. Regional therapy and other ablative therapies

IV. GLUCAGONOMA

A. DEMOGRAPHICS

1. Rare, approximately 20% associated with MEN1

B. PRESENTATION

1. Most commonly present with mild glucose intolerance (>90%) and weight loss

2. Necrolytic migratory erythema—cyclic migrations of legions with spreading margins and healing centers
   a. Occurs in 70% of patients
   b. Located on lower abdomen, perineum, perioral, or feet
   c. Due to low levels of amino acids
3. Other symptoms—depression, deep venous thrombosis, cachexia, hypoaminoacidemia, anemia, diarrhea, and stomatitis
4. Typically located in body and tail of pancreas
5. Tend to be large tumors with metastases

C. DIAGNOSIS
1. Biochemical tests
   a. Fasting serum glucagon level—positive if greater than 1000 pg/mL
2. Biopsy of skin rash has pathognomonic histology.
3. Localization
   a. Multiphasic CT scan—usually identifies tumor because often large and located in body and tail of the pancreas. Also can identify metastases
   b. MRI, EUS, and somatostatin receptor scintigraphy/PET alternatives
   c. Additional modalities—visceral angiography and portal venous sampling

D. MANAGEMENT
1. Reverse catabolic state with octreotide and amino acid supplementation, nutritional support
2. Resection if possible
3. Metastatic disease
   a. Found in more than half of patients
   b. As described previously for NET

V. VASOACTIVE INTESTINAL POLYPEPTIDOMA, VIPoma

A. DEMOGRAPHICS
1. Rare, approximately 5% association with MEN1; other neoplasms can secrete vasoactive intestinal peptide (VIP), including adrenal tumors

B. PRESENTATION
1. Usually presents with high-volume diarrhea exacerbated by enteral intake, but that does not resolve with fasting
2. Hypokalemia and acidosis from electrolyte imbalances
3. WDHA syndrome (watery diarrhea, hypokalemia, and achlorhydria), Verner-Morrison syndrome, or pancreatic cholera

C. DIAGNOSIS
1. Biochemical tests
   a. Serum fasting vasoactive intestinal polypeptide level greater than 75 pg/mL with secretory diarrhea and pancreatic mass
2. Localization
   a. Same as others described previously

D. MANAGEMENT
1. Initial resuscitation—rehydration and correct electrolytes
2. Control diarrhea
   a. Octreotide and other somatostatin analogs
   b. Additional agents—steroids, nonsteroidal antiinflammatories, phenothiazines
3. Surgery
   a. Complete resection via distal pancreatectomy if located in tail of pancreas, regional nodes
   b. Exploration for metastases
4. Metastatic disease
   a. As previously described for NET

VI. SOMATOSTATINOMA

A. DEMOGRAPHICS
1. Rare, approximately 50% associated with MEN1; 10% of neurofibromatosis type 1 (NF-1) patients may develop these tumors, characteristically in duodenum

B. PRESENTATION
1. Classic syndrome
   a. Diabetes mellitus (DM) or glucose intolerance, cholelithiasis, steatorrhea, and diarrhea and weight loss, hypochlorhydria
   b. Seen with pancreatic tumors but not duodenal tumors, which more often present with jaundice, weight loss, bleeding

C. DIAGNOSIS
1. Often incidental finding during invasive procedures, including cholecystectomy
2. Biochemical tests—serum somatostatin level greater than 10 ng/mL
3. Localization—as with other pancreatic NETs

D. MANAGEMENT
1. Exploration
   a. Resection—treatment of choice
   b. Cholecystectomy because of high incidence of cholelithiasis
2. Metastatic disease
   a. Found in majority of patients
   b. Somatostatin analogs as well as other treatments as described previously for other functional pancreatic NETs; however, prognosis poor

VII. PANCREATIC POLYPEPTIDOMAS

A. DEMOGRAPHICS
1. Rare

B. PRESENTATION
1. Nonspecific symptoms such as diarrhea and weigh loss

C. DIAGNOSIS
1. Increased serum pancreatic polypeptide (>300 pmol/L) and pancreatic mass
2. Localization as with other pancreatic NETs

D. MANAGEMENT
1. Exploration—resection is treatment of choice.
2. Metastatic disease
    a. Found in majority of patients
    b. As with other pancreatic NETs

RECOMMENDED READINGS

Eriksson B, Oberg K. Neuroendocrine tumors of the pancreas. *Br J Surg*. 2000;87:129.
Goldin SB, Aston J, Wahi MM. Sporadically occurring functional pancreatic endocrine tumors: review of recent literature. *Curr Opin Oncol*. 2008;20(1):25–33.
Oberg K. Chemotherapy and biotherapy in the treatment of neuroendocrine tumours. *Ann Oncol*. 2001;12(suppl 2):S111–S114.

52

NEUROENDOCRINE TUMORS

PART X

Vascular Surgery

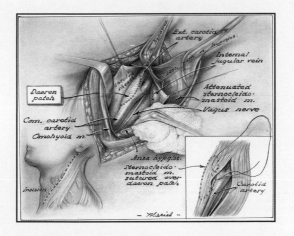

Thromboembolic Disease

Aaron Beckwith, MD

Who spends himself in a worthy cause; who at the best knows in the end the triumph of high achievement, and who at the worst, if he fails, at least fails while daring greatly, so that his place shall never be with those cold and timid souls who neither know victory nor defeat.

—Theodore Roosevelt

53

I. INTRODUCTION

A. EPIDEMIOLOGY

1. Deep vein thrombosis (DVT) and pulmonary embolism (PE) are two manifestations of venous thromboembolism (VTE). Despite advances in prevention and treatment of VTE, PE remains the most common preventable cause of hospital death, responsible for approximately 150,000–200,000 deaths per year in the United States.
   a. Prevention begins before surgery by considering the surgical procedure, its risks, and the patient's comorbidities.
   b. The physician must consider the length of hospitalization, postoperative course, and the patient's rehabilitation status.

B. CAUSATIVE FACTORS

1. Multiple predisposing factors contribute to development of DVTs, and contributing are the characteristics found in *Virchow triad:*
   a. Venous stasis—inactivity, cardiac factors (i.e., congestive heart failure), anesthesia induction
   b. Endothelial injury—all operative procedures in which blood flow is interrupted
   c. Hypercoagulability—medical conditions (cancer, pregnancy, inherited hematologic diseases)

C. OTHER RISK FACTORS FOR THE DEVELOPMENT OF DEEP VEIN THROMBOSIS

1. Age older than 40 years
2. Malignancy
3. History of DVT or PE
4. Obesity
5. Major surgery
6. Trauma
7. Pregnancy
8. Oral contraceptives (hormonal therapy)
9. Physical inactivity

D. CLINICAL PRESENTATION

Nonspecific and often detected only after PE has occurred

1. Signs include swelling, tenderness, calf pain elicited on passive dorsi-flexion of the ankle (Homan sign), or fever.
   a. Less than 50% of patients with DVTs will exhibit these signs.

E. DIFFERENTIAL DIAGNOSES

1. Achilles tendonitis, arterial insufficiency, arthritis, cellulitis, lymphangitis, varicose veins, superficial thrombophlebitis, Baker cyst

F. DIAGNOSIS

1. Best made by Doppler ultrasonography, but other methods include venography or impedance plethysmography (historically)

G. SEQUELAE

1. Death, as previously discussed
   a. DVTs from the iliofemoral, pelvic, ovarian, axillary, subclavian, and internal jugular veins, as well as the inferior vena cava and cavernous sinuses of the skull, can lead to PE.
   b. Clinical presentation is inconsistent but can include dyspnea, chest pain, hemoptysis, tachycardia, fever, increased central venous pressures, and electrocardiographic changes (arrhythmias, enlarged P waves, ST depression, T wave inversions notably in leads III, AVF, V1, V3 and V4).
      (1) Physical examination can be inconsistent and often nondiagnostic.
      (2) Most common symptoms according to Prospective Investigation of Pulmonary Embolism Diagnosis (PIOPED) study were dyspnea (73%), pleuritic chest pain (66%), cough (37%), and hemoptysis (13%).
   c. Diagnosis is established by radiographic imaging studies.
      (1) The gold standard test is pulmonary angiography.
         (a) Highly invasive, technically difficult to perform
      (2) Computed tomographic angiography is less invasive and offers nearly the same specificity and sensitivity as pulmonary angiography.
         (a) Has become the imaging modality of choice
      (3) High-probability ventilation/perfusion (V/Q) scan coupled with a high clinical suspicion for PE can also be diagnostic.
         (a) V/Q scans are not as frequently used, given the accuracy of computed tomographic angiography.
      (4) Chest radiographs initially are normal.
         (a) Rare findings include:
            (i) Westermark sign—dilatation of the pulmonary vessels proximal to an embolism with collapse of distal vessels
            (ii) Hampton hump—triangular, pleural-based infiltrate with the apex pointed toward the hilum, a rare late finding of pulmonary infarction

2. Postthrombotic syndrome—can occur in patients with acute DVT and signifies chronic venous insufficiency; classic findings include brawny, nonpitting edema and ulcer formation

3. Upper extremity DVT—presents with upper extremity swelling and/or pain and less commonly with superior vena cava syndrome
   a. Classification of upper extremity DVTs
      (1) Primary thrombosis—effort thrombosis (Paget-Schroetter syndrome) is thought to cause microtrauma to the venous intima, leading to initiation and propagation of the coagulation cascade
      (2) Secondary thrombosis—axillary or subclavian vein thrombosis caused by indwelling catheters

4. Other DVTs
   a. Superior vena cava obstruction—majority related to tumor invasion; other causes include mediastinal fibrosis, granulomatous disease, vasculitis, or aortic aneurysms
   b. Inferior vena cava thrombosis is generally related to the extension of thrombi from the pelvic or femoral veins.
   c. Tumor thrombus as a consequence of tumor invasion (e.g., renal, hepatic, adrenal) into the vena cava

II. METHODS OF PROPHYLAXIS AND TREATMENT OF DEEP VENOUS THROMBOSES AND PULMONARY EMBOLI

A. DEEP VEIN THROMBOSIS PROPHYLAXIS

1. Mechanical
   a. Leg elevation—no substantial evidence shown to improve clinical outcomes
   b. Graduated compression stockings (thromboembolism deterrent "TED" hose)—must be well-fitted; only marginal effect
   c. Early ambulation—simple and extremely effective
   d. Pneumatic compression boots or sequential compression devices
      (1) Promote venous return and activate the fibrinolytic system
      (2) Inexpensive and useful in patients who cannot be systemically anticoagulated

2. Pharmacologic agents (see the next section)

B. TREATMENT OF DEEP VEIN THROMBOSIS AND PULMONARY EMBOLI

1. Warfarin
   a. Disrupts the hepatic synthesis of vitamin K–dependent coagulation factors (II, VII, IX, and X, and proteins C and S). Patients should be systemically anticoagulated with heparin before initiation, given the prothrombotic state that occurs with depletion of proteins C and S.
   b. It is generally not used for prophylaxis of DVTs.
   c. Therapeutic levels vary depending on the reason for anticoagulation; however, the goal international normalized ratio is 2–3 for DVT.
      (1) Dosing must be individualized.

53

THROMBOEMBOLIC DISEASE

      (2) Multiple drug interactions

      (3) Effects reversed with the administration of vitamin K and fresh frozen plasma

  d. It is contraindicated in pregnancy and in patients at risk for recurrent hemorrhage (recent cerebrovascular accident [CVA] or head trauma).

  e. Therapy is maintained for at least 3 months.

2. **Unfractionated heparin**

  a. Increases the activity of antithrombin III and prevents conversion of fibrinogen to fibrin.

  b. Does not produce clot lysis but does inhibit active thrombogenesis.

  c. Prophylactic dosing is administered subcutaneously (SC) 2 to 3 times daily between 5000 and 8000 units, depending on the weight of the patient.

  d. Therapeutic dosing for systemic anticoagulation is based on weight with an 80-unit/kg intravenous bolus or can be initiated without bolus depending on the clinical situation, followed by 18-unit/kg per hour maintenance infusion, and titrated to maintain therapeutic partial thromboplastic time.

      (1) Reversed with the administration of protamine and fresh frozen plasma

  e. It is safe to use during pregnancy but contraindicated in patients with a history of heparin-induced thrombocytopenia (HIT).

3. **Low-molecular-weight heparin (LMWH; e.g., enoxaparin)**

  a. Binds to antithrombin III and accelerates activity, inhibiting thrombin and factor Xa

  b. Can be administered once or twice daily depending on indication and dosing (30–40 mg SC for prophylaxis or 1 mg/kg for therapeutic anticoagulation)

      (1) Does not require systemic monitoring

      (2) Cannot be reversed with fresh frozen plasma; however, protamine can be given

      (3) Dose adjustment required/precaution advised for CrCl less than 30 mL/min

  c. Contraindicated in patients with HIT but less likely to cause HIT

4. **Thrombolytics (tissue plasminogen activator)**

  a. Used therapeutically only

  b. Promote rapid clot lysis leading to prompt resolution of symptoms, restoration of normal venous circulation, and preservation of venous valvular function

      (1) Does not prevent clot propagation, rethrombosis, or subsequent embolization

      (2) Not effective if the thrombus is organized; will work only on the surface of the clot

      (3) Administered transvenously via a catheter-directed system to allow injection of the agent at the site of the clot

  c. Patients must be systemically anticoagulated after administration of thrombolytics

d. Multiple contraindications exist, including active internal hemorrhage, recent history of intracranial or intraspinal surgery or trauma, intracranial neoplasm, arteriovenous malformation or aneurysm, history of stroke in previous 2 months, and bleeding diathesis.

5. Special circumstances—HIT
   a. Prothrombotic disorder associated with a decrease in platelets, the administration of unfractionated heparin, and occasionally with LMWH
   b. Occurs typically within 2 weeks of heparin administration
   c. Subdivided into HIT types I and II
      (1) HIT I—transient decrease in platelet count that corrects after heparin is discontinued
         (a) Platelet counts rarely decline to less than 100/L.
         (b) It is not attributed to an immune reaction.
      (2) HIT II—autoimmune reaction with antibodies (mainly immunoglobulin G [IgG]) reactive to platelet factor 4 that form complexes with heparin
   d. Clinical diagnosis confirmed with HIT antibody panel; all heparin products should be stopped if suspected
   e. Alternatives for anticoagulation: argatroban (direct thrombin inhibitor), danaparoid, or bivalirudin

C. PROPHYLACTIC INFERIOR VENA CAVA FILTER PLACEMENT

1. Patients who develop DVTs despite being anticoagulated. Consider for high-risk patients (quadriplegics, severe closed head injury, etc.) who have contraindications to other forms of prophylaxis or cannot be anticoagulated.
2. The filter is designed to prevent embolization of a potentially fatal thrombus to the pulmonary circulation, not to prevent DVT.
3. Technical considerations
   a. Can be placed from either an internal jugular or femoral approach
4. Complications include malpositioning, persistent vena caval leak, filter thrombosis, filter migration, and caval thrombosis.

III. AN APPROACH TO PROPHYLAXIS

A. DETERMINE THE PATIENT'S RISK FACTORS

1. Low risk—age less than 40 years; ambulatory or minor surgery
2. Moderate risk—age greater than 40 years; abdominal, pelvic, or thoracic surgery
3. High risk—age greater than 40 years; prior DVT or PE, malignancy, hip and other orthopedic surgeries, immobility, hypercoagulable states

B. PROPHYLAXIS OF CHOICE

1. Encourage early ambulation in all patients, and get physical/occupational therapy involved early, if indicated.
2. CHEST guidelines for prevention of VTE in nonorthopedic surgical patients:
   a. Low risk for VTE (~1.5%)—suggest mechanical prophylaxis, preferably with intermittent pneumatic compression (IPC).

53

THROMBOEMBOLIC DISEASE

b. Moderate risk for VTE (~3%)—suggest LMWH, low-dose unfractionated heparin, or mechanical prophylaxis with IPC over no prophylaxis.
c. High risk for VTE (~6%)—recommend pharmacologic prophylaxis with LMWH or low-dose unfractionated heparin over no prophylaxis. In these patients, also recommend adding mechanical prophylaxis with IPC to pharmacologic prophylaxis.
3. Prophylaxis should be started before the initiation of anesthesia; low-dose SC unfractionated heparin is usually given in a dose of 5000 units 2 hours preoperatively and then every 8–12 hours postoperatively.
4. High-risk patients should be watched closely for clinical signs and symptoms of DVT. Duplex scanning is the least invasive method for screening.

IV. APPROACH TO THE PATIENT WITH PULMONARY EMBOLUS

A. PHYSIOLOGY

1. Respiratory consequences: Increased physiologic alveolar dead space secondary to V/Q mismatch leads to pneumoconstriction, hypoxemia, and hyperventilation.
2. Hemodynamic consequences: PE leads to vascular congestion secondary to a decreased pulmonary vascular bed, leading to increased resistance (pulmonary hypertension). In the cardiac compromised patient, this can lead to cardiac collapse secondary to increased right ventricular afterload.

B. TRANSFER PATIENT TO A MONITORED CARE SETTING/ INTENSIVE CARE UNIT.

1. Aggressive respiratory and hemodynamic monitoring often are obtainable only in an intensive care unit setting.
2. The patient may need to be intubated and require mechanical ventilatory support.

C. CONSIDER ANTICOAGULATION VERSUS THROMBOLYTIC THERAPY.

1. Initiation of anticoagulation should be considered early in a patient suspected of having a PE.
2. Thrombolytics should be reserved for patients who are hemodynamically unstable or have poor underlying cardiopulmonary reserve.
3. Refer to Section II for a description of treatment modalities.

D. SURGICAL TREATMENT OPTIONS

1. Pulmonary embolectomy
   a. Open embolectomy—performed through median sternotomy with cardiopulmonary bypass; associated with high morbidity and mortality
   b. Transvenous embolectomy with a suction cap–tipped catheter passed via jugular or femoral vein
      (1) Useful in massive PE in which there is a contraindication to fibrinolytic therapy

RECOMMENDED READINGS

Jundt JP, et al. Venous and lymphatic disease. In: Brunicardi FC, et al., eds. *Schwartz's Principles of Surgery*. 10th ed. New York, NY: McGraw-Hill; 2014.

Kearon C, Akl EA, Omelas J, et al. Antithrombotic therapy for VTE disease: chest guideline and expert panel report. *Chest*. 2016;149:315–352.

Aneurysms

Grace E. Martin, MD

I. EPIDEMIOLOGY

A. GENERAL

1. Aneurysm—permanent focal dilation of an artery to at least 1.5 times the normal diameter
   a. A normal adult male has an aorta that is approximately 2 cm in size (anything >3 cm is considered abnormal).
   b. Arterial dilation less than 50% increase in diameter = ectasia
   c. Diffuse enlargement of several arterial segments that are 50% greater than the normal diameter = arteriomegaly
2. Abdominal aortic aneurysm (AAA) is the most common type of aneurysm for which patients present for treatment.
3. Male predominance: male/female ratio of 3:1
4. Familial tendency (sex-linked and autosomal recessive)—Relative risk for first-degree relatives of affected individuals is 11.6 times greater than the general population.
5. Those with known popliteal or femoral aneurysms have a 50% likelihood of also having an AAA.

B. CASE REPORT

A 65-year-old man with a history of hypertension, hyperlipidemia, and diabetes mellitus presents with acute onset of back pain for the past 3 hours. He has smoked 1 purified protein derivative (PPD) for the past 50 years. His initial set of vital signs is as follows: heart rate 128, blood pressure 95/52 mm Hg, and respiratory rate 26. Abdominal examination reveals a tender pulsatile mass.

He exhibits the classic triad of ruptured AAA—abdominal/back/flank pain, pulsatile mass, and hypotension.

C. RISK FACTORS

1. Acquired factors
   a. Cigarette smoking—strongest modifiable risk factor associated with AAA development
   b. Hypertension
   c. Age greater than 50 years old
   d. Heart transplant recipient
2. Inheritable factors
   a. Connective tissue disorders—Marfan syndrome, type IV Ehlers–Danlos
   b. First-degree relative with an AAA

D. CAUSATIVE FACTORS

1. Arterial wall degeneration from atherosclerosis with concurrent loss of elastin caused by proteolysis and inflammation leads to a *fusiform (spindle-shaped) aneurysm.*
2. An infectious process in the arterial wall leads to a *mycotic aneurysm.*
   a. Most commonly caused by *Salmonella* or *Staphylococcal* infection

II. PATHOLOGY

A. LOCATION

1. Infrarenal—95% of cases
   a. Distribution factors include elastin/collagen ratio, reflected pulsatility from the aortic bifurcation, diminished vasa vasorum, possible localized autoimmune reaction, and increased metalloproteinase activity.
2. Juxtarenal—extends to the renal arteries
3. Suprarenal—extends to the superior mesenteric artery (SMA) or celiac artery
4. Thoracoabdominal—extends into both the thoracic and abdominal portions of the aorta

B. CHARACTERISTICS

1. Composition—AAAs are true aneurysms; the entire arterial wall is involved.
2. Extension—10%–20% of AAAs also involve the iliac arteries (usually the common iliacs and/or internal iliacs).

C. ASSOCIATED MANIFESTATIONS OF DIFFUSE ATHEROSCLEROSIS

1. Hypertension—40% of patients
2. Coronary artery disease—30% of patients
3. Associated occlusive arterial disease
   a. Iliac arteries—16%
   b. Carotid arteries—7%
   c. Renal arteries—2%
4. Other associated aneurysms
   a. Thoracic aorta—4%
   b. Femoral and popliteal arteries—2%–3%; up to 92% with common femoral artery aneurysm and 64% with a popliteal artery aneurysm have an AAA

III. NATURAL HISTORY

A. GENERAL CONSIDERATIONS

1. Diameter is the strongest predictor of rupture.
2. Increased size = increased rate of rupture
   a. Laplace law—A larger radius increases wall tension, which in turn increases the risk for rupture of the aneurysmal wall.
3. Average growth is 0.4 cm/year.
4. Growth is often staggered, and an aneurysm may be stable for one period and then grow rapidly in another period.

54

ANEURYSMS

TABLE 54.1

RISK OF RUPTURE BASED ON SIZE

AAA Diameter (cm)	Risk of Rupture per Year
<4	0
4–5	0.5–5
5–6	3–15
6–7	10–20
7–8	20–40
>8	30–50

AAA, Abdominal aortic aneurysm.

B. STATISTICS

1. Risk of rupture is based on size (Table 54.1).
2. UK small aneurysm trial suggested that women have a higher rate of rupture at smaller diameters.
3. Renal artery involvement, chronic obstructive pulmonary disease, and diastolic hypertension may also increase the rate of rupture.

IV. CLINICAL PRESENTATION

A. SYMPTOMS

1. Most AAAs are asymptomatic.
2. Two-thirds of known AAAs are incidental findings on imaging studies done for other reasons.
3. Most common symptoms include new-onset abdominal pain and low back pain. May also present as flank, inguinal, or genital pain.
4. Symptoms may be caused by compression of surrounding structures—inferior vena cava, ureter, duodenum.

B. PHYSICAL EXAMINATION

1. Palpation
   a. Presence of pulsatile mass on deep palpation—larger than 5-cm aneurysm palpable in up to 75% of patients
   b. In larger patients, it may be impossible to detect AAAs regardless of diameter.
2. Other pulses: It is important to evaluate peripheral arteries for associated occlusive disease (pulses and bruits) or additional aneurysmal disease.

V. DIAGNOSTIC STUDIES

A. PLAIN FILMS

1. Calcific rim ("egg shell") or large soft-tissue shadow is often visible projecting anterior to the spine.

B. B-MODE ULTRASOUND

1. Screening imaging test of choice because of ease of use and most cost-effective method of confirming and following AAAs

2. Can also evaluate blood flow in renal and visceral arteries
3. Difficult to evaluate the suprarenal aorta because of bowel gas or obesity

C. COMPUTED TOMOGRAPHY SCAN
1. Can provide accurate characterization of entire aorta—gold standard for preoperative planning and diagnosis of a ruptured AAA
2. Permits assessment of diameter, length, wall thickness, and thrombus
3. Three-dimensional reconstruction used for endograft evaluation and planning

D. MAGNETIC RESONANCE IMAGING
1. Comparable in accuracy with computed tomography (CT) scan but more expensive and less readily available
2. May have a role in patients in whom intravenous contrast is contraindicated
3. No role in ruptured patients, given the length of time needed to complete the examination

E. AORTOGRAPHY
1. Poor study for diagnosis or assessment of size, because mural thrombus within AAA can obscure actual aneurysm sac size
2. Expensive and invasive
3. Being replaced by CT and magnetic resonance angiograms that provide noninvasive three-dimensional images
4. Provides information regarding associated vascular lesions for renal arteries and distal runoff
5. Indications for aortography—evidence of accessory renal arteries, horseshoe kidneys, mesenteric ischemia, and peripheral arterial occlusive disease

VI. ELECTIVE MANAGEMENT OF ABDOMINAL AORTIC ANEURYSM

A. OPERATIVE INDICATIONS
1. Decision for repair is individualized—There is not a single threshold size.
2. Patients with AAAs larger than 4–5 cm are candidates for elective operation, unless medical comorbidities significantly increase the operative risk.
3. Surveillance is safe up to 5.5 cm, unless symptomatic or rapidly expanding more than 1 cm/year.
4. A region of 5.5 cm is likely appropriate for the average patient, but patient preference for those who are younger, with low operative risk, or female patients with high rupture risk may consider repair at 4.5–5.5 cm.

B. PREOPERATIVE WORK-UP
1. Every patient should undergo history and physical examination, electrocardiogram (EKG), chest x-ray (CXR), complete blood count (CBC), basic metabolic panel, and coagulation studies.

2. Physical examination should include a peripheral pulse examination with formal ABIs.
3. Anesthesia consultation

C. PREOPERATIVE PREPARATION

1. Severity of coronary artery disease, patient age, female gender, creatinine, and chronic obstructive pulmonary disease (COPD) are independent predictors of mortality.
2. All patients undergoing elective vascular procedures should be started/continued on a beta-blocker, aspirin, and statin. Those with known atherosclerotic cardiovascular disease should also be taking an angiotensin-converting enzyme (ACE) inhibitor.
3. Cardiac evaluation
   a. Patients with active cardiac problems (unstable coronary syndromes, decompensated congestive heart failure [CHF], arrhythmias, valvular disease) should be seen preoperatively by a cardiologist.
   b. Patients who can walk up a flight of stairs (>4 METS) may undergo vascular procedures without additional testing.
4. CT angiography with three-dimensional reconstruction is a valuable tool to both determine whether to proceed with an open or endovascular repair and to tailor grafts to the individual anatomy.
5. Bowel preparation is optional.
6. Epidural anesthesia may be a useful adjunct for postoperative pain management and compromised pulmonary status.
7. In the operating room (OR), an arterial line, adequate venous access (usually a central venous line), and Foley catheter should be placed.
8. In the OR, a peripheral pulse examination should be performed before any incisions for a baseline examination.
9. The antimicrobial preparation should be extended from the nipple line to the toes, and the patient should receive an adequate weight-based dose of either a first-generation cephalosporin (Cefazolin) or vancomycin.

VII. OPEN ABDOMINAL AORTIC ANEURYSM REPAIR

A. APPROACH

1. Midline incision—best for ruptured AAAs, as the aorta at the diaphragm can be easily accessed for proximal control
2. Bilateral subcostal incision—best for obese patients, extensive iliac artery aneurysms, and need for renal artery revascularization
3. Left flank incision (retroperitoneal approach)—best for patients with multiple prior abdominal surgeries, abdominal wall stomas, suprarenal aneurysms, and horseshoe kidneys

B. OPERATIVE STEPS

1. Identify and release the ligament of Treitz for adequate mobilization of the small bowel and duodenum.

2. The retroperitoneum overlying the infrarenal aorta is incised down to the iliac bifurcations.
3. Patient is systemically heparinized (100 units/kg), and control is obtained proximal and distal to the aneurysm sac.
4. Longitudinal arteriotomy is made along the length of the aneurysm sack. If both iliacs are involved, then the arteriotomy will only include one of the two arteries.
5. The proximal and distal anastomoses are end-to-end configurations and should not involve diseased or aneurysmal aortic segments.
6. The residual aneurysm sack is closed around the graft to prevent future aortoenteric fistulization.

C. INTRAOPERATIVE PROBLEMS

1. The inferior mesenteric artery (IMA) should be ligated from within the aneurysm to avoid injury to collateral vessels of the left colon.
2. Back-bleeding lumbar vessels should be suture ligated.
3. Excessive calcification of the iliacs makes it unsafe to cross-clamp. Instead, vascular control may be obtained with an intraluminal approach via a balloon thromboembolectomy catheter.
4. Reperfusion should occur one vessel at a time, to avoid hypotension and metabolic derangements associated with rapid reperfusion of ischemic tissue.
5. Prevent ischemia and ensure adequate perfusion by several intraoperative maneuvers:
   a. Palpate the root of the superior mesenteric artery for pulsatility.
   b. Doppler ultrasound—Audible flow decreases the risk for postoperative ischemic colitis.
   c. IMA back pressure greater than 40 mm Hg indicates adequate collateral retrograde flow.
   d. Fluorescein—Ultraviolet luminescence should show bowel viability.
   e. In those with decreased visceral blood supply and a patent IMA with back pressure greater than 40 mm Hg, consider reimplantation of the IMA into graft.

D. PROSTHETIC GRAFT

1. Tube graft if iliac arteries are normal; bifurcated graft if iliacs are aneurysmal
2. The arterial sites where the graft will be sewn into place cannot be involved by aneurysmal enlargement or mural thrombus.

E. POSTOPERATIVE COURSE

1. Patients are admitted to intensive care unit (ICU) initially; mean total hospitalization is 8 days.
2. Overall, 35% of patients experience a postoperative complication after open repair of an AAA.
3. CT scan is performed at 3 years after surgery for pseudoaneurysm surveillance.

54

ANEURYSMS

VIII. COMPLICATIONS

A. LOWER EXTREMITY ISCHEMIA
1. Found to occur in 3% of patients after open repair.
2. Causes are multiple and may include:
   a. Distal embolization of thrombus or atheromatous debris from the aneurysm sack
   b. Thrombosis from inadequate heparinization, hypercoagulable conditions, or inadequate arterial runoff
   c. Clamp injury/technical errors including anastomotic defects
3. Large emboli above the ankle can be removed with an embolectomy catheter.

B. CARDIAC EVENTS
1. Cardiac complications include ischemia, infarction, arrhythmias, and CHF.
2. Cardiac events occur in up to 25% of patients and are the leading cause of perioperative mortality.

C. RENAL INSUFFICIENCY
1. Causes include hypovolemia, contrast nephrotoxicity, atheroembolization, and inflammatory response from ischemia-reperfusion injury of the lower extremities.
2. Acute renal failure requiring dialysis is rare and occurs in less than 1% of patients.

D. STROKE
1. Stroke associated with AAA repair can be embolic or secondary to hypotension.

E. COLONIC ISCHEMIA
1. Suspect ischemia if patient has bowel movement during the first 24–72 hours after surgery.
2. Mucosal ischemia most common and usually manifested by mucosal sloughing; resolves spontaneously in most cases with bowel rest.
3. *Requires immediate flexible sigmoidoscopy* (or abdominal CT) to diagnose—most commonly affected location is the sigmoid colon
4. Transmural involvement requires reexploration and colonic resection.
5. Most common after emergent open AAA repair (25%–40% of patients)

F. SPINAL CORD ISCHEMIA
1. Anterior spinal artery syndrome—paraplegia with loss of light touch and pain sensation, and loss of sphincter control. Proprioception and temperature sensation are spared.
2. Occurs in 0.25% of patients; however, the effects are irreversible.

G. SEXUAL DYSFUNCTION
1. Retrograde ejaculation and/or inability to maintain erection

2. Caused by injury to sympathetic plexus around aorta or inadequate hypogastric perfusion
3. May occur in 5%–18% of men after open or endovascular repair; always counsel men regarding this risk

H. LATE COMPLICATIONS

1. Aortoenteric fistula
   a. Distal portion of the duodenum is the most common location.
   b. Presentation—gastrointestinal bleeding with associated abdominal and back pain; may have "herald bleed" of small amount of hematemesis, followed by exsanguinating hemorrhage per rectum
   c. Diagnosis—Perform endoscopy to rule out other sources.
   d. Treatment—remove graft, oversew aorta, repair enteric defect; drain retroperitoneum, extraanatomic bypass (axillary-bifemoral)
2. Late infection of prosthetic graft material requires extraanatomic bypass.

IX. ENDOVASCULAR ABDOMINAL AORTIC ANEURYSM REPAIR

A. INDICATIONS

1. Currently, most appropriate for patients at increased risk for conventional open repair
2. May be the preferred treatment method if vascular anatomy is appropriate, in older or higher risk patients, or in those with multiple prior abdominal surgeries
3. Patient preference is of great importance.
4. May not be eligible because of anatomic variability of the aneurysm, such as size and angulation of the proximal neck and extent of iliac aneurysmal or atherosclerotic disease

B. PROCEDURE

1. Preoperative preparation
   a. Similar to that of an open repair; however, multiple measurements with CT reconstructions of the aorta are necessary to determine the size and optimal placement of the endograft
   b. General anesthesia is most commonly used; however, several local anesthetic techniques have also been described.
   c. Nasogastric decompression is not necessary.
   d. The operation should be performed in an endovascular suite with a fixed fluoroscopic unit.
2. Operative steps
   a. Both femoral arteries are exposed and 2 cm of the vessels are dissected free.
   b. The femoral vessel that will be used for insertion of the endograft is then accessed using the Seldinger technique. A sheath is placed and a guidewire is advanced to the thoracic aorta.

ANEURYSMS

54

c. The opposite femoral vessel is then accessed in a similar manner and used to maintain heparinization and inject contrast agents.

d. Before graft deployment, the location of the renal arteries is confirmed and marked on the imaging screen.

e. The aortic endograft with a unilateral iliac gate is placed, followed by cannulation of this graft via the contralateral femoral artery to deploy the contralateral iliac gate.

f. An aortic occlusion balloon is then advanced over the ipsilateral wire to mold the graft to its multiple fixation sites.

3. Postoperative course

a. Diets are started within 12 hours, and patients are usually discharged on POD#1.

b. An abdominal x-ray is obtained on POD#1 to confirm the endograft placement.

C. LONG-TERM CARE

1. Patients should be followed, given the propensity for long-term complications associated with endografts.

2. A CT with intravenous (IV) contrast should be obtained 1 year postoperatively; then yearly CT scans without IV contrast are acceptable.

3. More frequent imaging is necessary if complications should occur, or there is evidence that the aneurysm continues to grow.

D. COMPLICATIONS

1. Endoleaks—perfusion of the aneurysm sack outside the lumen of the endograft

a. Approximately 10%–20% of patients develop an endoleak within 1 year of undergoing an endovascular repair (Table 54.2).

2. Iliac artery injuries from device insertion—rupture, dissection, limb occlusion

3. The same complications are seen as in open repairs and may be reviewed as noted previously.

TABLE 54.2
ENDOLEAKS

Endoleak Type	Definition	Notes
Type I	Originates at either the proximal or distal attachment sites of the graft	Needs urgent treatment/revision
Type II	Originates from the collateral circulation from the lumbar or IMA	Most common type of endoleak. Can usually be followed by imaging
Type III	Caused by fabric tears or problems at graft-graft interfaces	Needs urgent treatment/revision
Type IV	Transgraft extravasations from needle-holes or graft porosity	Usually transient leaks (<24 h)

IMA, Inferior mesenteric artery.

E. OUTCOMES

1. Most recent retrospective studies demonstrate comparable mortality rates between endovascular abdominal aortic aneurysm repair (EVAR) and open repair, with EVAR patients having lower 30-day and 1-year mortality rates, shorter ICU and inpatient stays, and earlier functional recovery.

X. OPERATIVE MORTALITY

A. OPEN REPAIR

1. Elective open repair mortality rate is 2.2%–9%; mortality risk increases with age.
2. Emergent open repair mortality rate: ranges from 20% to 80% (mean, 50%), depending on the condition of the patient at presentation

B. ENDOVASCULAR ABDOMINAL AORTIC ANEURYSM REPAIR

1. Elective endovascular repair mortality rate: 1.2%–1.7%
2. Emergent endovascular repair mortality rate: 24%

XI. RUPTURED ABDOMINAL AORTIC ANEURYSM

A. SYMPTOMS

1. Acute abdominal pain is the most common symptom.
2. Patient may present hemodynamically stable or in shock, depending on the body's ability to tamponade the bleeding.
3. Patients may also present with bleeding into the gastrointestinal (GI) tract secondary to an aortoenteric fistula (duodenum most common site).
4. Patients may also present with high-output congestive heart failure secondary to an aortocaval fistula.

B. PRINCIPLES OF MANAGEMENT

1. Hemodynamically unstable patients go directly to the operating room.
2. Stable patients with questionable presence of AAA may undergo emergent abdominal CT scan or ultrasound.
3. Aggressive fluid resuscitation is not indicated, and mild hypotension (SBP >80 mm Hg) is appropriate to avoid rupture into the peritoneal cavity.
4. Management of symptomatic/painful AAAs that are not ruptured:
   a. AAAs >5 cm: These patients should be admitted with the plan to repair the aneurysms within 48 hours.
   b. AAAs 4–5 cm: These patients should be admitted, and their pain should be further investigated. Risk of rupture is small.
   c. AAAs <4 cm: Additional sources of pain should be investigated. Risk of rupture is small.
5. Be prepared for incision on induction because of further hypotension with anesthetic agent.
6. Mortality rate of those who reach the hospital is 50%.
7. Overall mortality rate for AAA rupture is 80%–90%.

TABLE 54.3

SCREENING

Size of Aneurysm	Time Between Reimaging	Type of Imaging
<3 cm	5 years	Ultrasound
3.0–3.4 cm	3 years	Ultrasound
3.5–3.9 cm	1 year	Ultrasound
>4.0 cm	6 months	CT

CT, Computed tomography.

XII. ABDOMINAL AORTIC ANEURYSM SCREENING (TABLE 54.3)

A. ULTRASOUND

1. Men 65–75 years old with any smoking history should have a single screening ultrasound.
2. Screening in women, even those with a family history, is not thought to be beneficial.

RECOMMENDED READINGS

Badger SA, Harkin DW, Blair PH, Ellis PK, Kee F, Forster R. Endovascular repair or open repair for ruptured abdominal aortic aneurysm: a Cochrane systematic review. *BMJ Open.* 2016;6:e008391. http://dx.doi.org/10.1136/bmjopen-2015-008391.

Chang DC, Parina R, Wilson S. Survival after endovascular vs open aortic aneurysm repairs. *JAMA Surg.* 2015;150:1160–1166. http://dx.doi.org/10.1001/jamasurg.2015.2644.

Guirguis-Blake J, Beil T, Senger C, Whitlock E. Ultrasonography screening for abdominal aortic aneurysms: a systematic evidence review for the U.S. Preventative Services Task Force. *Ann Intern Med.* 2014;160:321–329. http://dx.doi.org/10.7326/M13-1844.

Li Y, Li Z, Wang S, et al. Endovascular versus open surgery repair of ruptured abdominal aortic aneurysms in hemodynamically unstable patients: literature review and meta-analysis. *Ann Vasc Surg.* 2016;32:135–144. http://dx.doi.org/10.1016/j.avsg.2015.09.025.

Peripheral Vascular Disease

Grace E. Martin, MD

Peripheral vascular disease is not a particularly recent phenomenon. Histological examination of the calf vessels of Egyptian mummies has shown changes indistinguishable from the degenerative arterial disease we see today.

—Vascular Medicine Review

I. DEFINITIONS

1. *Peripheral vascular disease* refers to multiple disorders that result from stenotic, occlusive, and aneurysmal diseases of the arteries and veins of the extremities.
2. *Peripheral arterial disease* (PAD) refers to atherosclerosis involving the aorta, iliac, and lower extremity arteries.

II. PERIPHERAL ARTERIAL DISEASE

A. EPIDEMIOLOGY

1. An estimated 200 million people worldwide live with PAD.
2. In the United States, it is estimated that 5.9% of adults older than 40 years have PAD.
3. The prevalence and severity of the disease are elevated in African Americans and Hispanics.

B. RISK FACTORS

1. Family history of PAD
2. Smoking—most important modifiable risk factor
3. Diabetes mellitus—increases risk by two- to fourfold
4. Hyperlipidemia
5. Hypertension
6. Chronic kidney disease

C. NATURAL HISTORY

1. Five percent of symptomatic patients will progress to critical limb ischemia (CLI).
2. In patients with CLI, 25% will require limb amputation at 1 year.
3. Severity of disease often depends on the presence of multilevel disease, concurrent diabetes, and smoking status.
4. Predictors for other vascular disease
   a. A decreased ankle/brachial index (ABI) predicts increased rates of overall mortality.
   b. At 5 years, 20% of patients with PAD will experience a nonfatal cardiovascular event, and 15%–20% will die from a cardiovascular event.

D. PATHOPHYSIOLOGY
1. **Atherosclerosis**
   a. Chronic immunoinflammatory, fibroproliferative disease of the large and medium-sized arteries
   b. Modified response to injury hypothesis
      (1) Endothelial injury caused by hyperlipidemia, smoking, shear injury, and hypertension
      (2) The leaky injured endothelium allows for low-density lipoprotein (LDL) migration. The lipoproteins further potentiate the immune response.
      (3) Monocytes (primarily) are recruited by LDL, and once within the intima, digest the lipoproteins, eventually becoming foam cells.
      (4) Apoptosis of the foam cells leads to a lipid-rich core within the intima, and plaque begins to accumulate.
      (5) Over time, smooth muscle cells secrete extracellular matrix and accumulate lipids.
   c. Plaque ulceration or rupture
      (1) Can induce thrombosis and possibly occlusion of the vessel if severe narrowing is already present
      (2) Induces recruitment of platelets and subsequent fibrin deposition
2. **Thromboembolic disease**
   a. Macroembolic—often from a cardiac source such as atrial fibrillation
   b. Microembolic—may be secondary to cardiac or arterial disease (plaque rupture, aneurysm debris, etc.)

E. SYMPTOMS
1. **Classic claudication**
   a. Cramping, tightness, or aching in the lower extremities (LEs) brought on by exertion and relieved by rest
      (1) Aortoiliac occlusive disease causes hip, buttock, and thigh pain.
      (2) Femoral and popliteal disease causes calf pain.
      (3) Tibial disease causes calf pain but also foot numbness and pain.
   b. Leriche syndrome—aortoiliac disease that causes the triad of buttock claudication, impotence, and muscular atrophy
   c. Rule out "pseudoclaudication," which may be caused by venous occlusive disease, chronic compartment syndrome, spinal stenosis, or radiculopathies.
2. **CLI**
   a. Limb pain that occurs at rest
   b. Often indicative of chronic, multilevel disease
   c. Patients with CLI have a high risk of eventual limb loss.
3. **Acute limb ischemia (ALI)**
   a. Rapid or sudden loss in limb perfusion that threatens tissue viability

b. Causes
   (1) Embolism
      (a) Sudden onset without previous symptoms
      (b) Known embolic source—atrial fibrillation, dilated cardiomyopathy
      (c) Usually lodged at arterial branch points where artery lumens narrow
   (2) Thrombosis
      (a) Often superimposed on an ulcerated mural thrombus
      (b) Thrombus often propagates distally.
      (c) Most commonly occurs at the superficial femoral artery
c. Often characterized by the 6 Ps and found in the first webspace
   (1) Pain out of proportion to stimuli
   (2) Paralysis
   (3) Paresthesias
   (4) Pulselessness
   (5) Pallor
   (6) Poikilothermia or cold limb
4. Atypical leg pain (20%–40% of patients with PAD)
5. Asymptomatic (50% of patients with PAD)
   a. Assess for compromised ambulation, impaired exercise tolerance, impaired balance

F. PHYSICAL EXAMINATION FINDINGS
1. Skin changes—dryness, cool temperature, and hair loss of the LEs
2. Pulse examination
   a. Decreased or absent LE pulses—Femoral artery can feel grossly calcified on palpation.
   b. Graded as absent, diminished, or normal (scale of 0–2) and compared bilaterally
   c. Pulses are often present in one limb but absent in the contralateral limb.
3. LE ulceration—found on the toes and feet, extremely painful, and often become infected, especially in individuals with diabetes

G. LAB WORK
1. Patients with PAD are often found to have hyperhomocysteinemia, impaired estimated GFR, and increased C-reactive protein levels.

H. DIAGNOSTIC STUDIES
1. ABI
   a. Should be performed in any patient with claudication symptoms
   b. LE systolic blood pressure (SBP) divided by the higher of two upper extremity (UE) SBPs: ABI = (LE SBP) / (UE SBP)
   c. A continuous wave Doppler probe is placed over either the dorsalis pedis (DP) or posterior tibial (PT), and a blood pressure cuff is

TABLE 55.1

ANKLE/BRACHIAL INDEX MEASUREMENTS AND ASSOCIATED DIAGNOSIS

Ankle/Brachial Index	Interpretation
>1.3	Highly calcified lower extremity vessels; identification of PAD is not accurate using the ankle/brachial index
0.9–1.1	Normal range
0.4–0.8	Claudication
0.2–0.4	Rest pain
<0.2	Tissue loss

PAD, Peripheral arterial disease.

inflated. The cuff is deflated, and the pressure reading when the Doppler signal returns is recorded. This is then compared with a manually obtained UE blood pressure measurement (Table 55.1).

  d. Advantages
   (1) Inexpensive
   (2) Able to monitor disease progression and predict limb survival
   (3) The magnitude of depression of the ABI correlates with an increased risk of cardiovascular death.
  e. Exercise testing
   (1) ABIs are measured after 5 minutes of walking on a treadmill and compared with ABIs measured at rest.
   (2) Used primarily to confirm the diagnosis of claudication in those with atypical symptoms
2. Segmental limb pressures
  a. Compares bilateral SBPs at several LE arterial levels, as well as the magnitude and contour of pulse volumes
  b. Four measurements are attempted on each leg—high-thigh, low-thigh, high-calf, and low-calf
  c. Advantages—can provide localization of anatomic lesions
  d. Limitations
   (1) Qualitative, not quantitative, evaluation of disease
   (2) May not be accurate in more distal arterial beds
3. Doppler waveform analysis
  a. Used in conjunction with segmental limb pressures, and measures arterial velocities and velocity waveforms at several sites along both LEs
  b. The waveforms change with increasing severity of proximal vessel narrowing
  c. Advantages
   (1) Able to assess patients with diabetes with calcified vessels
   (2) Able to assess PAD severity and progression
  d. Limitations
   (1) Highly operator dependent
   (2) Inability to pinpoint arterial lesion
   (3) Low accuracy in tortuous or overlapping segments

4. **Duplex ultrasound**
   a. Able to diagnose anatomic location and degree of stenosis from the infrarenal aorta to the distal tibial arteries
   b. Assesses the individual artery waveform, end-systolic and end-diastolic flow, and peak systolic velocity (PSV)
      (1) In nondiseased vessels, the triphasic waveform is maintained from the proximal to distal arteries.
      (2) The PSV decreases from the proximal to distal arteries in nondiseased arteries, but becomes elevated in diseased arteries.
      (3) A 50% or greater reduction in diameter of an artery correlates with a drop in pressure across that lesion.
   c. Used for the surveillance of LE vein graft patency and is recommended throughout the life of the graft
   d. Advantages
      (1) High sensitivity (80%–90%) and specificity (68%–90%), regardless of operator or multilevel disease
      (2) Delineates flow turbulence, vessel characteristics, and changes in velocity
   e. Disadvantages—unable to identify the best site for a distal graft anastomosis
5. **Computed tomographic angiography (CTA)**
   a. An angiographic image is created from multiple cross-sectional images that can then be rotated to any oblique view.
   b. Advantages
      (1) Delineates anatomy and significant stenoses
      (2) Evaluates associated soft tissue and arterial wall defects
      (3) Can be a helpful adjunct for operative planning
   c. Limitations
      (1) Spatial resolution improving with multidetector scanners, but still limited compared with angiography
      (2) Arterial phase may be obscured by venous filling or asymmetric contrast boluses.
6. **Magnetic resonance angiography**
   a. Advantages
      (1) Delineates anatomy and significant stenoses
      (2) Diagnostic accuracy similar to angiography
      (3) Can also be a helpful adjunct for operative planning
   b. Limitations—often overestimates the degree of stenosis caused by flow turbulence
7. **Contrast angiography**
   a. Most common diagnostic study to stratify patients before intervention
   b. Advantages
      (1) Gold standard—able to delineate inflow and outflow vasculature and to characterize lesion
      (2) Able to preoperatively treat selected lesions with endoluminal therapies

c. Disadvantages
  (1) Contrast load—contrast nephropathy, allergic reaction
  (2) Vascular access complications—aneurysm, dissection

III. MANAGEMENT OF ATHEROSCLEROTIC PERIPHERAL ARTERIAL DISEASE

A. MEDICAL MANAGEMENT

1. Decrease the risk of myocardial infarction, stroke, and cardiovascular death.
   a. Smoking cessation
   b. Walking program—walking 30–45 minutes, 3–5 days/week
   c. Blood pressure control—Beta-blockers and angiotensin-converting enzyme (ACE) inhibitors have been demonstrated to reduce cardiovascular risks in patients with PAD.
   d. High-dose statin therapy
   e. Antiplatelet therapy
      (1) Low-dose aspirin (81 or 325 mg/day) decreases cardiovascular events in patients with PAD.
      (2) Clopidogrel is an effective alternative to acetylsalicylic acid therapy.
      (3) Dual-platelet therapy with both aspirin and clopidogrel is only beneficial in those with symptomatic atherothrombotic events.
2. Improve symptoms and quality of life and prevent amputation.
   a. Smoking cessation
   b. Walking program—walking 30–45 minutes, 3–5 days/week
   c. Cilostazol—type III phosphodiesterase inhibitor. Contraindicated in patients with heart failure. Adherence low because of side effects (diarrhea, palpitations).
   d. Good foot care—moisturizing cream, nail care, treat and prevent tinea, orthotics to prevent abnormal pressure points

B. REVASCULARIZATION THERAPY

1. General principles
   a. Identification of patterns of arterial obstruction
      (1) Inflow disease—stenosis or occlusion of the suprainguinal vessels (infrarenal aorta and iliac arteries)
      (2) Outflow disease—stenosis or occlusion of the infrainguinal LE arterial tree (femoral, popliteal arteries)
      (3) Runoff disease—stenosis or occlusion in the trifurcation vessels (anterior tibial, PT, and peroneal arteries)
   b. When choosing endovascular therapy versus surgery, the surgeon should consider the following:
      (1) Anatomy of the lesion
      (2) Severity of patient symptoms
      (3) Comorbid conditions
      (4) Risks of surgical intervention

2. Indications
   a. CLI—Without revascularization, most patients will progress to limb loss.
   b. Recurrent or limb-threatening atheroembolism
   c. Patients with severe, lifestyle-limiting claudication symptoms
3. Endovascular therapy
   a. Includes a variety of therapies:
      (1) Angioplasty with balloon dilation
      (2) Stents
      (3) Catheter-directed thrombolysis
      (4) Thrombectomy
   b. Angioplasty
      (1) Better for proximal compared with distal vessel lesions
      (2) Patency decreases with the following conditions:
         (a) Long segment disease
         (b) Multiple lesions
         (c) Poor runoff
         (d) Multiple comorbid conditions
   c. Stenting
      (1) Most effective in:
         (a) A single stenosis of the common or external iliac arteries
         (b) A single stenosis of the superficial femoral or popliteal arteries less than 3 cm
      (2) Also used as salvage therapy for failed balloon angioplasty in the femoral, popliteal, and tibial arteries
      (3) Complications
         (a) Thrombosis, dissection, perforation, distal embolism
         (b) Complications are usually local.
      (4) Long-term results—depend on the initial extent of aortoiliac disease, but are usually not as good as open surgery
4. Surgical bypass therapy
   a. Indications
      (1) Lack of response to exercise and pharmacotherapy
      (2) Severe impairment in activities of daily living
      (3) Absence of other significant comorbid conditions
      (4) Suitable vascular anatomy
      (5) CLI
   b. Preoperative assessment
      (1) History and physical examination
      (2) Road map—The inflow, outflow, and runoff of the entire extremity must be evaluated with angiography or CTA.
      (3) Cardiovascular risk assessment must be performed to stratify patients.
         (a) Further testing such as electrocardiogram, chemical stress test, or coronary angiography may be necessary.
         (b) Coronary revascularization may be necessary before elective intermediate or high-risk surgery.

55

PERIPHERAL VASCULAR DISEASE

(4) All patients with cardiovascular disease should be started on the following if there are no contraindications:
  (a) ACE inhibitor
  (b) Beta-blocker
  (c) Statin
  (d) High-dose aspirin
c. Choice of bypass conduit
  (1) Autologous vein
    (a) Ipsilateral greater saphenous vein (GSV) most frequently harvested
    (b) Best choice if available, specifically for below knee bypass
    (c) Can become stenotic or aneurysmal at the midpoint and anastomotic sites
  (2) Synthetic material (Dacron, Gore-Tex)
    (a) Best for above knee bypass when vein is not available
d. Specific procedures
  (1) Inflow disease
    (a) Aortobifemoral bypass—for patients with aortoiliac disease
      (i) Abdominal incision to expose the infrarenal aorta down to the common iliacs
      (ii) Bilateral groin incisions to expose the common, deep, and superficial femoral arteries
      (iii) The aorta is transected, and the proximal graft is sewn in place (end to end or end to side).
      (iv) The distal limbs of the prosthesis are then tunneled through the retroperitoneum, and the distal anastomoses are performed.
    (b) Aortoiliac endarterectomy—less commonly performed since the development of bypass grafts
    (c) Axillofemoral bypass ("extraanatomic reconstruction")
      (i) Reserved for patients with no other options for revascularization—hostile abdomens, high-risk patients
      (ii) Graft is tunneled from the axillary artery to the ipsilateral femoral artery. A femoral-femoral bypass is then performed.
  (2) Outflow and runoff disease—for patients with femoral, popliteal, and tibial disease
    (a) Endarterectomy—used only in femoral arterial disease
    (b) Popliteal artery bypass—Vein conduit is preferred, whether bypassing to the above or below knee popliteal artery.
    (c) Distal artery bypass (e.g., femoral-tibial)
      (i) Prosthetic material should be avoided because of high failure rates.
      (ii) The least diseased tibial or pedal artery should be used as outflow.

C. CRITICAL LIMB ISCHEMIA
1. Natural history
   a. CLI is at the end of the PAD spectrum.
   b. One-year mortality rate for patients with nonrevascularizable CLI is 10%–40%.
   c. Six-month major amputation rate for patients with nonrevascularizable CLI is 10%–40%.
   d. Pharmacotherapy considerations
      (1) Cilostazol and pentoxifylline are not useful.
      (2) All patients should be considered for secondary cardiovascular prevention, which should include beta-blocker, ACE inhibitor, statin, and aspirin.
   e. Endovascular therapy—shows similar 1-year limb salvage rates but a higher need for reinterventions
2. Surgical therapy
   a. Multilevel disease is very common.
   b. In those with multilevel disease, inflow lesions should be addressed first.
   c. Sequential composite grafts (combination vein and prosthetic grafts, jump grafts) may be necessary.
   d. Infrainguinal revascularization is less durable than aortoiliac revascularization.
   e. If tissue loss or persistent infection is present, limb amputation may be the only surgical option.
3. Postoperative care
   a. Important to evaluate for recurrent disease and new arterial lesions
   b. Imaging
      (1) ABIs should be performed routinely at clinic visits
      (2) Duplex ultrasound of the graft
   c. Antiplatelet therapy

D. ACUTE LIMB ISCHEMIA
1. Overview
   a. ALI is a sudden decrease in limb perfusion causing a threat to limb viability, with a risk of major limb loss.
   b. Severity of ischemia depends on the following factors:
      (1) Location of occlusion
      (2) Extent of secondary thrombosis
      (3) Presence of preexisting collateralization
   c. Patients with ALI have a mortality rate of 13%, limb gangrene rate of 27%, and transformation to chronic limb ischemia in 18.3%.
   d. Irreversible ischemia (paralysis and rigor of the limb) may occur if arterial flow is not restored promptly.
2. Causes
   a. Traumatic occlusion or arterial disruption
   b. Embolism
      (1) Sudden onset without previous symptoms
      (2) Known embolic source—atrial fibrillation, dilated cardiomyopathy

(3) Usually lodge at arterial branch points where arterial lumen narrows

c. Thrombosis

(1) Often superimposed on an ulcerated mural thrombus

(2) Thrombus also often propagates distally

3. Diagnosis

a. Often diagnosed by history and acute onset of symptoms (see the six Ps earlier)

b. More difficult to diagnose in the elderly, as their pain threshold from chronic disease is often elevated

c. ABI: 0.0–0.2

d. If patient is not critically ill, can consider imaging with a CTA with runoff of the LEs and 3D reconstructions

4. Therapy—determined by limb viability (Table 55.2)

a. IV heparin should be administered on diagnosis for those with class II and III ALI; prevents secondary thrombosis

b. Local catheter-based thrombolysis for symptoms less than 14 days in duration

c. Open thromboembolectomy is the standard operation for type II ALI.

d. Decompressive fasciotomies may be required distal to the occlusion if compartment pressures (>30 mm Hg) are increased from muscle and soft tissue swelling.

e. All patients should be monitored for ischemia reperfusion injury, and creatine kinase (CK) and renal function should be measured often.

f. Anticoagulation should be maintained after an ALI event, as the incidence of recurrent emboli is as high as 45%.

IV. RENAL ARTERY DISEASE

A. EPIDEMIOLOGY

1. Renovascular disease is the cause in 5% of those with severe hypertension.

2. It is the second most common cause of hypertension in children (the first is aortic coarctation).

B. NATURAL HISTORY

1. A progressive disease. Progress to occlusion occurs more often in patients with hypertension and diabetes mellitus.

C. CLINICAL CONSEQUENCE

1. Hypertension

a. Stenosis or decreased flow through the renal arteries induces activation of the renin-angiotensin system (RAS).

(1) Renin hydrolyzes angiotensinogen to angiotensin I.

(2) ACE facilitates the enzymatic conversion of angiotensin I to angiotensin II

TABLE 55.2

THERAPY DETERMINED BY LIMB VIABILITY

Category	Prognosis	Sensory Loss	Arterial Doppler Signals	Management
I. Viable	Not immediately threatened	(−)	Audible	Medical therapy and exercise
II. Threatened	—	—	—	Emergent operation or catheter-directed thrombolysis
IIa. Marginally	Salvageable if promptly treated	(−)	Often inaudible	—
IIb. Immediately	Salvageable with immediate revascularization	Mild-to-moderate	Usually inaudible	—
III. Irreversible	Major tissue loss inevitable	Severe, paralysis, rigors	Inaudible	Conservative treatment, scheduled amputation

(3) Angiotensin II increases blood pressure via multiple mechanisms.
   (a) Arteriolar vasoconstriction
   (b) Works directly on the renal tubules to induce Na^+ reabsorption
   (c) Induces water reabsorption in the collecting ducts by inducing antidiuretic hormone (ADH) secretion from the posterior pituitary
   (d) Increases sympathetic activity
   (e) Increases aldosterone secretion from the adrenal cortex
(4) Aldosterone increases renal reabsorption and retention of Na^+ and water
2. Impaired kidney function and renal atrophy

D. PATHOPHYSIOLOGY
1. Type of disease
   a. Unilateral stenosis
      (1) Affected kidney hypersecretes renin with the contralateral kidney working to suppress the renin production.
         (a) Affected kidney secretes Na^+ with the contralateral kidney working to secrete Na^+.
         (b) Results in a relative intravascular volume depletion
         (c) Responds well to ACE inhibitors
      (2) Left and right renal arteries are affected at the same rate.
   b. Bilateral stenosis or unilateral disease of a solitary kidney
      (1) Over time, renin secretion decreases secondary to chronic sodium retention.
      (2) Seventy-five percent of patients with renal artery arteriosclerosis have bilateral lesions.

2. Causative factors
   a. Renal artery atherosclerosis—95% of reported cases of renovascular hypertension
      (1) Most commonly presents in patients 60–70 years old
      (2) Affects men more than women at a ratio of 2:1
      (3) Eighty percent of atherosclerotic lesions represent spillover of aortic atherosclerotic disease—a proximal third of the vessel is most commonly affected.
   b. Arteriofibrodysplasia—5% of reported cases of renovascular hypertension
      (1) May affect the intima or media (85% of cases)
      (2) Usually a systemic process, with the internal carotids being the most common extrarenal vessels affected
      (3) Almost exclusively affects women
      (4) String-of-beads appearance on angiography
   c. Renal artery aneurysms
   d. Developmental disease—renal artery ostial stenoses

E. DIAGNOSIS
1. History
   a. Onset of hypertension before the age of 30 years
   b. Presence of resistant (requiring more than three agents to control blood pressure) or malignant (evidence of end-organ damage) hypertension
   c. Unexplained atrophic kidney or discrepancy in size of kidneys greater than 1.5 cm
2. Physical examination
   a. Upper abdominal bruits during systole and diastole
3. Laboratory evaluation and physiologic testing
   a. Increased BUN/creatinine, especially after initiation of ACE or ARB therapy
   b. Renin activity comparisons
      (1) Used only when the risk of an intervention necessitates a confirmed diagnosis
      (2) Renal vein renin ratio (RVRR)—compares the renin activity of blood drawn from both renal veins
4. Imaging
   a. Noninvasive imaging
      (1) Duplex ultrasound—high sensitivity but operator dependent, and can be limited by the patient's body habitus and bowel gas
      (2) CT angiography—provides 3D angiographic images of renal arteries; does carry risk of contrast-induced nephrotoxicity
      (3) MRA—less effective in detecting subtle arterial wall deformities
   b. Catheter angiography—gold standard, but not used as a first-line study

5. Treatment
   a. Medical therapy
      (1) ACE inhibitors—effective for renovascular hypertension, but renal function must be closely monitored, as these drugs can have a deleterious effect on the kidneys
      (2) ARBs do not have good data in their use in renovascular hypertension.
      (3) Beta-blockers are also effective in the treatment of hypertension related to RAS.
   b. Endovascular therapy
      (1) Indications for endovascular therapies:
         (a) Asymptomatic bilateral or hemodynamically significant unilateral RAS
         (b) Accelerated, resistant, or malignant hypertension
      (2) Catheter-based intervention
         (a) Balloon angioplasty—recommended for arterial fibrodysplasia
         (b) Stent placement—indicated in atherosclerotic lesions
      (3) Complications—intima or media disruption (rare)
   c. Surgical therapy
      (1) Aortorenal bypass
         (a) Autologous reverse saphenous vein grafts used for arteriosclerotic and fibrodysplastic diseases
      (2) Nonanatomic bypass procedures—include hepatorenal and splenorenal bypasses
      (3) Endarterectomy
         (a) Bilateral disease—best treated with an aortic approach in which an excision is made from the SMA to below the renal arteries
         (b) Distal renal arterial disease—best treated with a direct renal endarterectomy with patch angioplasty
      (4) Complications
         (a) Nephrectomy is required in half of failed primary surgical procedures

F. RENAL ARTERY ANEURYSMS

1. Characteristics
   a. Often located at renal artery bifurcations and are saccular in nature
   b. Extraparenchymal (90%) aneurysms are more common than intraparenchymal.
   c. Typically associated with medial fibrodysplasia, although arteriosclerosis may also be a cause
2. Clinical consequences
   a. Rupture is the most feared and often necessitates nephrectomy; exsanguination occurs rarely

3. Treatment
   a. Indications for intervention
      (1) Aneurysms with functionally important renal artery stenosis
      (2) Aneurysms with thrombus and evidence of distal embolization
      (3) Aneurysms in women of childbearing age
      (4) Aneurysms with diameters >1.5 cm
      (5) Aneurysms causing flank pain
   b. Surgical treatment—Usually an open, extraperitoneal approach is used, and the aneurysm is resected and the artery primarily closed.
   c. Endovascular treatment
      (1) Stents may be placed across the aneurysms similar to in abdominal aortic aneurysm (AAA) therapy.
      (2) Intraparenchymal aneurysms may undergo embolization.
4. Surveillance
   a. Those aneurysms that do not undergo treatment should be followed long term with CTA, MRA, or abdominal ultrasonography.

V. LOWER EXTREMITY ANEURYSM DISEASE

A. EPIDEMIOLOGY
1. Male-to-female ratio in those with femoral or popliteal aneurysm is 30:1.
2. Femoral artery aneurysm
   a. Incidence—relatively uncommon; however, the incidence of pseudoaneurysms is on the rise
   b. Concurrent AAA in 85% of cases of true femoral aneurysms
3. Popliteal aneurysm
   a. Incidence rate of ~1% in men ages 65–80 years old
   b. Concurrent AAA in 40%–50% of cases

B. NATURAL HISTORY
1. Unlike AAAs, peripheral aneurysms do not often rupture; instead, they cause flow disturbances that lead to thrombosis and thromboembolism.

C. FEMORAL ARTERY ANEURYSMS
1. Characteristics
   a. Common femoral aneurysm is most prevalent.
   b. Majority of true aneurysms are due to atherosclerotic disease.
   c. False aneurysms are due to anastomotic, traumatic, and mycotic lesions.
   d. Patients with true femoral aneurysms often have multiple other aneurysms.
   e. Patients often have comorbidities that include cigarette smoking, hypertension, coronary artery disease, and diabetes mellitus.
2. Diagnosis:
   a. Presents as a thigh mass with compression of neighboring structures or with thromboembolic complaints
   b. Should be evaluated with duplex ultrasound, CT angiography, or MRA

3. **Management**
   a. Indications for intervention
      (1) Aneurysms that cause local symptoms
      (2) Patients who present with limb-threatening thromboembolic events or rupture
      (3) Aneurysms greater than 2.5 cm in greatest diameter
   b. Surgical repair
      (1) Elective repair
         (a) Femoral artery is usually accessed through a longitudinal groin cut-down.
         (b) The aneurysm sac is opened, and the atheromatous and thrombotic debris is removed.
         (c) Preferred repair with a Dacron or polytetrafluoroethylene (PTFE) interposition graft. Small aneurysms may be excised.
      (2) Repair of the ruptured aneurysm
         (a) Consider accessing the external iliac for proximal control.

D. **POPLITEAL ARTERY ANEURYSMS**
1. **Characteristics**
   a. Sixty percent to 70% of patients with one popliteal aneurysm will have a bilateral popliteal aneurysm.
   b. One-third of patients with asymptomatic popliteal aneurysms will develop complications requiring emergent intervention within 5 years of diagnosis.
   c. Typical comorbidities include smoking, hypertension, cardiac disease, and diabetes mellitus.
2. **Diagnosis**
   a. More than 50% of patients present with local ischemic or distal embolic complaints.
   b. Rupture occurs rarely and is confined to the popliteal space.
   c. Physical examination: Two-thirds of patients will have a pulsatile mass with the knee flexed.
   d. Evaluate with duplex ultrasonography and/or CT angiography; assess the contralateral limb as well.
3. **Management**
   a. Indications for intervention: Surgical treatment is indicated for all symptomatic and most asymptomatic popliteal aneurysms.
   b. Surgical repair
      (1) Popliteal artery is usually accessed by a medial thigh and calf incision.
      (2) A posterior approach may be used if the aneurysm is confined to the popliteal space.
      (3) Bypass grafting is preferred, and the aneurysm is ligated proximally and distally.
      (4) Endovascular therapies are reserved for high-risk patients and are not routinely used.

E. FEMORAL ARTERY PSEUDOANEURYSM
1. Characteristics
   a. Incidence rate of 0.3% after diagnostic catheterizations
   b. Incidence rate of 1.5% after therapeutic procedures. The use of percutaneous closure devices decreases the rate to 0.1%.
   c. Higher rate of anastomotic aneurysms with postoperative wound infections, smoking, and prosthetic grafts (compared with autologous vein grafts)
2. Pathophysiology—incomplete dilation of some but not all layers of the arterial wall
3. Diagnosis
   a. Frequently present as a pulsatile mass on a patient who has previously undergone a femoral artery reconstructive procedure
   b. Evaluate with duplex ultrasonography and/or CT angiography
4. Management
   a. Pseudoaneurysms less than 2 cm usually resolve spontaneously.
   b. Anastomotic pseudoaneurysms greater than 2 cm require surgical management similar to that of true aneurysms.
   c. Larger, symptomatic pseudoaneurysms can be managed with ultrasound-guided compression or thrombin injection.
   d. Pseudoaneurysms complicated by bleeding or acute compression of surrounding structures often need operative management.

F. MYCOTIC ANEURYSMS
1. Characteristics
   a. Refers to any infected aneurysm
   b. Typically the result of intravenous drug use, but may be secondary to arterial trauma (iatrogenic or otherwise)
   c. *Staphylococcus aureus* infections account for 65% of infected femoral artery aneurysms.
2. Causes and pathogenesis
   a. Septic emboli from endocarditis become lodged into normal arteries and cause weakening of the artery wall.
   b. Atherosclerotic plaques may house bacteria during episodes of bacteremia, weakening the walls further.
   c. Bacteria may spread to artery walls from a local abscess.
   d. Contamination during arterial trauma
3. Diagnosis
   a. Lab work—Patients may exhibit an elevated white blood cell count and positive blood cultures.
   b. Ultrasound and CT angiography are helpful but not always diagnostic.
   c. Diagnosis is usually confirmed at the time of surgery.
4. Management
   a. All mycotic aneurysms should be addressed surgically, as they have a propensity toward growth and rupture.
   b. Patient should be started on antibiotics before surgery and maintained on antibiotics for at least 6 weeks postoperatively.

c. Definitive surgical therapy includes complete removal of the infected aneurysm segment, as well as adjacent infected tissue.

VI. CHRONIC VENOUS INSUFFICIENCY

A. OVERVIEW

1. Anatomy
   a. Deep system—common femoral, deep femoral, femoral, popliteal, and tibial/peroneal veins
   b. Superficial system—great and lesser saphenous veins, veins outside the deep fascia
   c. Perforating system—veins that connect the deep and superficial systems
2. Physiology
   a. Large amounts of blood can build up in the LEs, as veins exhibit high compliance and extendability.
   b. Once the capacitance of the vein has been met, ongoing venous hypertension leads to edema of the surrounding tissues.
   c. During exercise, the calf muscle acts as a pump to propel the venous blood toward the trunk.
3. Pathophysiology and etiology
   a. Risk factors—advanced age, positive family history, obesity
   b. Three different problems with the venous system may exist that all lead to chronic venous insufficiency.
      (1) Venous obstruction—see the chapter addressing deep venous thrombosis.
      (2) Valvular insufficiency
         (a) Seventy percent of cases involve the superficial venous system, and 30% of cases involve the deep venous system.
         (b) Usually due to venous valve prolapse or deep venous thrombosis leading to high venous pressures
      (3) Calf muscle pump malfunction
         (a) Muscle disuse: paraplegia, traumatic injury, elderly or bedridden patients
         (b) Muscle fibrosis: muscular dystrophy, multiple sclerosis

B. DIAGNOSIS

1. Symptoms
   a. Venous claudication—pain and swelling experienced while walking, which is relieved by rest
2. Physical examination
   a. Skin changes—edema, hyperpigmentation, stasis dermatitis, eczema, telangiectasias
   b. Venous ulcers—Medial malleolus is the classic location.
3. Imaging
   a. Air and photoplethysmography
      (1) Both are used infrequently and cannot provide information regarding the anatomic location of disease.

b. Venous duplex scanning
   (1) Most commonly used imaging method before surgical intervention
   (2) Patient stands upright and multiple pneumatic cuffs are serially deflated.
   (3) Reflux lasting more than 0.5 seconds after cuff deflation indicates pathologic reflux.

C. MANAGEMENT

1. Medical management

a. Compression
   (1) Elastic compression—support stockings
   (2) Inelastic compression—Unna boots, four-layer bandage, and so on
   (3) Either type of compression should provide at least 25 mm Hg of compression to have a clinical effect.
   (4) Compression has been shown to decrease the rate of postthrombotic syndrome after deep vein thrombosis (DVT) and increase venous stasis ulcer healing rates.

2. Surgical management

a. Percutaneous laser ablation—used for telangiectasias up to 0.7 mm in diameter

b. Venous sclerotherapy
   (1) Needle injection of caustic substances directly into the vein to cause endoluminal damage and luminal collapse
   (2) Indications
       (a) Patients with branch varicosities without major saphenous reflux
       (b) Combination therapy along with GSV ablation to control branch varicosities in those with major saphenous reflux

c. Phlebectomy—Varicose veins are removed through small stab incisions with a hook instrument.

d. Saphenous vein stripping/ablation
   (1) The calf venous system should be evaluated, as deep venous occlusive disease is a relative contraindication to vein stripping.
   (2) The GSV is ligated at the saphenofemoral junction; then the vein is removed down to the level of the knee.
   (3) The vein can either be stripped with stripping wires or destroyed with thermal heat down the entirety of the vein.

e. Iliac vein stenting and bypass
   (1) Indicated for those with focal iliac venous occlusion/obstruction
   (2) Bypass procedures will use native saphenous vein or PTFE grafts

f. Venous valvuloplasty
   (1) Most commonly performed in the femoral or popliteal locations
   (2) Multiple approaches, including direct open repair, transmural valve repair, and valve transposition or transplantation

RECOMMENDED READINGS

Falk E. Pathogenesis of atherosclerosis. *J Am Coll Cardiol*. 2006;47(8):C7–C12.

Fukuda I, Chiyoya M, Taniguchi S, Fukuda W. Acute limb ischemia: contemporary approach. *Gen Thorac Coardiovasc Surg*. 2015;63(10):540–548. http://dx.doi.org/10.1007/s11748-015-0574-3.

Olin JW, White CJ, Armstrong EJ, Kadian-Dodov D, Hiatt WR. Peripheral artery disease: evolving role of exercise, medical therapy, and endovascular options. *J Am Coll Cardiol*. 2016;67(11):1338–1357. http://dx.doi.org/10.1016/j.jacc.2015.12.049.

Teraaa M, Conte MS, Moll FL, Verhaar MC. Critical limb ischemia: current trends and future directions. *J Am Heart Assoc*. 2016;5(2). Pii: e002938. http://dx.doi.org/10.1161/JAHA.115.002938.

Carotid Disease

Willythssa S. Pierre-Louis, MD

I. BACKGROUND: STROKE

1. Fourth most common cause of death in the United States
2. One million hospital admissions/year
3. Significant neurologic morbidity
4. Risk factors for stroke
   a. Nonmodifiable
      (1) Sex (male)
      (2) Age (>55 years)
      (3) Race (African American)
      (4) Family history
   b. Modifiable
      (1) Hypertension—preeminent risk factor
      (2) Smoking
      (3) Obesity
      (4) Physical inactivity
      (5) Diet
      (6) Diabetes
      (7) Hypercholesterolemia
      (8) Alcohol
      (9) Renal insufficiency
5. Etiologies of stroke
   a. Ischemic—insufficient blood supply
      (1) Embolic (two-thirds of ischemic strokes)—clot or plaque forma-
          tion outside of the cerebral vasculature
          (a) *Carotid embolization*—cholesterol or fibrin/platelet matter
          (b) Cardiogenic embolization—valvular disease, atrial fibrillation
          (c) Hematologic causes—hypercoagulability disorders
      (2) Thrombotic
          (a) Local in situ occlusion of cerebral vessels, *or*
          (b) *Carotid thrombosis*
              (i) Circle of Willis collateralizes in response.
              (ii) Chronicity and extent of thrombosis may determine
                   symptoms.
              (iii) Acute flow impairment may occur (e.g., a hypotensive
                    event).
   b. Hemorrhagic—10%–15% of strokes
      (1) Intracranial hemorrhage caused by trauma, among other factors
      (2) Rupture of cerebral aneurysm
6. Definition of transient ischemic attack
   a. Commonly referred to as mini-stroke
      (1) Strokelike symptoms lasting less than 24 hours

TABLE 56.1		
RELATION OF NEUROLOGIC IMPAIRMENT WITH VASCULAR LESION		
Symptoms	Vascular Distribution	Neurologic Distribution
Transient monocular blindness (amaurosis fugax)		
Visual field disturbances	Retinal artery	Limited to the ipsilateral retina/eye
Altered mental status		
Impaired judgment		
Contralateral motor weakness	Anterior cerebral artery	Cerebral hemisphere
Loss of sensation		
Speech/language deficits		
Visual field deficits	Middle cerebral artery	Cerebral hemisphere
Hemianopsia		
Impaired memory	Posterior cerebral artery	Cerebral hemisphere
Dysarthria, dysphagia, diplopia		
Limb or gait ataxia		
Simultaneous motor, sensory, and visual loss	Vertebrobasilar	Brainstem, cerebellum, cerebrum

56

CAROTID DISEASE

b. Warning signs for stroke
   (1) A total of 30% of patients with a transient ischemic attack (TIA) will go on to develop an ischemic stroke in 5 years.
   (2) Although often lasting much less than 24 hours, infarction may have occurred.

II. DIAGNOSIS

A. HISTORY

1. Characteristics of neurologic symptoms—can localize a circulatory impairment (see Table 56.1 for a more complete review)
   a. Onset—left leg weakness and speech difficulty
   b. Provoking factors—none, onset is sudden and unexplained
   c. Palliative factors—none, resolves with time
   d. Timing differentiates between TIA and stroke—majority of TIAs last less then 6 hours.
   e. Associated symptoms
   f. Pertinent negatives—denies nausea, vomiting, fevers, chest pain, or chest palpitation
2. Medical history—risk factor assessment including hypertension, diabetes, and coronary disease
3. Surgical history
   a. Three-vessel coronary artery bypass grafting 2 years ago
   b. Guidelines recommend carotid evaluation in the preoperative work-up of selected high-risk potential coronary bypass patients.

4. Allergies/medications—no known drug allergies; currently taking atenolol, metformin, lisinopril, and aspirin
5. Social history—nonsmoker, quit 10 years ago; drinks alcohol socially; no recent travel

B. PHYSICAL EXAMINATION

1. HEENT (head, eyes—presence of Hollenhorst plaque does not increase the risk of TIA or stroke, ears, nose, and throat)
   a. There are no carotid bruits bilaterally.
   b. *The presence of a carotid bruit has low sensitivity for detecting more than 70% stenosis.*
   Amaurosis fugax alone is associated with the same stroke risk as a TIA.
2. Cardiovascular
   a. Rate and rhythm are regular, with no murmurs.
   b. *Evaluate pulse and murmurs for possible cardiac sources of emboli.*
3. Pulmonary—clear bilaterally
4. Abdomen—no palpable masses or audible periumbilical bruits
5. Vascular
   a. Two plus carotid, radial, femoral, popliteal, and dorsalis pedis pulses bilaterally
   b. *A full vascular examination is important to diagnose other possible pathologic conditions, including aneurysms.*
6. Neurologic
   a. Cranial nerves II–XII intact. 5 of 5 strength in all upper and lower extremity muscle groups. No evidence of hyperreflexia
   b. *A full neurologic examination may help to identify symptoms in active stroke and localize a lesion.*

C. IMAGING

1. Carotid duplex ultrasound (Fig. 56.1)
   a. Advantages
      (1) Noninvasive
      (2) Can give information on velocities, anatomy, and plaque morphology
      (3) Can achieve high sensitivity (>75%) and specificity (>95%) if combinations of parameters are measured (Table 56.2). Contralateral stenosis/occlusion can falsely elevate velocities; low cardiac output can influence velocities
   b. Disadvantages: Ultrasound is limited by the following factors:
      (1) Operator dependence
      (2) Tortuous vessels
      (3) Visualizations of proximal common carotid or intracranial branches
      (4) Arterial calcification

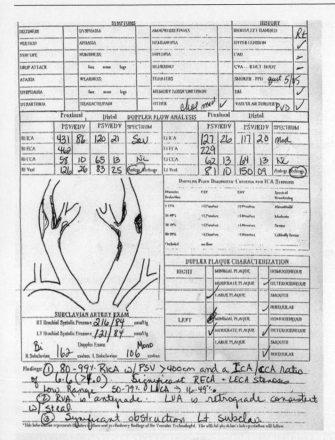

FIG. 56.1
Report of carotid duplex ultrasound.

TABLE 56.2

CAROTID STENOSIS VELOCITY CRITERIA BY CAROTID DUPLEX ULTRASOUND

Degree of Stenosis of the Internal Carotid Artery	Peak Systolic Velocity	End-Diastolic Velocity	Internal Carotid Artery/Common Carotid Artery Ratio
Normal <50%	<125	<40	<2.0
Between 50%–70%	125–230	40–100	2.0–4.0
>70%	>230	>100	>4.0
Occluded	Undetectable	N/A	N/A

2. Computed tomographic angiography
   a. Advantages
      (1) Anatomy of the arch—important planning for carotid stenting
      (2) Demonstrates relative position of calcifications and stenosis near the carotid bifurcation
      (3) Provides an estimate of the residual lumen and less likely to overestimate stenosis
   b. Disadvantage—requires a contrast bolus comparable to that of angiography
3. Magnetic resonance angiography
   a. Advantages
      (1) Avoids nephrotoxic contrast agents
      (2) May allow characterization of plaque morphology
   b. Disadvantages
      (1) Can overestimate stenosis
      (2) Incompatible with implanted metallic devices
      (3) Claustrophobia
4. Angiography—no longer the gold standard
   a. Advantages
      (1) Used mostly in the case of conflicting results between two other imaging techniques
      (2) Evaluation of entire carotid system including collaterals and the aortic arch
      (3) Necessary for patients undergoing carotid artery stenting (CAS)
   b. Disadvantages
      (1) Invasiveness and cost
      (2) Neurologic and vascular morbidity (risk of stroke or TIA can be as high as 1.3%)
      (3) Limited views

III. DIFFERENTIAL DIAGNOSIS OF STROKE/TRANSIENT ISCHEMIC ATTACKS

A. ATHEROSCLEROTIC DISEASE
1. Comprises 90% of carotid occlusive disease cases
2. Anatomy influences hemodynamics—formation of plaque on lateral walls
3. Pathophysiology
   a. Hyperlipidemia, hypertension, diabetes, and so on, lead to endothelial injury.
   b. Monocytes driven by more low-density lipoproteins adhere to and invade the damaged endothelium.
   c. Plaque size increases.
   d. Increased platelet activity furthers endothelial damage.
   e. Platelets stimulate intimal smooth muscle cells to secrete extracellular matrix.

f. Muscle cells accumulate lipids, and the plaque center becomes necrotic.

g. Plaque ulceration and rupture are similar to acute coronary syndrome.

B. FIBROMUSCULAR DYSPLASIA

1. Replacement of normal tissue, most often the media, by extracellular matrix leading to a stenosis or aneurysms, or both.
   a. "String of beads"—pathognomonic
   b. Commonly affect other vascular beds, such as the renal arteries
   c. Can also be associated with intracranial aneurysm or occlusive disease
   d. Treatment: medical management with antiplatelets, angioplasty, versus open surgical dilation

C. COILS AND KINKS BECAUSE OF ANATOMIC VARIATION

1. Often require open surgical repair
   a. True coil usually congenital
   b. Kinks often acquired lesions related to gradual lengthening of the artery with gradual shortening of the cervical spine with age
2. Turbulent flow or focal narrowing resulting in accelerated atherosclerotic degeneration

D. CAROTID ANEURYSMS

1. False—blunt trauma, iatrogenic injury versus pseudoaneurysm
2. True—as with other anatomic arterial sites, mycotic, underlying connective tissue disorders
   a. Treatment: antiplatelet therapy, endovascular versus open surgical repair

E. CAROTID DISSECTION

1. Intimal tear followed by intimal dissection
   a. Previous history of minor trauma
   b. Treatment: often medical management with antiplatelet or anticoagulation if asymptomatic

F. RADIATION ARTERITIS

1. Highest incidence of carotid stenosis tends to occur 15 years after exposure.

G. TAKAYASU ARTERITIS

1. Rare vasculitis of unknown etiology causing inflammation leading to stenoses or aneurysms of the aorta and its major branches, affecting all three layers
   a. Most common second or third decade of life
   b. Treatment: immunosuppression

56

CAROTID DISEASE

H. GIANT CELL ARTERITIS

1. Mostly transmural inflammation of unknown etiology, often affects the temporal artery (hence temporal arteritis)
   a. Most commonly affects women older than 50 years
   b. Treatment: immunosuppression

IV. MANAGEMENT

A. MEDICAL

1. Risk factor modification
   a. Hypertension therapy
      (1) Systolic/diastolic goals based on presence of concomitant diabetes and chronic kidney disease
   b. Smoking cessation
   c. Treatment of hypercholesterolemia
      (1) Statins
         (a) Lower cholesterol
         (b) Antiinflammatory—decrease cell/endothelial interaction and decrease number of inflammatory cells
   d. Treatment of diabetes
   e. Obesity—weight loss and physical activity
2. Antiplatelet therapy
   a. Aspirin
      (1) Provides overall cardiovascular health benefits
      (2) Beneficial as secondary prevention in patients with a history of TIA and stroke at low dose (81 mg or 325 mg)
   b. Dipyridamole—useful in secondary prevention after TIA or stroke
   c. Clopidogrel
      (1) Also effective in secondary prevention
      (2) Aspirin plus clopidogrel—increased risk for bleeding without improved benefit as compared with aspirin alone

B. SURGICAL—CAROTID ENDARTERECTOMY

1. Indications
   a. Symptomatic disease with greater than 70% stenosis
   b. Asymptomatic disease with greater than 80% stenosis
   c. The clinical trials that drive these recommendations may now be outdated, given new "best" medical therapies (e.g., statins, angiotensin-converting enzyme inhibitors).
      (1) North American Symptomatic Carotid Endarterectomy Trial (NASCET): In symptomatic patients with greater than 50% stenosis, carotid endarterectomy (CEA) provides risk reduction of 10.1% over 5 years.
      (2) European Carotid Surgery Trial (ECST): In symptomatic patients with greater than 70% stenosis, CEA provides risk reductions of 9.6% over 3 years.

    (3) Asymptomatic Carotid Atherosclerosis Surgery (ACAS): In asymptomatic patients with greater than 60% stenosis, CEA provides risk reductions of 5.4% over 5 years.

2. Contraindications
   a. Severe neurologic manifestations after stroke may lead to high rates of mortality.
   b. Completely occluded carotid
   c. Concurrent morbid illness
   d. Anatomic considerations
3. Conventional CEA: vertical arteriotomy and closure with patch angioplasty
4. Alternative CEA: eversion endarterectomy
   a. Transection of the bifurcation
   b. Mobilization and then eversion of the entire circumference of the adventitia off the plaque
   c. End-to-end anastomosis of the previously transected carotid bifurcation
5. Cerebral perfusion monitoring
   a. Options
      (1) General anesthesia with electroencephalographic monitoring
      (2) Local nerve block with conscious monitoring
      (3) Cerebral oximetry—noninvasive method that can approximate electroencephalographic/neurologic evaluation
   b. Anesthetic choice governed by surgeon's choice and patient comorbidity
   c. Shunting
      (1) Routine shunting in all cases
      (2) Selective shunting after intraoperative measurement of stump pressure after clamping, any sort of neurologic change in an awake patient or if changes on cerebrovascular monitoring

C. ENDOVASCULAR—CAROTID ARTERY STENTING
1. Indications
   a. Recurrent stenosis
   b. Severe comorbidities
      (1) Severe cardiopulmonary disease
   c. Surgically hostile neck status
   d. History of prior radiation therapy—relative indication
   e. A very experienced center/practitioner
2. Use of an embolization protection device recommended
3. Intraoperative complications
   a. Bradycardia—atropine
   b. Hypotension—volume replacement, phenylephrine, or both
   c. Stroke—increased stroke risk in patients older than 80 years

V. POSTOPERATIVE COMPLICATIONS
Similar between the CEA and CAS.

56

CAROTID DISEASE

A. CARDIOVASCULAR
1. Myocardial infarction—most common postoperative complication
2. Hemodynamic instability
   a. Hypotension—use of phenylephrine (Neo-Synephrine)
   b. Hypertension—use of nitroprusside

B. NEUROLOGIC
1. Stroke
   a. Temporary internal carotid artery occlusion
   b. Embolization—platelet
   c. Thrombosis—flap dislodgement
   d. Recurrent stenosis
2. Cranial nerve dysfunction—2%–7%, most often cranial nerves X and XII (unique to CEA)
3. Cerebral hyperperfusion syndrome
   a. Increased regional blood flow in the setting of disordered intracerebral autoregulation after revascularization
      (1) Increased risk of cerebral palsy if contralateral carotid artery severe stenosis or occlusion
   b. Symptoms—migrainelike headache that may progress to seizures
   c. Seen typically several days after CEA or CAS
   d. Can lead to intracerebral hemorrhage—very high mortality

VI. POSTOPERATIVE CARE
1. Lifetime aspirin
2. Clopidogrel for 30 days after procedure
3. Screening carotid duplex ultrasound at 1 month, 6 months, and annually after procedure
4. Continued risk factor modification

RECOMMENDED READINGS
Cronenwett J, Johnston KW. *Rutherford's Vascular Surgery*. Philadelphia: Elsevier Saunders; 2014.

Ferguson GG, Eliasziw M, Barr HWK, Clagett GP, Barnes RW, Wallace MC, Taylor DW, Haynes RB, Finan JW, Hachinski VC, Barnett HJM; and for the North American Symptomatic Carotid Endarterectomy Trial (NASCET) Collaborators. The North American symptomatic carotid endarterectomy trial: surgical results in 1415 patients. *Stroke*. 1999;30:1751–1758. http://dx.doi.org/10.1161/01.STR.30.9.1751.

Ricotta JJ, et al. Updated Society for Vascular Surgery guidelines for management of extracranial carotid disease. *J Vasc Surg*. 2011;54:e1–e31.

Walker MD, Marler JR, Goldstein M, et al. Endarterectomy for asymptomatic carotid artery stenosis. *JAMA*. 1995;273:1421–1428. http://dx.doi.org/10.1001/jama.1995.03520420037035.

Mesenteric Ischemia

Aaron Beckwith, MD

The credit belongs to the man who is actually in the arena, whose face is marred by dust and sweat and blood.

—Theodore Roosevelt

Mesenteric ischemia is defined by insufficient perfusion to meet the metabolic needs of the end organs (small intestine and colon) supplied by the mesenteric vasculature. Successful treatment requires a high index of suspicion, early recognition of both acute and chronic presentations, and prompt treatment before the onset of irreversible intestinal ischemia and infarction.

I. ANATOMY AND PHYSIOLOGY

A. VASCULAR SUPPLY
Circulation deficits in the gastrointestinal tract are uncommon because of abundant collateral circulation among the following:
1. Celiac axis
   a. Supplies foregut (stomach to second portion of duodenum)
2. Superior mesenteric artery (SMA)
   a. Supplies midgut (second portion of duodenum to proximal two-thirds of transverse colon)
3. Inferior mesenteric artery (IMA)
   a. Supplies hindgut (distal third of transverse colon to rectum)

B. COLLATERAL VESSELS
1. Pancreaticoduodenal arcade (celiac artery and SMA)
2. Marginal artery of Drummond (SMA and IMA)
3. Arc of Riolan (SMA and IMA)
4. Areas prone to ischemia are the splenic flexure (Griffith point) and the rectosigmoid junction (Sudeck point).

C. PHYSIOLOGY
1. Occlusive (macrovascular)
   a. Acute ischemia—thrombotic and embolic
   b. Chronic ischemia
2. Nonocclusive
   a. Low-flow state caused by microvascular vasospasm in response to systemic physiologic stress
   b. Sympathetic stimulation
   c. Decreased blood flow
   d. Drugs—digitalis and others
3. Less common causes
   a. Mesenteric venous thrombosis
   b. Median arcuate ligament syndrome

    c. Iatrogenic (i.e., ligation of IMA during aortic surgery)
      (1) Acute symptoms
      (2) Absence of adequate collateral circulation
    d. Aortic dissection involving mesenteric arteries
      (1) Acute symptoms
    e. Mesenteric arteritis, polyarteritis nodosa, lupus erythematosus, Kawasaki disease, fibromuscular dysplasia, other vascular pathologies
    f. Radiation arteritis
    g. Cholesterol emboli

II. EPIDEMIOLOGY

1. One in every 1000 hospital admissions in the United States
2. Increasing prevalence because of increased awareness, improved imaging, and advancing age of population with multiple comorbidities

III. ACUTE MESENTERIC ISCHEMIA

A. RISK FACTORS

1. Any process that increases the potential for embolism from heart or proximal vasculature (cardiac arrhythmias, low cardiac output states, valvular heart disease, myocardial infarction)

B. CLINICAL PRESENTATION

1. Hallmark of mesenteric ischemia is severe, acute abdominal pain out of proportion to examination
2. Early
    a. Sudden onset of abdominal cramps; nausea, vomiting, diarrhea; diffuse abdominal tenderness without peritoneal signs
3. Late
    a. Symptoms of intestinal infarction
    b. Bloody diarrhea caused by mucosal sloughing and intestinal spasm from ischemia
    c. Fever and peritonitis develop late and are ominous findings indicative of bowel infarction.
    d. Hypotension and acidosis eventually lead to shock.
    e. Despite intervention, 80%–85% mortality rate at this point

C. CAUSATIVE FACTORS

1. Embolization of SMA
    a. Occurs in 40% of cases
    b. Occurs in one-third of patients with antecedent embolic episodes (lower extremity embolus, cerebrovascular accident)
    c. Most emboli lodge 3–10 cm distal to SMA origin, in tapered segment distal to takeoff of middle colic artery
      (1) "Meniscus sign" with abrupt cutoff of normal proximal SMA seen on mesenteric angiography

2. Thrombosis of SMA
   a. Occurs in 40% of cases
   b. Thrombus formation on atherosclerotic plaque or stenotic lesion
      (1) Collateral vasculature usually well developed because of chronicity of mesenteric atherosclerosis
   c. More insidious presentation compared with embolic ischemia
   d. Often preceded by symptoms of chronic mesenteric ischemia (abdominal angina); for example, postprandial pain, weight loss, bloating, diarrhea
   e. Mesenteric angiogram shows occlusion at most proximal SMA, with tapering seen 1–2 cm from origin with collateral circulation.
3. Nonocclusive ischemia
   a. Occurs in 20% of cases
   b. Vasoconstriction of mesenteric vasculature caused by low flow
      (1) Common predisposing conditions include myocardial infarction, congestive heart failure, renal or hepatic disease, medications (e.g., digoxin, epinephrine), trauma, sepsis, hypovolemia, or hypotension.
   c. Mesenteric angiogram shows segmental vasospasm with relatively normal appearing main SMA trunk.

D. DIAGNOSIS
1. Computed tomography (CT) angiography with lateral views
   a. Typically demonstrates occlusion or near occlusion of celiac artery or SMA
2. Laboratory findings
   a. Increased hematocrit consistent with hemoconcentration.
   b. Leukocytosis with left shift
   c. Possible increase in amylase, lactate dehydrogenase, creatine phosphokinase, or alkaline phosphatase
   d. Evidence of metabolic acidosis with persistent base deficit
3. Radiographs nonspecific
   a. Can exclude pneumoperitoneum, obstruction, or volvulus
   b. Commonly see adynamic ileus with gasless abdomen

E. MANAGEMENT
1. Expeditious evaluation and diagnosis are essential.
2. Aggressive fluid resuscitation
3. Nasogastric tube, Foley catheter
4. Evaluate and treat hemodynamics (central venous catheter, arterial line).
5. Parenteral antibiotics
6. With peritonitis or evidence of intestinal infarction, immediate abdominal exploration is warranted.
7. Systemic anticoagulation with heparin to prevent further thrombus propagation

57

MESENTERIC ISCHEMIA

8. Embolus
   a. Immediate exploration after adequate resuscitation
      (1) Primary goal—restore arterial perfusion with open surgical embolectomy.
   b. SMA exposure
      (1) Reflection of transverse colon superiorly and retraction of small bowel into right upper quadrant
         (a) SMA located at root of small bowel mesentery passing over third/fourth portion of duodenum as it emerges beneath pancreas
      (2) Retraction of duodenum medially after incision of retroperitoneum lateral to fourth portion of duodenum
   c. Embolectomy is performed via transverse arteriotomy in proximal SMA using standard balloon embolectomy catheters.
      (1) Arteriotomy may be closed with or without a vein patch.
   d. For more distal SMA emboli, individual jejunal and ileal branches can be isolated at root of small bowel mesentery.
   e. After SMA blood flow restored, assess bowel viability by direct inspection/palpation, Doppler assessment, or fluorescein examination.
      (1) Resect all nonviable bowel.
      (2) Assess bowel supplied by SMA from mid-jejunum to ascending/transverse colon.
      (3) Doppler assessment of intestinal arterial flow
   f. Consider second-look operation 24–48 hours after embolectomy to reinspect bowel with questionable viability with resection of all nonviable bowel.
9. Thrombosis
   a. Perform immediate exploration after adequate resuscitation.
   b. Resect all nonviable bowel.
   c. Revascularization may be required with aortomesenteric bypass graft (prosthetic or saphenous vein) to distal SMA, bypassing proximal SMA lesion.
      (1) Saphenous vein or prosthetic grafts (prosthetic grafts should be avoided in presence of nonviable bowel)
      (2) Origin of graft
         (a) Aorta
            (i) Supraceliac infradiaphragmatic aorta may have less atherosclerotic disease, decreasing risk for embolic complications with cross-clamping of aorta compared with more atherosclerotic infrarenal aorta.
            (ii) Allows antegrade graft placement—less prone to kinking
         (b) Iliac artery
   d. Resect nonviable bowel after revascularization.
   e. Consider a second-look operation.
10. Nonocclusive
   a. Arteriography may demonstrate narrowing or spasm of mesenteric vessels.

b. Goal of treatment is to restore blood flow as quickly as possible, which may be accomplished by removing inciting factors (minimize or stop vasoconstricting agents), and to treat underlying causes (sepsis, heart failure, etc.).

c. Only other possible intervention is angiographic catheter at SMA orifice with infusion of vasodilating agents (i.e., papaverine, tolazoline), but there are not robust data that demonstrate the benefit of this therapy.

d. Perform exploratory laparotomy if peritoneal signs develop.
   (1) Be sure to maintain adequate body temperature in operating room with use of warm irrigation fluid and laparotomy pads in an attempt to reduce intestinal vasoconstriction.

IV. CHRONIC MESENTERIC ISCHEMIA

57

MESENTERIC ISCHEMIA

A. CAUSATIVE FACTORS

1. Atherosclerosis may lead to chronic episodic or constant hypoperfusion in patients with multivessel mesenteric occlusion or stenosis.
2. It may be precipitated by illness, resulting in dehydration (i.e., nausea, vomiting, diarrhea).

B. DIAGNOSIS

1. Often present with chronic postprandial epigastric abdominal pain—colicky, dull, and crampy in nature, occurring 30–60 minutes after meal
2. A total of 70% of cases have history of abdominal angina.
3. Involuntary weight loss because of "food fear"
4. CT angiography or magnetic resonance (MR) angiography

C. TREATMENT

1. Open surgical revascularization has superior long-term patency rates.
   a. Transaortic endarterectomy
      (1) Indicated for ostial lesions of patent celiac artery and SMA
      (2) Approach via left medial visceral rotation exposing aorta with mesenteric branches.
      (3) Lateral aortotomy encompassing both celiac artery and SMA
      (4) Careful not to create intimal flap—must visualize termination site of endarterectomy
   b. Mesenteric artery bypass
      (1) Indicated for occlusive lesions 1–2 cm distal to mesenteric origin
      (2) Antegrade from supraceliac aorta
      (3) Retrograde from infrarenal aorta or iliac artery
      (4) Can use autologous saphenous vein grafts or prosthetic material
2. Percutaneous angioplasty with or without stenting
   a. Lower risk of periprocedural morbidity and mortality but higher rate of restenosis

D. PROGNOSIS

1. Best long-term results with multivessel revascularization
2. Recurrence rates variable

V. MESENTERIC VENOUS THROMBOSIS

A. **CAUSATIVE FACTORS—VENOUS THROMBOSIS PREDOMINANTLY A RESULT OF STAGNATION OF BLOOD FLOW, HYPERCOAGULABILITY, AND VASCULAR INJURY**
1. Acquired, local factors
   a. Pancreatitis, trauma, malignancy, portal hypertension
2. Inherited hypercoagulable states
   a. Protein C and S deficiency, myeloproliferative disorders, Factor V Leiden mutation, antithrombin III deficiency, etc.
3. Idiopathic

B. **CLINICAL PRESENTATION**
1. A total of 5%–10% of acute mesenteric ischemia cases
2. Acute mesenteric venous thrombosis will present like other forms of acute mesenteric ischemia, with colicky abdominal pain that is out of proportion to physical examination.
   a. Diarrhea, nausea, and vomiting
3. Subacute and chronic mesenteric venous thrombosis may have a more insidious onset of symptoms.

C. **DIAGNOSIS**
1. Labs—complete blood count (CBC) with differential, serum electrolytes, serum lactic acid, and monitoring for signs of bowel ischemia, metabolic acidosis, or sepsis
2. CT scan
   a. Study of choice
   b. Visualization of intraluminal thrombus, enlargement of thrombosed vein, focal or segmental bowel wall thickening
   c. Can also detect portal and ovarian vein thrombosis
3. MR venography most accurate but CT is recommended because of its widespread availability
4. Duplex ultrasound scan of mesenteric and portal veins
   a. Often limited by distended bowel gas pattern

D. **TREATMENT**
1. Fluid resuscitation
2. Early heparinization for suspected thrombosis
3. Nasogastric tube with bowel rest
4. Foley catheter
5. Broad-spectrum antibiotics
6. Laparotomy for peritonitis or suspected infarction
   a. Often find edema and cyanotic discoloration of mesentery and bowel wall with thrombus of distal mesenteric veins
   b. Arterial supply usually intact
   c. Wide resection of nonviable bowel followed by reanastomosis
   d. Thrombectomy considered for large segments of compromised bowel
   e. Consider second-look operation.

7. Postoperative care
   a. Continue anticoagulation for 6 months and possibly for life.
8. Evaluate cause of thrombosis including work-up for hypercoagulable state.

E. PROGNOSIS
1. Better prognosis than other forms of acute mesenteric ischemia

VI. MEDIAN ARCUATE LIGAMENT SYNDROME (CELIAC ARTERY COMPRESSION SYNDROME)

A. CAUSATIVE FACTORS
1. Narrowed celiac artery origin caused by extrinsic compression or impingement by median arcuate ligament

B. PRESENTATION
1. Nonspecific abdominal pain usually located in upper abdomen and precipitated by meals
2. Often in young women between 20 and 40 years of age

C. DIAGNOSIS
1. CT angiography or MR angiography
2. Mesenteric duplex of celiac artery and SMA with inspiration and expiration
3. Aortogram
   a. Lateral views show significant celiac artery compression
   b. Imaging with inspiration and expiration

D. TREATMENT
1. Patient must be counseled that relief of celiac compression may not relieve symptoms.
2. Release of ligament compressing proximal celiac artery with possible bypass graft to correct any persistent stricture

RECOMMENDED READING
Tavakkoli A, et al. Small intestine: mesenteric ischemia. In: Brunicardi FC, et al., (eds). *Schwartz's Principles of Surgery*. 10th ed. New York: McGraw-Hill; 2014.

57

MESENTERIC ISCHEMIA

Dialysis Access

Gillian Goddard, MD

It's a beautiful day to save lives.
—Derek Shepherd, *Grey's Anatomy* (TV show)

I. INTRODUCTION

1. In the first quarter of 2014, 671,851 patients were treated for end-stage renal disease (ESRD).
2. In 2013, the number of people on the kidney transplant list was 5 times greater than the number of people who received a transplant.
3. 2006 National Kidney Disease Outcomes Quality Initiative (K/DOQI)
   a. An initiative that set a goal of arteriovenous (AV) fistula target rate greater than 65% with catheter rate less than 10%
   b. Due to fact that AV fistula has best long-term primary patency rates, has lowest rates of thrombosis, requires fewest secondary interventions, and has the lowest overall morbidity and mortality when compared with other modalities of dialysis access
4. All patients on dialysis should be considered for kidney transplant and referred to a transplant program for evaluation, especially if dialysis access sites become limited.

II. GENERAL OVERVIEW OF DIALYSIS ACCESS TYPES

A. SHORT-TERM/EMERGENT ACCESS

1. Can be used immediately for dialysis
   a. Nontunneled (uncuffed catheters)
   b. Tunneled (cuffed catheters)
   c. Early cannulation grafts (e.g., Acuseal graft)
   d. Peritoneal dialysis catheters

B. LONG-TERM ACCESS

2. Have to wait for maturation time before initiating dialysis
   a. AV fistula
   b. AV graft
   c. HeRO graft
   d. Peritoneal dialysis catheters

III. DIALYSIS CATHETERS

A. NONTUNNELED (NONCUFFED CATHETERS)

1. A temporary intravenous (IV) catheter placed into a central vein
2. Internal jugular vein > subclavian vein > femoral vein

    a. The right internal jugular vein is best because it offers a more direct route to superior vena cava (SVC) than does a left-sided catheter.

    b. Internal jugular vein has less risk of catheter-associated central venous stenosis than subclavian vein.

    c. Femoral nontunneled catheters have a high rate of infection and should be used only if access is unable to be obtained via internal jugular or subclavian veins.

3. Duration—used in hospitalized patients
4. Pros: can be placed at bedside and used immediately because there is no maturation time
5. Cons: high infection rates and short duration of use

B. TUNNELED CATHETERS (CUFFED)

1. An IV catheter is placed into a central vein and is tunneled under the subcutaneous tissue before exiting the skin surface. The cuff is typically 1–2 cm away from the skin insertion site and helps to form a fibrin sheath around the catheter, which decreases the rate of infection.
2. Preferred placement site—same as nontunneled catheters (see earlier)
3. Duration—should be removed as soon as possible; no longer than a year
4. Pros—can be used immediately because there is no maturation time
5. Cons—high infection rates and must be kept clean and dry because it is outside of the body (e.g., no swimming)
6. Things to consider: Tunneled catheters can be placed at the time of fistula placement and used while waiting for the fistula to mature. However, tunneled catheters should not be placed on the same side as the maturing AV access.

IV. ARTERIOVENOUS FISTULAS AND GRAFTS

A. ARTERIOVENOUS FISTULA

1. A connection between an artery and a vein that allows for vascular access for hemodialysis
2. Pros—best long-term patency rates, low rates of thrombosis, require fewest secondary interventions, and overall lowest morbidity and mortality when compared with AV grafts or catheters
3. Cons—longest maturation time with a high risk of primary failure. Primary failure is the inability of the graft to be successfully used for dialysis, typically due to lack of graft maturation or early thrombosis of the graft. However, AV fistulas have superior patency rates compared with AV grafts after being successfully used for dialysis.

B. ARTERIOVENOUS GRAFT

1. A synthetic material, such as polytetrafluoroethylene (PTFE), is used to connect the artery and vein and when the native vessels are not suitable for creating an AV fistula.

58

DIALYSIS ACCESS

2. Pros—lower rates of infection when compared with dialysis catheters, shorter maturation time compared with AV fistula. Some AV grafts can be used in 24 hours, such as an Acuseal graft.
3. Cons—higher risk of infection, seroma formation, and thrombosis when compared with an AV fistula
   a. The higher rate of thrombosis leads to lower patency rates compared with AV fistulas.
4. In the setting of central venous stenosis, you can consider placing an HeRO graft, which has an arterial inflow anastomosis in either the brachial or axillary artery with the venous outflow component in the right atrium, much like a tunneled central line and effectively bypassing the area of central venous stenosis.

C. PREOPERATIVE CONSIDERATIONS FOR ARTERIOVENOUS FISTULA PLACEMENT

1. Vascular mapping
   a. Arterial requirements: unobstructed inflow to the AV fistula, patent palmar arch (Allen test), and luminal diameter of 2.0 mm or greater at the anastomosis site
   b. Venous requirements: unobstructed outflow from fistula, luminal diameter greater than 2.5 mm, straight segment for cannulation, vein depth less than 1 cm from skin surface, direct continuity of the outflow vein with central veins
2. If arterial and venous requirements are not met, consider placing an AV graft.

D. PREFERRED LOCATIONS OF PLACEMENT OF ARTERIOVENOUS FISTULAS AND GRAFTS

1. Start distally to preserve more proximal veins for later use.
   a. Radial-cephalic > brachial-cephalic > brachial-basilic
2. Nondominant > dominant arm
3. Native AV fistula > AV graft

V. ARTERIOVENOUS FISTULA MATURATION

1. The process by which a fistula becomes ready for cannulation. This occurs when the vein undergoes arterialization and develops adequate blood flow, wall thickness, and diameter.
2. An AV fistula or graft must be mature before hemodialysis initiation. Failure of the AV fistula to mature is a cause of primary graft failure.
3. "Rule of 6s" from KDOQI for fistula maturation
   a. At 6 weeks the fistula should:
      (1) Be able to support a blood flow of 600 mL/min
      (2) Be a maximum of 6 mm from skin surface
      (3) Have a diameter greater than 6 mm

      (a) If a fistula fails to mature by 6 weeks, a fistulogram or other imaging study should be performed to determine the cause of the problem

4. **Maturation times**
   a. AV fistula—6 weeks before hemodialysis use
   b. AV graft—3–6 weeks before use, although some AV grafts can be used in 24 hours
5. **Physical examination of mature fistula**
   a. Palpable thrill—caused by the turbulent blood flow of arterial blood into venous circulation; ensures that the fistula is patent
   b. Pulsatile thrill—indicates venous stenosis
   c. Palpate arterial pulse to ensure there is adequate inflow into the fistula
6. **Primary failure**
   a. An AV fistula or graft that does not mature and is never used for dialysis access
   b. AV fistulas have higher rates of primary failure but have superior long-term patency rates when compared with AV grafts.
   c. Risk factors of primary failure—peripheral location of fistula, female gender, diabetes mellitus, surgical expertise

VI. COMPLICATIONS OF ARTERIOVENOUS FISTULAS AND GRAFTS

1. **Aneurysm or pseuodoaneurysm formation**
   a. Leads to overlying skin changes and possible rupture
   b. Risk of formation reduced by rotating cannulation sites
   c. Treatment—surgical resection, aneurysmectomy, or placement of an interposition graft
2. **Infection**
   a. Treatment for infected AV fistulas—treat similar to subacute bacterial endocarditis with 6 weeks of antibiotics. However, if septic emboli occur because of infected fistula, the fistula will need to be surgically excised.
   b. Treatment for infected AV graft—if mild overlying cellulitis, treat with antibiotics. Part of the graft or the entire graft may have to be surgically excised, depending on the severity of the infection.
3. **Thrombosis**
   a. Treatment—percutaneous versus surgical thrombectomy; be sure to order a venogram ± arteriogram to determine cause
4. **Stenosis**
   a. Typically occurs near the anastomosis due to neointimal hyperplasia and can lead to thrombosis
   b. Indicated by pulsatile thrill on physical examination
   c. Treatment—interventional angioplasty/stenting versus surgical revision
5. **Steal syndrome**
   a. Diversion of arterial blood flow away from the distal extremity due to AV fistula

  b. Symptoms—cyanotic, cold, and ischemic extremity with numbness and tingling
  c. Ischemic monomelic neuropathy (IMN)—complication of steal syndrome that causes axonal nerve injury secondary to low blood flow to the radial, ulnar, or median nerves
  d. Most commonly seen when the brachial artery is used (e.g., brachiocephalic fistula)
  e. Treatment—distal revascularization and interval ligation (DRIL procedure), proximalization of the arterial inflow, or banding

6. **High-output congestive heart failure (CHF)**
  a. Occurs in less than 1% of fistulas; associated with high fistula flow rate
  b. History of severe CHF is a contraindication of fistula placement.
  c. Treatment—ligate the fistula.

7. **Venous hypertension in the extremity of the fistula/graft**
  a. Usually due to central venous stenosis
  b. Can eventually cause skin changes that can lead to edema and nonhealing skin ulceration

VII. PERITONEAL DIALYSIS

1. A dialysate solution is injected into the peritoneal cavity and then allows the peritoneum to act as a membrane across which fluids/substances are exchanged from the blood via osmosis and diffusion.

2. Typically a Tenckhoff catheter is placed into the peritoneal cavity laparoscopically.
  a. This consists of two cuffs and is associated with a lower risk of peritonitis.
  b. The deep cuff is placed above peritoneum and below rectus muscle, whereas the superficial cuff is placed 2 cm from skin insertion site.

3. After placement of the peritoneal dialysis catheter, the typical wait time is 2 weeks before initiating peritoneal dialysis, although it can be earlier with some peritoneal dialysis.

4. It is the most common type of dialysis in children.

5. Peritoneal dialysis can be placed at the time of an AV fistula to prevent the use of tunneled dialysis catheters while waiting for fistula maturation, thereby potentially saving a future access site.

6. Pros: allows for at-home nightly dialysis while the patient sleeping, have to wait only 2 weeks or less before use compared with prolonged maturation times for AV fistulas/grafts, allows for a less restrictive diet

7. Cons: patient must undergo training in how to use it properly, must be kept sterile, risk of peritonitis, harder to achieve rapid metabolic control compared with hemodialysis, can lead to hernia formation and peritoneal fluid leaks

RECOMMENDED READINGS

Sidawy AN, Spergel LM, Allon M, et al. The Society for Vascular Surgery: clinical practice guidelines for the surgical placement and maintenance of arteriovenous hemodialysis access. *J Vasc Surg*. 2008;48(Suppl 5):2S–25S.

Stone PA, Mousa AY, Campbell JE, et al. Dialysis access. *Ann Vasc Surg*. 2012;26: 747–753.

United States Kidney Disease Outcomes Quality Initiative (NKF KDOQI) Guidelines. 2006 updates. Available at http://kidneyfoundation.cachefly.net/professionals/KDOQI/guideline_upHD_PD_VA/index.htm. Accessed August 2017.

The Diabetic Patient

Jennifer Baker, MD

One in four kids have either pre-diabetes or diabetes—what I like to call diabesity. How did this happen?

—Mark Hyman, MD

I. DEFINITIONS

A. DIABETES

1. Diagnosis of diabetes is made by a random glucose level ≥200 mg/dL with concurrent symptoms of hyperglycemia (blurry vision, thirst, polyuria, weight loss) or any two of the following tests performed on the same day or any one of the following tests performed on different occasions:
   a. Fasting blood glucose level (after 8-hour fasting) ≥126 mg/dL
   b. Oral glucose tolerance test (highest sensitivity)—8-hour fasting, followed by drinking 75 g glucose; check blood glucose 2 hours later, glucose level ≥200 mg/dL
   c. Hemoglobin A1c level ≥6.5 % (lowest sensitivity)
2. Impaired glucose tolerance (prediabetes) is diagnosed by fasting blood glucose between 110 and 125 mg/dL or oral glucose tolerance test between 140 and 200 mg/dL.
3. Type 1 diabetes (5%–10% of total) is caused by autoimmune destruction of beta cells in the islets of Langerhans; insulin supplementation is required.
4. Type 2 diabetes (90%–95% of total) is caused by a combination of peripheral insulin resistance and relative insulin deficiency; it is treated by weight loss, diet modification, oral agents, or insulin.

B. METABOLIC SYNDROME

1. Diagnosis is made by possessing any three of the following traits:
   a. Serum triglycerides ≥150 mg/dL or treatment for high triglycerides
   b. High-density lipoprotein (HDL) less than 40 mg/dL in men or less than 50 mg/dL in women, or treatment for low HDL
   c. Abdominal obesity (waist circumference ≥102 cm in men or ≥88 cm in women)
   d. Blood pressure ≥130/85 mm Hg, or treatment for hypertension
   e. Fasting blood glucose greater than 100 mg/dL or treatment for hyperglycemia
2. Treatment involves treating the underlying cause (obesity) and cardiovascular risk factors (lipid-lowering agents and antihypertensive therapy).

II. MEDICAL THERAPIES

A. ORAL ANTIHYPERGLYCEMICS

1. Sulfonylureas (glipizide [Glucotrol], chlorpropamide, glimepiride, glyburide, tolazamide, tolbutamide)—stimulate insulin release from beta cells by inhibiting the adenosine triphosphate (ATP)-dependent potassium channel in the pancreatic beta cells
   a. Can cause hypoglycemia (notably glyburide and chlorpropamide) and weight gain
2. Short-acting insulin secretagogues (repaglinide [Prandin], nateglinide)—similar mechanism to sulfonylureas, shorter acting; less risk for hypoglycemia
3. Thiazolidinediones (pioglitazone [Actos], rosiglitazone)—increase peripheral insulin sensitivity by binding to peroxisome-proliferator-activated receptor gamma in the nucleus, which alters DNA transcription
   a. Can cause edema and weight gain and induce heart failure
4. Biguanides (metformin [Glucophage])—decrease hepatic glucose production by suppressing gluconeogenesis (inhibits mitochondrial glycerophosphate dehydrogenase) and increase insulin sensitivity in peripheral tissue
   a. Less hypoglycemia than sulfonylureas
   b. Higher risk for lactic acidosis and may cause gastrointestinal upset; contraindicated in renal failure, hepatic dysfunction, congestive heart failure (CHF), metabolic acidosis, alcoholism, and dehydration
   c. Hold before administration of intravenous (IV) contrast, in acute illness, and surgery.
5. α-Glucosidase inhibitors (acarbose [Precose], miglitol)—delayed glucose absorption from intestine by competitive inhibition of α-glucosidase
   a. Can cause flatulence, abdominal discomfort, and diarrhea
6. Dipeptidyl peptidase 4 (DPP-4) inhibitors (sitagliptin [Januvia], saxagliptin, linagliptin, alogliptin)—inhibit DPP-4, resulting in prolonged glucagon-like peptide-1 levels and increased insulin synthesis
7. Glucagon-like peptide receptor agonists (liraglutide [Victoza], albiglutide, dulaglutide)—similar mechanism to DDP-4 inhibitors; not considered initial therapy

B. INSULIN

1. Rapid-acting—lispro (Humalog), aspart (NovoLog)
   a. Onset 15–30 minutes, peak 30–90 minutes, duration 3–4 hours
   b. Used in continuous subcutaneous insulin pumps; can be given IV
2. Fast-acting—regular (Humulin R, Novolin R)
   a. Onset 30–60 minutes, peak 2–4 hours, duration 6–10 hours
   b. Used in continuous IV infusions and more immediate when IV
3. Intermediate-acting—NPH (Humulin N, Novolin N)
   a. Onset 1–4 hours, peak 4–12 hours, duration 12–24 hours
   b. Subcutaneously; cannot be given IV

59

THE DIABETIC PATIENT

4. Long-acting—glargine (Lantus), degludec (Tresiba), detemir (Levemir pen)
   a. Onset 1–2 hours, peak 3–20 hours, duration 24–30 hours
   b. Subcutaneously; cannot be given IV

C. ORDERING AN INSULIN REGIMEN IN A PATIENT WITH HYPERGLYCEMIA

1. Goal blood glucose varies, usually 80–130 mg/dL before meal and 90–140 mg/dL at bedtime.
2. Weight-based estimation of insulin need
   a. Type 1 diabetic will require 0.4–0.7 unit/kg per day.
   b. Type 2 diabetic will require 0.3–1 unit/kg per day.
3. Traditional subcutaneous sliding scale insulin
   a. Fast- or rapid-acting insulin is dosed before every meal and at bedtime, or every 6 hours schedule for patients not eating, based on blood glucose level checked at that time.
   b. When 24-hour insulin requirement is known, either after conversion from continuous IV infusion or after doses of subcutaneous sliding scale given for 1 day, may add long-acting insulin to regimen totaling 50%–66% of daily requirement.
   c. Advantages include being commonly used and relatively easy to order and administer.
   d. Disadvantages include being nonphysiologic and reactive in treating hyperglycemia.
4. Basal-bolus-correction subcutaneous dosing
   a. Goal is to administer 50% of daily insulin in a long-acting form to mimic physiologic continuous basal insulin secretion and 50% as three subcutaneous boluses of fast- or rapid-acting insulin to mimic physiologic prandial insulin peaks.
   b. Based on premeal blood glucose levels, subcutaneous "correction" dose of fast- or rapid-acting insulin may be given with scheduled bolus. Basal and bolus doses are then adjusted for the next day's orders to try to eliminate need for correction doses.
   c. Bolus doses are given on every 6 hours schedule for patient who is not eating and receiving continuous tube feeds.
   d. Advantages include being more physiologic.
   e. Disadvantages include being a more confusing regimen to order and administer.
5. Continuous IV insulin infusion (insulin drip)
   a. In most hospitals, it is used only in intensive care unit (ICU) setting.
   b. Most commonly regular insulin is used.
   c. Target glucose is 140–180 mg/dL.
   d. Intense glycemic control (80–110 mg/dL) has shown no survival benefit and has greater risk of hypoglycemia and greater mortality.
   e. Blood glucose level checks are every hour to minimize hypoglycemia (associated with increased morbidity and mortality).

   f. When transitioning from insulin infusion to subcutaneous insulin injection, there must be at least a 2-hour overlap of the infusion and injection.

D. ADJUSTING MEDICATIONS FOR SURGERY

1. Preoperative adjustments

   a. Hold chlorpropamide, glyburide, glipizide 48–72 hours before surgery (long half-life).

   b. All other oral agents may be taken until the day before or day of surgery.

   c. One-half usual dose of intermediate- or long-acting insulin given the morning of surgery.

2. Intraoperative adjustments

   a. Patients with type 2 diabetes undergoing short procedure can be managed with glucose checks and doses of subcutaneous rapid- or short-acting insulin to obtain a level less than 200 mg/dL.

   b. For other patients with type 2 and all with type 1 diabetes, use continuous IV infusion intraoperatively for goal blood glucose levels of 120–180 mg/dL.

   c. Monitor blood glucose levels every 1–2 hours intraoperatively. If the patient is requiring high amounts of insulin, monitor potassium levels every 4 hours.

   d. Subcutaneous insulin pumps should be turned off and IV infusion substituted.

3. Postoperative adjustments

   a. Hold metformin after surgery for 72 hours until normal diet is resumed and until normal renal function has been documented.

   b. Other oral agents may be restarted after surgery when patient resumes normal diet; continue coverage with subcutaneous insulin until oral agents restarted.

   c. Ideally can maintain continuous IV infusion until patient starts eating regular diet.

4. Discharge adjustments

   a. Any patient requiring insulin while hospitalized should have follow-up with primary care physician to be evaluated or treated for diabetes.

   b. Patients requiring less than 20 units/day of insulin may be discharged without insulin or oral therapy.

   c. Patients requiring 20–35 units/day of insulin should be discharged on an oral antihyperglycemic medication, with glucometer, diabetes teaching, and appropriate follow-up.

   d. Patients requiring more than 35 units/day of insulin should be discharged on their in-hospital insulin regimen, with glucometer, diabetes teaching, and appropriate follow-up.

E. HYPOGLYCEMIA (BLOOD GLUCOSE LEVEL LESS THAN 70 MG/DL)

1. Therapies that increase risk for hypoglycemia

   a. Discontinuation of glucose source without adjustment of insulin dose

   b. Administration of regular insulin every 4 hours (half-life is 6 hours, leads to "stacking")

59

THE DIABETIC PATIENT

   c. Continuous venovenous hemodialysis with bicarbonate substitution fluid
   d. Inotropic support
   e. Octreotide therapy
2. **Initial therapy**
   a. If patient is awake and able to swallow, give 15 g oral glucose (as glucose tablets, 4 ounces juice or soda, or 8 ounces milk).
   b. If patient is unconscious or unable to swallow, give 15 g IV glucose (30 mL dextrose 50%).
   c. Recheck blood glucose in 15 minutes.
   d. Repeat process until blood sugar level is greater than 70 mg/dL.
3. **Prevent recurrence**
   a. If more than 1 hour until next meal, give snack with 15 g carbohydrate and protein/fat.
   b. If the patient is unconscious, give additional 15 g glucose if blood glucose level is less than 90 mg/dL.
   c. Do NOT hold dose of intermediate- or long-acting insulin for single episode of hypoglycemia. If multiple episodes occur, decrease dose as appropriate.

F. DIABETIC KETOACIDOSIS
1. **Definition:** hyperglycemia (250–800 mg/dL) with an anion-gap metabolic acidosis, serum ketones, and urine ketones
2. **Can occur in type 1 or 2 diabetics (more common in type 1) and is secondary to insulin deficiency**
   a. It is often secondary to gross lack of insulin or relative lack of insulin in catabolic states (increased catecholamines, cortisol, glucagon, and growth hormone).
   b. Common conditions that precipitate diabetic ketoacidosis (DKA) include trauma, infection, insulin errors, and myocardial infarction.
3. **Clinical features**
   a. Dehydration and thirst
   b. "Pear drop," "nail varnish," or "musty apple" breath secondary to ketone bodies
   c. Kussmaul respirations in the setting of severe metabolic acidosis
   d. Abdominal pain and vomiting
4. **Treatment**
   a. The goal of treatment is to correct the metabolic abnormalities and inhibit the generation of ketones.
   b. Administer insulin at 0.1 unit/kg per hour IV infusion and decrease it to 50% of rate when bicarbonate increases to greater than 16 mEq/L.
   c. Administer fluids (normal saline) at 1 L/h for 2 hours, then change to half-normal saline at 250–500 mL/h. Add dextrose to fluids when serum glucose level is less than 200 mg/dL and decrease rate to 100 to 250 mL/h.

d. Expect profound potassium and phosphate deficits with correction of acidosis and hyperglycemia.
  (1) If serum potassium falls below 3.3 mEq/L, insulin infusion should be stopped and potassium corrected to avoid cardiac arrhythmias secondary to hypokalemia.

G. NONKETOTIC HYPEROSMOLAR HYPERGLYCEMIA
1. Definition: hyperglycemia (≥600 mg/dL) with hypertonic serum and osmotic diuresis
2. Usually occurs in patients with type 2 diabetes and is most often precipitated by infection
3. Treatment similar to that for hypovolemic hypernatremia
   a. Fluids (normal saline) to replace calculated free water deficit (with correction of plasma sodium level, which will be falsely reduced by hyperglycemia); dehydration more severe than in DKA
   b. Insulin therapy only after hypovolemia is corrected

III. GLYCEMIC CONTROL IN THE CRITICALLY ILL PATIENT
A. HYPERGLYCEMIC RESPONSE TO SURGERY AND ANESTHESIA
1. Upregulation of sympathomimetic and hypothalamo-pituitary-adrenal axis leads to high levels of catecholamines and glucocorticoids, resulting in hyperglycemia.
2. Counterregulatory hormones (glucagons, corticotropin, growth hormone), upregulated in response to stress, promote hepatic gluconeogenesis and peripheral lipolysis and glycolysis (insulin resistance).
3. Proinflammatory cytokines (tumor necrosis factor-α and interleukin-6) induce peripheral insulin resistance by blocking expression of insulin-dependent (GLUT 4) membrane glucose transporters.

B. IATROGENIC HYPERGLYCEMIA
1. Can be exacerbated by IV dextrose infusions, parenteral or enteral nutrition, or steroid administration. Immobility alone also leads to insulin resistance in skeletal muscles.

C. GLYCEMIC CONTROL
1. Blood glucose between 140 and 180 mg/dL demonstrated less hypoglycemia than intensive insulin therapy regimen (blood glucose between 80 and 110 mg/dL).
2. Many ICUs have established insulin protocols.

D. SPECIAL POPULATIONS
1. Trauma patients
   a. Hyperglycemia on admission (blood glucose ≥200 mg/dL) associated with higher infection rates, longer hospitalizations, and greater mortality
   b. Prolonged hyperglycemia associated with greater mortality

59

THE DIABETIC PATIENT

   c. Preexisting type 2 diabetes associated with longer ICU stays, increased
      ventilator support, and greater morbidity
2. Burn patients
   a. Hyperglycemia associated with increased infection rates, reduced
      skin graft viability, and increased mortality
3. Cardiac surgery patients
   a. Hyperglycemia in the first 2 postoperative days associated with
      greater mortality, deep sternal wound infections, and increased
      length of stay
   b. Intraoperative hyperglycemia associated with greater mortality and
      increased wound infection

IV. COMPLICATIONS OF DIABETES

A. TISSUE HYPOXIA CAUSED BY MICROVASCULAR DISEASE
1. Endothelial cell dysfunction
   a. Production of glyoxal, 3-deoxyglucosone, and methylglyoxal (ad-
      vanced glycogen end [AGE] products) secondary to intracellular
      autoxidation of glucose causes damage to target tissue leading to
      metabolic alterations (changes in cytokines and growth factors)
      and extracellular matrix protein modifications resulting in abnormal
      interactions.
   b. Hyperglycemia increases flux through the polyol pathway consuming
      nicotinamide adenine dinucleotide phosphate (NADPH) leading to
      increased intracellular oxidative stress and cell injury.
2. Thickening of capillary basement membrane
   a. Hyperglycemia leads to increased microvascular blood flow and
      capillary hypertension, which increase shear stress on the vascular
      wall causing the accumulation of fibronectin decreasing capillary
      permeability.
3. Dysregulation of microvascular circulation
   a. Rigid basement membrane prevents local vasodilatation in response
      to tissue damage, leading to hypoxia and tissue breakdown.
4. The process is responsible for retinopathy and nephropathy and contributes to poor wound healing associated with diabetes.

B. INCREASED RISK FOR INFECTION AND SLOW WOUND HEALING BECAUSE OF IMPAIRED IMMUNE FUNCTION
1. Chemotaxis of leukocytes and macrophages is impaired by hypergly-
   cemia, leading to prolonged inflammatory phase of wound healing by
   slowing rates of collagen synthesis and decreased granulation tissue
   formation.
2. Patients with diabetes are at increased risk for perioperative infections,
   including wound infections.
3. They are also at increased risk for staphylococcal infections, Fournier
   gangrene, and candidiasis.
4. Risk for infection can be decreased with good glycemic control, but
   poor healing occurs even in patients with well-controlled disease.

C. **INCREASED RATE OF ATHEROSCLEROSIS LEADS TO MACROVASCULAR DISEASE.**
1. Enhanced thrombotic potential in patients with diabetes because of endothelial dysfunction, secondary decreased nitric oxide (NO) production, and upregulation of platelet aggregation
   a. It is thought to be secondary to generation of reactive oxygen species and superoxide anion production.
   b. Superoxide anions increase the hexosamine pathway, which ultimately decreases nitric oxide synthase (NOS) activation.
2. Diabetes elevates circulating levels of fatty acids, causing liver to produce more very-low-density lipoprotein (VLDL), resulting in hypertriglyceridemia.
3. Diabetes causes abnormal platelet function secondary to increased glycoprotein Ib and IIb/IIIa.
4. Plasma coagulation factors (factor VII and thrombin) are increased, whereas anticoagulation factors (thrombomodulin and protein C) are decreased in diabetes.
5. Peripheral vascular disease (PVD) and diabetes
   a. Patients with diabetes with PVD are at greater risk for amputation, cardiovascular events, and cerebrovascular events than patients without diabetes with PVD.
   b. Patients with diabetes with PVD may not suffer from claudication, due to peripheral neuropathy, leading to delayed diagnosis.
   c. Pattern of occlusive disease typically involves medium-sized arteries (popliteal trifurcation and tibial vessels) and spares proximal (large) vessels.
   d. Diagnostic studies—ankle/brachial indices (often falsely increased because of artery calcification), exercise ankle/brachial indices, segmental pressure, pulse volume recordings (more reliable in calcific vessels), and toe pressures

D. **NEUROPATHIES OCCUR IN MOTOR, SENSORY, AND AUTONOMIC NERVES.**
1. Charcot neuroarthropathy (Charcot foot)
   a. Motor neuropathy leads to muscle weakness, atrophy, and paresis.
   b. Sensory neuropathy leads to loss of protective sensations and development of deformities.
   c. Autonomic neuropathy leads to vasodilatation and decreased sweating, causing warm feet and dry skin.
2. Gastroparesis results in need for nasogastric decompression or promotility agent (metoclopramide) perioperatively.

V. DIABETIC FOOT ULCERS
1. Occurrence
   a. Risk for patients with diabetes experiencing development of an ulcer is 12%–25% over lifetime.
   b. Incidence of amputation is 0.5–5.0 per 1000 people with diabetes.

    c. Location and symptoms can differentiate arterial and venous ulcers.

      (1) Diabetic ulcers are located on high-weight-bearing areas (metatarsal heads), dry or weeping, and painless unless infected.

      (2) Arterial ulcers (10% of foot ulcers) are located on distal toes, dry, painful, and surrounded by shiny skin; pain is relieved with dependent positioning.

      (3) Venous ulcers (70% of foot ulcers) are located superior to medial (or lateral) malleolus, weeping, painless unless infected, and surrounded by dry, discolored skin with lower extremity edema.

2. **Pathophysiology**

    a. Neuropathy (Charcot foot, as described previously)

    b. Ischemia—secondary to both microvascular and macrovascular dysfunction

    c. Decreased immune response with difficulty recruiting inflammatory cells

    d. Most commonly secondary to accidental trauma as inciting factor

    e. Infection typically not a cause of ulceration but may potentiate ulcer and delay healing

3. **Prevention**

    a. Routine foot care

      (1) Inspection for skin breakdown daily.

      (2) Promptly remove (debride) any callus.

      (3) Treatment of onychomycosis (nail fungus) with topical or oral agents. Brittle diseased nails present less of a barrier to bacterial infection.

      (4) Fitting with orthotic shoes minimizes daily trauma to feet.

    b. Diabetes management with somatosensory (monofilament) testing annually to detect diminished sensation

    c. Early detection of PVD (annual ankle/brachial indices in individual with diabetes older than 50 years, with follow-up studies for falsely increased results) and early revascularization procedures

    d. Smoking cessation

4. **Management**

    a. Treat infection first. Establish if revascularization is necessary/warranted. Decrease weight/forces applied to ulceration. Lastly, surgically debride hyperkeratotic (callused), necrotic, and infected tissue (including bone) to healthy bleeding wound bed.

    b. Assessment for infection—purulent or foul-smelling drainage, warmth, erythema, tenderness

      (1) Failure of wound to heal after proper debridement may also indicate infection.

      (2) Deep tissue cultures (not superficial wound swabs) should be obtained at time of debridement or in nonhealing wounds after debridement.

      (3) It is typically polymicrobial, but *Staphylococcus aureus* is most common pathogen.

      (4) IV antibiotic therapy is often required for optimal tissue penetration, and antibiotic regimen should be tailored to culture results.

    c. Osteomyelitis treated by surgical removal of infected bone, followed by IV antibiotics for remaining infection in surrounding soft tissue (usually 6 weeks)

      (1) Classic radiographic findings (demineralization, periosteal reaction, bony destruction) take up to 2 weeks to appear (30%–50% of bone has been destroyed).

      (2) Other imaging modalities include magnetic resonance imaging (most sensitive and specific), bone scan, and bone probe.

      (3) Often a clinical diagnosis is made at time of debridement, with appearance of purulent material around bone and spongy texture of bone when removed.

    d. Off-loading of pressure from wound is necessary for healing of ulcer.

      (1) Elevate foot above level of heart when sitting or in bed.

      (2) Cast-walkers and half shoes, which are tailored specifically for the involved foot to keep weight distributed to all parts of foot except ulcer, allow patient to remain active.

    e. Dressings should be designed to keep wound bed moist to promote migration of fibroblasts and epithelialization of wound.

      (1) Wet-to-dry dressings also allow for mechanical debridement of fibrinous exudate and devitalized tissue with dressing changes.

      (2) Packing of deeper tracts with moist packing gauze allows for healing by secondary intention.

      (3) Wounds with large amounts of exudate usually require dry dressings and frequent changes.

      (4) Multiple different dressings chosen based on ulcer appearance; include hydrogels, foams, hydrocolloid, polymer films, alginates, and negative pressure wound therapy.

    f. Weekly measurements of wound size to objectively document healing (shrinking).

5. **All diabetic foot wounds without ischemia or infection (including osteo-myelitis) should heal.**

RECOMMENDED READINGS

Chadwick P, Edmonds M, McCardle J, Armstron D. International best practice guidelines: wound management in diabetic foot ulcers. *Wounds Int*. 2013. Available from <www.woundsinternational.com>.

Creager MA, Luscher TF, Cosentino F, Beckman JA. Diabetes and vascular disease pathophysiology. *Circulation*. 2003;108:1527–1532.

Kavanagh BP, McCowen KC. Glycemic control in the ICU. *N Engl J Med*. 2010; 363:2540–2546.

Joshi GP, Chung F, Vann MA, et al. Society for ambulatory anesthesia consensus statement on perioperative blood glucose management in diabetic patients undergoing ambulatory surgery. *AnesthAnalg*. 2010;111:1378–1387.

PART XI

Cardiothoracic Surgery

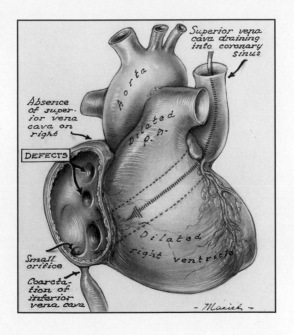

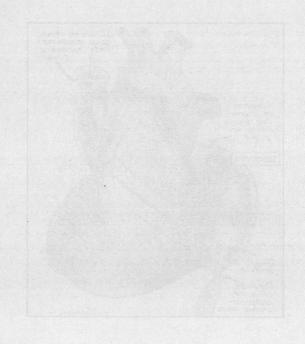

Benign Tumors of the Lung

Audrey E. Ertel, MD

Another glorious day, the air as delicious to the lungs as nectar to the tongue.

—John Muir

I. OVERVIEW

1. These tumors account for less than 1% of all resected lung tumors.
2. They may be derived from epithelial, mesodermal, or endodermal cell lines.
3. Hamartomas account for greater than 75% of benign tumors of the lung.
4. Endobronchial tumors present with signs and symptoms related to airway obstruction (most often pneumonia) and bleeding.
5. Peripheral airway and parenchymal tumors usually present as incidental solitary pulmonary nodules.

II. HISTORY

1. The probability of malignancy rises with age; greater than 50 years of age raises risk of malignancy significantly.
2. Only 5% of all radiographically detected lung nodules prove to be malignant.
3. Smoking, family history, female sex, emphysema, chemical exposure, asbestos, or coal mining are risk factors for malignancy.

III. PHYSICAL EXAMINATION

1. Lymph node assessment—cervical, supraclavicular, and axillary
2. Dyspnea/shortness of breath (SOB)
3. Chest pain
4. Cough
5. Weight loss
6. Hemoptysis
7. Most commonly, nodules are asymptomatic and found incidentally.

IV. INITIAL EVALUATION

1. Characterize the mass through imaging, that is, dedicated chest computed tomography (CT) scan, which is respiratory gated.
2. Based on features (nodule vs. mass), determine to monitor or establish a histologic diagnosis.

a. Nodule; ≤3 cm, regular borders and surrounded by normal parenchyma
b. Mass; greater than 3 cm, irregular (particularly speculated), extensions to pleura or adjacent structures or other associated abnormalities

V. IMAGING

1. Comparison radiographs are essential.
2. Tumor doubling time
   a. Malignant tumors double in weeks to months.
   b. Benign tumors double over years or remain unchanged (solid nodules are followed for 2 years if unchanged as doubling time is inconsistent with malignancy).
3. Computed tomography
   a. CT scanning is the standard modality to assess lung lesions and provides the following features:
      (1) Location—upper lobe lesions are more often malignant.
      (2) Size less than 1 cm have a 2%–6% risk of malignancy
      (3) Attenuation—solid, mixed attenuation (partially solid) or ground-glass opacity (no solid component)
      (4) Rate of growth
      (5) Border—smooth (often benign) versus irregular (spiculation is statistically correlated with malignancy)
      (6) Calcification—popcorn, laminated, central, and diffuse—all point to benign etiology
      (7) Invasiveness into adjacent structures
      (8) Hilar or mediastinal adenopathy (a smooth-edged lesion is considered a mass if associated with lymphadenopathy)
      (9) Presence suspicious lesions that could herald metastatic spread
4. Positron emission tomography (PET) scan
   a. Determines metabolic rate of tissues based on the uptake of fluorode-oxyglucose (FDG)
   b. The intensity of uptake is measured in standardized uptake value (SUV), with a threshold of 2.5 or greater correlating with malignancy.
   c. Inflammation (sarcoidosis) and infection (fungal granuloma) can be PET positive, typically less than 2.5 SUV.
   d. When performed for patients with benign-appearing lesions, the PET scan helps to further determine probability of benign disease if negative. In the setting of a mass (higher suspicion of malignancy), the PET is most useful to assess mediastinal or distant areas for abnormal FDG uptake.

VI. BIOPSY OPTIONS

1. Sputum cytology—not used routinely, should be considered on a case-by-case basis
2. Flexible bronchoscopy with direct biopsy or transbronchial needle aspiration (TBNA)

3. Endobronchial ultrasound–guided transbronchial biopsy (EBUS-TBNA)
4. Percutaneous fine-needle aspiration, CT guided
5. Surgical biopsy—diagnostic wedge resection via video-assisted thoracic surgery (VATS)

VII. EPITHELIAL TUMORS

A. POLYPS
1. Can be solitary or multiple
2. Polypoid areas of bronchial mucosa with a fibrous stalk
3. Covered by ciliated columnar epithelium with possible areas of squamous metaplasia
4. Thought to be secondary to a chronic inflammatory process
5. Benign but may be symptomatic because of their bronchial obstruction effect

B. PAPILLOMA
1. Classified as squamous, glandular, or mixed
2. Can be solitary or multiple
3. Multiple papillomatosis is usually a childhood disease with multiple papillomas of the vocal cords and trachea.
4. Most commonly located in the more proximal airway
5. Squamous papillomas are composed of a thin central fibrovascular core covered by stratified squamous epithelium.
6. Typically associated with the human papillomavirus (HPV)
   a. Most squamous papillomas are benign neoplasm of squamous epithelium (often associated with HPV 6 and 11).
   b. Malignant degeneration to squamous cell carcinoma (often associated with HPV 16 and 18)
7. Treatment usually based on laser ablation
8. May require endoscopic removal or bronchotomy for direct resection. A sleeve resection may be required.
9. Avoid bleeding because it can spread and seed the papillomatosis to unaffected areas.

C. MUCOUS GLAND ADENOMA
1. This benign tumor of the bronchus is derived from bronchial mucous glands.
2. It is composed of small, mucus-filled cysts lined with well-differentiated mucous epithelium.
3. Unlike mucoepidermoid carcinoma, there are no squamous or intermediate cells present.
4. Patient age ranges from 25 to 67 years in reported cases.
5. Symptoms are cough, fever, recurrent pneumonia, and hemoptysis.
6. Chest radiograph often demonstrates obstructive pneumonia or postobstructive atelectasis.
7. It is most often found in the major bronchi of the middle and lower lobes.

8. Grossly, tumors vary in size and can project into the bronchial lumen and are encapsulated by a thin membrane.
9. It rarely has a stalk but can be completely removed endoscopically.
10. Surgical resection is indicated when the distal lung has been extensively damaged or if endoscopic removal is contraindicated or incomplete.
11. Complete surgical resection results in cure.

VIII. MESENCHYMAL TUMORS

A. VESSEL ORIGIN

1. Sclerosing hemangioma
   a. It is a rare, benign tumor occurring at an average age of 50 years.
   b. Most patients are asymptomatic with a solitary nodule usually in a lower lobe.
   c. Average size range is from 3 to 5 cm.
   d. Histologically it is of two cell types—cuboidal surface cells and round cells within the surface layer.
   e. Calcifications are present in one-third of tumors.
   f. Architecture is a combination of papillary, sclerotic, solid, and hemorrhagic patterns.
   g. It may be derived from type 2 alveolar pneumocytes.
   h. Magnetic resonance is particularly useful for diagnosis.
   i. Surgical excision is the treatment of choice if bleeding or obstruction occurs.

2. Lymphangioma
   a. Four basic types:
      (1) Lymphangioma
      (2) Lymphangiectasis
      (3) Lymphangiomatosis
      (4) Lymphatic dysplasia
   b. Usually small and peripheral
   c. CT shows the lesion to have a smooth border.
   d. May be associated with dyspnea or hemoptysis
   e. Surgical resection has excellent outcomes.

3. Nerve
   a. Granular cell tumor
      (1) Derived from Schwann cells
      (2) Average age of patient is 40 years, with male predominance.
      (3) Found incidentally in greater than 50% of cases; otherwise, usually present with symptoms of obstruction
      (4) Chest radiograph shows lobar infiltration, coin lesions, and lobar atelectasis.
      (5) Solitary lesions are present in 75% of cases, less than 10% are multiple; remainder are solitary lesions with multiple skin lesions.
      (6) Gross tumors vary from 0.5 to 5 cm.

      (7) Commonly present as an endobronchial lesion

      (8) Microscopically composed of large cells with abundant pink granular cytoplasm

      (9) Conservative treatment except with a malignant association

    (10) Complete resection is curative, but tumors may recur.

    (11) Laser treatment may be appropriate in certain cases.

    (12) With associated damaged lung, surgical resection is indicated.

  b. Neurilemoma

      (1) Equal sex distribution

      (2) May occur in a major bronchus, but majority are seen in the lung parenchyma

      (3) May be difficult to classify because of degenerative changes

  c. Neurofibroma

      (1) Most occur in an endobronchial location

      (2) Seen in young to middle-aged adults

      (3) Surgical resection or endobronchial ablation is indicated as dictated by the extent and location of the tumor.

4. Muscle

  a. Leiomyoma

      (1) These tumors account for 2% of benign tumors.

      (2) May occur in the trachea, bronchus, or parenchyma. Usually equally distributed.

      (3) Seen in young to middle-aged adults

      (4) More common in women than men

      (5) In women who have had a uterine leiomyoma removed in the past, it is difficult to differentiate a true pulmonary leiomyoma from a benign metastasizing leiomyoma from the original uterine tumor.

      (6) These tumors may be managed by laser resection and close monitoring.

IX. MISCELLANEOUS TUMORS

A. FIBROMA

1. Most commonly found arising from visceral pleura
2. Found in the mediastinum, retroperitoneum, external surface of the stomach, and small intestine
3. Tumors are composed of spindle cells with dense bundles of collagen.
4. Complete resection is curative.
5. Commonly presents as an endobronchial lesion

B. HAMARTOMA

1. It is the most common benign tumor of the lung.
2. Hamartomas consist of abnormal arrangements of normal cells and demonstrate slow growth patterns.
3. Cartilage is the most common mesenchymal tissue present in the lesions; fatty tissue is also a frequent component.

4. It presents as a well-circumscribed, solitary pulmonary nodule 90% of the time (contains popcorn calcifications 30% of the time).
5. It is usually 1–2 cm.
6. It is most common in middle-aged adults, with a male dominance.
7. When symptomatic, patients may present with hemoptysis, cough, or chest pain.
8. Biopsy is indicated in any patient with symptoms.
9. Transthoracic needle biopsy is diagnostic in 85% of lesions.
10. There is a 50% incidence rate of postbiopsy pneumothorax that is twice the incidence of biopsy of other peripheral lesions.
11. When the diagnosis is made by needle biopsy, observation is safe.
12. Endobronchial lesions are not detectable radiographically except when distal lung changes are observed.
13. Endobronchial lesions are best treated by laser ablation.
14. Reports of malignancy in a hamartoma are rare; however, no real evidence exists that these tumors arise from the underlying hamartoma.
15. Surgical excision only if symptomatic or when located more proximally with endobronchial compression; also when carcinoma cannot be ruled out

C. TERATOMA
1. Occurs rarely as primary lung tumor. Most common location is the anterior mediastinum.
2. Of those found in the lung, most are found in the anterior segment of the left upper lobe.
   a. Clear cell (sugar) tumor
3. Unknown histogenesis
4. Equally distributed between the sexes
5. Most patients are asymptomatic.
6. The lesions are solitary, peripheral, and 1.5–3 cm.
7. Excision is curative.

X. OTHER TUMORS
A. LIPOMA
1. These tumors arise from the wall of the bronchus in 80% of cases.
2. They are more common in male than in female individuals.
3. They may cause obstruction with pulmonary complications.
4. Bronchial laser vaporization is the treatment of choice when possible.

B. CHONDROMA
1. These are true pulmonary mesenchymal tumors.
2. They are often confused with hamartomas.
3. Most chondromas are endobronchial in location and most often occur in men.
4. Extension requires surgical resection, which is curative.

5. There is a subgroup of tumors that occurs in women that are associated with gastric sarcomas or an extraadrenal paraganglioma (located in the neck, thorax, or abdomen—association is known as Carney triad).
6. The location of these tumors is primarily parenchymal.
7. They have a tendency to be multiple.
8. In more than half of cases they contain areas that are calcified and need to be differentiated from hamartomas.
9. Microscopically mature bone and cartilage are seen peripherally with degenerative changes centrally.
10. The triad is a chronic persistent indolent disease. Treatment consists of repeated resections of respective tumors. (*Note:* Refers to Carney syndrome, inherited autosomal disorder, melanotic schwannoma, multiple myomas, multiple areas of skin pigmentation, and one or more endocrine disorders; this is not the same as Carney triad.)

XI. INFLAMMATORY PSEUDOTUMORS
A. PLASMA CELL GRANULOMA
1. This tumor has been called a variety of names, including fibrous histiocytoma, inflammatory pseudotumor, and fibroxanthoma.
2. Because of the low-grade malignant potential of these tumors, radical resection is recommended (lobectomy, including sleeve lobectomy).

B. PULMONARY HYALINIZING GRANULOMA
1. It is a tumor of dense hyalinized connective tissue that occurs as the result of inflammatory or postinflammatory changes.
2. Patients are asymptomatic or present with cough, shortness of breath, chest pain, and weight loss.
3. Lesions are nodular and vary from a few millimeters to 15 cm.
4. Many patients have multiple lesions, with most being bilateral.
5. Half of the patients have a history of an autoimmune disorder or past fungal or mycobacterial disease.

XII. OTHER BENIGN TUMORS
A. MUCINOUS CYSTADENOMA
1. Defined as a unilocular cystic lesion whose fibrous wall is lined by well-differentiated, presumably benign, columnar mucinous epithelium
2. Usually occurs in smokers in their 50s–60s; equal distribution between the sexes
3. Usually located at or near the periphery of the lung
4. Filled with clear gelatinous material
5. The cysts may have areas of borderline malignancy or adenocarcinoma.
6. Treatment is complete resection.

60

BENIGN TUMORS OF THE LUNG

B. NODULAR AMYLOID

1. These occur in three types—tracheobronchial, nodular pulmonary, and diffuse (interstitial) pulmonary.
2. Nodular pulmonary amyloidosis is a focal collection of amyloid in the lung, usually with a giant cell reaction around it.
3. It may be solitary or multiple nodules.
4. Most patients are in their 70s.
5. Most patients are asymptomatic and are discovered incidentally.
6. Long-term follow-up is needed because of the possibility of malignant lymphoma.
7. These lymphomas are identified by lymphatic tracking of the lympho-cytic infiltrate, pleural infiltration, and sheetlike masses of plasma cells.

RECOMMENDED READINGS

Chang AC, Lin J. Lung neoplasms. In: Mulholland MW, Lillemoe KD, Doherty GM, et al., eds. *Surgery, Scientific Principles & Practice*. 5th ed. Philadelphia: Lippincott Williams & Wilkins; 2010.

Shields TW, Robinson PG. Benign tumors of the lung. In: Shields TW, Locicero J, Reed CE, Feins RH, eds. *General Thoracic Surgery*. 7th ed. Philadelphia: Lippincott Williams & Wilkins; 2009:171569–171590.

Malignant Tumors of the Lung

Audrey E. Ertel, MD

Smoking is one of the leading causes of statistics.

—Anonymous

I. EPIDEMIOLOGY

A. GENERAL

1. Incidence of lung cancer in the United States has been declining among men and only recently began decreasing in women.
2. Overall prevalence is approximately 125 per 100,000 people per year.
3. Estimated new cases per year in the United States: 212,584 (111,907 male and 100,677 female)

B. MORTALITY

1. Primary lung malignancies are the leading cause of cancer deaths, accounting for 13% of all new cancers and 26.5% of all cancer deaths.
2. Estimated deaths per year in the United States: 158,080
3. Remains by far the leading cause of cancer-related deaths in both sexes in the United States
4. Overall 5-year survival rate is 17.8%; for localized disease this increases to 54%.

II. ETIOLOGY

A. CIGARETTE SMOKING

1. Overall risk for lung cancer in smokers versus nonsmokers is 20–25 times greater.
2. Only 10% of patients with lung cancer are nonsmokers, but 25%–50% of these patients have significant second hand smoke exposure.
3. The current downtrend in national incidence of smoking reflects the decline in the incidence of lung cancer diagnosis.
4. Importantly, the increasing incidence of lung cancer in never-smokers, particularly women, is a serious public health issue.

B. EXPOSURE

1. Radon
2. Asbestos (more common cause of lung cancer than mesothelioma)
3. Ionizing radiation
4. Arsenic
5. Nickel
6. Chromium
7. Mustard gas
8. Chloromethyl ethers

III. SCREENING

A. GENERAL

1. No proper screening method was available until results of the National Lung Screening Trial (NLST) were published in 2011.
2. Lung cancer has a high morbidity and mortality, significant prevalence, identifiable risk factors, and evidence that therapy is more effective in early stages.
3. NLST demonstrated at least 20% reduction in lung cancer–specific death in high-risk patients (i.e., >55 years of age with >30 pack-years of smoking).

B. SCREENING MODALITIES

1. Chest x-ray (CXR) and/or sputum culture—no longer recommended. No impact on mortality
2. Low-dose chest computed tomography (LDCT)—multidetector CT scanners use low-dose radiation (10 times less than diagnostic scans) to generate high-resolution imaging.
   a. Imperative to understand that this is a process rather than a test (i.e., patients have to commit to follow-up as needed to achieve reduced mortality)
   b. NLST—LDCT in high-risk patients yearly for at least 3 years
      (1) Participants aged 55–74 years with a history of at least 30 pack-years, including current smokers and those who had quit within 15 years
      (2) Demonstrated that LDCT screening reduced mortality in high-risk population compared with CXR screening—at least 20% reduction in mortality (trial was stopped early given substantial results).
      (3) A total of 96.4% of scans were positive, making a multidisciplinary approach an essential component of the process to minimize unwarranted interventions.
   c. Societies recommending the implementation of the NLST guidelines
      (1) American Association for Thoracic Surgery (AATS)—recommend LDCT screening in high-risk patients between ages 55 and 79 years.
      (2) National Comprehensive Cancer Network (NCCN)—annual LDCT screening for high-risk patients aged 55–74 years or age ≥50 with a history of 20 pack-years with additional risk factor (other than second hand smoke exposure)
   d. Centers for Medicare and Medicaid Services (CMS) started covering LDCT screening of lung cancer in 2015.
3. Positron emission tomography (PET) scans—not a recommended screening modality
   a. Sensitivity 96%, specificity 79%
   b. False negative—tumors with low metabolic activity such as carcinoma in situ, carcinoid tumors, tumors with sizes below the resolution (typically <10 mm), and patients with uncontrolled hyperglycemia

c. False positive—inflammation or infection, typically with standardized uptake value (SUV) less than 2.5
d. LDCT followed by PET scan in patients with noncalcified lesions ≥7 mm had sensitivity of 61% and specificity of 91%, with a negative predictive value (NPV) of 71%. If then followed by a repeat CT, NPV increased to 100%.

IV. SOLITARY PULMONARY NODULE

A. GENERAL
1. A solitary pulmonary nodule (SPN) is defined as ≤3 cm surrounded by normal lung parenchyma and without adenopathy, atelectasis, or pleural effusion.
2. A lesion greater than 3 cm is defined as a mass.
3. Patients with an SPN undergo evaluation based on the suspicion for malignancy, whereas those with a mass undergo work-up for suspected malignancy.

B. DIFFERENTIAL DIAGNOSIS
1. Lung malignancy, primary or metastatic
2. Inflammation—sarcoidosis
3. Infection—granulomas, fungal balls
4. Congenital lesion—hamartoma
5. Vascular—pulmonary vascular arteriovenous malformations (PVMs)
6. Previous trauma

C. RADIOGRAPHIC CHARACTERISTICS OF BENIGN NODULE
1. Small (<3 cm), smooth with sharply circumscribed margins
2. Benign calcification—laminar, central, diffuse/homogeneous, and popcorn patterns
3. Stable in size on CT imaging over 2-year period (solid), 3 years for a subsolid nodule—doubling time is 20–400 days for malignant tumors.

D. MANAGEMENT OF SOLITARY PULMONARY NODULE
1. Depends greatly on size of the lesion and if the lesion has increased in size, patient's age, and smoking history, as well as additional characteristics on CT scan (calcifications, spiculations)

V. CLINICAL FEATURES

A. RESPIRATORY
1. Cough—usually dry, persistent (50%–75%)
2. Dyspnea with or without wheezing (25%–40%)
3. Hemoptysis—may be small and recurrent or sudden and massive (20%–50%)
4. Symptoms of acute pneumonia (that is slow to resolve)
5. No symptoms in early stages

61

MALIGNANT TUMORS OF THE LUNG

B. ASSOCIATED SYNDROMES
1. Endocrine abnormalities
   a. Syndrome of inappropriate secretion of antidiuretic hormone
   b. Hypercalcemia
   c. Ectopic adrenocorticotropic hormone (Cushing syndrome)
2. Neurologic—peripheral neuropathies, cerebellar degeneration, degeneration of the cerebral cortex, pseudodementia
   a. Lambert-Eaton syndrome—proximal muscle group wasting
3. Musculoskeletal—clubbing, hypertrophic pulmonary osteoarthropathy (progressive ankle pain), polymyositis
4. Vascular—anemia, leukocytosis, thrombocytosis, hypercoagulable disorders
5. Cutaneous—dermatomyositis, acanthosis nigricans

C. EVIDENCE OF METASTATIC OR LOCALLY ADVANCED DISEASE
1. Mediastinal invasion
   a. Tracheal obstruction with stridor and dyspnea
   b. Dysphagia
   c. Hoarseness (ipsilateral involvement of recurrent laryngeal nerve)
   d. Horner syndrome
      (1) Tumor involving cervical and first thoracic segment of sympathetic trunk (Pancoast tumors)
      (2) Ptosis, meiosis, anhidrosis of the affected side
   e. Superior vena cava syndrome
      (1) Compression or direct invasion of great veins of thoracic outlet
      (2) Dyspnea, severe headaches, and periorbital, facial, and neck edema
2. Metastatic disease/locally advanced disease
   a. Malignant pleural effusions
   b. Bone pain
   c. Weight loss
   d. Neurologic symptoms
   e. Chest pain and chest wall involvement

D. METHOD OF SPREAD
1. Invades lymphatics and blood vessels, resulting in early metastasis
2. A total of 30%–50% of patients with lung cancer have lymphatic or hematogenous spread at initial presentation.
3. Metastases in order of frequency—regional lymph nodes, liver, bone, adrenals, and brain
4. Contralateral pulmonary metastases at postmortem examination—10%–14%

VI. PATHOLOGY

A. HISTOLOGIC CLASSIFICATION
Malignant epithelial lung tumors according to World Health Organization (2015):
1. Adenocarcinoma—40%
2. Squamous cell carcinoma (SCC)—20%

3. Large cell carcinoma (LCC)—10%
4. Neuroendocrine carcinoma—20%–25%
5. Sarcomatoid carcinoma—5%–10%

B. LOCATION OF PRIMARY TUMORS
1. "Central" tumors—most frequently SCC, also small cell carcinomas and carcinoids
2. "Peripheral" tumors—adenocarcinoma and LCCs

VII. ADENOCARCINOMA—40%

A. GENERAL
1. Increased incidence due to low-tar filtered cigarettes
2. Characterized by glandular differentiation, mucin production, or pneumocyte marker expression
3. Markers: CK7$^+$ and CK20$^-$ indicate adenocarcinoma (cytokeratins), TTF-1 limits it to the lung
4. Accounts for greater than 70% of surgically resected cases
5. Subtypes include: lepidic, acinar, papillary, micropapillary, solid, invasive mucinous, colloid, fetal, enteric, and minimally invasive

B. PATHOLOGIC FEATURES
1. Often peripherally located with central fibrosis and pleural puckering

VIII. SQUAMOUS CELL CARCINOMA—20%

A. GENERAL
1. Incidence has declined, likely due to changes in smoking behavior.
2. Relatively slow growing and late to metastasize; survival rate better than adenocarcinoma
3. Marker: p63 is commonly used to confirm diagnosis and distinguish from adenocarcinoma.
4. Adenosquamous carcinoma consists of tumors composed of more than 10% malignant glandular and squamous components.

B. PATHOLOGIC FEATURES
1. Occurs in the segmental, lobar, or main stem bronchi in 90% of cases
2. Characterized by keratinization, keratin pearl formation, and intercellular bridges
3. Spread pattern is as follows:
   a. Endobronchial growth and invasion of peribronchial lung parenchyma, soft tissue, and lymph nodes
   b. Peripheral tumors commonly invade chest wall.

IX. LARGE CELL CARCINOMA—10%

A. GENERAL
1. Most tumors occur in a peripheral and subpleural location.
2. Rapid growth and early metastasis
3. Poor prognosis

61

MALIGNANT TUMORS OF THE LUNG

B. PATHOLOGIC FEATURES
1. Do not show definitive squamous or glandular differentiation
2. Grow in sheets without organization or pattern
3. Necrosis and hemorrhage are dominant features of these tumors.
4. Most LCCs defined by morphologic criteria can be reclassified as adenocarcinoma and SCC using lineage-specific markers.

X. NEUROENDOCRINE CARCINOMA—20%–25%

A. GENERAL
1. Characterized by organoid growth pattern, "salt-and-pepper" chromatin distribution, and expression of neuroendocrine markers
2. Histologic differentiation is determined by tumor proliferation rate, which correlates with tumor aggressiveness and prognosis.
3. Separated into four groups: typical, atypical, small cell, and large cell neuroendocrine tumor
   a. Typical and atypical carcinoids are low and intermediate grade, respectively. SCC and LCNT are deemed high-grade tumors.
   b. Typical carcinoid is treated conservatively with wedge resection and clear margins; all others are indications for lobectomy.

XI. OTHER—5%–10%

A. GENERAL
1. Sarcomatoid carcinoma
   a. Include the following types: pleomorphic, spindle cell, giant cell, carcinosarcoma, and pulmonary blastoma

XII. DIAGNOSIS
1. Radiology

A. CHEST RADIOGRAPH
Findings that raise suspicion of malignancy include the following:
1. New or enlarging focal lesion, particularly if spiculated
2. Pleural effusion, same side as lung lesion
3. Noncalcified pleural nodularity
4. Enlarged hilar or mediastinal nodes

B. CHEST COMPUTED TOMOGRAPHY SCAN
The standard image modality to assess lung pathology
1. May show additional pulmonary nodules—small satellite lesions often indicate an infectious etiology.
2. Evaluate spread to pleural and mediastinal structures.
3. Assess borders, exact location, and consistency (solid, mixed-attenuation, or ground-glass opacity).
4. Measure precise growth when comparing with previous scans.
5. Standard diagnostic scan = 100 anteroposterior (AP) CXRs, LDCT scans = 10 x-rays (may vary based on equipment)

C. POSITRON EMISSION TOMOGRAPHY SCAN

1. Uses fluorodeoxyglucose (FDG) to capture tissue metabolism by the nuclear medicine camera, most often then fused with a whole body CT for anatomic detail; standard component of the clinical staging of lung cancer (even not tissue-proven in preparation for wedge biopsy immediately followed by lobectomy if confirmed malignant)
2. Most useful to raise or lower suspicion of lymph node involvement and distant metastasis
3. Although not a "cancer test," an SUV greater than 2.5 has statistical correlation with malignancy prediction.

D. CLINICAL STAGING

Determine the highest radiographic stage to facilitate the selection of proper biopsy modality.

1. CT scan (diagnostic or LDCT)—Dedicated chest scan uses respiratory gating to enhance visualization versus whole body scan (PET/CT) not timed with respiration.
2. PET/CT scan—best at assessing distant metastasis, followed by regional nodal spread and lastly to assess lung mass activity
3. CT abdomen to evaluate liver and adrenal glands if PET/CT scan raises suspicion

E. TISSUE BIOPSY

1. Sputum cytology
   a. A total of 70%–80% sensitive with multiple specimens with central tumors
   b. Cytology most diagnostic for SCC, intermediate for adenocarcinoma, and least for small cell carcinoma
   c. Not routinely used as part of the work-up of a patient with a lung mass; consider on a case-by-case basis
2. Bronchoscopy
   a. Best for central tumors (diagnostic yield decreases the more peripheral the mass is)—Segmental tumors can be directly visualized and biopsied while subsegmental masses can undergo high-yield washings and brushings.
   b. More distal tumors, if visualized by fluoroscopy, can be reached via transbronchial biopsy with reasonable results.
   c. Complications are rare, and this procedure is routinely performed as outpatient.
   d. For subsegmental and more peripheral lesions, consider the use of electromagnetic navigational bronchoscopy (ENB), which raises biopsy yield significantly.
   e. Endobronchial ultrasound (EBUS) bronchoscopy is becoming the most common modality for diagnosing and staging of lung cancer, being able to biopsy mediastinal stations (2R, 2L, 4R, 4L, and 7) in addition to hilar stations (10, 11, 12), which are not reached by mediastinoscopy.

61

MALIGNANT TUMORS OF THE LUNG

f. Rapid on-site examination cytology (ROSE) is very effective in confirming the adequacy of the biopsies.

3. **Mediastinoscopy**
   a. Up to 50% of patients have involved mediastinal lymph nodes at initial presentation.
   b. Mediastinoscopy is used in patients with lymphadenopathy (>1 cm) before a planned pulmonary resection to evaluate resectability and confirm staging.
   c. Provides access to stations 2R, 2L, 4R, 4L, and 7, which are all key to determine N2 disease.
   d. At our institution we favor performing a mediastinoscopy in patients with critical suspicion of N2 disease, even in the face of a negative EBUS.
   e. We typically do not biopsy the mediastinum in clinical stage I (no abnormalities on CT and PET scans). However, any tumor greater than 4 cm, more centrally located, or with any lymphadenopathy (>1 cm) requires tissue staging of the mediastinum.

4. **Needle biopsy**
   a. False-negative result in 10% of patients
   b. Provides cytology assessment and, in selected patients, a core needle biopsy can be considered (significantly increases rate of complications)
   c. May be performed transbronchoscopically (TBNA) or via percutaneous approach with CT guidance
      (1) TBNA approach is indicated for extrabronchial tumors without bronchial wall abnormalities with a tumor visualized on fluoroscopy.
      (2) ENB increases the yield significantly, typically in lesions that are too small or not peripheral enough for a percutaneous biopsy.
      (3) CT guidance is used for peripheral lesions greater than 2 cm (varies by institution).
   d. Contraindications
      (1) Bleeding disorders or anticoagulation
      (2) Bullous disease near the lesion
      (3) Inappropriate window relative to size and location
   e. Complications
      (1) Pneumothorax—20%–25% of cases; 10% require chest tube placement
      (2) Minor hemoptysis—6% of cases

5. **Video-assisted thoracoscopic surgery (VATS)**
   a. Provides an excisional biopsy of peripheral nodules, allows biopsy of lymph nodes (particularly the hard-to-reach level 5), and evaluates pleural implants and effusions
   b. Frozen section pathology is greater than 90% accurate in confirming or ruling out malignancy.
   c. Permits immediately proceeding to lobectomy and mediastinal lymph node resection if mass is malignant (procedure is both diagnostic and therapeutic)

d. Requires general anesthesia and single-lung ventilation, therefore making patient selection of critical importance

e. This strategy requires a complete clinical staging, as well as preoperative risk stratification (including pulmonary function tests) before the VATS procedure.

F. CLASSIFICATION AND STAGING

1. Determines treatment options and prognosis
2. Tumor/node/metastasis (TNM) classification for lung carcinoma (2010 International Staging System published in the 7th American Joint Committee on Cancer [AJCC] Manual)

   a. Primary tumor (T)

   T0: No tumor

   Tx: Positive cytology

   Tis: Carcinoma in situ

   T1: Less than 3 cm, no main bronchial invasion, no invasion of visceral pleura

   T1a: ≤2 cm

   T1b: Greater than 2 cm but ≤3 cm

   T2: Greater than 3 cm but *less than 7 cm* or any size that invades visceral pleura, or main bronchus greater than 2 cm from carina, atelectasis extending to hilum

   T2a: Greater than 3 cm but ≤5 cm

   T2b: Greater than 5 cm but ≤7 cm

   T3: Greater than 7 cm or directly invades main bronchus less than 2 cm from carina, parietal pleura, phrenic nerve, diaphragm, or pericardium

   T4: Invades mediastinum, heart, great vessels, trachea, recurrent laryngeal nerve, esophagus, carina, vertebral body, malignant effusion, or satellite tumor nodule in the same lobe

   b. Regional lymph nodes (N)

   N0: No nodes

   N1: Ipsilateral nodes (peribronchial or hilar) and intrapulmonary nodes

   N2: Ipsilateral nodes (mediastinal) or subcarinal nodes

   N3: Contralateral nodes (mediastinal) or hilar; ipsilateral or contralateral scalene or supraclavicular nodes

   c. Distant metastases (M)

   M0: No metastasis

   M1: Metastasis

   M1a: Separate tumor nodule(s) in a contralateral lobe, pleural nodes, or malignant effusion

   M1b: Distant metastasis

3. Staging for lung cancer:

   Occult carcinoma: Tx N0 M0

   Stage Ia: T1a–T1b N0 M0

   Stage Ib: T2a N0 M0

Stage IIa: T1a–T1b N1 M0, T2a N1 M0, T2b N0 M0
Stage IIb: T2b N1 M0, T3 N0 M0
Stage IIIa: T1–T3 N2 M0, T3–T4 N1 M0
Stage IIIb: any T N3 M0, T4 N2 M0
Stage IV: any T, any N, M1a or M1b

4. Regional lymph node stations (American Thoracic Society):
   2R: Right upper paratracheal (suprainnominate) nodes
   2L: Left upper paratracheal (supraaortic) nodes
   4R: Right lower paratracheal nodes
   4L: Left lower paratracheal nodes
   5: Aortopulmonary nodes
   6: Anterior mediastinal nodes
   7: Subcarinal nodes
   8: Paraesophageal nodes
   9: Pulmonary ligament nodes
   10R: Right main bronchial nodes
   10L: Left main bronchial nodes
   11: Intrapulmonary nodes

XIII. TREATMENT

1. Preoperative evaluation
   a. Assess resectability if primary tumor
   b. Rule out regional and distant metastasis
   c. Assess mediastinal lymph node spread
      (1) Staging
         (a) Noninvasive
            (i) Chest CT (lymph node >1 cm suspicious): 57% sensitive, 82% specific
            (ii) PET scan
         (b) Mediastinoscopy
            (i) Traditionally the gold standard; in some practices replaced by EBUS in most routine staging cases
            (ii) Remains an essential procedure that at our institution is performed on a case-by-case basis even with negative EBUS results
      (3) False-negative results in 8% of tests
      (4) Less than 1% rate of major complications
         (c) Endoscopic ultrasound with fine-needle aspiration, further enhanced if a radial US probe is used. Adequacy of staging requires the pathologic report of lymphocytes in the samples.
         (d) VATS wedge biopsy
      (5) MUST obtain tissue:
         (a) Positive lymph nodes (N1–N3) on CT, PET, or both
         (b) Negative N2/N3 lymph nodes on CT and PET, but:
            (i) T2–T4 lesion
            (ii) Suspicious N1 lymph nodes

       (iii) Synchronous primary cancers

       (iv) Solitary brain and adrenal metastasis

  d. Assess patient's ability to tolerate resection.

    (1) Pulmonary function tests: FEV_1 (forced expiratory volume in 1 second) and DLCO (diffusing capacity of the lung for carbon monoxide), for the patient to tolerate a lobectomy, the postoperative predicted values needed are greater than 40% ($POFEV_1$, PODLCO)

2. Surgical resection

  a. General

    (1) Clinical stage I and II cancers/pathologic stage III

    (2) Five-year survival rate after resection: 50%

    (3) Adjuvant chemotherapy in stage II; there is evidence of negative effect in stage I

    (4) Role for surgery in stage IIIA disease:

      (a) Single level N2 disease

      (b) Induction chemoradiation followed by surgery

      (c) Good risk patients

      (d) Surgically resectable primary

      (e) Absence of bulky N2 disease

      (f) Absence of progression of disease after induction therapy

  b. Lobectomy and mediastinal lymph node resection/sampling

    (1) Procedure of choice for disease confined to one lobe

      (a) In Lung Cancer Study Group (1995), lobectomy versus limited resection showed 75% increase in local recurrence and 50% increase in cancer-related death when limited resection performed.

    (2) Includes entire first-level lobar lymphatics

    (3) Mortality rate of 0%–8%

    (4) Still being debated whether mediastinal resection versus sampling should be offered—no benefits of resection proven yet

    (5) Sleeve lobectomy for peribronchial tumor or lymph node involvement at resection site

    (6) VATS/robotic lobectomy

      (a) Same operation as when done open (thoracotomy), with no difference in cancer-free survival

      (b) Robotic lobectomy allows a more thorough mediastinal nodal resection.

      (c) No data yet that determine that the VATS or robotic approach is superior—improved pain and faster recovery data based on VATS versus thoracotomy reports

      (d) Advantages

        (i) No rib spreading means less postoperative pain.

        (ii) Shorter hospital stay

        (iii) Improved pulmonary function

        (iv) Decreased inflammatory response

      (e) Contraindications
         (i) Central tumors
         (ii) Tumor greater than 6 cm
         (iii) Extensive hilar calcification
         (iv) T3 lesions
         (v) N2 disease
    c. Pneumonectomy
      (1) Indications—hilar involvement or tumor extension across oblique fissure
      (2) Can result in poor pulmonary reserve with significant change in lifestyle
      (3) Mortality rate of 5%–10%

3. Nonsurgical therapy
    a. Stage III
      (1) Radiation and chemotherapy (cisplatin based)
      (2) Five-year survival rate of 10%
      (3) Median survival of 12–14 months
    b. Stage IV
      (1) Chemotherapy only
      (2) Five-year survival rate of less than 1%
      (3) Surgical resection in very select patient—oligometastatic disease appears to behave differently than stage 4 disease:
         (a) Isolated adrenal or brain metastasis
         (b) No involvement of N2 lymph nodes (requires tissue staging)

4. Surveillance after curative-intent therapy
    a. Most lung cancer recurrences present during the first 2 years after curative treatment.
    b. Patient will have 1%–2% yearly risk for development of a new primary lung cancer.
    c. Follow-up includes the following: radiograph study (chest CT or chest radiograph), history, and physical examination every 6 months for 2 years, then annually.

XIV. THE FUTURE

1. Diagnostic modalities are evolving rapidly: lung cancer markers will be detected in the blood (liquid biopsy) and likely in the breath.
2. Tumor markers are being studied with the expectation that lung cancer will eventually transition from pathology classification to biological (markers) grouping.
3. Tumor markers currently play a role in the treatment of adenocarcinoma (ALK, EGFR), with many more being defined resulting in targeted therapy.
4. Surgical technology will continue to evolve, allowing for smaller incision across fewer intercostal spaces improving recovery.
5. Percutaneous and bronchoscopic technology will provide treatment alternatives by using cryotherapy and radiofrequency ablation.

RECOMMENDED READINGS

Carcinoma of the lungs. In: Shields TW, Locicero J, Reed CE, Feins RH, eds. *General Thoracic Surgery*. 6th ed. Philadelphia: Lippincott Williams & Wilkins; 2009:1281–1664.

Chang AC, Martin J, Rusch VW. Lung neoplasms. In: Mulholland MW, Lillemoe KD, Doherty GM, et al., eds. *Surgery, Scientific Principles & Practice*. 4th ed. Philadelphia: Lippincott Williams & Wilkins; 2006:1367–1395.

Kramer BS, Berg CD, Aberle DR, Prorok PC. Lung cancer screening with low-dose helical CT: results from the National Lung Screening Trial (NLST). *J Med Screen*. 2011;18:109–111.

Thymus and Mediastinal Tumors

Winifred Lo, MD

We are here to add what we can to life, not to get what we can from life.

—William Osler

I. ANATOMY AND EMBRYOLOGY

1. The thymus gland originates from the third and fourth pharyngeal pouches (along with the lower parathyroid glands) and typically descends into the anterior mediastinum.
2. The Shields three-compartment model is the most anatomic model and widely used by thoracic surgeons.
3. Anterior compartment is bordered by sternum (anterior), pericardium (posterior), and pleura (lateral).
   a. Contains thymus, internal mammary arteries, connective tissue, lymph nodes, fat
4. Visceral compartment is bordered by thoracic inlet (superior), pericardium (anterior), and anterior surface of vertebrae (posterior).
   a. Contains heart, pericardium, great vessels, airway, esophagus
5. Posterior compartment/paravertebral sulci are bordered by anterior aspect of vertebral bodies (posterior) and costophrenic angles (laterally).
   a. Contains spine, proximal intercostal neurovascular bundles, sympathetic chain, lymphatic tissue, connective tissue

II. ASSESSMENT OF MEDIASTINAL MASSES

Differential diagnosis for mediastinal masses depends on patient age, gender, the compartment of the mass, computed tomography (CT) characteristics, and symptoms. The appropriate evaluation for mediastinal masses is therefore highly variable and specific to the lesion in question.

III. ANTERIOR MEDIASTINAL MASSES

Despite being the smallest compartment, 50% of mediastinal tumors are located in the anterior mediastinum.

A. THYMOMAS

1. Epidemiology
   a. Most common mediastinal neoplasm (20%) in adults, most common neoplasm in anterior mediastinal compartment
   b. Most common in the 40–60-year-old age group
2. Presentation
   a. Symptoms are typically secondary to mass effect and may include dyspnea, chest pain, and cough.

(1) At time of presentation, $^1/_3 - ^1/_2$ are asymptomatic.

(2) A total of 40% have symptoms related to mass effect.

(3) A total of 30% have systemic symptoms.

(4) Locally invasive tumors may present with phrenic nerve paralysis or superior vena cava (SVC) syndrome.

b. Several autoimmune disorders are associated with thymoma.

    (1) Myasthenia gravis (MG) is the most common autoimmune disorder (45%).

        (a) Etiology: Autoantibodies block acetylcholine receptors at neuromuscular junction.

        (b) Presentation: diplopia, ptosis, dysphagia, weakness, fatigue

        (c) A total of 30%–50% of patients with thymoma will have MG, so it is critical to rule out myasthenia when evaluating a patient with a suspected thymoma; only 10%–15% of patients with MG will have concomitant thymoma.

        (d) Thymectomy improves symptoms in up to 60% of patients (symptoms improve slowly).

    (2) Red cell aplasia (2%–5%)

    (3) Hypogammaglobulinemia (2%–5%)

    (4) Systemic lupus erythematosus, polymyositis, rheumatoid arthritis, and other syndromes are less commonly associated

3. **Evaluation**

a. Differential: intrathoracic thyroid, parathyroid tumors, lymphoma, germ cell tumors

b. Imaging

    (1) CT chest demonstrates a homogeneous mass with possible calcification. It is used to delineate the size and extent of the lesion, invasion of neighboring structures, and distant metastases.

    (2) Chest MRI is typically not necessary but can be helpful to determine vascular or neural involvement.

    (3) Fluorodeoxyglucose-positron emission tomography (FDG-PET) is used in some centers; however, most thymomas are slow growing and rarely metastasize, making its clinical utility unclear. It is more useful for thymic carcinoma.

c. Labs: α-fetoprotein (AFP), β-human chorionic gonadotropin (β-hCG) to rule out germ cell tumors in appropriate situations

d. Biopsy

    (1) Diagnosis: truly needed for advanced tumors in which induction therapy or nonoperative approach is being considered OR when lymphoma is high on differential

    (2) Small lesions (stage I/II): complete excision for diagnosis

    (3) Large lesions: CT-guided core needle biopsy, anterior mediastinotomy (Chamberlain procedure), thoracoscopic biopsy

4. Staging: The most common staging systems for thymoma is the Koga modification of the Masaoka staging system.
   a. Stage I: completely encapsulated
   b. Stage IIa: microscopic extracapsular extension
   c. Stage IIb: macroscopic invasion into surrounding fatty tissue
   d. Stage III: macroscopic invasion into neighboring organs
   e. Stage IVa: pleural or pericardial metastasis
   f. Stage IVb: lymphogenous or hematogenous metastasis

5. Treatment
   a. Stage I: complete resection, adjuvant therapy not recommended
   b. Stage II: complete resection, adjuvant radiation therapy controversial
      (1) Radiation therapy may be recommended for close or positive margins or for higher-risk pathology (World Health Organization [WHO] type B2, B3, or C).
   c. Stage III: patients typically treated with multimodality therapy
      (1) Induction chemotherapy (cisplatin based) typically given if suspected preoperative
      (2) Complete resection 4–6 weeks after completion of chemotherapy
      (3) Adjuvant radiation therapy
   d. Stage IV
      (1) In patients with limited stage IVa disease, a combination of induction chemotherapy followed by complete resection and adjuvant radiation can be considered.
      (2) Unresectable patients are typically treated with chemotherapy.
   e. Prognostic factors for overall survival: completeness of resection, Masaoka stage, and WHO classification.
   f. Ten-year survival by stage
      (1) Stage I: 100%
      (2) Stage II: 98%
      (3) Stage III: 78%
      (4) Stage IV: 47%

6. Surgical approach
   a. Complete resection through a median sternotomy is the most common surgical approach.
   b. Resection should be from the phrenic nerves laterally to the thoracic inlet (including the thymic horns) superiorly and down to the diaphragm inferiorly.
   c. En bloc resection of locally invaded structures should be done to get a complete resection: pericardium, lung, unilateral phrenic nerve, SVC, innominate vein.
   d. Phrenic nerve resection should be avoided in patients with myasthenia.
   e. Minimally invasive techniques (i.e., thoracoscopic, robotic, transcervical) are being increasingly used for smaller tumors.

B. THYMIC CARCINOMA
1. Epidemiology: more common in men, fifth decade
2. Presentation: cough, shortness of breath, chest pain, fatigue, weight loss
3. Chest CT: heterogeneous appearing soft tissue mass; local invasion common
4. Histology: squamous cell carcinoma most common
5. Treatment
   a. Complete surgical resection
   b. Induction chemotherapy given for larger tumors
   c. Adjuvant radiation
   d. Unresectable tumors treated with chemotherapy and radiation
6. Five-year survival: approximately 40%

C. GERM CELL TUMORS
1. Comprise 15% of anterior mediastinal masses
2. Etiology: from primitive germ cells that fail to migrate appropriately during embryonic development
3. These can be divided into benign and malignant types
   a. Benign: teratoma
   b. Malignant
      (1) Seminoma
      (2) Nonseminomatous germ cell tumor
   c. Malignant germ cell tumors can be of primary mediastinal origin (located in the anterior mediastinum) or metastasis from testicular cancer (usually located in the visceral compartment)
   d. Serum tumor markers used in the evaluation: AFP, β-hCG
4. Benign teratomas
   a. Most common mediastinal germ cell tumors (account for 85% of cases)
   b. Composed of at least two of three primitive germ layers (i.e., endoderm, mesoderm, ectoderm tissues)
   c. Epidemiology
      (1) Second to fourth decades
      (2) Equal distribution between genders
   d. Presentation: mostly asymptomatic; some experience cough, dyspnea, chest pain
   e. Evaluation
      (1) Chest CT shows a well-defined, lobulated mass; may have cystic areas and/or calcifications (i.e., bone, teeth)
      (2) Serum tumor markers: AFP and β-hCG negative
   f. Treatment
      (1) Surgical excision
      (2) Histology demonstrates normal tissue (i.e., teeth, calcifications, fatty tumors) abnormally present in the mediastinum
5. Seminomas: 25%–50% of all malignant mediastinal germ cell tumors (GCTs)
   a. Epidemiology: males in third to fourth decades

62

THYMUS AND MEDIASTINAL TUMORS

   b. Presentation: most patients symptomatic, typically associated with mechanical effects of tumor on adjacent mediastinal structures
      (1) Dyspnea, substernal chest pain, weakness, cough, weight loss
      (2) SVC syndrome present in 10%–20% of patients
   c. Evaluation
      (1) Chest CT: bulky, lobulated, homogeneous masses (local invasion rare)
      (2) Serum tumor markers: AFP negative; may have minor elevation of β-hCG
      (3) Biopsy: CT-guided needle biopsy, anterior mediastinotomy
   d. Treatment
      (1) Chemotherapy
      (2) Radiation can be used for local recurrence or residual disease
      (3) Surgery rarely indicated
6. **Nonseminomatous germ cell tumors**
   a. Epidemiology: males in third to fourth decades
   b. Presentation
      (1) Many patients are symptomatic: chest pain, hemoptysis, cough, fever, dyspnea, tachycardia
      (2) A total of 10% develop hematologic malignancies
      (3) Klinefelter syndrome 5%–20%
   c. Histology
      (1) Nonseminomatous elements, such as choriocarcinomas, embryonal cell carcinomas, yolk sac
      (2) Other elements may be present: seminoma, teratoma, degenerative cancer (primitive neuroectodermal tumor, sarcoma)
   d. Diagnosis
      (1) Chest CT: nonhomogeneous mass, areas of necrosis, and/or hemorrhage
      (2) Serum tumor markers
         (a) A total of 95% produce β-hCG or AFP.
   Pearl: *Any elevation of AFP is diagnostic of nonseminoma.*
      (3) Biopsy not indicated if serum tumor markers elevated
   e. Treatment
      (1) Chemotherapy
         (a) Bleomycin, etoposide, cisplatin (BEP)
         (b) May substitute ifosfamide for bleomycin (etoposide, ifosfamide, cisplatin [VIP]): less toxic
      (2) Postchemotherapy CT and tumor markers obtained
      (3) Surgical resection of residual disease
      (4) Five-year survival: approximately 60%

D. LYMPHOMAS

Although lymphoma commonly involves the mediastinum, primary mediastinal lymphoma is uncommon and accounts for only 10% of lymphomas. To obtain a diagnosis, biopsies should be done with at least a core needle biopsy. Other biopsy options are anterior mediastinotomy or thoracoscopic. All tissue should be sent fresh for possible flow cytometry (most important for non-Hodgkin lymphoma). The most common primary mediastinal lymphomas are:

1. Hodgkin lymphoma
   a. Bimodal distribution: young adulthood, greater than 50 years
   b. Nodular sclerosing type accounts for greater than two-thirds of cases
   c. Presentation: constitutional B symptoms (fevers, night sweats, weight loss), cough, dyspnea, chest pain, pleural effusions
   d. Histology: Reed-Sternberg cell
   e. Treatment: chemotherapy (+ local field radiation therapy for early stage disease)
2. Non-Hodgkin lymphoma
   a. Mean age for primary mediastinal 30–35 years
   b. Common histologies
      (1) Lymphoblastic lymphoma (aggressive)
      (2) Large B-cell lymphoma (most common primary mediastinal non-Hodgkin lymphoma)
         (a) Rapidly growing mass
         (b) SVC syndrome 30% of patients
   c. Treatment: chemotherapy ± radiation

Pearl: *The most common lesions include "terrible Ts": thymoma, teratoma/germ cell tumor, (terrible) lymphoma, thyroid tissue.*

IV. VISCERAL MEDIASTINAL COMPARTMENT MASSES

A. BRONCHOGENIC CYSTS
1. A total of 60% of mediastinal cysts
   a. Formed from ventral foregut, rarely have connection to bronchial tree
   b. Most associated with a major airway: subcarinal, perihilar
   c. Approximately 15% intrapulmonary
2. Presentation
   a. Approximately 50% asymptomatic
   b. Symptoms due to compression of adjacent organs: dyspnea, cough, dysphagia, may become infected
3. Diagnosis
   a. Chest CT: homogeneous mass, may have increased density due to mucoid material
   b. MRI: can help to distinguish cystic from solid lesions
   c. Endoscopic biopsy should be avoided as infection may occur.
4. Treatment
   a. Resection recommended because most patients have or will develop symptoms or complications, such as secondary infection
   b. Thoracotomy or thoracoscopy
   c. Complete resection of mucosal lining to prevent recurrence

62

THYMUS AND MEDIASTINAL TUMORS

B. ENTERIC (DUPLICATION) CYSTS

1. Approximately 5%–15% of mediastinal cysts
2. From primitive dorsal foregut, usually derived from esophagus
3. Most common in lower one-third of esophagus
4. Associated congenital malformation in 10%
5. Presentation
   a. Common symptoms: chest pain, dysphagia
   b. Complications: bleeding, perforation, infection
6. Diagnosis
   a. Barium swallow: filling defect with normal mucosa
   b. Chest CT: homogeneous mass, low attenuation
7. Treatment
   a. Resection recommended because most patients have or will develop symptoms or complications, such as secondary infection
   b. Thoracotomy or thoracoscopy

C. NEUROENTERIC CYSTS

1. Rare, due to failure of separation of notochord from primitive gut
2. Most diagnosed in infancy due to tracheobronchial compression
3. Histology: presence of both enteric and neural tissue in surgical specimens
4. Associated with vertebral anomalies (scoliosis, spina bifida)
5. Treatment: complete surgical resection (curative), may require laminectomy

D. PERICARDIAL CYSTS

1. Occur mostly in the right cardiophrenic angle (70%)
2. Mostly asymptomatic
3. Usually do not communicate with pericardium
4. Chest CT: unilocular cyst with fluid attenuation
5. Treatment: resection only if symptomatic or uncertainty of diagnosis

V. POSTERIOR MEDIASTINAL MASSES

Neurogenic tumors are the most common and typically arise from sympathetic ganglia, intercostal nerves, and paraganglia cells. A total of 70%–80% of these tumors are benign (Table 62.1).

A. NERVE SHEATH TUMORS

1. Most common neurogenic tumors
2. Arise from the intercostal nerve sheaths
   a. Neurilemomas (schwannomas)
   b. Neurofibromas
3. Presentation
   a. Most asymptomatic
   b. Pleuritic chest pain, dyspnea

TABLE 62.1

NEUROGENIC TUMORS

Tumor Origin	Benign	Malignant
Nerve sheath	Schwannoma	Neurofibrosarcoma
	Neurofibroma	
	Granular cell	
Ganglion cell	Ganglioneuroma	Ganglioneuroblastoma
		Neuroblastoma
Paraganglionic	Pheochromocytoma	Pheochromocytoma
	Chemodectoma	Chemodectoma

4. Diagnosis:
   a. Chest CT: smooth or lobulated homogeneous mass paraspinal location
   b. MRI: rule out intraspinal extension (10%)
5. Treatment
   a. Complete excision
   b. Most can be approached thoracoscopically.
   c. Laminectomy for those with intraspinal extension

RECOMMENDED READINGS

Detterbeck F, Nicholson A, Kondo K, Van Schil P, Moran C. The Masaoka-Koga Stage classification for thymic malignancies: clarification and definition of terms. *J Thorac Oncol*. 2011;6(7):S1710–S1716.

Detterbeck F, Parsons A. Thymic tumors. *Ann Thorac Surg*. 2004;77(5):1860–1869.

Kondo K, Monden Y. Therapy for thymic epithelial tumors: a clinical study of 1,320 patients from Japan. *Ann Thorac Surg*. 2003;76(3):878–884.

62

THYMUS AND MEDIASTINAL TUMORS

Cardiac Surgery

Heather Palomino, MD

Never let the skin stand between you and the diagnosis.

I. PREOPERATIVE EVALUATION

A. HISTORY
1. History of present illness—detailed account of symptom chronology: acute versus chronic
   a. Angina—stable or unstable, arrhythmia, congestive heart failure
   b. Timing of recent intervention
   c. Dyspnea: New York Heart Association (NYHA) functional classification for heart failure
      (1) Class I: no limitations during ordinary activity, asymptomatic
      (2) Class II: slight limitation during ordinary activity
      (3) Class III: marked limitation of ordinary activity
      (4) Class IV: no physical activity without symptoms
   d. Arrhythmia, palpitations, peripheral edema
2. Medical and surgical history—detailed
   a. Prior sternotomy
   b. Recent percutaneous coronary intervention (PCI)
3. Medications and allergies—detailed list and dosages
   a. Current anticoagulation use; clopidogrel should be stopped 5 days before surgery
4. Social history, including tobacco, ethyl alcohol, and drug use
5. Family history
6. Review of symptoms

B. PHYSICAL EXAMINATION—COMPLETE AND SYSTEMS BASED
1. Neurologic—cranial nerves, strength, and motor bilaterally
2. Pulmonary—rales, rhonchi, wheezing (pneumonia, congestive heart failure, chronic obstructive pulmonary disease)
3. Cardiovascular
   a. Signs or symptoms of congestive heart failure—jugular venous distention, rales, S3 gallop
   b. Arrhythmias, presence of a pacemaker, and/or defibrillator
   c. Previous sternotomy/thoracotomy incisions, chest tubes
   d. Vascular examination
      (1) Documentation of peripheral pulses—radial, ulnar, femoral, dorsalis pedis
      (2) Evidence of tissue loss or ischemic extremities
      (3) Evaluation of carotid disease, bruits
      (4) Evaluation of neck/groin for potential internal jugular/femoral cannulation

     (5) Evaluation of conduit suitability (radial arteries, saphenous veins, blood pressure in both arms)

  e. Heart murmurs

     (1) Systolic ejection: aortic stenosis (AS) (radiates to carotids), pulmonary stenosis, atrial septal defect (ASD), innocent flow murmurs

     (2) Pansystolic: mitral regurgitation (MR) (radiates to axilla), tricuspid regurgitation, ventricular septal defect (VSD), patent ductus arteriosus (PDA)

     (3) Early diastolic: aortic insufficiency (AI), pulmonary regurgitation

4. Gastrointestinal—old incisions, hernia
5. Musculoskeletal—strength, sensation, gait, among others

C. PREOPERATIVE TESTING

1. Electrocardiogram—arrhythmias, ischemic changes, conduction delays, chamber enlargement
2. Laboratory—complete blood cell count, electrolytes, coagulation profile, type and crossmatch for 2 units of packed red blood cells
3. Posteroanterior and lateral chest radiograph—visualize plane between sternum and heart on lateral
4. Nuclear perfusion testing
  a. Myocardial reserve—hibernating myocardium that may benefit from revascularization
  b. Functional significance of coronary lesion
5. Cardiac catheterization and echocardiogram
  a. Distribution of coronary artery disease
  b. Evaluation of ventricular wall motion and ejection fraction function and wall motion
  c. Presence of valvular dysfunction
6. Risk calculator (STS, EuroScore, Seattle Heart Failure Models)

D. PREOPERATIVE ORDERS

1. Accurate height and weight recorded in chart to calculate body surface area
2. Twelve-lead electrocardiogram
3. Posteroanterior and lateral chest radiograph (recent)
4. Hibiclens scrub and clipper prep to chest the night before surgery
5. Nothing by mouth (NPO) after midnight
6. Antibiotics on call—cefuroxime 1.5 g intravenous (IV) on call or use vancomycin 1 g IV for reoperative/valve patients
7. Medications
  a. In general, medications are continued until surgery, especially antianginal agents, antihypertensive agents with the exception of angiotensin-converting enzyme (ACE) inhibitors, nitroglycerin, and heparin drips (hold hours before surgery).
  b. Continue all antiarrhythmic agents.

c. Perioperative steroid and insulin coverage is per routine.

d. Ensure appropriate discontinuation of anticoagulants.

8. **Perioperative monitors generally placed immediately before operation**

   a. Right radial/brachial radial/brachial arterial line

   b. Swan-Ganz catheter (some institutions omit this step for straightforward procedures)

II. OPERATIVE PROCEDURES

A. CORONARY ARTERY BYPASS GRAFTING

1. Indications

   a. Chronic stable angina unrelieved by medication/asymptomatic angina—left main disease, left main equivalent disease (proximal left anterior descending [LAD] and proximal circumflex arteries), three-vessel disease

   b. Unstable angina despite treatment/stable angina—left main disease, left main equivalent, three-vessel disease, two-vessel disease with proximal LAD and reduced ventricular function (left ventricular ejection fraction [LVEF] <50%)

   c. Acute myocardial infarction—if significant coronary disease exists beyond the area of infarction, ongoing angina after infarction, or unstable hemodynamic status. Controversy exists on the timing of surgical intervention. Unstable angina/non–ST elevation myocardial infarction (NSTEMI)—left main, left main equivalent disease

   d. Ventricular arrhythmias with coronary disease/ST elevation myocardial infarction (STEMI)—failed PCI or anatomically not a PCI candidate

   e. Failed percutaneous transluminal coronary angioplasty/poor LV function—left main disease, left main equivalent, proximal LAD and two-vessel disease

   f. Life-threatening ventricular arrhythmias—left main, three-vessel disease

   g. Failed PCI—shock with ongoing ischemia

2. **Coronary artery bypass grafting (CABG) has been shown to be superior to medical treatment of coronary disease in the following situations:**

   a. In patients with asymptomatic or mild angina and the following conditions:

      (1) Significant left main disease (Veterans Affairs Cooperative Study 1972–74)

      (2) Three-vessel coronary artery disease with proximal left anterior descending disease or double-vessel disease in conjunction with left main disease (European Coronary Surgery Study Group 1973–76)

      (3) Three-vessel disease and ventricular dysfunction (Coronary Artery Surgery Study 1975–79)

   b. In patients with chronic moderate-to-severe angina

   c. Unstable angina despite full medical therapy

    d. Failed percutaneous transluminal coronary angioplasty with reasonable targets

    e. Persistent ventricular arrhythmias in patients with coronary artery disease

    f. Patients with diabetes with double-vessel disease—reduced ventricular function

3. There is no difference in rates of myocardial infarction in CABG and medically treated patients.

4. PCI is acceptable treatment option for single-vessel disease or two-vessel disease. CABG has been shown to be superior to drug-eluting stent (DES) PCI in patients with complex coronary disease, such as left main or three-vessel disease. CABG has been shown to have lower incidence of revascularization and myocardial infarction (MI) in the Synergy Between Percutaneous Coronary Intervention with Taxus and Cardiac Surgery (SYNTAX) trial.

5. Internal mammary artery grafts are the conduit of choice because of superior patency rates compared with saphenous vein grafts (in situ and free grafts) (90%–95% vs. 50%–60% at 10 years). Patency rates for the internal mammary artery compared with the great saphenous vein graft at 10 and 15 years are 95% and 88% and 61% and 32%, respectively. Radial artery and less commonly gastroepiploic artery may be used as conduit.

6. Off-pump CABG is an approach used to minimize aortic manipulation and avoid the systemic effects of cardiopulmonary bypass. On-pump versus off-pump CABG shows no difference in outcomes, with off-pump surgery conferring a lower initial stroke risk that was not clinically significant and a trend toward lower number of target vessels grafted.

B. VALVE REPLACEMENT OR REPAIR

1. AS

    a. It is commonly caused by bicuspid valve, rheumatic disease, or calcific/degenerative AS.

    b. Symptoms include triad of dyspnea, angina, and syncope.

    c. AS severity

       (1) Mild AS: aortic valve area greater than $1.5\ cm^2$, mean pressure gradient less than 25 mm Hg, peak jet velocity less than 3.0 m/s

       (2) Moderate AS: aortic valve area 1.0–$1.5\ cm^2$, mean pressure gradient 25–40 mm Hg, peak jet velocity 3.0–4.0 m/s

       (3) Severe AS: aortic valve area less than $1.0\ cm^2$, mean pressure gradient greater than 40 mm Hg, peak jet velocity greater than 4.0 m/s

    d. Indications for surgery

       (1) Symptomatic patients with severe AS valve gradient of greater than 50 mm Hg or valve area less than $0.8\ cm^2/m^2$

       (2) Asymptomatic patients with significant stenosis and left ventricular hypertrophy should be considered who are undergoing CABG.

63

CARDIAC SURGERY

(3) Asymptomatic patients with evidence of decreased systolic function should also be considered.

e. Coronary angiography is performed before surgery because of high rate of concomitant coronary artery disease.

2. **AI**

a. Causative factors include rheumatic disease, annular ectasia, endocarditis, aortic dissection, and aortitis.

b. Frequently asymptomatic unless acute or decompensated

c. Acute AI presents with syncope, pulmonary edema, classic "water hammer" pulse, and Austin Flint murmur (late diastolic) from blood flow regurgitant jet hitting the anterior mitral valve leaflet.

d. Indications for surgery

(1) Symptomatic patients

(2) Patients with cardiomegaly or deteriorating systolic function as assessed by echocardiography asymptomatic; patients with severe AI and reduced systolic function less than 50% as assessed by echocardiography

(3) Asymptomatic patients and left ventricular diameter at end diastole (LVEDD) greater than 75 mm or left ventricular diameter at end systole (LVESD) greater than 55 mm

3. **Mitral stenosis**

a. Primarily rheumatic—leaflet thickening with calcification and fusion

b. Symptoms—dyspnea, orthopnea, and paroxysmal nocturnal dyspnea, atrial fibrillation. Loud S1, opening snap. Radiographs may demonstrate left atrial enlargement and pulmonary venous hypertension.

c. Indications for surgery—presence of chronic symptoms or acute episodes of pulmonary venous hypertension. Mitral valve area less than 1.5 cm^2 and NYHA class III–IV symptoms

d. Chronic atrial fibrillation—a complication of progressive left atrial enlargement

4. **Mitral regurgitation**

a. Causative factors—rheumatic disease, myxomatous valve structure, endocarditis, ischemia or papillary muscle dysfunction, and congenital structural defects

b. Severity and development of symptoms—varies with causative factor; rheumatic disease is more insidious in onset, whereas ischemic mitral regurgitation is often acute in onset.

c. Carpentier classification

(1) Type I—normal leaflet motion: endocarditis, dilated cardiomyopathy with annular dilation

(2) Type II—excessive leaflet motion: prolapse, chordal rupture, papillary muscle rupture

(3) Type III—restricted leaflet motion

(a) IIIa: restricted opening: rheumatic disease

(b) IIIb: restricted closing: ischemic MR

d. As with mitral stenosis, indications for surgery depend on the severity of symptoms. Indications for surgery:
   (1) Symptomatic severe MR and NYHA class II–IV LV dysfunction
   (2) Asymptomatic severe MR with normal LV if repair greater than 90% likely, or new atrial fibrillation, or pulmonary artery pressure (PAP) greater than 50 mm Hg at rest
e. Ischemic mitral regurgitation is usually corrected at the time of coronary bypass, with either valve replacement or annuloplasty. Often mild ischemic mitral regurgitation may improve by coronary bypass only.
f. Rheumatic or myxomatous valve disease may be corrected by valve repair or replacement. The advantages of repair versus replacement are the low rate of endocarditis and lack of need for long-term anticoagulation. Mitral valve repair is associated with favorable outcomes over replacement.

C. INFECTIVE ENDOCARDITIS

1. Incidence 6.2 per 100,000 people per year
2. Etiology—indwelling catheters, IV drug use in the setting of damaged cardiac endothelium results in platelet and fibrin deposition and allows bacteria or fungus to adhere
3. Mitral > aortic > tricuspid (most common in IV drug users), may also have prosthetic valve endocarditis
4. Microbiology
   a. *Streptococcus viridans*, *Staphylococcus aureus*, *Staphylococcus epidermidis*, enterococci
5. Clinical findings
   a. Fevers, new murmur, Roth spots, Osler nodes, Janeway lesions, petechiae
6. Duke criteria
   a. Major criteria (2): positive blood cultures (*S. viridans*, *Streptococcus bovis*, HACEK [*Haemophilus* species, *Aggregatibacter* species, *Cardiobacterium hominis*, *Eikenella corrodens*, and *Kingella* species], enteroccoci, *S. aureus*), evidence for endocardial involvement on echocardiogram
   b. Minor criteria (5): fever less than 38°C, vascular phenomena, immunologic phenomena, positive blood culture not previous meeting requirement, new-onset heart failure, new conduction disturbances, predisposing heart condition or IV drug use
7. Echocardiography—Transesophageal is 90% specific and 95% sensitive for detecting endocardial vegetations or lesions, versus transthoracic (90% specific and 50% sensitive).
8. Indications for surgery—new-onset heart failure, new heart block, continued sepsis despite optimal medical management, valve dehiscence, and fungal infection

D. AORTIC DISSECTION

1. Causative factors—hypertension, atherosclerosis, connective tissue disorders, cystic medial necrosis (e.g., Marfan syndrome, Ehlers-Danlos, Turner syndrome), infections, trauma, pregnancy, age greater than 60 years are risk factors.

2. Clinical considerations
   a. Dissections diagnosed within 2 weeks from onset of symptoms are acute.
   b. Mortality secondary to acute dissection ranges from 30% to 40%.
   c. Clinical presentation—sudden sharp tearing chest pain that radiates to the back; other symptoms can include stroke, MI, hemopericardium/tamponade, severe AI, renal/mesenteric ischemia, limb ischemia, paraplegia

3. DeBakey classification
   a. Type I—intimal disruption of ascending aorta that extends to involve the entire descending thoracic aorta and abdominal aorta
   b. Type II—involves the ascending aorta only (stops at the innominate artery)
   c. Type III—involves the descending thoracic and abdominal aorta only (distal to left subclavian artery)

4. Stanford classification
   a. Type A—any dissection that involves the ascending aorta
   b. Type B—any dissection that involves only the descending aorta, distal to the left subclavian artery

5. Diagnosis is usually made by aortogram, chest computed tomography scan, or echocardiogram (transesophageal echocardiogram [TEE] or transthoracic echocardiogram [TTE]). Preoperative control of hypertension with nitroprusside and beta-blockers is an essential part of management.

6. Initial management
   a. Start beta-blockade first to decrease heart rate and aortic wall dP/dt.
   b. Nitroprusside can then decrease the blood pressure (if sodium nitroprusside [SNP] given first, it actually increases cardiac work and the dP/dt; this theoretically can increase propagation of the dissection).

7. Dissection may advance proximally, disrupting coronary blood flow or inducing aortic valve incompetence, or distally, causing stroke, renal failure, paraplegia, or intestinal ischemia.

8. Indications for emergent operative repair
   a. Acute type A dissection
      (1) Operative repair involves replacement of the affected aorta with a prosthetic graft.
      (2) Cardiopulmonary bypass is required, and hypothermic circulatory arrest is often used for transverse arch dissections.
      (3) Aortic valve replacement (AVR) and coronary reimplantation may be required for type A aneurysms that involve the aortic root.

b. Type B dissection with failed medical therapy such as hypertension, inadequate pain control, progressive dissection by radiographic studies, impaired organ perfusion, or impending aortic rupture
   (1) Type B dissections can be medically managed unless expansion, rupture, or compromise of branch arteries develops or hypertension becomes refractory.
9. Postoperative complications include renal failure, intestinal ischemia, stroke, and paraplegia.

E. TRAUMATIC AORTIC DISRUPTION
1. This injury results from deceleration injury and usually occurs just distal to the left subclavian artery, at the level of the ligamentum arteriosum.
2. Chest radiograph findings include widened mediastinum, pleural capping, associated first and second rib fractures, loss of the aortic knob, hemothorax, deviation of the trachea or nasogastric tube, and associated thoracic injuries (scapular and clavicular fractures).
3. Definitive diagnosis is made by aortogram, but chest computed tomography and transesophageal echocardiography also aid in the diagnosis.
4. Imperative that immediate life-threatening injuries (e.g., positive diagnostic peritoneal lavage) be treated before repair.

F. AORTIC ANEURYSMS
1. Ascending aortic aneurysm greater than 5.5 cm or greater than 4.0–5.0 cm with a known connective tissue disorder or bicuspid valve (depending on the diagnosis)
   a. Interposition graft or aortic root enlargement (if root involved); valve-sparing techniques available
2. Aortic arch greater than 5.5 cm or enlargement by 0.5 cm/year
   a. Requires deep hypothermic circulatory arrest (DHCA) to 15°C
   b. Trifurcated Dacron interposition graft
3. Descending aorta greater than 6.5 cm or enlargement by 0.5 cm/year
   a. Crawford classification
      (1) Type I—from the origin of the left subclavian to the suprarenal abdominal aorta
      (2) Type II—from the origin of the left subclavian to the aortoiliac bifurcation
      (3) Type III—mid-descending thoracic aorta to the aortoiliac bifurcation
      (4) Type IV—distal thoracic aorta below the diaphragm to the aortoiliac bifurcation
   b. Surgical repair requires lateral thoracotomy extended to a midline laparotomy; full cardiopulmonary bypass or partial left heart bypass

63

CARDIAC SURGERY

G. CONGENITAL HEART SURGERY

Numerous congenital anomalies have been described, but in general, most congenital heart diseases can be broken down according to the physiologic disturbances.

1. Obstructive lesions: Lesions include valvular stenoses and coarctation of the aorta. Long-term sequelae include concentric cardiac hypertrophy and subsequent failure because of ventricular pressure overload. Repair or replacement of the involved valve or segment is the mainstay of operative treatment.

2. Left-to-right shunts (acyanotic): ASD and VSD make up most patients in this group. Also included are PDA and truncus arteriosus. Symptoms are due to chronic volume overload of the pulmonary circulation, which eventually leads to pulmonary hypertension. Cyanosis is a late finding in these anomalies because of right-sided heart pressures exceeding left-sided heart pressures (Eisenmenger syndrome). Operative repair involves patch closure of the septal defect or ductal ligation.

3. Right-to-left shunts (cyanotic): These defects include tetralogy of Fallot, transposition of the great arteries, tricuspid atresia, total anomalous pulmonary venous drainage, and Ebstein anomaly. These defects involve complex repairs that are usually performed during infancy. Palliative procedures include Blalock-Taussig shunts (subclavian artery to pulmonary artery) and aortopulmonary artery shunts.

III. POSTOPERATIVE CARE

A. HEMODYNAMICS

1. Invasive monitors include arterial lines, pulmonary artery catheters (PACs), and occasionally left atrial catheters.
   a. PAC:
      (1) Direct pressure monitoring of right arterial pressure (RAP), right ventricular pressure (RVP), PAP, pulmonary artery wedge pressure (PAWP)
      (2) Derived pressure parameters: systemic vascular resistance (SVR), pulmonary vascular resistance (PVR), systemic vascular resistance index (SVRI), PVR, oxygen consumption per unit time (Vo_2), oxygen delivery (DO_2)
      (3) Derive CO by Fick equation or thermodilution.

2. Every effort should be made to optimize ventricular filling pressures and systemic blood pressures. In general, up to 2 L of crystalloid is used; after that, blood or colloid is used to increase filling pressures. Hypertension aggravates bleeding along suture lines and is controlled by a nitroprusside drip. Lower blood pressures are preferred as long as a mean blood pressure greater than 60 mm Hg is maintained. There are numerous causes for hypotension after surgery; before beginning specific treatment, know the filling pressures, cardiac rhythm, cardiac index (CI), and SVR.

3. Goal CI >2.2, mixed venous oxygen saturation (Svo$_2$) >65%–80%, central venous pressure (CVP) <12–15 mm Hg, mean arterial pressure (MAP) >65 mm Hg

B. ARRHYTHMIAS

1. Nodal or junctional rhythm
   a. May not need treatment for asymptomatic, normotensive patient
   b. Due to nodal tissue edema after valve repair or replacement, often self-limiting
   c. May require atrioventricular pacing if hypotension occurs
2. Supraventricular tachycardia—includes atrial fibrillation and flutter. One-third of all cardiac patients develop atrial fibrillation in the postoperative setting.
   a. Onset may be preceded by multiple premature atrial contractions.
   b. Atrial electrocardiogram using atrial pacing leads is often helpful in distinguishing fibrillation from flutter during rapid rates.
   c. Atrial fibrillation—IV beta-blockade, diltiazem, amiodarone
   d. In both instances, if any significant decline in blood pressure or cardiac output occurs, the arrhythmia should be treated with synchronous direct current cardioversion at 50–100 joules. This may be repeated with increasing energy levels (100–200–360 J).
   e. Adenosine can be used initially as a diagnostic and therapeutic intervention. Transient bradycardia/asystole allows interpretation of rhythm.

C. ANTIARRHYTHMICS

1. Digoxin is not routinely used unless patient has been taking it previously.
2. After patient has been weaned from postoperative drips, metoprolol is started and titrated to effect.
3. Atrial fibrillation may be treated with IV beta-blockade, calcium channel blockade, or amiodarone, depending on surgeon preference.
   a. Amiodarone is often loaded as a 150-mg bolus and started on a gtt (drops/min) of 1 mg/min for 6 hours. The gtt is then decreased to 0.5 mg/min for the next 18 hours.
   b. Conversion to oral dosing is usually done when gtt is finished, continued for 6 weeks, and then weaned off.
4. Ventricular arrhythmias are often treated with amiodarone.

D. ANTICOAGULATION

1. Aspirin is given to all CABG patients.
2. Clopidogrel (Plavix) is restarted in all patients with recent stents.
   a. Patients with fresh stents may need to undergo intervention. It must be continued in patients with bare-metal stents within the past 30 days and drug-eluting stents within the past 6 months if not protected by a coronary bypass graft.
   b. Sometimes Plavix is continued intraoperatively.

3. Patients with bioprosthetic valves may be started on warfarin therapy and kept therapeutic (international normalized ratio [INR], 2–3) for 3 months.
4. Patients with mechanical valve replacements (MVRs) are given warfarin starting postoperative day 1, and the dosage is adjusted to maintain INR between 2.0 to 3.0 (AVR) and 2.5 to 3.5 (MVR) for lifelong anticoagulation.

E. HARDWARE

1. Mediastinal tubes are discontinued when drainage is less than 200 mL/8 hours and no air leak is present.
2. Antibiotics are discontinued according to perioperative guidelines after the mediastinal tubes are removed or at 24 hours (depending on surgeon preference).
3. Pacing wires are (by convention) atrial on right side and ventricular on left side. They are removed at 3 days or the day before discharge.

IV. POSTOPERATIVE COMPLICATIONS

A. ARRHYTHMIAS

1. Ventricular ectopy is the most common complication.
   a. For frequent (>6–10/min) or multifocal premature ventricular complexes, treat with lidocaine bolus of 1 mg/kg, followed by drip at 2–4 mg/min.
   b. Cardioversion is needed if it progresses to symptomatic ventricular tachycardia or if ventricular fibrillation develops.
   c. Atrial or atrioventricular pacing at a slightly greater rate may suppress ectopy.
2. Nodal or junctional rhythm
   a. Asymptomatic, normotensive patient may not need treatment.
   b. Rule out digoxin toxicity; make certain serum K^+ level greater than 4.5; rule out hypomagnesemia.
   c. It may require atrioventricular sequential pacing if loss of atrial kick has significant hemodynamic sequelae.
3. Supraventricular tachycardia—includes atrial fibrillation and flutter
   a. Onset may be preceded by multiple premature atrial contractions.
   b. Atrial electrocardiogram using atrial pacing leads is often helpful in distinguishing fibrillation from flutter during rapid rates.
   c. Atrial fibrillation—may consider IV beta-blockade, calcium channel blockade, or amiodarone
   d. Atrial flutter may be treated by the following:
      (1) Rapid atrial pacing greater than 400 beats/min
      (2) IV beta-blocker or calcium channel blocker. Calcium channel blockers must be given judiciously because wide complex supraventricular tachycardia can mimic ventricular tachycardia.
      (3) IV amiodarone
   e. In both instances, if any significant decline in blood pressure or cardiac output occurs, the arrhythmia should be treated with synchronous

direct current cardioversion at 50–100 J. This may be repeated with increasing energy levels (100–200–360 J).

f. Adenosine can be used initially as a diagnostic and therapeutic intervention. Transient bradycardia/asystole allows interpretation of rhythm and may be therapeutic.

B. BLEEDING

1. Causative factors—include medications, clotting deficits, reoperation, prolonged operation, technical factors, hypothermia, and transfusion reactions
2. Treatment
   a. Ensure normothermia.
   b. Measure clotting factors—prothrombin time, partial thromboplastin time, fibrinogen, platelet count, activated clotting time, and thromboelastogram.
   c. Correction
      (1) Fresh frozen plasma, cryoprecipitate, platelets
      (2) Protamine for prolonged heparinization
   d. Transfusion reaction protocol if suspected
3. Exploration for postoperative hemorrhage—indications include mediastinal tube output of greater than 300 mL/h over 1 hour, greater than 200 mL/h over 2 hours, or greater than 100 mL/h over 3 hours, despite correction of clotting factors, greater than 200 mL/h despite correction of clotting factors. Technical factors are found as cause greater than 50% of the time.

C. CARDIAC TAMPONADE

1. Hypotension with increasing filling pressures and decreased cardiac output; decreasing urine output, quiet distant heart sounds, and eventual equalization of right- and left-sided atrial pressures.
2. High degree of suspicion that coincides with excessive postoperative bleeding
3. Tamponade is a clinical diagnosis, and all confirmatory studies are adjuncts!
4. Chest radiograph may demonstrate wide mediastinum; echocardiogram if readily available or diagnosis uncertain
5. Treatment—emergent for sudden reexploration is treatment of choice and may be indicated at bedside for sudden hemodynamic decompensation.
   Transfusion to optimize preload and inotropic support; avoid increased positive end-expiratory pressure.

D. RENAL FAILURE

1. Incidence rate of 1%–30%
2. Diagnosis—renal versus prerenal azotemia

63

CARDIAC SURGERY

3. **Management**
   a. Optimize volume status and cardiac output.
   b. Discontinue nephrotoxic drugs.
   c. Maintain urine output >30 mL/h (low-dose dopamine, furosemide, ethacrynic acid as indicated; furosemide (Lasix) or furosemide/chlorothiazide (Diuril) drips for persistent oliguria)
   d. Dialysis—either continuous venovenous or hemodialysis may be used.
   e. Outcome—mortality rate of 0.3%–23% depending on the degree of azotemia; if dialysis is required, mortality rate ranges from 27% to 53%.

E. RESPIRATORY FAILURE

1. **Mechanical**—mucus plugging, malpositioned endotracheal tube, pneumothorax
2. **Intrinsic**—volume overload, pulmonary edema, atelectasis, acute respiratory distress syndrome (ARDS), chronic obstructive pulmonary disease (COPD), pneumonia, pulmonary embolus (uncommon)

F. LOW CARDIAC OUTPUT SYNDROME

CI less than 2.0 L/min per m^2

1. **Signs**—decreased urine output, acidosis, hypothermia, altered sensorium cardiogenic shock
   a. Hemodynamics
      (1) CI less than 1.8 L/min per m^2
      (2) Stroke volume index less than 20 mL/h
      (3) Pulmonary capillary wedge pressure greater than 18 mm Hg
      (4) SVR greater than 2400 dyn × seconds/cm^5
2. **Assessment**—heart rate and rhythm (electrocardiogram: possible acute myocardial infarction), preload and afterload states (pulmonary artery catheter readings), measurement of cardiac output
3. **Etiology**—ischemia/hypoxemia, acidosis, pump failure, arrhythmias, hypovolemia
4. **States of impaired myocardium due to pump failure**
   a. Infarcted—irreversible
   b. Hibernating myocardium—impaired myocardium that can be reversed if blood flow is restored; chronic contractility depressed stated that improves immediately with revascularization
   c. Stunned myocardium—LV dysfunction without cell death that occurs after restoration of blood flow from an ischemic insult, fully reversible
5. **Treatment**
   a. Stabilize rate and rhythm.
   b. Optimize volume status, preload, afterload, and systemic vascular resistance.
   c. Correct acidosis, hypoxemia if present (chest radiograph for pneumothorax)

d. Administer inotropic agents (e.g., dobutamine or milrinone drips).

e. Persistent low cardiac output despite inotropic support requires placement of intraaortic balloon pump, which inflates in early diastole and deflates just before systole, decreasing afterload and improving coronary perfusion.

G. CARDIAC TAMPONADE

1. Onset—suggested by increasing filling pressures with decreased cardiac output; decreasing urine output and hypotension; quiet, distant heart sounds; and eventual equalization of right- and left-sided atrial pressures

2. High degree of suspicion that coincides with excessive postoperative bleeding

3. Chest radiograph may demonstrate wide mediastinum; echocardiogram if readily available or diagnosis uncertain

4. Treatment—emergent reexploration is treatment of choice and may be needed at bedside for sudden hemodynamic decompensation. Transfusion to optimize volume status and inotropic support; avoid increased positive end-expiratory pressure

H. PERIOPERATIVE MYOCARDIAL INFARCTION AFTER REVASCULARIZATION

1. Incidence rate of 5%–20%

2. Diagnosis—new-onset Q waves after surgery; heart block, decreasing cardiac output, serial isoenzymes, increased myoglobin (MB) fractions; segmental wall motion abnormalities by TTE or TEE

3. Etiology—kinking of conduits, vasospasm, or graft thrombosis

4. Treatment—vasodilation (IV nitroglycerin is preferred to nitroprusside). Continued hemodynamic deterioration should be treated with immediate intraaortic balloon counterpulsation. This "unloads" the ventricle and may preserve nonischemic adjacent myocardium. Reexploration if surgical etiology

5. Outcome—associated with increased morbidity and mortality, as well as poorer long-term results

V. PHARMACOLOGY

A. INOTROPES

1. Epinephrine—direct α, $\beta1$, $\beta2$ agonist

   a. Per Advanced Cardiac Life Support (ACLS) protocol, 1-mg bolus for cardiac arrest

2. Milrinone—phosphodiesterase inhibitor, increases contractility and decreases afterload

3. Dobutamine—direct $\beta1$ agonist greater than $\beta2$ agonist, increases contractility

4. Dopamine—low-dose dopamine receptors, moderate dose $\beta1$ and $\beta2$ receptors, high-dose $\alpha1$ receptors, used at low/moderate dose to increase cardiac contractility and decrease afterload

CARDIAC SURGERY

63

B. VASOPRESSORS

1. Norepinephine (Levophed)—direct $\alpha 1$ agonist greater than $\beta 1$ agonist, increases both afterload and contractility, caution with end-organ ischemia and ischemia of limbs/digits
2. Phenylephrine (Neo-Synephrine)—$\alpha 1$ agonist, reflex bradycardia, increases afterload, decreases heart rate

C. VASODILATORS

1. Nitroglycerine—venodilator, decreases preload and oxygen demand on the heart
2. Labetalol—beta-blocker, alpha1-blocker, decreases heart rate and after load
3. Nitroprusside (Nipride)—nitric oxide (NO) prodrug, increases cyclic guanosine monophosphate (cGMP), venodilator, decreases preload, caution with overdose

D. POSTOPERATIVE FEVER

1. Common in the first 24 hours after surgery; most commonly cytokine storm; however, it may be associated with pyrogens introduced during cardiopulmonary bypass. Treat pyrexia with acetaminophen and cooling blankets because associated hypermetabolism and vasodilation can be detrimental to hemodynamic status and increase myocardial work.
2. Postoperative fevers in valve patients should be followed closely with cultures. CABG patients should have full fever work-up on fifth postoperative day if still febrile.
3. Special attention should be paid to invasive monitors and should be changed if infection is suspected.
4. Sternal wound—daily inspection for drainage and stability. Sternal infections are disastrous in the cardiac patient, and early evidence of postoperative infection should be treated with operative debridement.
5. Postpericardiotomy syndrome—characterized by low-grade fever, leukocytosis, chest pain, malaise, and pericardial rub on auscultation. Usually occurs 2–3 weeks after surgery and is treated with nonsteroidal antiinflammatory agents. Steroids are necessary for some cases.

E. CENTRAL NERVOUS SYSTEM COMPLICATIONS

1. Causative factors—preexisting cerebrovascular disease, prolonged cardiopulmonary bypass, intraoperative hypotension, and emboli (either air or particulate matter)
2. Transient neurologic deficit—occurs in up to 12% of patients. Improvement usually within several days
3. Permanent deficit—suspect in patients with delayed awakening postoperatively; may have pathologic reflexes present
4. Postcardiotomy psychosis syndrome—incidence rate of 10%–24%. Starts around postoperative day 2 with anxiety and confusion; may progress to disorientation and hallucinations. Treat with rest and quiet

environment; antipsychotics may be given as necessary. It is essential to rule out organic cause of delirium (e.g., substance withdrawal, hypoxemia, hypoglycemia, and electrolyte abnormality).

5. Computed tomography scan early for suspected localized lesions; electroencephalogram in patients with extensive dysfunction

6. Treatment—optimize cerebral blood flow and avoid hypercapnia.
   a. Postoperative seizures are treated with lorazepam and phenytoin.
   b. Mannitol may be needed in presence of increased intracranial pressure, depending on hemodynamic status.

RECOMMENDED READINGS

Booth DC, Deupree RH, Hultgren HN, DeMaria AN, Scott SM, Luchi RJ. Quality of life after bypass surgery for unstable angina: five-year follow up results of a Veterans Affairs Cooperative Study. *Circulation*. 1991;83:87.

DeBakey ME, McCollum CH, Crawford ES, et al. Dissection and dissecting aneurysm of the aorta: twenty-year follow up of five hundred twenty-seven patients treated surgically. *Surgery*. 1982;92:1118.

Emergency Cardiac Care Committee and Subcommittees. American Heart Association. Guidelines for resuscitation and emergency cardiac care. *JAMA*. 1992;268:2171.

Gersh BJ, Califf RM, Loop FD, Akins CW, Pryor DB, Takaro TC. Coronary bypass surgery in chronic stable angina. *Circulation*. 1989;79(suppl I):46.

Mohr FW, Morice MC, Kappetein AP, et al. Coronary artery bypass graft surgery versus percutaneous coronary intervention in patients with three-vessel disease and left main coronary disease: 5-year follow-up of the randomized, clinical SYNTAX trial. *Lancet*. 2013;381(9867):629–638.

63

CARDIAC SURGERY

Cardiac Transplantation

Dennis Wells, MD

The tree of liberty must be refreshed from time to time with the blood of patriots and tyrants.

—Thomas Jefferson

I. HISTORY

1. The techniques for heart transplantation were developed by Norm Shumway and Richard Lower at Stanford University in the 1960s.
2. James Hardy performed the first heart transplant into a human with a chimpanzee xenograft in 1964 at the University of Mississippi.
   a. The patient died immediately of acute rejection.
3. Christiaan Barnard performed the first allograft human heart transplant in December 1967 in Durbin, South Africa.
   a. The patient, a 54-year-old man, received the heart of a 25-year-old woman and survived 18 days until he died of pneumonia.
4. Three days later, Adrian Kantrowitz performed the first transplant in the United States at Maimonides Medical Center in Brooklyn, New York.
   a. He transplanted the heart of a 2-day-old anencephalic male into an 18-day-old male infant, who survived 6.5 hours before dying of acidosis.
5. Initial results continued to be poor, and the procedure fell from favor.
6. Shumway and the team at Stanford continued their research, and with the availability of cyclosporine in 1981, heart transplantation subsequently became widely accepted.
7. A total of 2804 heart transplants were performed in the United States in 2016. This number is relatively unchanged in the previous 15 years.

II. INDICATIONS

1. Heart failure due to ischemic disease, dilated cardiomyopathy, valvular heart disease, hypertensive cardiomyopathy, etc.
2. Intractable angina despite revascularization attempts and maximal medical therapy, or in a patient who is not a candidate for revascularization
3. Intractable arrhythmia uncontrolled with medical therapy, pacemaker, and ablative therapies, or in a patient who is not a candidate for ablative therapy
4. Hypertrophic cardiomyopathy with New York Heart Association (NYHA) class IV heart failure symptoms despite therapeutic interventions and maximal medical therapy
5. Congenital heart disease
6. Primary cardiac malignancy confined to the myocardium and without evidence of metastatic disease

III. CONTRAINDICATIONS

A. ABSOLUTE CONTRAINDICATIONS

1. Older than 70 years (specific age limit is institution specific)
2. Fixed pulmonary hypertension evidenced by pulmonary vascular resistance greater than 5 Wood units or transpulmonary gradient greater than 15 mm Hg
3. Systemic illness limiting life expectancy regardless of heart transplant; examples include:
   a. Malignancy (with the exception of primary cardiac tumors as mentioned previously) other than skin cancer, with a disease-free survival of less than 5 years
   b. Irreversible organ dysfunction (may be considered for heart-kidney, or heart-liver transplant)

B. RELATIVE CONTRAINDICATIONS

1. Diabetes mellitus with end-organ damage
2. Severe chronic obstructive pulmonary disease (COPD)
3. Recent pulmonary embolism
4. Severe peripheral and cerebrovascular disease
5. Obesity (body mass index [BMI] >35 kg/m^2)
6. Alcohol or drug abuse
7. Active tobacco use or within the past 6 months
8. Lack of social support
9. Proven record of noncompliance with medical therapies
10. Psychiatric illness preventing adequate compliance with medical therapies
11. Amyloidosis and human immunodeficiency virus (HIV): previously considered absolute contraindications but now listing is considered at some specialized institutions with multidisciplinary teams and protocols to guide therapy in the appropriately selected patient

IV. PREOPERATIVE EVALUATION

1. Thorough evaluation by a multidisciplinary heart failure and transplant team must be performed prior to listing.
2. Preoperative work-up should include at minimum the following:
   a. Complete laboratory profile: complete blood count (CBC), comprehensive medical panel (CMP), liver function tests (LFTs), coagulation studies, thyroid panel, iron panel, blood type, etc.
   b. Infectious work-up, including blood and urine cultures and evaluation for cytomegalovirus (CMV), herpes simplex virus (HSV), HIV, varicella, viral hepatitis, toxoplasmosis, tuberculosis
   c. Urinalysis and 24-hour urine studies

64

CARDIAC TRANSPLANTATION

d. Cardiac studies, including electrocardiogram (EKG), Holter monitor, echocardiogram, viability studies, cardiopulmonary exercise testing (CPET), right and left heart catheterization, myocardial biopsy if indicated to determine etiology of heart failure

e. Pulmonary function tests, chest x-ray (CXR), and computed tomography (CT) chest

f. Carotid duplex, additional vascular studies, such as ABIs or angiography if indicated

g. Renal ultrasound

h. Esophagogastroduodenoscopy (EGD), colonoscopy

i. Liver biopsy if indicated

j. Dual energy x-ray absorptiometry (DEXA) scan to assess for osteoporosis

k. Neurologic and psychiatric evaluation including dementia and depression screening

l. Dental evaluation

m. Assessment of social support system, prior history of medical compliance, financial resources, and evaluation of literacy and educational needs

V. LISTING CRITERIA

1. CPET should include respiratory exchange ratio greater than 1.05 and achievement of anaerobic threshold on optimal medical therapy.

   a. Oxygen consumption (Vo_2) with a maximum of less than or equal to 14 mL/kg per minute in absence of beta-blocker or less than or equal to 12 mL/kg per minute in presence of beta-blocker as determined by CPET

2. Right heart catheterization must be performed and repeated at 3–6-month intervals for assessment of pulmonary vascular resistance (PVR).

   a. If transpulmonary gradient is greater than 15 mm Hg or PVR is greater than 3 Wood units, a vasodilator challenge should be performed.

   b. If pulmonary hypertension is unable to be reversed with maximal medical therapy and/or mechanical support for the left ventricle (LV)

      (1) Pulmonary hypertension is then considered "fixed," and is a contraindication to transplant.

3. Heart failure prognosis score indicating 1-year estimated survival less than 80%. (These criteria must be used in conjunction with Vo_2 maximum and not as standalone criteria for listing.)

   a. Based on Seattle Heart Failure Model or a heart failure survival score in the high- to medium-risk range

VI. LISTING STATUS ACCORDING TO WHOM IT MAY CONCERN: ORGAN PROCUREMENT AND TRANSPLANTATION NETWORK POLICIES

1. Adult status 1A includes those patients 18 years old and who meet at least one of the following criteria:

a. Requires mechanical circulatory support device, including total artificial heart (TAH), intraaortic balloon pump, extracorporeal membrane oxygenation (ECMO)

b. Requires continuous mechanical ventilation

c. Requires continuous infusion of a single high-dose intravenous inotrope or multiple intravenous inotropes, and requires continuous hemodynamic monitoring of left ventricular filling pressures

d. Patients who are undergoing mechanical circulatory support and there is medical evidence of significant device-related complications, such as thromboembolism, device infection, mechanical failure, or life-threatening ventricular arrhythmias

e. Patients may also be listed as status 1A for 30 total days any time after insertion of a mechanical circulatory support device, even if they are stable and outpatients. These 30 days do not have to be consecutive.

2. **Adult status 1B:**
   a. Patients with a mechanical circulatory assist device in place, or
   b. Patients on continuous infusion of intravenous inotropes (including outpatient inotrope infusions)

3. **Adult status 2:**
   a. All other patients listed for cardiac transplant who do not meet any status 1 criteria

4. **Adult status 7:**
   a. Inactive

5. **Pediatric heart status 1A includes those patients less than 18 years old and who meet at least one of the following criteria:**
   a. Requires continuous mechanical ventilation
   b. Requires assistance of an intraaortic balloon pump
   c. Has ductal dependent pulmonary or systemic circulation, with ductal patency maintained by stent or prostaglandin infusion
   d. Has a hemodynamically significant congenital heart disease diagnosis and requires infusion of multiple intravenous inotropes or a high dose of a single intravenous inotrope
   e. Requires assistance of a mechanical circulatory support device

6. **Pediatric heart status 1B includes those patients who meet at least one of the following criteria:**
   a. Requires infusion of one or more inotropic agents but does not qualify for pediatric status 1A
   b. Is less than 1 year old at the time of the candidate's initial registration and has a diagnosis of hypertrophic or restrictive cardiomyopathy

7. **Pediatric heart status 2 includes pediatric patients listed for transplant who do not meet status 1 criteria.**

VII. MEDICAL AND MECHANICAL BRIDGES TO TRANSPLANT

1. Advanced pharmacologic support in heart failure patients awaiting transplant includes continuous infusion of intravenous inotropic agents.

64

CARDIAC TRANSPLANTATION

2. Mechanical circulatory support devices include the intraaortic balloon pump, which is almost universally confined to inpatient, nonambulatory use, as well as long-term options of left ventricular assist devices (LVADs), right ventricular assist devices (RVADs), and a TAH.

3. Patients with biventricular heart failure may require LVAD and RVAD support or TAH.

4. Although ambulatory and outpatient use of LVADs has become quite common, most patients requiring an RVAD remain in the hospital.

5. The TAH system now has an ambulatory driver that allows for outpatient use.

   a. One of the essential differences in ventricular assist devices and the TAH is that insertion of the TAH requires removal of the native heart. Although recovery and bridge to explant is uncommon in patients with a ventricular assist device, it is not an option with the TAH, and therefore the patient must be screened to have unrecoverable heart failure and be a candidate for heart transplant before insertion of the TAH.

VIII. DONOR SELECTION, EVALUATION, AND MANAGEMENT

A. DONOR SELECTION

1. Brain-dead donors are screened for being an appropriate cardiac donor.

2. Although expanded criteria are being used for donor selection at some centers, particularly those transplanting higher risk or more elderly patients, some suggested criteria for donor selection include:

   a. Age less than 55 years

   b. Absence of cardiac disease, cardiac arrest, prolonged hypotension, cardiac trauma

   c. Absence of sepsis, bacteremia, transmittable infections, such as HIV, hepatitis B or C

   d. Absence of malignancy

   e. Hemodynamic stability without requirement of high-dose inotropic or vasopressor agents

B. DONOR EVALUATION

1. Diagnostics should include the following:

   a. Laboratory studies for blood typing and infectious work-up

   b. Arterial blood gas

   c. CXR

   d. EKG

   e. Echocardiography

   f. Right heart catheterization as indicated

   g. Coronary angiography in males older than 45, females older than 50, or in those with risk factors for coronary disease or history of cocaine use

h. ABO matching must be performed to avoid hyperacute rejection.

2. Donor height and weight is an important factor in cardiac donor selection and should be within 30% of the recipient's. A larger donor heart is preferable for recipients with higher PVR to reduce the risk of post-transplant right heart failure.

3. Intraoperative evaluation of the donor heart at the time of organ procurement is the most critical step and must include palpation of the coronary arteries to assess for calcification, as well as visual inspection for ventricular dysfunction and evidence of infarction or trauma. Visual inspection of the heart valves must be performed after removal of the donor heart.

4. Care should be taken to avoid volume overload, which can cause ventricular distention.

5. A mean arterial pressure greater than 60 mm Hg should be maintained with use of inotropes or vasopressor agents if indicated.

6. Central venous pressure (CVP) should be maintained between 6 and 10 mm Hg and pulmonary capillary wedge pressure (PCWP) between 8 and 12 mm Hg.

7. The goal should be to maintain normal oxygenation, temperature, pH and electrolyte concentrations, and glucose levels.

8. Brain-dead patients undergo significant neurohormonal changes, and hormonal resuscitation with insulin, corticosteroids, triiodothyronine, vasopressin, and methylprednisolone can improve hemodynamic state and reduce the need for vasopressors.

IX. DONOR HEART PROCUREMENT

1. Exposure is through a median sternotomy, and the pericardium is incised longitudinally.

2. Inspection of the heart and palpation of the coronaries should be performed.

3. The superior vena cava (SVC) is mobilized and encircled with ties; the azygous vein is ligated and divided. The aorta and pulmonary artery are dissected, and adequate exposure of the inferior vena cava (IVC) is ensured.

4. After preparation for procurement of the abdominal organs is complete, the patient is fully heparinized and the SVC is ligated superior to the azygous vein.

5. The IVC is incised, exsanguinating the patient.

6. A cross-clamp is placed on the ascending aorta and cold preservation solution is administered into the ascending aorta to arrest the heart, which is surrounded by ice slush for cooling.

a. Various preservation solutions are available that differ in their ionic concentrations; some common examples include University of Wisconsin, St. Thomas Hospital, and Custodiol HTK solutions.

64

CARDIAC TRANSPLANTATION

7. The LV is vented by an incision in the left atrial appendage, or right superior pulmonary vein.
8. All efforts are made to avoid distension of the ventricles, overpressurization of the ascending aorta, or intracoronary air.
9. The IVC is divided in consult with the abdominal team, followed by the pulmonary veins (or left atrium), the aorta proximal to the innominate, the pulmonary artery, and SVC.
10. Inspection for a patent foramen ovale is performed and, if present, should be closed.
11. Preservation of the donor heart should continue with immediate transfer of the heart to a cold preservation solution to maintain a temperature of 4°C–10°C.
12. An ischemic period of ideally less than 4 hours, but no longer than 6 hours, is considered safe.

X. OPERATIVE TECHNIQUE FOR CARDIAC TRANSPLANTATION

1. Orthotopic implantation with bicaval anastomosis has become the most common technique for cardiac transplantation.
   a. Biatrial anastomosis is associated with decreased long-term survival and is not recommended unless specific anatomic reasons dictate its use. Many transplant recipients are currently being transplanted with a mechanical circulatory assist device in place, and adequate time must be allotted for recipient preparation to allow for removal of the mechanical device as well.
2. A median sternotomy is performed, and the patient is placed on cardiopulmonary bypass via standard aortic and bicaval cannulation.
3. Recipient cardiectomy is performed just before actual arrival of the donor heart by transecting the aorta and pulmonary arteries just above the aortic and pulmonic valves. The SVC and IVC are transected, and the left atrium is cut to leave a left atrial cuff around the orifices of the pulmonary veins.
4. The donor heart is prepared by trimming the left atrium to fit the left atrial cuff of the recipient heart.
5. The left atrial anastomosis is performed with a running suture.
6. The aortic anastomosis is completed in an end-to-end fashion, allowing early reperfusion of the donor heart, reducing warm ischemic time.
7. The IVC and SVC are anastomosed end to end.
8. The pulmonary artery anastomosis is end to end (care must be taken to avoid kinking from a too long donor pulmonary artery).
9. Routine steps are taken to de-air, and the patient is weaned from cardiopulmonary bypass.
10. Inhaled nitric oxide may be used routinely or if indicated because of evidence of pulmonary hypertension and right ventricular failure.

XI. POSTOPERATIVE MANAGEMENT

1. Early graft failure
   a. It is often due to right ventricular failure, left heart dysfunction due to ischemic injury, and improper preservation and occasionally due to acute rejection.
   b. Support for primary graft dysfunction includes pharmacologic methods, such as inotropes and inhaled nitric oxide, as well as mechanical circulatory support including intraaortic balloon pump, RVAD, and ECMO.
2. Arrhythmias can be a difficult problem because of autonomic denervation that occurs with cardiectomy.
3. Arrhythmias are less common after bicaval transplant technique than after biatrial techniques.
4. A heart rate of 90–110 beats/min is targeted, and bradycardia can be addressed.
   a. Temporary epicardial pacing
   b. Inotropes
   c. Specific agents to increase heart rate, such as isoproterenol or theophylline, the latter of which can be taken orally
5. Supraventricular tachycardias may be treated similarly to the standard patient, but these and ventricular arrhythmias should be treated seriously and investigated for rejection or ischemic injury with myocardial biopsy.

XII. IMMUNOSUPPRESSION AND LONG-TERM MANAGEMENT

1. The donor and recipient must be ABO compatible.
2. A panel reactive antibody (PRA) test is performed preoperatively to determine sensitization of the recipient to alloantigens.
   a. If the PRA test is greater than 10%, prospective crossmatching should be performed before transplant.
3. After transplantation, immunosuppression is initiated with a combination of corticosteroids, mycophenolate, and calcineurin inhibitors.
4. Acute rejection is often insidious and must be monitored for by routine endomyocardial biopsy. A biopsy is taken via a catheter-based approach through the right internal jugular vein with biopsy of the right ventricle. This is performed weekly for several weeks and then spread out to intervals of 3–6 months.
5. Grading of rejection is based on pattern of lymphocytic infiltrate and presence of myocyte necrosis.
6. The majority of cases of acute rejection can be managed medically. Mild cases may not require changes in therapy unless there is evidence of graft dysfunction. Resumption of intravenous steroids and adjustment of immunosuppression therapy is the typical therapy for acute rejection with frequent monitoring for reversal of rejection with endomyocardial biopsy.

64

CARDIAC TRANSPLANTATION

7. Vascular rejection is a humoral immune response and is more difficult to address than acute cellular rejection and likely plays a role in cardiac allograft vasculopathy (CAV), which can cause a rapidly developing coronary atherosclerosis and is the most common cause of death after the first year posttransplant. Patients typically have annual coronary angiography to monitor for this complication, but there is no specific treatment that is effective at preventing or reversing the process. Retransplantation is indicated for CAV.

XIII. PREVENTION OF OPPORTUNISTIC INFECTION

1. As with other solid organ transplants, prophylaxis to prevent bacterial, viral, and fungal infectious diseases in the posttransplant patient includes the following:
   a. Trimethoprim-sulfamethoxazole for pneumocystis
   b. Nystatin for candida
   c. Gancyclovir or acyclovir for CMV, unless the donor and recipient were both CMV negative, and acyclovir for HSV and varicella zoster
2. Immunizations should be administered in the preoperative and postoperative setting, as appropriate.

XIV. SURVIVAL

1. Expected 1-year survival from a heart transplant in the modern era is 90%. Of those surviving the first year, 50% are alive at 13 years after transplant.

RECOMMENDED READINGS

Allen JG, Shah AS, Conte JV, Baumgartner WA. Heart transplantation. In: Cohn LH, ed. *Cardiac Surgery in the Adult*. 4th ed. New York: McGraw-Hill; 2012. chap 64.

Organ Procurement and Transplantation Network (OPTN) Policies. Effective Date: 7/7/2016, Page 61–65, Policy 6: Allocation of Hearts and Heart-Lungs. 6.1 Status Assignments. <https://optn.transplant.hrsa.gov/> Accessed October 17, 2016.

Mehra MR, Canter CE, Hannan MM, on behalf of the International Society for Heart Lung Transplantation (ISHLT) Infectious Diseases, et al. Pediatric and Heart Failure and Transplantation Councils. The 2016 International Society for Heart Lung Transplantation listing criteria for heart transplantation: a 10-year update. *J Heart Lung Transplant*. 2016;35:1–23.

UNOS. <https://www.unos.org/> Accessed November 7, 2016.

PART XII

Surgical Subspecialties

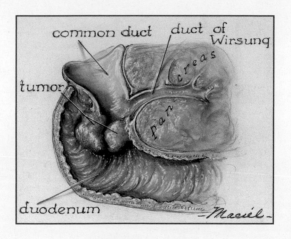

Surgical Subspecialties

General Pediatric Surgery

Ashley Walther, MD

Nobody cares how much you know, until they know how much you care.

—Theodore Roosevelt

I. FLUIDS AND NUTRITION

A. MAINTENANCE FLUIDS

1. Neonates—fluid requirement is 65 mL/kg over 24 hours.
2. By the end of the first week of life—fluid requirements increase to 100 mL/kg over 24 hours.
3. To calculate based on weight:
   a. [100 mL/kg per 24 hours (4 mL/kg per hour) for first 10 kg] + [50 mL/kg per 24 hours (2 mL/kg per hour) for each kg 11–20] + 25 mL/kg per 24 hours (1 mL/kg per hour) for each additional kilogram over 20]
4. Maintenance fluid—dextrose 5% in ¼ normal saline

B. RESUSCITATION FLUIDS

1. Crystalloid: lactated Ringer or 0.9% normal saline
   a. Ten to 20 mL/kg bolus
   b. For ongoing fluid loss (high nasogastric output, protracted vomiting or diarrhea), replace 1 mL fluid loss with 1 mL replacement every 4 hours using D5 ½ normal saline + 20 mEq KCl/L
2. Blood product replacement
   a. Packed red blood cells (pRBCs): 10–15 mL/kg
   b. Fresh frozen plasma (FFP): 10–15 mL/kg
   c. Platelets: 1 unit/5 kg body weight

C. FLUID BALANCE

1. Clinical signs of dehydration
   a. Lethargy, decreased feeding
   b. Tachycardia, reduced urine output, depressed fontanelle
2. Clinical signs of fluid overload
   a. New/increased oxygen requirement, respiratory distress
   b. Tachypnea, tachycardia

D. ACID-BASE ANOMALIES

1. Metabolic acidosis—inadequate tissue perfusion
   a. Causes
      (1) Intestinal ischemia (necrotizing enterocolitis, midgut volvulus, incarcerated hernia)
      (2) Bicarbonate loss from gastrointestinal (GI) tract (diarrhea)

65

771

        (3) Chronic renal failure with acid accumulation

        (4) Diabetic ketoacidosis

        (5) Ingestion (methanol, ethylene glycol, salicylates, paraldehyde, formaldehyde)

   b. Treatment—treat underlying cause

        (1) Sodium bicarbonate indicated if pH less than 7.1, bicarbonate less than 10

        (2) Replacement = base deficit × weight (kg) × 0.3

        (3) Administer half of calculated replacement amount over several hours then recheck pH

2. Metabolic alkalosis—gastric acid loss (pyloric stenosis: hypokalemic, hypochloremic), overaggressive diuresis

3. Respiratory acidosis—hypoventilation

4. Respiratory alkalosis—hyperventilation

E. TOTAL PARENTERAL NUTRITION

1. Indications: prolonged ileus, GI fistulas, gastroschisis/omphalocele, intestinal atresia, necrotizing enterocolitis, supplementation of enteral feeds in short bowel syndrome and malabsorption states, prematurity/very low birth weight

   a. Enteral nutrition preferred whenever possible to promote growth and function of GI tract

2. Complications

   a. Parenteral nutrition–associated liver disease (PNALD)

        (1) Cholestasis, can progress to end-stage hepatic fibrosis and cirrhosis

        (2) Treatment: decrease dose, modify/restrict lipids, or stop treatment; may require transplantation

   b. Sepsis—central line–related infections; prevent with meticulous care and aggressive treatment of all infections

II. LESIONS OF THE HEAD AND NECK

A. THRYOGLOSSAL DUCT CYST

1. Most common midline congenital cervical anomaly

2. Cause

   a. Thyroglossal tract arises from base of tongue (foramen cecum); residual thyroid tissue from descent may persist in midline.

   b. Pockets can fill with fluid and mucus, enlarging when infected, presenting as a nodule.

3. Symptoms

   a. Most present in first 5 years of life.

   b. Rounded, cystic mass of varying size in midline of neck; 60% adjacent to hyoid bone

   c. Moves cephalad with swallowing and tongue protrusion

   d. Often asymptomatic; may cause dysphagia, pain; drainage if infected

4. Work-up: thyroid-stimulating hormone (TSH) level, ultrasound; if hypothyroid or concern for lack of normal thyroid gland, obtain thyroid scan

5. Treatment
   a. Resection to avoid recurrent infection and rule out underlying malignancy
      (1) Sistrunk procedure: complete resection of cyst and its tract in continuity with the central hyoid bone
      (2) Recurrence (10%) from incomplete excision or intraoperative rupture
   b. Incision and drainage of abscess, antibiotic administration; definitive resection after resolution of inflammation

B. BRANCHIAL CLEFT ANOMALIES

1. Most arise from second cleft/pouch
2. Cause: incomplete obliteration of paired branchial clefts and arches during development
3. Symptoms: usually discovered in first decade, present as fistulae, sinus tract, cartilaginous remnants
   a. Second branchial cleft sinus presents with clear fluid draining from anterior border of lower $^1/_3$ of sternocleidomastoid muscle (SCM).
   b. Cysts are nontender soft tissue masses beneath SCM; may become infected; risk of in situ carcinoma in adults
4. Work-up: ultrasound to identify cystic nature of mass if not apparent on physical examination
5. Treatment
   a. Complete excision of cyst and tract
      (1) Use lacrimal probe to identify tract; may dip in methylene blue to stain tract
      (2) Multiple small transverse "stepladder" incisions used if tract is long
   b. Aspiration and systemic antibiotics if infected, resect when inflammation resolves

III. THORACIC DISORDERS

A. PULMONARY SEQUESTRATION

1. Nonfunctioning lung tissue, has anomalous arterial supply (systemic artery, not pulmonary artery) and absent or abnormal bronchial communication
2. Male predominance (3:1), left lower side more common
3. Associated with congenital diaphragmatic hernia (CDH), vertebral anomalies, and congenital heart disease
4. Two forms
   a. Extralobar: completely separate from normal lung, separate pleural covering
      (1) Often asymptomatic and found incidentally
      (2) May become infected by hematogenous spread of bacteria
   b. Intralobar: Incorporated into normal surrounding lung
      (1) Present with recurrent pneumonia and abscess formation in same bronchopulmonary segment

5. Diagnosis:
   a. Prenatal: ultrasound with Doppler flow, magnetic resonance imaging (MRI)
   b. Chest radiograph, ultrasound with Doppler flow, computed tomography (CT) chest
6. Surgical treatment
   a. Symptomatic sequestrations require resection
      (1) Extralobar—simple excision
      (2) Intralobar—lobectomy
      (3) Must find and ligate feeding systemic arterial vessel, usually in inferior pulmonary ligament

B. CONGENITAL CYSTIC ADENOMATOID MALFORMATION
1. Cystic proliferation of terminal respiratory bronchioles that form cysts
   a. Mucus-producing respiratory epithelium, increase in smooth muscle and elastic tissue within cyst walls, absence of cartilage
   b. Does not function in gas exchange but connects to tracheobronchial tree, leading to gas trapping
2. Most commonly arises from lower lobes (right and left equally); can be bilateral (rare)
3. Symptoms
   a. May be diagnosed as fetus or newborn
   b. Usual delayed presentation is infection in congenital cystic adenomatoid malformation (CCAM) area; pneumothorax, reactive airway disease, failure to thrive
4. Diagnosis
   a. Fetal: ultrasound, MRI, fetal echocardiogram (ECHO)
   b. Infant: chest x-ray (CXR), CT chest, ultrasound
5. Treatment: lobectomy
6. Prognosis
   a. Excellent, resection is curative
   b. Risk factors for poor outcome: hydrops fetalis, microcystic lesion, large size

C. CONGENITAL DIAPHRAGMATIC HERNIA
1. Embryology
   a. Failure of fusion of the transverse septum and the pleuroperitoneal folds during the eighth week of fetal development
   b. Right side closes before left
   c. Posterolateral portion of diaphragm last to complete fusion
   d. Affects ipsilateral and contralateral pulmonary development, resulting in pulmonary hypoplasia
2. Incidence: 1 in 3000 births, associated congenital defects (trisomies 18 and 21, cardiac malformations)
3. Types of defect

a. Bochdalek—most common (90%–95%), posterolateral location, more common on left side (80%–85%)
   (1) Herniated contents often include left lobe of liver, spleen, and almost entire GI tract.
b. Morgagni—rare (5%–10%), anterior midline through sternocostal hiatus of diaphragm, more common on right side (90%)

4. Symptoms
   a. Often detected on prenatal ultrasound
   b. Respiratory distress (dyspnea, cyanosis, hypoxemia, hypercarbia, metabolic acidosis)
      (1) Caused by intrathoracic bowel compressing the mediastinum; with swallowed air, bowel distends and further compresses the pulmonary parenchyma worsening symptoms
   c. Scaphoid abdomen, asymmetric distended chest; auscultation of bowel sounds in chest
   d. Persistent fetal circulation
   e. Symptoms may develop immediately or within first 24 hours of life

5. Diagnosis
   a. Prenatal ultrasound—mean age at discovery is 24 weeks
      (1) Evidence of herniated viscera, abnormal intraabdominal anatomy, mediastinal shift away from herniated viscera
      (2) Lung-to-head ratio (predictor of severity of left CDH)
         (a) Product of right lung length and width at level of cardiac atria divided by head circumference
         (b) Ratio less than 1 = poor prognosis; ratio greater than 1 = more favorable outcome
   b. Prenatal MRI—determines liver position in relation to the diaphragm, accurately assess lung volume
   c. CXR at birth—demonstrates loops of intestine in chest, assess gastric location with placement of orogastric tube

6. Treatment
   a. Physiologic emergency, not a surgical emergency
   b. Cardiopulmonary stabilization—intubation and mechanical ventilation with permissive hypercapnia, may require oscillator
      (1) Administration of inhaled nitric oxide
      (2) ECHO to assess pulmonary hypertension
      (3) May require extracorporeal membrane oxygenation (ECMO)—used until pulmonary hypertension reversed and lung function (compliance) improves
   c. Vascular access—arterial and venous access through umbilicus, additional preductal arterial monitoring (right radial arterial catheter or transcutaneous saturation probe)
   d. Nasogastric tube for decompression
   e. Temperature regulation, glucose homeostasis, volume monitoring
   f. Surgical intervention

(1) Subcostal incision or thoracotomy
(2) Reduction of abdominal contents, evisceration for adequate visualization
(3) Excise hernia sac if present to minimize recurrence
(4) Primary repair—if adequate tissue present using interrupted nonabsorbable suture
(5) Patch closure—prosthetic material, provides tension-free repair
    (a) Risks: infection, dislodgement, reherniation
(6) Abdominal wall closure difficulty due to loss of domain—simple skin closure, repair hernia later versus temporary closure with prosthetic material (silo)

7. Prognosis—improved with improvements in management, survival as high as 80%

IV. ESOPHAGEAL ANOMALIES

A. TRACHEOESOPHAGEAL FISTULA

1. Embryology: failure of separation of trachea from esophagus, pathogenesis heterogeneous and multifactorial
2. Incidence: 1 in 3500 live births
3. Associated congenital anomalies
   a. VATER or VACTERL syndrome
      (1) Vertebral (missing vertebrae)
      (2) Anorectal (imperforate anus)
      (3) Cardiac (several congenital cardiac diseases)
      (4) Tracheoesophageal fistula (TEF)
      (5) Renal agenesis
      (6) Radial limb hyperplasia
   b. "Nonsyndromic"—cardiovascular (24%), urogenital (21%), digestive (21%), musculoskeletal (14%), central nervous system (CNS; 7%)
4. Anatomic variations
   a. Esophageal atresia (EA) with distal TEF—type C (84%)
   b. EA with proximal TEF—type B (5%)
   c. TEF without EA—type E (or "H-type"; 4%)
   d. EA with proximal TEF and distal TEF—type D (1%)
5. Symptoms
   a. Type B, C, and D: excessive salivation, feeding intolerance (choking/coughing immediately after feeding), gagging from aspiration via fistulous tract
   b. Type C and D:
      (1) With coughing or crying, air passes into stomach causing abdominal distention and respiratory difficulty.
      (2) With refluxed gastric contents into tracheobronchial tree, more susceptible to chemical pneumonitis
   c. Type E: may have delayed presentation with recurrent pneumonia, bronchospasm, and failure to thrive

6. Work-up
   a. Prenatal ultrasound—small or absent stomach bubble, maternal polyhydramnios due to inability to swallow amniotic fluid
   b. Inability to pass orogastric tube beyond the esophagus
   c. Chest radiograph (frontal and lateral)
      (1) Dilated proximal pouch (air injected through tube distends pouch)
      (2) Coiled orogastric feeding tube in proximal pouch
      (3) Air in stomach and bowel confirms presence of distal TEF
   d. Contrast esophagram—diluted barium delineates pouch, confirms diagnosis and often TEF
   e. Bronchoscopy—evaluate for TEF
   f. Associated anomalies: ECHO, vertebral radiographs with spinal ultrasound if abnormal, clinical examination for patent anus, abdominal ultrasound of kidneys, plain films of anomalous extremities
   g. Initial management
7. Operative treatment
   a. Rarely an emergency, often delayed 24–48 hours for full assessment
   b. Open thoracotomy or thoracoscopic division of the fistula and primary anastomosis of fistula
      (1) Left lateral decubitus position, right posterolateral incision
      (2) Extrapleural approach
      (3) TEF ligation, oversewing of tracheal defect
      (4) Primary esophagoesophagostomy under low tension
      (5) Leave transanastomotic feeding tube and retropleural chest tube
   c. In setting of large TEF with severe respiratory distress syndrome, may require intubation and emergency operative intervention

B. ISOLATED ESOPHAGEAL ATRESIA—TYPE A (6%)

1. Occur in setting of prematurity, Down syndrome, associated duodenal atresia
2. Symptoms: inability to swallow (excessive salivation, feeding intolerance), scaphoid abdomen
3. Work-up: abdominal radiographs—no air in GI tract
4. Treatment
   a. Placement of gastrostomy tube in first 24–48 hours of life—early enteral feeds, stretching of stomach and distal esophageal remnant
   b. Esophageal elongation of upper remnant (8–12 weeks): upper pouch bougienage, multistage extrathoracic elongation with cervical esophagostomy, use of traction suture or magnets
   c. Delayed primary repair
      (1) Thoracotomy or thoracoscopic approach, dissection and mobilization of the proximal and distal esophageal segments
      (2) If unable to perform primary anastomosis, gastric transposition to cervical esophagus or colonic interposition

C. SURVIVAL
1. Overall survival 85%–95%
2. Worse prognosis in setting of EA
   a. Early complications: anastomotic leak, esophageal stricture (requiring dilation in up to 80%), recurrent TEF
   b. Late complications: gastroesophageal reflux disease (GERD), tracheomalacia, dysphagia/dysmotility

V. GASTROINTESTINAL TRACT

A. HYPERTROPHIC PYLORIC STENOSIS
1. Gastric outlet obstruction caused by hypertrophied pyloric muscle
2. Incidence: 2–4 per 1000 live births; male-to-female ratio is 4:1, with 30% of patients being first-born males
3. Usually occurs in the first 2 months of life, with average age of clinical presentation 2–12 weeks
4. Symptoms: nonbilious, postprandial, projectile emesis that increases in volume and frequency. Infant is hungry after emesis.
5. Lab values: "contraction" alkalosis (hypokalemia, hypochloremia, metabolic alkalosis, "paradoxical aciduria"). Unconjugated hyperbilirubinemia may also be present.
6. Physical examination: classic palpable pyloric tumor ("olive") in the midepigastrium to right upper quadrant seen in up to 80% of infants; examination is facilitated by nasogastric decompression and calming with dextrose/water solution
7. Work-up: Ultrasound is study of choice for confirming diagnosis (>3 mm thick, >14 mm long) when pyloric tumor is not palpable or equivocal.
8. Preoperative management
   a. Operation is never an emergency; adequate preoperative preparation is necessary for low morbidity.
   b. Nothing by mouth (NPO) and nasogastric decompression may be needed if there is continued emesis.
   c. Fluid resuscitation (20 mL/kg crystalloid) and electrolyte correction including potassium repletion (after urine output ensured) are mandatory before operative repair. Correct HCO_3 to less than 30.
   d. D5 $1/2$ normal saline at 125%–150% maintenance fluids
9. Surgical treatment: Ramstedt pyloromyotomy via right upper quadrant, periumbilical, or laparoscopic approach
   a. Splitting of the antropyloric mass, leaving mucosal layer intact with blunt spread of muscle fibers
   b. Pyloromyotomy incision length of approximately 2 cm is sufficient
10. Postoperative management
    a. Nasogastric tube removed in operating room
    b. Continued intravenous (IV) hydration until tolerating oral intake
    c. NPO × 4 hours then initiate ad libitum bottle feeds with full strength breast milk or formula

    d. Emesis common; if clinically significant, hold feeds for 2 hours and then restart PO ad libitum

B. INTESTINAL OBSTRUCTION IN THE NEONATE

1. Suspect obstruction with history of maternal polyhydramnios, bilious emesis, abdominal distention, or failure to pass meconium within first 24 hours of life.
2. Bilious vomiting in an infant is a surgical emergency and requires emergent evaluation to rule out malrotation and midgut volvulus.
3. Intrinsic duodenal obstruction
   a. Frequent association with other anomalies
   b. May be caused by duodenal web, atresia, or stenosis
   c. Symptoms: bilious vomiting, minimal abdominal distention (only proximal bowel and stomach)
   d. Work-up: abdominal radiographs—reveal "double bubble" sign
   e. Surgical treatment: excision of webs or duodenostomy for atresia/stenosis; evaluation of distal bowel for concurrent atresias
   f. Ampulla of Vater at the level of the web—at risk for injury
4. Extrinsic duodenal obstruction: malrotation
   a. Narrow base and lack of fixation for the midgut mesentery, with predisposition to volvulus and intestinal infarction
   b. Volvulus frequently results in significant vascular compromise and intestinal necrosis.
   c. Symptoms: sudden onset of bilious vomiting as newborn (bilious emesis in child <1 year is volvulus until proven otherwise)
   d. Work-up: upper GI series to visualize malpositioned ligament of Treitz versus immediate laparotomy if index of suspicion is high
   e. Surgical treatment: Ladd procedure
      (1) Emergent laparotomy, evisceration, reduction of volvulus by counterclockwise rotation ("turning back the hands of time"), division of "Ladd bands," thereby widening the mesenteric base between the duodenum and the colon
      (2) Appendectomy, placement of small bowel in right side and colon in left side of the peritoneal cavity
      (3) Resect nonviable bowel; questionably viable bowel should remain with a planned 24-hour second-look laparotomy
      (4) Delay in diagnosis can lead to significant loss of bowel length resulting in short gut syndrome
5. Jejunoileal obstruction—atresia and stenosis
   a. Frequently result of late mesenteric vascular accidents in utero
   b. Work-up
      (1) Abdominal radiographs show dilated loops of small bowel
      (2) Contrast barium enema to rule out colonic atresia, may show small, unused "microcolon"
   c. Classification of jejunoileal atresia:

65

GENERAL PEDIATRIC SURGERY

(1) **Type I**—single mucosal atresia, bowel wall and mesentery in continuity, and normal bowel length

(2) **Type II**—single atresia with discontinuity of bowel and gap in mesentery (blind ends joined by fibrous cord running on intact mesentery)

(3) **Type IIIa**—disconnected blind ends as in type II but no cord connecting and a mesenteric gap

(4) **Type IIIb**— "apple peel" or "Christmas tree" deformity with markedly decreased bowel length with vascular supply from the ileocolic vessels

(5) **Type IV**—multiple atresias resulting in short bowel length

d. Surgical treatment: individualized, depending on number and length of atresias

(1) Resection with anastomosis, tapering enteroplasty, and exteriorization in the presence of compromised bowel

(2) Resection of proximal dilated bowel with end-to-end anastomosis

6. **Meconium ileus**

a. Associated with cystic fibrosis

b. Obstruction of the distal ileum from inspissated meconium

c. Simple meconium ileus: bowel is impacted with pellets of meconium, with proximally dilated ileum packed with thick, tarlike meconium.

(1) Presentation: progressive abdominal distention, failure to pass meconium

d. Complicated meconium ileus: associated with meconium cysts, atresia, perforation, meconium peritonitis, volvulus, or intestinal necrosis

(1) Presentation: sepsis, distention, respiratory distress

e. Work-up

(1) Abdominal radiograph: no air-fluid levels, "soap bubble" appearance in proximal colon

(2) Contrast enema: microcolon with inspissated plugs of meconium

f. Medical treatment: Gastrografin enemas after hydration, nasogastric decompression, empiric antibiotics, and vitamin K to correct coagulopathy

g. Surgical treatment: indicated for complicated cases and where nonoperative therapy fails

(1) Simple enterotomy and irrigation of bowel with *N*-acetylcysteine (Mucomyst)

(2) Bowel resection with primary anastomosis or temporary diverting colostomy or distal chimney enterostomy

7. **Hirschsprung disease**

a. Absence of parasympathetic ganglion cells in the affected segment of intestine; rectum and rectosigmoid most common

b. Familial forms of Hirschsprung disease associated with mutations in RET (REarranged during Transfection) proto-oncogene, endothelin receptor B, and endothelin-3 genes

   c. Symptoms: failure to pass meconium in first 24 hours, abdominal
      distension, and vomiting; suspected in any infant who has chronic
      constipation during the first year of life
   d. Work-up
      (1) Barium enema with transition point (rectum of small to normal
          size with proximal colorectal dilation)
      (2) Suction rectal biopsy to confirm (absence of ganglion cells in
          Meissner [submucosal] and Auerbach [intermuscular] plexus;
          increase in acetylcholinesterase staining in hypertrophic nerve
          trunks)
   e. Surgical treatment: one-stage pull-through operation, laparoscopic
      versus open versus transanal
      (1) Previous standard was a multistage approach, starting with
          diverting colostomy proximal to the aganglionic segment (leveling
          colostomy) followed by a definitive pull-through procedure at
          9–12 months of age.
   f. Morbidity and mortality: enterocolitis (10%–30%), anastomotic leak
      (1%–5%), and stricture (3%–5%)

C. INTESTINAL OBSTRUCTION IN THE INFANT (2 MONTHS TO 2 YEARS)

1. Intussusception
   a. Most common cause of bowel obstruction in 2-month to 2-year age
      range
   b. Documented recent viral infection (adenovirus, rotavirus, enterovirus)
      in >50%
   c. Caused by telescoping of one segment of bowel (intussusceptum)
      into another (intussuscipiens)
      (1) Most frequently at ileocecal region
   d. Symptoms: sudden onset of recurring severe, crampy abdominal
      pain, vomiting, drawing up of legs
      (1) Bloody ("currant jelly") stools in 60%
      (2) An elongated sausage-shaped mass may be palpable in right
          upper quadrant with an "empty" right lower quadrant (RLQ)
   e. Work-up: contrast enema—air or barium
      (1) Diagnostic and therapeutic: initial treatment by attempted hydro-
          static/pneumatic reduction during air/contrast enema if peritonitis
          or free air has been ruled out first (50%–90% success rate). May
          require repeated attempts
   f. Surgical treatment: if air enema reduction is unsuccessful or if perito-
      nitis is present
      (1) Laparoscopic approach with gentle reduction by traction on the
          proximal bowel. Consider conversion to open with failure to
          reduce.
      (2) If manual reduction is not possible or if lead point is identified,
          resection is indicated.

65

GENERAL PEDIATRIC SURGERY

2. Incarcerated inguinal hernia
   a. Indirect hernia
   b. Presentation: bulge in the groin or within the scrotum, may or may not cause pain
   c. Work-up: physical examination, ultrasound to differentiate between hernia and hydrocele
      (1) Manual reduction at presentation
   d. Surgical treatment: elective high ligation and excision of patent sac
      (1) If strangulated or unable to manually reduce, needs urgent operative repair with possible bowel resection

D. NECROTIZING ENTEROCOLITIS

1. Most common GI emergency in the premature neonate
2. More than 90% of cases are found in premature or low-birth-weight infants; occurs in 5% of neonatal intensive care admissions
3. Etiology multifactorial: ischemia/reperfusion injury, activation of proinflammatory cascade, infectious
4. Symptoms
   a. Early: vomiting, bloody bowel movements, ileus, delayed gastric emptying, abdominal distention
   b. Late: abdominal wall discoloration, lethargy, apnea, bradycardia, hypothermia, shock, acidosis, and neutropenia
5. Work-up
   a. Abdominal radiograph = pneumatosis intestinalis (air in bowel wall), may have portal venous gas
      (1) Late findings include "fixed" loop of bowel (suggests gangrenous changes) or free air.
   b. Paracentesis under ultrasound guidance, positive if greater than 0.5 mL brownish fluid, contains bacteria on Gram stain
6. Medical treatment
   a. Fluid resuscitation with correction of acidosis
   b. Nasogastric decompression, NPO, parenteral nutrition
   c. Systemic antibiotics, serial complete blood count (CBC)
   d. Serial examinations and abdominal radiographs (every 4–6 hours)
7. Indications for surgery
   a. Pneumoperitoneum, portal venous gas (relative indication)
   b. Diffuse peritonitis, abdominal wall erythema or induration
   c. Clinical deterioration—persistent/worsening acidosis, thrombocytopenia, and leukopenia
8. Surgical treatment
   a. Small bowel resection; goal is maximal preservation, leave questionable bowel and perform second-look to assess viability
   b. Bedside peritoneal drain placement an option for critically ill premature neonates

E. MECKEL DIVERTICULUM

1. Most common form of congenital malformation of small bowel
   a. Persistent vitelline duct remnant
   b. Less commonly—persistent vitelline duct with sinus, persistent omphalomesenteric band, and vitelline duct cyst
2. Occurs on antimesenteric border of ileum within 60 cm of ileocecal valve
3. Symptoms/complications
   a. Bleeding—usually painless, caused by ulceration of adjacent tissue from ectopic gastric mucosa
      (1) Usually stops spontaneously but can be massive
   b. Obstruction—intussusception or secondary to internal hernia around persistent omphalomesenteric band
   c. Inflammation—mimics acute appendicitis
   d. Perforation
4. Work-up: high degree of suspicion
   a. "Meckel scan": technetium 99m–pertechnetate scan—pertechnetate taken up by heterotopic gastric mucosa
      (1) False-positive results with enteric duplications
      (2) False-negative results with small amounts of gastric mucosa, recent barium study, or pelvic Meckel hidden behind the bladder
5. Surgical management
   a. Laparoscopic versus open resection
   b. Diverticulectomy, wedge resection of diverticulum and adjacent ileum with primary anastomosis
   c. Incidental finding: most perform prophylactic removal to prevent morbidity and mortality associated with complications
6. "Rule of 2s"—occurs in 2% of the population, 2% symptomatic, 2 feet from the ileocecal valve, 2 inches in length, 2 types of mucosa (gastric/pancreatic), 2:1 male to female ratio, often found in children less than 2 years old

F. APPENDICITIS

1. Most common emergent abdominal operation in children
2. Symptoms: anorexia and vague abdominal pain, migration of pain to the RLQ, onset of fever and vomiting
   a. Typical symptoms not always present, vary by patient age and position of appendix
   b. Delay in diagnosis and treatment is associated with rupture; pain relief followed by development of generalized abdominal pain and peritonitis
      (1) Incidence of perforation 20%–35% in children, increased frequency in younger age
3. Physical examination: pain in RLQ at McBurney point
   a. Rovsing sign: RLQ pain with palpation in left lower quadrant (LLQ)

65

GENERAL PEDIATRIC SURGERY

b. Psoas sign: pain with hyperextension of the right leg at the hip in the left lateral decubitus position

c. Obturator sign: pain with flexion and internal rotation of the right hip

4. **Lab findings**
   a. CBC with differential—leukocytosis with elevated neutrophils or band cells
   b. Urinalysis—grossly abnormal results suggests alternative source of abdominal pain.

5. **Work-up**
   a. Ultrasound—noncompressible structure in RLQ, greater than 6 mm wide; tenderness (sonographic McBurney)
   b. CT scan—thickened appendiceal wall, periappendiceal fat stranding
      (1) Perforated appendix: periappendiceal or pericecal air, abscess, phlegmon, extensive free fluid

6. **Medical management**
   a. Nonoperative treatment with antibiotics for perforated appendicitis, drain placement for abscess—interval appendectomy after 6 weeks
   b. Nonoperative treatment with antibiotics for acute, nonperforated appendicitis—ongoing research

7. **Surgical management: Appendectomy is the definitive treatment.**

G. GASTROESOPHAGEAL REFLUX

1. **Immature lower esophageal sphincter function with prolonged relaxation**

2. **Symptoms: crying/irritability, malnutrition and failure to thrive, emesis, esophagitis, apnea/bradycardia**

3. **Work-up**
   a. Esophagogastroduodenoscopy with biopsy for pathology
   b. Esophageal manometry
   c. Twenty-four-hour pH, impedance probe (most sensitive and specific for pathologic reflux)
   d. Upper GI imaging series (exclude gastric outlet obstruction and malrotation)—poor test for reflux
   e. Technetium gastric emptying scan (rule out delayed gastric emptying or outlet obstruction)

4. **Medical management**
   a. Ninety percent resolve spontaneously.
   b. Small, frequent feeds
   c. In infants—upright positioning after feeds; thickened feeds; elevate head of bed
   d. In children—avoid tomato and citrus products, fruit juices and caffeine; low-fat diet
   e. Medications: antacids, H_2 blockers, proton pump inhibitors

5. **Surgical management**
   a. Indication: failure of medical therapy, stricture, bleeding, severe esophagitis, weight loss, Barrett esophagus with intestinal metaplasia

b. Often performed in combination with gastrostomy tube when feeding access required
c. Laparoscopic fundoplication
   (1) Most common: Nissen (360 degrees)
   (2) Alternatives: Toupet (posterior 270 degrees) or Thal (anterior 270 degrees)
   (3) Pyloroplasty in setting of delayed gastric emptying
d. Complications: wrap herniation, dysphagia, recurrent GERD, vagus nerve injury (delayed gastric emptying)

VI. ABDOMINAL WALL DEFECTS

A. OMPHALOCELE

1. Midline umbilical ring defect, range in size (4–12 cm), eviscerated contents covered by sac (peritoneum and amnion)
   a. Sac contains stomach, small bowel, liver, and colon
2. Incidence: 1 in 5000 live births
3. Associated anomalies: malrotation; trisomy 13, trisomy 18, Beckwith-Wiedemann syndrome, pentalogy of Cantrell (epigastric omphalocele, anterior diaphragmatic hernia, distal sternal cleft, pericardial defects, congenital heart disease)
   a. Congenital heart disease, cardiac defects—tetralogy of Fallot, ventricular septal defect (VSD), atrial septal defect (ASD), pulmonary hypertension
   b. Genitourinary anomalies—OEIS complex (omphalocele, exstrophy, imperforate anus, spinal defects)
4. Work-up: seen on antenatal ultrasound, serial ultrasounds, MRI if inconclusive
   a. Labs: elevated alpha fetoprotein (AFP) in amniotic fluid and maternal serum
5. Mode of delivery (vaginal vs. C-section) determined by obstetric indications; term delivery
6. Medical management
   a. Resuscitation begins at delivery, gastric decompression
   b. Wrap sac in saline-soaked gauze and impervious dressing.
   c. Place in incubator or under radiant heater.
7. Surgical management
   a. Goal is reduction of herniated viscera, closure of fascia and skin
      (1) Primary closure: stable neonate, small defect
      (2) Staged closure: allow sac to epithelialize versus place silo, perform gradual reduction or serial reduction and excision of sac
8. Mortality: up to 30% in setting of coexisting congenital anomalies

B. GASTROSCHISIS

1. Abdominal wall defect, generally less than 5 cm and located to right of umbilical cord, evisceration of bowel, covered by inflammatory peel, no sac

65

GENERAL PEDIATRIC SURGERY

2. Incidence: 1 in 2000 live births
3. Associated anomalies: malrotation, intestinal atresia (10%–20%)
4. Work-up: seen on antenatal ultrasound, serial ultrasounds, MRI if inconclusive
5. Labs: elevated AFP and acetylcholinesterase in amniotic fluid; higher maternal serum AFP
6. Mode of delivery (vaginal vs. C-section) determined by obstetric indications; term delivery
7. Medical management
   a. Identical to omphalocele
   b. Strict glucose monitoring—at risk for hypoglycemia
8. Surgical management
   a. Enlarge defect in setting of bowel compromise, untwist to restore circulation if needed
   b. Inspect bowel for atresia, necrosis, or perforation; do not remove intestinal peel.
      (1) Consider primary anastomosis of healthy bowel if atresia present
   c. Goal is return of bowel into abdomen without damage to other viscera.
      (1) Primary reduction and fascial closure
      (2) Silo placement, serial reduction, delayed fascial closure
      (3) Primary or delayed reduction without fascial closure
9. Mortality: approximately 10%

C. UMBILICAL HERNIA
1. Defect in umbilical ring; most close spontaneously in the first 3–5 years of life
2. Incidence: higher in African-American and premature/low-birth-weight infants
3. Management: observe until 3–5 years of age; if no improvement in size, consider repair
   a. Absolute indications are rare: incarceration, strangulation, perforation, evisceration.
   b. Larger defects (>1.5 cm) persisting past 5 years of age should be repaired.
4. Repair: transverse closure, inversion of umbilical skin

D. INGUINAL HERNIA
1. Patent processus vaginalis, 10% bilateral, majority are indirect
2. Incidence: higher in preterm infants and males
3. Signs/symptoms: asymptomatic, intermittent bulge with increased intraabdominal pressure (crying, straining)
   a. Found by parents at bathing or pediatrician during well-child check
   b. Incarcerated with obstruction: pain, distention, vomiting, obstipation
4. Work-up: physical examination, ultrasound

5. Surgical management: will not resolve spontaneously and high risk of incarceration; surgical repair required, uses high ligation of the sac
   a. Laparoscopic repair, evaluate contralateral side
   b. Attempt reduction of incarcerated bowel; if strangulation suspected or unable to reduce, urgent repair indicated

E. SHORT BOWEL SYNDROME

1. Deficiency or removal of large portion of small bowel resulting in insufficient absorptive surface area to sustain growth, hydration, or electrolyte balance
2. Etiology: necrotizing enterocolitis (most common), intestinal atresia, gastroschisis, malrotation with volvulus
3. Incidence: 1%; survival: 90%
4. Symptoms: malnutrition, weight loss or inadequate weight gain, diarrhea, steatorrhea
5. Medical management: enteral feeds favored, parenteral nutrition as needed for adequate supplementation
   a. H_2 blockers (treats hypersecretion), loperamide (treats diarrhea), and erythromycin (for dysmotility)
   b. Antibiotics: broad-spectrum IV antibiotics for catheter-associated blood stream infections; Cipro/Flagyl for bacterial overgrowth
   c. Omegaven (IV fish oil formula) in the setting of intestinal failure–associated liver disease
6. Surgical management
   a. Longitudinal intestinal lengthening and tailoring (LILT) operation
   b. Iowa I operation (two stage, lengthening procedure)
   c. Serial transverse enteroplasty (STEP) operation—alternating transverse application of surgical stapling device
   d. Intestinal transplantation

VII. ANORECTAL MALFORMATIONS

1. Large spectrum of defects, ranging from mild anal anomalies to complex cloacal malformations
2. Incidence: 1 in 5000 live births
   a. Most common defect in males: rectourethral fistula
   b. Most common defect in females: rectovestibular fistula
   c. Imperforate anus without fistula associated with Down syndrome
3. Diagnosis: physical examination
   a. Meconium visualized on perineum confirms rectoperineal fistula; in urine confirms rectourinary fistula
   b. Assess for associated defects—VATER symptom complex: vertebral, anorectal, tracheal, esophageal, renal
   c. Imaging: cross-table lateral x-ray to assess position of rectum
4. Medical management: IV fluids, antibiotics, gastric decompression

65

GENERAL PEDIATRIC SURGERY

5. Surgical management
   a. Presence of a perineal fistula, anal stenosis, or rectum below coccyx: posterior sagittal anorectoplasty
   b. Significant associated defects, premature, meconium in urine, or rectal gas above the coccyx: colostomy, staged repair
6. Complications: infection, dehiscence, strictures, rectal mucosal prolapse
   a. Constipation—most common, treat with bowel regimen
   b. Fecal incontinence—due to sphincter dysfunction versus constipation versus increased motility, treat with bowel management programs
   c. Urinary incontinence—intermittent catheterization

VIII. NEOPLASMS

A. NEUROBLASTOMA

1. Neoplasm of neural crest origin, most common malignant abdominal tumor in children
2. More than half less than 2 years old at diagnosis
3. Symptoms—metabolically active from catecholamines causing hypertension (25%) or vasoactive intestinal peptide excess
   a. Abdominal primary—abdominal mass (50%–75%); can occur in retroperitoneum, adrenal medulla, paraspinal ganglia
   b. Thoracic primary—respiratory distress, spinal cord compression
   c. Cervical primary—Horner syndrome
4. Diagnosis
   a. Abdominal radiograph (finely stippled tumor calcification), ultrasound (determine solid vs. cystic lesion)
   b. CT and MRI to determine resectability
   c. Metaiodobenzylguanidine (MIBG) scintigraphy—most sensitive and specific, shows primary tumor and bone involvement
   d. Urinary catecholamine breakdown products
5. Management—based on biologic features (karyotype, *MYCN* oncogene amplification status) and clinical stage
   a. Fetal diagnosis or less than 6 months old with small tumor—observe
   b. Low risk (stages 1 and 2a/b)—surgical excision alone
   c. Intermediate risk (stage 3)—surgery and chemotherapy
   d. High risk (stage 3 with amplified MYCN status, stage 4)—chemotherapy followed by complete (>90%) surgical resection if possible, radiotherapy for local control, myeloablative treatment with autologous stem cell rescue, and biologic therapies
6. Prognosis—inversely related to age; varies with site of primary, tumor histology, and MYCN status

B. WILMS TUMOR

1. Most common primary malignant renal tumor of childhood; second most common malignant abdominal tumor
2. Embryonal renal neoplasm

3. Presentation
   a. Mean age at diagnosis: 36 months
   b. Asymptomatic abdominal mass, hematuria, hypertension, 10% bilateral
   c. Associated congenital anomalies in 10%: WAGR (Wilms tumor, Aniridia, Genitourinary malformation, mental Retardation), Beckwith-Wiedemann syndrome, and Denys-Dash syndrome
4. Diagnosis:
   a. Ultrasound—determine site of origin, possible vascular or ureteral involvement
   b. CT abdomen—confirm renal origin, evaluate for bilateral tumors and metastatic disease (to liver)
   c. CT chest (metastatic lesions in lungs)
5. Surgical management:
   a. Surgical resection is primary component of treatment
   b. Requires safe resection, accurate staging, avoiding of complications that will upstage tumor (rupture, spillage)
   c. Hilar and regional lymph node sampling (bilateral)
   d. Remove tumor thrombus if extension into renal vein
6. Medical management:
   a. Neoadjuvant chemotherapy and radiation may enable operative resection if initially too large, intravascular extension of tumor thrombus to IVC, right atrium or bilateral tumors
   b. Adjuvant chemotherapy and radiation are beneficial and used in most cases
   c. Surgery alone for well-differentiated tumors less than 500 g
7. Prognosis: histology and stage of the tumor (most important factors), rapid response to treatment, loss of heterozygosity of 1p and 16q
   a. Worse with anaplasia, sarcomatous changes, positive nodes, higher staging, and older age

RECOMMENDED READINGS

Coran AG, Adzick NS, Krummel TM, Laberge JM, Shamberger RC, Caldamone AA, eds. *Pediatric Surgery*. 7th ed. Philadelphia: Elsevier; 2012.

Spitz L, Coran AG, eds. *Operative Pediatric Surgery*. 7th ed. Boca Raton, FL: CRC Press, Taylor&Francis Group; 2013.

65

GENERAL PEDIATRIC SURGERY

Neurosurgery

Christopher P. Carroll, MD

There are many nontraumatic neurosurgical conditions that pose an immediate threat to neurologic function or life. Due to the sensitivity of neurologic structures to insult and the relative lack of regenerative capacity in the central nervous system (CNS), the early recognition of such conditions is critical to prevent disabling neurologic deficit and loss of life. The high morbidity and mortality attributable to these conditions warrant their consideration as neurosurgical urgencies and emergencies. Although not meant to be exhaustive, this chapter provides an introduction to those nontraumatic neurosurgical urgencies or emergencies that will likely be encountered through the course of general surgical training and practice.

66

I. CRANIAL URGENCIES AND EMERGENCIES

A. SPONTANEOUS SUBARACHNOID HEMORRHAGE

1. Causative factors
   a. It may be traumatic or spontaneous (nontraumatic), with most common etiology being trauma.
   b. Spontaneous (e.g., nontraumatic) subarachnoid hemorrhage (SAH) is most commonly due to ruptured cerebral aneurysm (75%–80%).
      (1) Rupture of arteriovenous malformation (5%) is second most common nontraumatic etiology.
      (2) Mycotic/infectious aneurysm, CNS vasculitis, cerebrovascular dissection, and hemorrhagic tumors are less common etiologies.
         (a) The etiology is indeterminate in approximately 15% of spontaneous SAH.
   c. It can be accompanied by other intracranial hemorrhages.
      (1) Intracerebral hemorrhage (ICH) (20%–40%); intraventricular hemorrhage (IVH) (13%–28%); acute subdural hemorrhage (SDH) (2%–5%)
2. Clinical presentation
   a. Frequently present with "worst headache (HA) of life," nausea, vomiting, meningismus (neck stiffness), photophobia, and altered level of consciousness
      (1) Risk factors include prior aneurysm rupture, hypertension, cigarette smoking, alcohol abuse, and use of sympathomimetics (ephedrine, amphetamine, cocaine); there is slight predilection for females, and rates are higher with Japanese ancestry.
   b. May have neurologic deficit from cranial nerve (CN) compression, hydrocephalus if accompanied by IVH, or signs of herniation if accompanied by ICH or SDH
   c. Patients graded at presentation with Hunt and Hess (Table 66.1) or World Federation of Neurological Surgeons (WFNS) grade (Table 66.2).

TABLE 66.1

HUNT AND HESS CLASSIFICATION OF SUBARACHNOID HEMORRHAGE

Grade[a]	Description	Clinical Vasospasm (%)
1	Mild headache and meningismus; or asymptomatic	22
2	Moderate to severe headache and meningismus; fixed cranial nerve deficit	33
3	Confusion; somnolence, or mild focal deficit (e.g., weakness)	52
4	Obtundation; stupor; moderate to severe hemiparesis; decerebrate rigidity	53
5	Coma; decerebrate posturing; grave condition	74

[a]Add one grade for severe vasospasm on initial imaging or sever systemic illness.

TABLE 66.2

WORLD FEDERATION OF NEUROLOGICAL SURGEONS CLASSIFICATION OF SUBARACHNOID HEMORRHAGE

Grade	GCS Score	Major Focal Deficit
0	N/A (unruptured aneurysm)	N/A
1	15	Absent
2	13–14	Absent
3	13–14	Present
4	7–12	Present or absent
5	3–6	Present or absent

66

NEUROSURGERY

3. Evaluation
   a. Clinical evaluation: Stabilize ABCs (airway, breathing, circulation), and then perform rapid assessment of neurologic function, focusing on mental status, CN evaluation, and any motor or sensory deficits.
   b. Radiographic evaluation: Noncontrast computed tomography (CT) head is the imaging modality of choice and when performed within 48 hours of symptom onset has sensitivity of approximately 90%.
      (1) Radiographic findings include hyperdense subarachnoid blood concentrated in subarachnoid spaces; may also see ICH, IVH, SDH, hydrocephalus, or signs of herniation (Fig. 66.1)
      (2) If SAH is clinically suspected *and* CT head is negative, a lumbar puncture should be performed.
         (a) SAH suggested by high red blood cell (RBC) count (generally >10,000) that does not clear between tubes; differentiate from a traumatic tap with lower RBC count (generally <5000) and decreasing RBC count between tubes
         (b) Xanthrochromia (yellow cerebrospinal fluid [CSF] supernatant after centrifugation) can be seen as early as 2–4 hours after rupture and is ubiquitous (almost 100% of patients) by 12 hours; persists for approximately 2–3 weeks in majority of patients

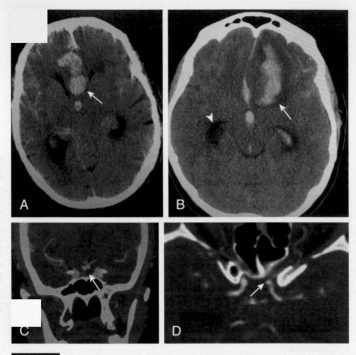

FIG. 66.1

(A) Acute subarachnoid hemorrhage involving interhemispheric fissure with intraventricular hemorrhage and early hydrocephalus *(arrow)*. (B) Acute subarachnoid hemorrhage of interhemispheric fissure with intraparenchymal hemorrhage of gyrus rectus and early hydrocephalus *(arrow)* (enlarged temporal horns *[arrowhead]*). (C) Anterior communicating artery aneurysm *(arrow)* identified in A. (D) Small left ophthalmic artery aneurysm *(arrow)* identified in B.

   c. If CT or lumbar puncture confirms SAH, focused vascular imaging is indicated.
   (1) Diagnostic cerebral angiography is the gold standard; invasive procedure with small (~1%) risk of arterial dissection or stroke
   (2) CT angiography is increasingly becoming the test of choice (sensitivity ~95%); rapid, noninvasive with primary risk being contrast nephropathy
      (a) If CT angiography is negative, proceed with diagnostic cerebral angiogram.
   (3) Magnetic resonance (MR) angiography has high sensitivity for subarachnoid blood (gradient echo/susceptibility-weighted angiography [GRE/SWAN] sequences) but lower overall sensitivity (~87%) for aneurysms; particularly poor for aneurysms less than 3 mm

d. If aneurysm is identified, be vigilant for additional lesions because approximately 20%–30% of patients with cerebral aneurysms have multiple.

(1) A total of 85%–90% of aneurysms are seen in the internal carotid circulation, with anterior communicating artery (30%), posterior communicating artery (25%), and middle cerebral artery (MCA) (20%) being the most common locations.

4. Initial management

a. Secure ABCs: Intubate as indicated (use short-acting paralytics to limit confounding neurologic examination for prolonged period); maintain systolic blood pressure (SBP) less than 160 mm Hg with goal SBP less than 140 mm Hg; and target mean arterial pressure (MAP) greater than 65 mm Hg to maintain cerebral perfusion.

(1) Strict blood pressure control reduces risk of re-rupture due to hypertension.

(2) Monitor creatine kinase MB (CKMB) and troponin for phenomena of posthemorrhagic stunned myocardium.

b. Provide antiepileptic medication for early seizure prophylaxis (e.g., levetiracetam or phenytoin twice a day [BID] × 7 days).

c. All spontaneous SAH patients should be started on nimodipine 60 mg every 4 (q4) hours orally for 21 days.

(1) Neuroprotective: improves morbidity and mortality without radiographic improvement in vasospasm (level I)

d. If acute hydrocephalus is seen, prompt placement of either ventriculostomy (extraventricular drain [EVD]) or lumbar drain to treat hydrocephalus.

(1) Acute hydrocephalus is a common treatable cause of acute deterioration after rupture and is life-threatening if untreated.

e. Treat elevated intracranial pressure (see page 268).

f. Maintain euvolemia and eunatremia—patients will often experience cerebral salt wasting or syndrome of inappropriate antidiuretic hormone secretion.

5. Surgical management

a. Prompt neurosurgical consultation is essential for evaluation and treatment of acute spontaneous SAH.

b. Aneurysms can be treated with either open or endovascular surgery.

(1) Open procedures: craniotomy for clipping, aneurysm trapping with or without cerebrovascular bypass, and parent vessel sacrifice

(2) Endovascular procedures: coil embolization, flow diverting stent, stent-assisted coiling, or parent vessel sacrifice

c. If feasible vis-à-vis clinical status and operative risk factors, early intervention (first 48–72 hours) is favored.

(1) Reduces risk window for re-rupture while aneurysm is unsecured

(2) Allows for hyperdynamic therapy of potential vasospasm (especially vasopressor regimen) when aneurysm is secured

66

NEUROSURGERY

TABLE 66.3			

MODIFIED FISHER SCALE CLASSIFICATION OF SUBARACHNOID HEMORRHAGE

Score	SAH on CT[a]	IVH on CT	Clinical Vasospasm (%)
N/A	No SAH	No IVH	
1	Thin SAH, focal or diffuse	No IVH	24
2	Thin SAH, focal or diffuse	IVH present	33
3	Thick SAH, focal or diffuse	No IVH	33
4	Thick SAH, focal or diffuse	IVH present	40

[a]Measurement made of largest axial and longitudinal dimension on axial computed tomography (CT) within 5 days of hemorrhage.

IVH, Intraventricular hemorrhage; *SAH,* subarachnoid hemorrhage.

6. **Vasospasm: delayed cerebrovascular changes, including vasoconstriction and vascular smooth muscle remodeling, which may result in delayed cerebral ischemia**
   a. Angiographic vasospasm is common in aneurysmal SAH (50%–70%), but clinical vasospasm is seen only in approximately 30% of aneurysmal SAH patients.
      (1) Less commonly seen in other SAH etiologies such as trauma; exception is penetrating brain injury (~20%–30%)
   b. It is rarely seen in first 48–72 hours; risk window is primarily days 3–14 post hemorrhage.
      (1) Peak incidence is at day 6–8 post hemorrhage; it is rarely seen beyond day 21 post hemorrhage.
      (2) Primary risk factor is amount of subarachnoid blood, which is graded with modified Fisher scale score (Table 66.3).
   c. Treatment is targeted at maintaining cerebral perfusion and opening critically vasoconstricted vessels.
      (1) Diagnosed clinically or angiographically; often perform surveillance regimen of transcranial Doppler studies
      (2) Clinically maintain euvolemia, hyperdynamic therapy, and modification of blood rheology ("triple H" therapy: hypervolemia, induced hypertension, and hemodilution).
      (3) Endovascular treatment options include intraarterial vasodilator administration (e.g., verapamil), angioplasty with or without stenting, or combination thereof.
7. **Outcome of SAH**
   a. Thirty-day mortality is frequently cited as 40%–60%.
      (1) A total of 10%–15% of patients will die before reaching medical care.
      (2) A total of 10% of patients die within first 72 hours, frequently due to rebleeding.
         (a) Rebleeding risk for unsecured aneurysm is 15%–20% in first 14 days and approximately 4% in first 24 hours.

(3) Approximately 25% die from medical complications of hemorrhage (e.g., myocardial infarction [MI], pneumonia (PNA), pulmonary embolism [PE]); 7% die due to complications of vasospasm.

b. Of those surviving their SAH, approximately one-third will have moderate or severe disability and approximately one-third return to their baseline functional status and quality of life.

c. Age (≥70 years) and presentation WFNS grade are best predictors of long-term outcome.

B. SPONTANEOUS INTRACEREBRAL/INTRAPARENCHYMAL HEMORRHAGE

1. Epidemiology
   a. ICH is the second most common form of stroke (15%–30%) but also has the highest mortality.
   b. Risk factors include age, male gender, previous stroke, hypertension (particularly uncontrolled), cigarette smoking, alcohol abuse, liver dysfunction, and sympathomimetic use.
   c. It is commonly seen in basal ganglia (50%), thalamus (15%), pons (10%–15%), hemispheric (10%–20%), and cerebellum (10%).
   d. Common etiologies include hypertensive urgency/emergency, sympathomimetic abuse (e.g., cocaine, amphetamine, ephedrine), coagulopathy (primary or iatrogenic), vascular abnormality (e.g., arteriovenous malformation [AVM], aneurysm), hemorrhagic transformation of prior stroke, tumor, and angiopathy.

2. Clinical presentation
   a. Generally hemorrhagic stroke (ICH) patients present with progressive symptom onset; compare with acute/immediate maximal deficit of ischemic or embolic stroke.
   b. Symptoms may be mild (HA, nausea, vomiting) or severe (coma, hemiplegia, herniation syndromes) and depend on both size and location of hemorrhage.

3. Evaluation
   a. CT head without contrast is the test of choice; it readily demonstrates all but the smallest ICHs (Fig. 66.2).
      (1) It may be associated with intraventricular, subarachnoid, or SDH if it transgresses pia/ependymal boundaries.
      (2) Location often narrows probable etiologies of the bleed.
         (a) Hypertensive ICH is most frequently seen in basal ganglia, thalamus, pons, and cerebellar hemispheres.
      (3) Repeat CT head often performed to establish stability of bleed; 30% will progress.
   b. Delayed MRI with and without contrast is often performed after patient is clinically stable to evaluate for underlying tumor or vascular malformation.
   c. Cerebral angiography may be pursued to rule out AVM, aneurysm, or angiopathy associated with ICH.

66

NEUROSURGERY

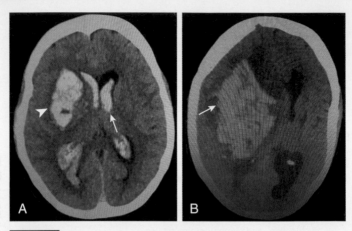

FIG. 66.2
(A) Acute intracerebral hemorrhage of the right basal ganglia *(arrowhead)* with intraventricular extension *(arrow)*. (B) Large acute right frontotemporoparietal intracerebral
hemorrhage with subfalcine herniation *(arrow)*.

4. Treatment
   a. Largely supportive and similar to acute SAH
      (1) Secure ABCs; blood pressure control (maintain SBP <160 mm
          Hg with goal SBP <140 mm Hg and target MAP >65 mm Hg);
          provide seizure prophylaxis for 7 days; prompt placement of
          ventriculostomy (EVD) for acute hydrocephalus; treat elevated
          intracranial pressure (see page 268)
   b. Surgical intervention remains controversial and under active inves-
      tigation with randomized controlled trials; results of prior trials and
      meta-analyses are often conflicting.
      (1) Surgery is generally thought to offer mortality benefit without
          significant benefit for neurologic recovery.
      (2) Lesions amenable to surgical evacuation include those approach-
          ing the cortical surface and cerebellar hemorrhages.
      (3) Surgical decompression and evacuation may be indicated
          in life-threatening herniation syndromes and cerebellar
          hemorrhages.
          (a) Surgery likely of little benefit in: minimally symptomatic
              lesions, massive ICH or large ICH of dominant hemisphere;
              patients With Glasgow Coma Scale (GCS) ≤5 or loss of
              brainstem reflexes; and elderly patients (age ≥75).
5. ICH outcomes
   a. Patients may be evaluated at admission using ICH score (30-day
      mortality, Table 66.4) or Functional Outcome in Patients With
      Primary Intracerebral Hemorrhage (FUNC) score (90-day functional

TABLE 66.4
INTRACEREBRAL HEMORRHAGE SCORE

Parameter	Finding	Points	Total ICH Score	30-Day Mortality (%)
GCS score (see	3–4	2	0	0
Table 20.1)	5–12	1	1	13
	13–15	0	2	26
Patient age	≥80 years	1	3	72
	<80 years	0	4	97
ICH location	Infratentorial	1	5	100
	Supratentorial	0	6	N/R ($n = 0$)
ICH volume[a]	≥30 mL	1		
	<30 mL	0		
IVH	Present	1		
	Absent	0		
Total score		0–6		

[a]Measurement made as ($L \times W \times H$)/2 on computed tomography (CT).
GCS, Glasgow Coma Scale; *ICH,* intracerebral hemorrhage; *IVH,* intraventricular hemorrhage; *N/R,* not recorded.

TABLE 66.5
FUNC SCORE FOR INTRACEREBRAL HEMORRHAGE

Parameter	Finding	Points	Total FUNC Score	90-Day Functional Independence	
				All Patients (%)	Survivors Only (%)
ICH volume[a]	<30 cc	4			
	30–60 cc	2	11	82	95
	>60 cc	0	9–10	66	75
Patient age	<70 years	2	8	42	48
	70–80 years	1	5–7	13	29
	>80 years	0	0–4	0	0
ICH location	Lobar	2			
	Deep	1			
	Infratentorial	0			
GCS (see	≥9	2			
Table 20.1)	≤8	0			
Pre-ICH cognitive impairment	Absent	1			
	Present	0			
Total score		0–11			

[a]Measurement made as ($L \times W \times H$)/2 on CT.
ICH, Intracerebral hemorrhage.

independence, Table 66.5); some controversy surrounds the use of these scores to guide management decisions.

b. Overall 30-day mortality is 40%–50% but is highly dependent on patient age, location and size of lesion, and etiology of hemorrhage.

c. Due to frequent location in basal ganglia and thalamus, it often results in disability due to hemiparesis; severity varies widely.

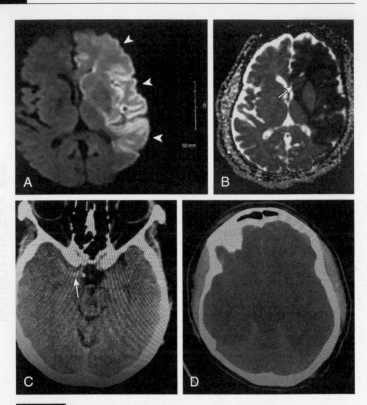

FIG. 66.3
(A) Acute middle cerebral artery (MCA) stroke on magnetic resonance imaging (MRI) apparent diffusion coefficient (ADC) sequence *(arrowheads)*. (B) Acute MCA stroke of A on MRI diffusion-weighted imaging (DWI) sequence, note sparing of the caudate *(arrow)*. (C) Hyperdense MCA seen in acute MCA thrombosis on CT *(arrow)*. (D) Bilateral acute strokes of the internal carotid artery (ICA) territories; note absence of gray-weight differentiation and loss of sulcal-gyral pattern due to edema.

C. MALIGNANT STROKE (Fig. 66.3)

1. A stroke or cerebral infarction entails irreversible neuron cell death due to inadequate cerebral perfusion; so-called malignant strokes threaten herniation due to mass effect by acute cerebral edema.
   a. Most commonly seen in MCA strokes involving greater than 50% of the MCA territory, resulting in subfalcine and uncal herniation
   b. Can be seen less commonly in complete posterior cerebral artery (PCA) strokes due to edema of the medial temporal lobe and resultant uncal herniation

   c. Also seen in large hemispheric cerebellar strokes where cerebellar edema results in brainstem compression and rapid neurologic decline

2. **Treatment of malignant stroke is similar to that of an expanding mass lesion and herniation syndrome.**
   a. Secure ABCs and stabilize vital signs.
   b. Hypertonic therapy or hyperventilation may be used as temporizing maneuver.
   c. Malignant stroke with clinical or radiographic progression, from neurologic decline to frank evidence of herniation, often requires surgical decompression via craniectomy.
     (1) Decompressive hemicraniectomy may reduce malignant MCA stroke mortality from approximately 80% to 37%; evidence for both improved mortality and functional outcomes
     (2) No strict indications, but generally decompression is considered for patients younger than 70 years; clinical or radiographic evidence of complete MCA stroke; clinical or radiographic evidence of large internal carotid artery (ICA), MCA, PCA, or cerebellar stroke resulting in clinical or radiographic evidence of herniation; and less than 72 hours from stroke onset (ICA/MCA/PCA) or less than 96 hours from stroke onset for cerebellar stroke.

D. HYDROCEPHALUS

Hydrocephalus is the abnormal accumulation of CSF within the ventricular system of the brain due to either obstruction of CSF circulation, abnormal CSF reabsorption at arachnoid granulations, or overproduction of CSF as in tumors of choroid plexus (rare). It is often described as either obstructive or noncommunicating or communicating.

1. **Acute hydrocephalus**
   a. Obstructive or noncommunicating hydrocephalus involves disruption of CSF circulation before the arachnoid granulations.
     (1) Classically seen with intraventricular and tectal tumors
     (2) Leads to CSF trapped in ventricular system proximal to lesion (e.g., biventricular hydrocephalus as seen with tumor obstructing foramina of Monro while third and fourth ventricles remain within normal limits) **(Fig. 66.4)**
     (3) Acute obstructive hydrocephalus may be seen with extensive IVH, leading to obstructive hydrocephalus.
   b. Communicating hydrocephalus is due to abnormal reabsorption of CSF at arachnoid granulations.
     (1) It is classically seen with posthemorrhagic or postinfectious etiologies.
     (2) All ventricles are enlarged by accumulating CSF.
     (3) Acute communicating hydrocephalus may be seen in the posthemorrhagic period (SAH or IVH) or after infectious meningitis.

66

NEUROSURGERY

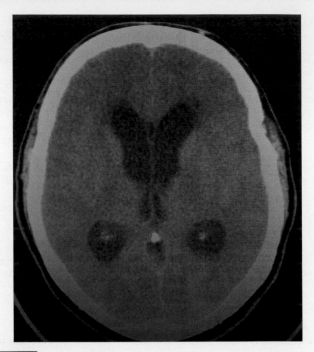

FIG. 66.4
Acute hydrocephalus with enlargement of both lateral ventricles.

   c. Presentation typically is that of elevated intracranial pressure (ICP): HA, nausea, emesis, blurring of vision, papilledema, ataxia, upgaze, or abducens palsies.

     (1) Acute hydrocephalus is rarely asymptomatic; chronic ventricular enlargement may be asymptomatic.

   d. Treatment of patients with acute neurologic decline often necessitates CSF diversion by EVD placement or, if communicating, by serial lumbar puncture or lumbar drain placement.

     (1) May be transient, especially in posthemorrhagic hydrocephalus but those who are reliant on CSF diversion will eventually need CSF shunt placement or third ventriculostomy.

     (2) Shunt may be placed from ventricles or lumbar cistern (communicating) to peritoneal cavity, pleural space, right atrium (via external jugular or facial vein), gallbladder, or bladder.

       (a) Ventriculoperitoneal shunts are the most common by far.

   e. Shunt infection is a frequent complication, seen in 5%–10% of new shunt placements.

(1) Most infections occur in first 2 months after placement.
(2) Spontaneous primary shunt infection becomes exceedingly unlikely at 12–24 months after placement.
  (a) Evaluation of a patient with a "mature" shunt infection should include evaluation for an extraventricular source (often seen with bacteremia in setting of urinary tract infection [UTI] or soft tissue infections).

2. **Shunted hydrocephalus and shunt malfunction**
   a. A common clinical scenario is that of a patient with known shunted hydrocephalus who presents with symptoms of elevated ICP due to shunt malfunction.
   b. Malfunction is commonly due to inadvertent reprogramming of programmable shunts, infection, occlusion of proximal or distal catheter, disconnection, or ventricular trapping.
   c. Evaluation generally involves plain x-ray (XR) shunt series of the skull, neck, chest, and abdomen to confirm valve type; shunt location and continuity; and, if adjustable, valve setting in addition to a CT of head to evaluate ventricular system.
   d. Treatment of decompensating shunt malfunction is shunt revision, although in the case of infection patients may first need externalization (as in abdominal pseudocyst formation) or EVD placement.

II. SPINAL URGENCIES AND EMERGENCIES

Vascular, congenital, and degenerative disease of the spinal column are often considered subacute or chronic pathologies. Degenerative spondylosis of the cervical, thoracic, and lumbar spine is exceedingly common such that the majority of patients of middle or advanced age will have clinical or radiographic evidence of degenerative spinal disease. Although often chronic in nature, there are a subset of nontraumatic spinal pathologies that warrant prompt evaluation and urgent or emergent intervention to preserve neurologic function.

A. DEGENERATIVE SPINAL DISEASE

Chronic neck (cervicalgia) or back pain (lumbago) are frequent complaints in outpatient, ambulatory, and emergency settings. Pain may or may not be accompanied by clinical neurologic deficit or radiographic abnormality. While most spinal pathologies are nonurgent, the recognition of those few urgent/emergent presentations of spinal pathology is essential to prevent significant morbidity including paralysis.

1. **Cauda equina syndrome**
   a. A clinical syndrome presenting with a combination of significant weakness of the lower extremities, bilateral paresthesias/anesthesia, disturbance of sphincter function, low back pain (LBP) or radiculopathy, hyporeflexia or areflexia, and sexual dysfunction.

(1) Some or all symptoms may be present, although it is classically seen as combination of LBP/radiculopathy, "saddle anesthesia," bilateral lower extremity weakness, and urinary retention with or without overflow incontinence.

(2) Autonomic dysfunction is a late symptom (urinary retention, impotence).

(3) Depressed or absent patella and Achilles reflexes are often seen.

b. Due to compression of multiple lumbosacral nerve roots of the cauda equina

(1) Usually bilateral symptoms across multiple spinal levels, typically L2 or lower

(2) Pain is often a dominant symptom, severe, and helps to differentiate from conus medullaris syndrome.

c. Most frequently due to large herniation of lumbar intervertebral disc, most commonly at L4–L5 or L5–S1

(1) Also seen with high-grade spondylolisthesis, tumors of the lumbar spine; postoperatively after lumbar spine surgery (e.g., hematoma or free graft material); and with spontaneous epidural hematoma (rare)

d. Usually will either develop acutely (e.g., large acute disc herniation) or indolently. The latter carries a worse prognosis.

e. Evaluation is typically urgent spine service consultation and obtaining CT/magnetic resonance imaging (MRI) of the lumbar spine.

(1) MRI is often the imaging modality of choice, given its demonstration of soft tissue pathologies often occult on CT.

f. Treatment is surgical decompression.

(1) Timing of surgery is controversial and a frequent topic in litigation. In general, strive to perform surgery within first 24 hours, although up to 48 hours may be done for preoperative medical optimization or in setting of irreversible anticoagulants.

(2) There is no statistically significant evidence of worsened neurologic outcome with delay up to 48 hours.

2. Conus medullaris syndrome

a. Clinical syndrome presenting with combination of weakness (often symmetric), saddle anesthesia, sphincter dysfunction (urinary retention with overflow incontinence and fecal incontinence), and loss of the Achilles reflex

(1) Pain is a rare component, which helps to differentiate from cauda equina syndrome. When present, typically in perineum or inner thighs

(2) Typically acute with sudden or rapid onset of bilateral symptoms

(3) Patellar reflex usually spared

(4) Fasciculations may be seen

b. Frequently due to disc herniation at level of conus medullaris, typically L1–L2

      (1) May also be seen in nontraumatic compression fractures, spinal tumors, postoperatively, or abscesses

  c. Evaluation is the same as for cauda equina syndrome: urgent spine service consultation and appropriate imaging guided by neurologic deficits on examination (typically cervical, thoracic, or both will be imaged).

  d. As with cauda equina syndrome, treatment is urgent surgical decompression.

3. **Myelopathy**

  a. Myelopathy results from compression of the spinal cord in the cervical or thoracic spine.

  b. Typically patients present with combination of bilateral extremity weakness (upper and lower extremities may both be affected) and sensory change with or without pain.

    (1) Sphincter or autonomic dysfunction may also be seen, and gait abnormalities (wide-based gait) are frequent.

    (2) It is often chronic or indolent in nature; acute presentations raise likelihood of disc herniation or pathologic fracture.

  c. It may be seen with a number of degenerative cervicothoracic conditions.

    (1) Frequently seen with cervicothoracic disc herniations or degenerative spinal stenosis of the cervical or thoracic spine

    (2) Less frequently seen in association with kyphoscoliosis, epidural lipomatosis (proliferation of epidural fat resulting in compression of thecal sac), and tumors of spinal column or canal

  d. Evaluation is typically performed with CT/MRI of the cervicothoracic spine.

  e. Treatment is typically surgical decompression with or without fixation and fusion, dependent on pathology and spinal level.

4. **Radiculopathy**

  a. It is characterized by pain and/or sensory disturbance in the distribution of a single dermatome and may be accompanied by weakness or disturbed reflexes.

  b. Often due to spinal intervertebral disc herniations, degenerative spondylosis, or degenerative spondylolisthesis resulting in nerve root impingement, although many other pathologies are possible

  c. Patients will typically improve with conservative treatment within 6 months of symptom onset.

  d. Imaging is based on severity of clinical presentation, but with persistent radiculopathy or weakness MRI of the suspected spinal region without contrast is often obtained. Lateral plain XRs can be obtained but are often limited.

    (1) Degenerative spinal pathology is seen in the majority of patients older than 50 years and is frequently asymptomatic.

  e. Indications for early imaging or spinal service consultation include cauda equina syndrome (see earlier); progressive neurologic deficit (e.g., weakness); failure of conservative management; or severe disabling radicular pain with conservative management of greater than 6–12 weeks.

III. CNS TUMORS

Although an exhaustive review of neurooncology is beyond the scope of this text, a general introduction to tumors of the brain and spine is essential for the general surgery house officer as mass effect, edema, and hemorrhage from brain tumors can lead to neurosurgical emergencies.

A. BRAIN TUMORS (FIG. 66.5)

1. Many brain tumors have an indolent course up to presentation, whereas others may progress rapidly and be accompanied by a rapid development and progression of neurologic symptoms, often without regard for their benign or malignant features.

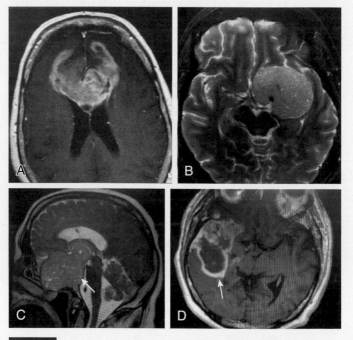

FIG. 66.5

(A) Bifrontal (also known as "butterfly") glioblastoma multiforme on post-contrast T1 magnetic resonance imaging (MRI). (B) Large left sphenoid wing meningioma encapsulating the left internal carotid artery. (C) Large pituitary adenoma eroding into upper nasopharynx *(arrow)*. (D) Right temporal lobe glioblastoma multiforme *(arrow)*.

a. The most common presenting symptom is progressive neurologic deficit, such as hemiparesis, hemianesthesia, aphasia, memory impairment, visual field deficit, or cranial nerve palsies with sellar and posterior fossa lesions.
   (1) It may be occult to patient and subtle on examination.
   (2) Motor weakness is the most common at presentation (~40%).
b. HAs are frequent with or without elevation of ICP and present in approximately 50% of patients who present with a brain tumor, primary or metastatic.
   (1) Severity often worsens with Valsalva and other maneuvers that elevate ICP (such as bending forward or down).
   (2) It is frequently accompanied by nausea and/or vomiting.
   (3) There are no features that reliably differentiate HA of brain tumor from much more common tension-type HA.
c. Seizure, often acute onset with or without secondary generalization, is the presenting symptom in approximately one-quarter of patients with brain tumor.
   (1) New onset seizures in atraumatic patient older than 40 years should be considered secondary to an intracranial mass lesion (hemorrhage, infection, tumor, etc.) until proven otherwise.
   (2) Seizures are rarely seen with posterior fossa tumors.
d. Elevated intracranial pressure is a common presentation of posterior fossa tumors, given the increased comorbidity of hydrocephalus.
   (1) Often present with HA, nausea, vomiting, and papilledema (>50%)
e. A posterior fossa tumor in an adult should be considered a metastasis until proven otherwise, and a systemic evaluation for primary malignancy should be promptly undertaken.
   (1) Often biopsy of primary site carries lower morbidity than does brain biopsy/resection.

2. **Evaluation of suspected brain tumors**
   a. Initial evaluation in adults is often a noncontrast CT of the head, which discloses the lesion and may also demonstrate evidence of mass effect or herniation, hemorrhage, and/or cerebral edema (Fig. 66.6).
   b. A high-quality MRI with and without contrast of the brain is the imaging modality of choice to better discriminate features of the lesion, as well as evaluate for multiple lesions (which may be occult on CT).
      (1) Not all brain tumors are enhancing, particularly low-grade gliomas.
   c. Systemic evaluation with CT of chest, abdomen, and pelvis is often performed in adults to evaluate for extracranial primary malignancy and should be performed promptly if history, examination, or radiographic features are suggestive of metastatic disease.
   d. MRI of spine is obtained for particular types of tumors to rule out "drop" metastases of primary tumors or spinal metastases in diffusely metastatic disease.

3. Initial management
    a. Early neurosurgical consultation is essential.
    b. Often will start seizure prophylaxis (supratentorial tumors); oral steroid regimen (cerebral edema and low suspicion for lymphoma), and nausea regimen
    c. Patients with progressive hydrocephalus, neurologic deficit, or hemorrhagic tumors may require urgent neurosurgical intervention.
4. Pediatric brain tumors are the second most common malignancy in children after leukemia (2–5 per 100,000).
    a. Commonly gliomas, germ cell tumors, and primitive neuroectodermal tumors (PNETs)
        (1) Cerebellar astrocytoma (a glioma) and medulloblastoma (a PNET) are the most common
    b. Predilection for posterior fossa tumors as compared with adults where supratentorial primary brain tumors far outweigh infratentorial

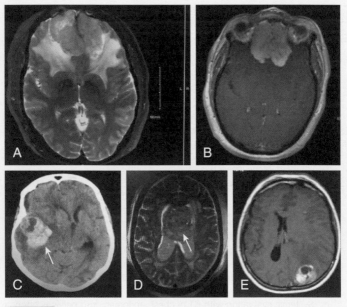

FIG. 66.6

(A and B) Large olfactory groove meningioma with significant surrounding edema on T2 FLAIR (A) and compression of the bilateral frontal lobes. (C) Hemorrhagic metastasis of the right temporal lobe with associated uncal and subfalcine herniation. (D) Central neurocytoma resulting in hydrocephalus of the bilateral ventricles *(arrow)*. (E) Left parietal glioblastoma multiforme with cerebral edema resulting in midline shift and compression of the left lateral ventricle.

   c. Neurocutaneous disorders (also known as phakomatoses), such as neurofibromatosis 1, neurofibromatosis 2, tuberous sclerosis, and von Hippel-Lindau, often present in childhood.

     (1) Characterized by common constellations of symptoms and cutaneous stigmata often present in childhood

5. Primary brain tumors

   a. Astrocytoma is the most common variety of primary intraaxial brain tumor, with glioblastoma multiforme (World Health Organization [WHO] Grade IV) being the most common primary brain tumor and also the astrocytoma with the highest number of malignant characteristics.

     (1) Surgical resection followed by the Stupp regimen (stereotactic radiotherapy, and temozolomide) has become the current standard for glioblastoma multiforme treatment at many centers with a median survival of 14.6 months.

     (2) New molecular markers and targets as well as immunotherapies are being actively researched to improve outcomes.

       (a) O^6-methylguanine-DNA-methyltransferase (MGMT) promoter methylation leads to a median survival of 18.2 months, with 34% 2-year survival versus 7.8% 2-year survival in unmethylated tumors.

   b. Meningiomas are slow-growing extraaxial tumors; they are the most common intracranial tumor, approximately 3% in autopsy series; and they are often slow growing and benign.

     (1) Small percentage (~2%) may have intraaxial (brain) invasion and malignant features.

     (2) Approximately one-third of incidental meningiomas will have no radiographic evidence of growth on 3-year follow up.

     (3) Due to slow growth and benign features, they may grow to be giant before creating symptoms due to mass effect.

     (4) Surgical resection, when complete, is often curative but not always feasible.

     (5) Other treatment options include observation (often indicated for small or incidental tumors) and stereotactic radiosurgery (smaller lesions).

   c. Nerve tumors of the cranial nerves are often benign, with the most common being vestibular schwannoma.

     (1) It frequently presents with combination of hearing loss, tinnitus, and dysequilibrium.

     (2) Audiogram is essential to preoperative work-up.

     (3) Treatment options include observation, stereotactic radiosurgery, and open resection with choice dependent on tumor size, location, hearing stats on audiogram, facial nerve function, and presence of neurofibromatosis 2 (bilateral vestibular schwannomas).

   d. Pituitary tumors are most often benign adenomas arising from the anterior pituitary gland, most commonly nonsecretory but frequently present with endocrine disturbance due to secretion or compression of the pituitary stalk.

(1) Large sellar tumors may compress the optic chiasm, resulting in visual field deficits (classically bitemporal hemianopsia), and can invade the cavernous sinus, resulting in cranial nerve palsies (lateral rectus palsy [CNVI] is the most common).

(2) Work up as previously mentioned plus endocrine evaluation.

   (a) Hypocortisolism can be life threatening when severe in the form of addisonian crisis and requires immediate supplementation with glucocorticoids.

   (b) Prolactinomas are unique in that they are highly susceptible to medical management with dopamine agonists.

(3) Pituitary apoplexy is a neurologic and/or endocrine deterioration due to rapid expansion of a pituitary mass, usually due to necrosis or hemorrhage.

   (a) Frequently presents as severe abrupt onset HA with fixed neurologic deficit (visual loss or opthalmoplegia are most common) or endocrine deficit in patients with pituitary mass.

   (b) Managed with urgent administration of glucocorticoids (addisonian crisis is the endocrine deficit that kills) and surgical resection.

(4) It is often managed with observation, medical management (prolactinoma), stereotactic radiosurgery, or resection.

   (a) Resection can be open cranial resection or endoscopic endonasal resection via transsphenoidal approach.

6. Cerebral metastases

   a. Cerebral metastases are the most common form of brain tumor and are frequently multiple (~70%) at the time of diagnosis.

   b. Evaluation is similar to that of primary brain tumors: high-quality MRI with and without contrast of brain as well as systemic imaging to identify primary malignancy and any extracranial metastases.

   (1) Identification of primary malignancy and extracranial metastases is often critical for staging and identifying lower risk site for biopsy.

   (2) A solitary intracranial lesion in setting of known primary often will require biopsy because approximately 10% will be primary brain neoplasms.

   c. The most common primary malignancies seen as cerebral metastases are lung carcinoma (40%), breast carcinoma (10%), renal cell carcinoma (7%), colorectal cancers (6%), and melanoma (3%).

   (1) Almost any primary malignancy may metastasize to the brain such that a brain lesion in setting of any primary malignancy should be considered a metastasis until proven otherwise.

   (2) A posterior fossa lesion in an adult is a metastasis until proven otherwise.

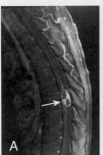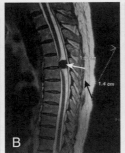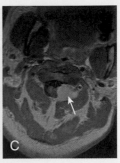

FIG. 66.7

(A) Intradural-extramedullary thoracic metastasis. (B) Intradural-extramedullary thoracic meningioma *(white arrow)*. (C) Intradural-extramedullary left C2 spinal schwannoma *(white arrow)*.

   d. Treatment varies with neurologic symptoms, status of primary malignancy, size, number/volume of metastases, and location.

     (1) Biopsy with possible resection is indicated when no primary malignancy is identified.

     (2) Surgical resection is often considered for large solitary lesions, symptomatic lesions, lesions with mass effect or resulting hydrocephalus, hemorrhagic lesions, and posterior fossa lesions but varies case by case.

B. SPINAL TUMORS (FIG. 66.7)

Spinal tumors can be primary (spinal cord, meninges, or peripheral nerves) or metastatic (vertebral, dural, parenchymal, or peripheral nerve). Tumors can be considered as extradural versus intradural and intradural-extramedullary versus intradural-intramedullary. Such a classification can help to guide differential diagnoses.

1. **Primary spinal tumors**
   a. Approximately 10%–15% of all primary CNS tumors involve the spine or spinal cord; most primary spinal tumors are benign.
   b. The majority of spinal tumors are either extradural (~50%–60%) or intradural-extramedullary (30%–40%).
      (1) Only 5% are intramedullary spinal cord tumors.
         (a) In adults, approximately one-third of primary intramedullary tumors are low-grade astrocytomas and one-third are ependymomas.
         (b) The remaining 40% include glioblastoma, germ cell tumors, and dermoid and epidermoid tumors, among others.
      (2) Primary extradural tumors are rare (chordoma, osteoblastoma, chondrosarcoma, osteosarcoma).

(3) The majority of primary intradural-extramedullary tumors are meningiomas or peripheral nerve tumors (schwannoma, neurofibroma).

c. Presentation of spinal tumors is often with pain and myelopathy, although many may start with radiculopathy (especially schwannomas) that progresses to myelopathy as the mass compresses the spinal cord.

   (1) Symptom onset is usually gradual but may progress rapidly in cases of tumor hemorrhage, associated syringomyelia, or parenchymal edema.

d. Evaluation often consists of systemic survey for primary malignancy and high-quality MRI with or without contrast of the spinal column (as multifocal metastases or multifocal benign primary tumors are not infrequent).

e. Treatment for asymptomatic lesions is often observation with intervention or even biopsy often outweighed by the potential risk of neurologic deficit after surgery.

f. Treatment for symptomatic lesions begins with biopsy and resection (as feasible) as soon as possible after symptom onset.

   (1) In low-grade intradural lesions a plane may be developed between the tumor and cord, allowing total excision.

      (a) For intradural-extramedullary low-grade tumors, if a plane is present a complete resection may be attempted, but one always sides toward partial resection in favor of possible transgression into the spinal cord parenchyma.

      (b) In intramedullary lesions the objective is tissue diagnosis and decompression of the spinal cord; partial resection is performed as feasible.

   (2) Intraoperative spinal monitoring is frequently used, and tumor resection may be aborted for significant changes versus baseline that persist after anesthetic/hemodynamic maneuvers.

2. Metastatic spinal tumors

a. Metastatic tumors are the most common neoplasm seen in the bony spinal column and extradural space.

   (1) Less than 5% of metastatic tumors have intradural-extramedullary involvement.

   (2) Metastatic intramedullary tumors are uncommon (<2% of all intramedullary tumors).

   (3) Metastatic bone tumors far outweigh primary bone tumors in the spine.

b. The most common spinal metastases are lymphoma (primary CNS non-Hodgkin lymphoma is rare in both the epidural and intramedullary spaces); metastatic lung carcinoma; metastatic breast carcinoma; and metastatic prostate carcinoma.

   (1) Most spinal metastases have radiographic evidence of osteolytic processes.

   (2) Breast carcinoma and prostate carcinoma may have osteoblastic findings.

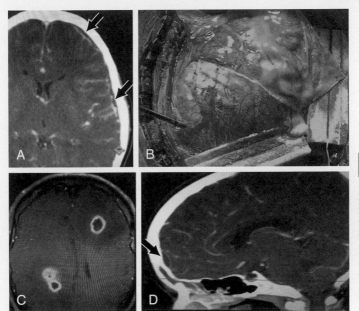

FIG. 66.8
(A and B) Subdural empyema *(arrows)* represented by enlargement of the subdural space (A) and intraoperative photo demonstrating frank pus beneath dura (B). (C) Multifocal abscesses and surrounding edema. (D) Frontal epidural abscess *(arrow)* due to direct extension of frontal sinusitis.

  c. If no primary location is available, biopsy is often the first treatment modality for asymptomatic lesions and followed with radiosurgery/chemotherapy.
    (1) In symptomatic lesions, open surgical biopsy, decompression, and resection as feasible is often the treatment of choice and followed with adjuvant chemotherapy and radiation as indicated.
    (2) Surgery is often not recommended, due to lack of benefit, in patients with paralysis greater than 8 hours; nonambulatory greater than 24 hours; prognosis of less than 3 months; medical frailty; or in cases of highly radiosensitive tumors.

IV. CNS INFECTIOUS URGENCIES AND EMERGENCIES (FIG. 66.8)
A. EPIDURAL ABSCESS
1. Epidural abscess can be seen in both the cranial compartment and spinal column, although it is more frequently seen in the spine.

2. Cranial epidural abscesses frequently arise from contiguous spread from adjacent osteomyelitis, mastoiditis, or sinusitis.
   a. It can also be seen in open skull fractures, penetrating trauma, and as postoperative infection after craniotomy.
   b. *Staphylococcus aureus* and *epidermidis* are the most common organisms, although anaerobes are also seen.
      (1) Chronic osteomyelitis of the skull can lead to edema and swelling of the overlying soft tissues and associated epidural extension, termed "Pott's puffy tumor."
   c. Patients may be neurologically nonfocal, and systemic evaluation may not disclose leukocytosis or elevated inflammatory markers.
      (1) HA is the most common presenting symptom.
   d. Small cranial epidural abscesses may be treated with antibiotics; however, antibiotics alone rarely eliminate the abscess.
      (1) They often require surgical irrigation and debridement, including of compromised bone.
      (2) In postoperative epidural abscess, an infected craniotomy flap may need to be removed and discarded to prevent subsequent recrudescence of infection.
      (3) Antibiotics are usually continued for 6–12 weeks based on infectious disease consultant recommendations.
3. Spinal epidural abscesses can arise from hematogenous spread, contiguous spread, or direct inoculation as in postoperative infections.
   a. Patients at risk include those with immune compromise, intravenous (IV) drug users, poorly controlled diabetics, patients with renal failure, and chronic alcoholics.
   b. Presentation is usually with complaint of exquisite back pain and tenderness at the affected level.
      (1) Pain and tenderness with pain-limited weakness may be the only symptoms and are commonly seen in osteomyelitis-discitis.
      (2) With epidural abscess, symptoms often progress to include radiculopathy from nerve irritation and then myelopathy due to cord compression.
   c. Organisms identified most frequently are *S. aureus*, streptococci, *Escherichia coli*, and *Pseudomonas*.
      (1) Chronic epidural abscess or osteomyelitis is most commonly due to *Mycobacterium tuberculosis*, especially outside the developed world.
      (2) Fungal infections are also commonly seen in chronic infection.
   d. Evaluation with systemic inflammatory work-up (white blood cell count [WBC], erythrocyte sedimentation rate [ESR], C-reactive protein [CRP]), blood and urine cultures, and imaging is often indicated.
      (1) Noncontrast CT may demonstrate osteolysis or free air, suggestive of osteomyelitis, discitis, or epidural abscess; contrast may or may not demonstrate an abscess.
      (2) Contrasted MRI is sensitive for epidural abscess and is the imaging modality of choice.

e. Osteomyelitis-discitis is treated medically with antibiotics after stereotactic or interventional radiology (IR)–guided biopsy; neurosurgical intervention is rarely indicated.

f. Small noncompressive abscesses with symptoms of pain and radiculopathy may be observed with antibiotic treatment.

   (1) Compressive abscesses with symptoms of myelopathy, extensive epidural abscesses, or abscesses with progressively worsening symptoms may require surgical irrigation and debridement plus antibiotics.

g. Patients with severe neurologic deficit before surgery may see only minimal improvement, even with surgery within 12 hours of symptom onset.

   (1) Patients with paralysis at presentation rarely see complete recovery.

   (2) Most cases of death are due to systemic complications of infectious process or as complications of paralysis.

B. SUBDURAL EMPYEMA

1. **A neurosurgical emergency in which abscess forms in subdural space, usually intracranial, although it can be seen in spine after surgery, penetrating trauma, or lumbar puncture**

a. Subdural space allows spread along entire convexity, interhemispheric fissure, and to contralateral hemisphere.

b. It may result from rupture of cerebral abscess at cortical surface, via contiguous spread of epidural abscess, or primarily.

   (1) Most often arises from contiguous spread; classically seen with otitis media or mastoiditis and more frequently with sinusitis or as a postoperative infection

c. Subdural abscess creates robust cortical reaction (cerebritis), which can lead to cortical venous thrombosis and ischemia.

d. Symptom onset is often abrupt and rapidly progressive due to mass effect and cortical inflammatory process.

   (1) Often begins with fever and HA, progressing rapidly to altered mental status, seizures, and/or focal neurologic deficit

e. Contrasted CT is often the first imaging modality used, although it may miss some small empyemas; MRI with and without contrast is highly sensitive.

2. **Urgent/emergent surgical evacuation is usually indicated and followed by broad antibiotic coverage until culture results are available.**

a. Dura must be opened to evacuate underlying pus; underlying brain is often friable with visible ischemic change.

b. Antiseizure prophylaxis is indicated, given the high risk for infarction and venous thrombosis.

3. **Mortality rates remain high, approximately 10%, and although neurologic deficits tend to improve after surgery and antibiotics, more than half will have persistent symptoms at discharge.**

66

NEUROSURGERY

a. Most fatalities are due to diffuse cerebral ischemia from cerebritis or venous thrombosis.

C. PARENCHYMAL ABSCESS

1. **Parenchymal abscesses are most commonly seen in the cerebrum and are relatively rare in the spinal cord.**
   a. Most cerebral abscesses arise by direct inoculation (as in penetrating traumatic brain injury [TBI]), contiguous spread (as in mastoiditis), or via hematogenous spread (as in bacteremia).
      (1) Primary cerebral abscesses are less common.
      (2) Risk factors include chronic sinusitis, chronic otitis, pulmonary abscesses, cardiac vegetations, immune compromise, and IV drug use.
   b. Presentation is similar to that of other mass lesions (e.g., tumors) but progression tends to be rapid due to the exponential growth and often marked cerebral edema.
      (1) Systemic evaluation may disclose a normal or minimally elevated leukocyte count, whereas ESR/CRP are usually abnormally elevated.
   c. The most common organisms are streptococci, anaerobes, staphylococci, and frequently polymicrobial.
      (1) A total of 20%–25% of abscess cultures will be sterile.
      (2) It is also seen with fungal infections (*Nocardia, Candida, Aspergillus*), toxoplasmosis, and mycobacteria.
   d. Evaluation includes cranial imaging with contrasted CT or MRI, the latter being more sensitive.
      (1) Often appears as ring-enhancing lesion with central hypointensity on contrasted T1, often restricted diffusion on diffusion-weighted imaging (DWI), and marked associated edema is frequent on T2-weighted fluid-attenuated inversion recovery (FLAIR)
      (2) Multifocal in many cases; MRI is more sensitive than CT
2. **The staple of treatment is appropriate IV antibiotic coverage, dexamethasone for marked cerebral edema and neurologic deterioration, and infectious disease consultation.**
   a. Small abscesses may be treated with stereotactic needle aspiration if culture needed is followed by antibiotics.
   b. Surgical excision is indicated in large abscesses, abscesses with neurologic deterioration due to mass effect, traumatic abscesses or cases of suspected CSF fistula, or in case of retained foreign body (abscess around impaled bone or projectile in accessible region).

V. OTHER NEUROSURGICAL URGENCIES/EMERGENCIES

A. SEIZURES AND STATUS EPILEPTICUS

1. Seizure is characterized by abnormal, disordered firing of neurons leading to neurologic dysfunction, either focal or diffuse.

2. They are categorized based on presence or absence of impaired consciousness.
   a. Simple partial seizure (50%–60%): focal motor, sensory, autonomic, visual, auditory, etc. seizure originating from one hemisphere *without* impairment of consciousness
   b. Complex partial seizure (0%–10%): partial seizure with impaired consciousness
      (1) Often characterized by automatisms (e.g., lip smacking)
      (2) May progress to secondarily generalized seizure
   c. Generalized seizures (40%): originate from bilateral hemispheric process that results in loss of consciousness (complex by definition)
      (1) Generalized tonic-clonic seizure (also known as grand mal): generalized seizure characterized by progression from tonic to clonic motor manifestation
         (a) Tonic seizure: sustained rigid contraction of muscles (hypertonic state)
         (b) Clonic seizure: bilateral, often rhythmic contractions of the upper and lower extremities, often symmetric
      (2) Absence seizure (also known as petite mal): characterized by impaired consciousness with little or no motor manifestation
      (3) Myoclonic seizure: abrupt jerking movement of body, isolated or in succession with associated electroencephalogram (EEG) abnormality
      (4) Atonic seizure (also known as drop attack): sudden loss of postural tone

3. Management of suspected seizures
   a. Stabilization of ABCs; early neurology consultation; EEG; and beginning antiepileptic drug (AED) regimen
   b. New-onset seizure in adult is acute intracranial process (tumor, hemorrhage, meningitis, cerebritis, etc.) until proven otherwise.

4. Status epilepticus
   a. A neurologic emergency
      (1) Mortality rate approximately 10%; approximately 2% directly attributable to seizure
      (2) Permanent CNS injury or death can occur if seizures are not controlled.
      (3) May lead to secondary cardiovascular, respiratory, or acid-base derangements, which can be life threatening
   b. Defined as a single seizure lasting longer than 5 minutes or seizure activity persisting after administration of first and second line antiepileptic drugs
      (1) Most commonly seen in patients with known seizure disorder who have inadequate anticonvulsant levels (noncompliance, drug interaction, etc.)
   c. Management
      (1) Evaluate ABCs: place on O_2; secure airway if threatened or if seizures persist; electrocardiogram (EKG); crash labs; IV access and give IV fluids

(a) Laboratory evaluation: complete blood count (CBC), electrolytes including Ca^{2+} and Mg^{2+}, arterial blood gas, blood glucose, liver function tests (LFTs), AED levels (if history of seizures)

(2) Perform neurologic assessment; place neurology consultation on confirming status epilepticus.

(3) Thiamine 100 mg IV and 50 mL D50 IV

(4) First line AED (adult): lorazepam 4 mg IV q10 min (classically 2 mg IV q5 min) until seizures abate

    (a) Alternatives: midazolam 10 mg intramuscular (IM) q10 min; diazepam 10 mg IV q20 min

(5) Second line AED (if seizures persist): Load with fosphenytoin 15–20 mg phenytoin equivalents (PEq)/kg IV at rate of 150 mg PEq/min OR phenytoin 15–20 mg/kg IV at rate of 50 mg/min (more potential for hypotension with infusion).

    (a) Maintain with 100 mg PEq q8 hours and check level; may adjust in 10-mg PEq increments

(6) Third line AED (if seizures persist): lorazepam gtt, propofol gtt, or phenobarbital gtt

B. BACLOFEN TOXICITY AND WITHDRAWAL

1. Used to treat chronic spasticity resulting from spinal cord lesions (e.g., multiple sclerosis [MS], tumor, spinal cord injury) refractory to other medications
2. Spasticity may be treated with implanted intrathecal baclofen pump.
3. Baclofen toxicity
   a. Neurologic emergency characterized by depression of CNS: confusion, delirium, lethargy, pupillary dilation, nausea/vomiting
   b. Severe toxicity/overdose results in bradycardia, hypotension or hypertension, hypothermia, seizures, coma, and death
   c. Treatment
      (1) ABCs with intubation if needed
      (2) Physostigmine 0.5–1 mg IV/IM q15–30 minutes given at less than 1 mg/min
      (3) Contact neurosurgery consultant or pump manufacturer in pump in place: aspirate pump reservoir and interrogate pump.
4. Baclofen withdrawal
   a. Often results from noncompliance with oral regimen or, in cases of intrathecal pump, empty baclofen reservoir or disrupted system
   b. Characterized by recrudescence of spasticity, agitation, tachycardia, and piloerection that can progress to seizures and delirium
   c. Severe withdrawal symptoms include rigidity, fever, hypotension or hypertension, neuroleptic malignant syndrome, rhabdomyolysis, disseminated intravascular coagulation (DIC), and death.
   d. Treatment
      (1) ABCs, intubation as needed
      (2) Baclofen PO/PE replacement

      (a) For patients with pump, ≥20 mg q6 hours may be required; often inadequate on its own for those with pump

      (b) Consider diazepam or midazolam IV if refractory to PO baclofen.

    (3) Pump evaluation; attempt to restore intrathecal regimen.

C. IDIOPATHIC INTRACRANIAL HYPERTENSION (ALSO KNOWN AS PSEUDOTUMOR CEREBRI)

1. Symptomatic ICP elevation greater than 20 mm Hg and papilledema on ophthalmology evaluation without evidence of intracranial mass or infection
   a. Typical patient is obese female of childbearing age (10–20 times more common than in general population).
   b. Often self-limited flare-up, recurrence common
   c. May be associated with dural venous sinus thrombosis or stenosis
2. Treatment, nonurgent except in cases of new visual deficit
   a. Consultation to ophthalmology for formal visual field, visual acuity, and optic nerve evaluation
   b. Acetazolamide and weight loss are first line therapies
   c. Surgery (optic nerve sheath fenestration and/or CSF diversion) reserved for cases with refractory visual loss or severe optic disc changes; often managed medically if HAs alone, although CSF diversion is therapeutic option

VI. HERNIATION SYNDROMES AND BRAIN DEATH

A. HERNIATION SYNDROMES CAN RESULT FROM A VARIETY OF BOTH TRAUMATIC AND NONTRAUMATIC CRANIAL PATHOLOGIES; THERE ARE FOUR COMMON HERNIATION SYNDROMES WITH WHICH ONE MUST BE FAMILIAR.

1. Subfalcine herniation
   a. Cingulate gyrus herniates under falx cerebri, resulting in "midline shift"; may be asymptomatic but herniation can compress the anterior cerebral arteries (ACAs), resulting in bilateral infarcts of the ACA territories (frontal parafalcine)
   b. May be herald of subsequent transtentorial herniation
2. Uncal herniation
   a. Uncus of temporal lobe herniates from its position on the tentorium to compress the crural cistern and midbrain
   b. Results in progressive compression of oculomotor nerve (CN III), PCA, and midbrain/superior pons
      (1) CN III and PCA normally course medial to uncus in crural cistern
      (2) Results in ipsilateral CN III palsy (dilated pupil), contralateral Babinski reflex, contralateral hemiparesis (cerebral peduncle), and PCA territory strokes (occipital lobe and medial temporal lobe)
         (a) Kernohan phenomenon: massive uncal or transtentorial herniation displaces midbrain such that *contralateral* cerebral

66

NEUROSURGERY

peduncle and, less often, CN III are compressed; results in *ipsilateral* hemiparesis and, less commonly, contralateral pupillary dilation

3. **Transtentorial herniation**
   a. Downward transtentorial herniation: due to supratentorial mass lesion, often preceded by uncal or subfalcine herniation; can be seen with CSF diversion with lumbar drain.
      (1) Results in compression of thalamus, midbrain, pons, and then brainstem, leading to depressed level of consciousness, posturing, cranial nerve deficits
   b. Upward transtentorial herniation: infrequently seen, often in setting of posterior fossa mass or CSF diversion with EVD
      (1) Results from cerebellar vermis pushing upward to compress the midbrain tectum, cerebral aqueduct, and, occasionally, superior cerebellar arteries (SCAs)
         (a) Compression of midbrain tectum may result in CN palsies or obstructive hydrocephalus.

4. **Tonsillar herniation**
   a. Cerebellar tonsils herniate through foramen magnum, compressing the medulla and spinal cord at craniocervical junction.
      (1) Results in brainstem compression leading to CN palsies and respiratory depression, which progresses to central respiratory arrest
      (2) May be accompanied by Cushing triad of hypertension, bradycardia, and disordered respiratory pattern
   b. Often seen with intracranial masses, particularly of posterior fossa, or elevated ICP
      (1) Can be precipitated by lumbar puncture in setting of posterior fossa mass or elevated ICP
   c. If acute, often rapidly fatal if not promptly recognized and treated
      (1) Differentiates from chronic herniation of cerebellar tonsils or cerebellum as seen in Chiari syndromes

B. BRAIN DEATH

Standards for establishing brain death vary state by state and institutionally but are generally guided by the Uniform Determination of Death Act (1980), which includes the provision that an individual can be declared as dead if he or she is determined to have, within reasonable medical standards, "irreversible cessation of all functions of the entire brain, including the brain stem." We present the criteria for brain death implemented at our institution.

1. **Establish absence of potentially confounding factors.**
   a. Confirm negative toxicology examination and absence of all sedative, narcotic, and paralytic agents or their effects.
   b. Maintain hemodynamic parameters within physiologic norms: temperature ≥96.5°F, SBP greater than 90 mm Hg, pH on arterial blood gas 7.35–7.45.

2. Neurologic examination is performed by two separate physicians.
   a. This can be performed simultaneously or independently; generally a specialist from neurology, neurosurgery, or neurocritical care is involved.
   b. Establish absence of response to central painful stimulation at three locations (GCS = 3).
      (1) Sternal rub, supraorbital pressure, temporomandibular joint pressure ("jaw thrust"), pectoralis tendon, etc.
   c. Establish absence of brainstem function bilaterally.
      (1) Absent pupillary light response—CNs II, III
      (2) Absent corneal reflex—CNs V, VII
      (3) Absent oculocephalic reflex (doll's eyes reflex)—CNs VI, VIII
      (4) Absent oculovestibular reflex (cold calorics test)—CN VI, VIII
      (5) Absent gag reflex—CNs IX, X
      (6) Absent cough reflex—CN X
   d. Establish failed apnea challenge—performed only if above are all absent
      (1) Arterial blood gas is obtained as baseline; baseline pH (7.35–7.45) and $Paco_2$ (35–40) should be within physiologic norms.
      (2) After preoxygenating, the patient is taken off ventilator; high-flow O_2 at 10–15 L/min is placed to endotracheal tube; and apnea is observed for 10 minutes.
          (a) Test is aborted if patient breathes, experiences cardiovascular or hemodynamic instability, or drops O_2 saturation below 80% by pulse oximetry.
      (3) Apnea challenge is failed if
          (a) No spontaneous respirations are observed (e.g., no tidal volumes on spirometer or no functional chest or abdominal movements to generate a breath).
          (b) Post apnea challenge arterial blood gas demonstrates $Paco_2$ greater than 60 mm Hg *OR* greater than 20 mm Hg increase over baseline.
   e. Absence of response to painful stimuli and cranial nerve function and failed apnea challenge constitute brain death.
3. At our institution no confirmatory testing is required, but this may vary.
   a. Common ancillary studies performed to confirm the clinical diagnosis of brain death may include electroencephalography (isoelectric EEG); cerebral angiography (absence of cerebral blood flow); or cerebral radionuclide angiogram (CRAG, absence of technetium 99m [^{99m}Tc] signal from parenchyma, also known as "hollow skull").

66

NEUROSURGERY

RECOMMENDED READINGS

Bakker NA, Metzemaekers JD, Groen RJ, Mooij JJ, Van Dijk JM. International subarachnoid aneurysm trial 2009: endovascular coiling of ruptured intracranial aneurysms has no significant advantage over neurosurgical clipping. *Neurosurgery*. 2010;66:961–962.
Britt RH, Enzmann DR. Clinical stages of human brain abscesses on serial CT scans after contrast infusion. *J Neurosurg*. 1983;59:972–989.

Connolly ES Jr, Rabinstein AA, Carhuapoma JR, et al. Guidelines for the management of aneurysmal subarachnoid hemorrhage: a guideline for healthcare professionals from the American Heart Association/American Stroke Association. *Stroke*. 2012;43:1711–1737.

Glantz MJ, Cole BF, Forsyth PA, et al. Practice parameter: anticonvulsant prophylaxis in patients with newly diagnosed brain tumors. Report of the Quality Standards Subcommittee of the American Academy of Neurology. *Neurology*. 2000;54:1886–1893.

Hemphill JC 3rd, Bonovich DC, Besmertis L, Manley GT, Johnston SC. The ICH score: a simple, reliable grading scale for intracerebral hemorrhage. *Stroke*. 2001;32:891–897.

Keles GE, Anderson B, Berger MS. The effect of extent of tumor resection on time to tumor progression and survival in patients with glioblastoma multiforme of the cerebral hemisphere. *Surg Neurol*. 1999;52:371–379.

McDougall CG, Spetzler RF, Zabramski JM, et al. The Barrow ruptured aneurysm trial (BRAT). *J Neurosurg*. 2012;116:135–144.

Molyneux AJ, Kerr RS, Birks J, et al. Risk of recurrent subarachnoid hemorrhage, death, or dependence and standardized mortality ratios after clipping or coiling of an intracranial aneurysm in the International Subarachnoid Aneurysm Trial (ISAT): long-term follow-up. *Lancet Neurol*. 2009;8:427–443.

Rost NS, Smith EE, Chang Y, et al. Prediction of functional outcome in patients with primary intracerebral hemorrhage: the FUNC score. *Stroke*. 2008;39:2304–2309.

Stupp R, Mason WP, van den Bent MJ, et al. Radiotherapy plus concomitant and adjuvant temozolomide for glioblastoma. *N Engl J Med*. 2005;352:987–996.

Webster J, Piscitelli G, Polli A, Ferrari CI, Ismail I, Scanlon MF. A comparison of cabergoline and bromocriptine in the treatment of hyperprolactinemic amenorrhea. *N Engl J Med*. 1994;331:904–909.

Wijdicks EFM, Varelas PN, Gronseth GS, Greer DM. Evidence-based guideline update: determining brain death in adults: report of the Quality Standards subcommittee of the American Academy of Neurology. *Neurology*. 2010;74:1911–1918.

Orthopedic Surgery

Ashley R. Miller, MD, and Tonya Dixon, MD

Sticks and stones may break my bones, but words will never hurt me.

—Proverb

No problem is ever so bad, that surgery cannot make it worse.

—Jack C. Hughston, MD

I. ASSESSMENT OF THE ORTHOPEDIC PATIENT

A. BASIC ADVANCED TRAUMA LIFE SUPPORT PRINCIPLES

1. Airway/breathing/circulation initial assessment
2. Disability/exposure
   a. Secondary examination of extremities
      (1) Appearance of abrasions and deep lacerations
      (2) Range of motion of all joints
      (3) Presence of crepitance at level of joint or extremity
      (4) Palpate extremities for areas of tenderness
         (a) High incidence of missed injuries secondary to distracting injuries
      (5) Evaluation of soft tissue envelope
   b. Obtain full-length imaging of injured bone, including joint above and below.

II. ORTHOPEDIC EMERGENCIES

A. HEMODYNAMICALLY UNSTABLE PELVIC FRACTURES

1. Usually high-energy mechanisms
   a. Hemodynamically unstable from intrapelvic hemorrhage: 15%–30%
   b. Overall mortality of 6%–35% in high-energy pelvic fractures
2. High incidence of concurrent trauma
   a. Head, abdominal, thoracic injuries
   b. A total of 60%–80% incidence of other musculoskeletal injuries
   c. Incidence of urogenital injuries: 12%
   d. Incidence of lumbosacral plexus injuries: 8%
3. Interdisciplinary approach
   a. General trauma surgeon
   b. Orthopedic surgeon
   c. Interventional radiologist
   d. Blood bank representative
4. Anatomy
   a. Pelvic ring
      (1) Sacrum and two innominate bones
      (2) Two sacroiliac joints and pubic symphysis

b. Vascular supply
   (1) Common iliac artery divides.
   (2) External iliac artery exits pelvis anteriorly over pelvic brim.
   (3) Internal iliac artery lies over pelvic brim close to sacroiliac joint.
       (a) Anterior branches: obturator, umbilical, vesical, pudendal, inferior gluteal, rectal, hemorrhoidal arteries
           (i) Pudendal and obturator arteries can be injured in pubic rami injuries.
       (b) Posterior branches: iliolumbar, superior gluteal, lateral sacral arteries

5. Evaluation of patient
   a. Airway/breathing/circulation as part of basic Advanced Trauma Life Support (ATLS) guidelines takes initial preference
   b. Concurrent evaluation for hemodynamic instability
   c. Disability/exposure
   d. Radiographic evaluation
      (1) Anteroposterior (AP) pelvic radiograph as initial primary assessment
      (2) Inlet/outlet radiographs to evaluate pelvic ring only when hemodynamically stable
      (3) CT scan of abdomen/pelvis with contrast to evaluate for active pelvic hemorrhage (sensitivity 84%, specificity 85%)
      (4) Young-Burgess classification of pelvic ring injuries
          (a) Anteroposterior compression (APC)
              (i) Anterior impact with disruption of pubic symphysis and anterior sacroiliac ligaments
                  (a) "Open book" type injuries
                  (b) Increased resuscitative requirements with increased severity of classification
          (b) Lateral compression (LC)
              (i) Lateral impact that rotates pelvis toward midline
                  (a) Rarely associated with hemodynamic instability
          (c) Vertical shear (VS)
              (i) Vertical translation of hemipelvis
                  (a) Severe local vascular injury
          (d) Combined mechanism (CM)
              (i) Multiple force vectors
   e. Treatment
      (1) Pelvic binder or sheet
          (a) Decreases intrapelvic volume
          (b) Applied during transport or resuscitation
          (c) Most effective in APC-type injuries
              (i) Reduced transfusion requirement, hospital length of stay, and mortality

(d) Correct application is centered over the greater trochanters of the femurs, not the iliac crests.
(e) Reduction of pelvis through internal rotation of knees and feet of patient
(2) Pelvic external fixation
(a) Anterior external fixator
(b) Posterior C-clamp
(3) Angiography
(a) Indicated in ongoing hemodynamic instability despite pelvic immobilization
(4) Pelvic packing
(a) Pelvic packing through exploratory laparotomy
(b) Retroperitoneal packing
(5) Fluid resuscitation/blood products

B. OPEN FRACTURES
1. Overview
a. Fracture with exposure to the external environment
b. Often high-energy mechanisms (motor vehicle crash, motorcycle accident, fall from height)
c. Risk of infection and wound healing complications
2. Gustilo-Anderson classification (Table 67.1)
a. Evaluation and classification of soft tissue envelope associated with fracture
(1) Type I
(a) Open wound less than 1 cm
(b) Minimal soft tissue injury
(2) Type II
(a) Open wound 1–10 cm
(b) Moderate soft tissue injury
(3) Type IIIA
(a) Open wound greater than 10 cm
(b) Extensive soft tissue injury

TABLE 67.1

GUSTILO CLASSIFICATION OF OPEN FRACTURES

Type	Description
I	Clean wound <1 cm in length
II	Clean wound >1 cm in length without extensive soft tissue damage, flaps, or avulsions
IIIA	Adequate soft tissue coverage despite extensive soft tissue damage, flaps, or high-energy trauma irrespective of wound size
IIIB	Inadequate soft tissue coverage with periosteal stripping, often associated with massive contamination
IIIC	Arterial injury requiring repair

From Melvin JS, Dombroski DG, Torbert JT, Kovach SJ, Esterhai JL, Mehta S. Open tibial shaft fractures: evaluation and initial wound management. *J Am Acad Orthop Surg*. 2010;18:10–19.

      (c) Often heavy contamination

      (d) Periosteal stripping

      (e) Adequate soft tissue coverage allowing for closure of wound

   (4) Type IIIB

      (a) Open wound greater than 10 cm

      (b) Extensive soft tissue injury

      (c) Heavy contamination

      (d) Periosteal stripping

      (e) Requires soft tissue flap for coverage

   (5) Type IIIC

      (a) Open wound greater than 10 cm

      (b) Extensive soft tissue injury

      (c) Often heavy contamination

      (d) Periosteal stripping

      (e) Associated vascular injury necessitating repair

      (f) May require soft tissue flap for coverage

3. Initial treatment

  a. Tetanus prophylaxis

  b. Antibiotics

   (1) Therapeutic antibiotic administration

      (a) Initiation as soon as possible

      (b) Within 3 hours of injury ideal

      (c) Duration: 24–72 hours, or until wounds are closed

   (2) Commonly gram-positive and gram-negative organisms

   (3) First-generation cephalosporin for gram-positive coverage

      (a) Cefazolin

   (4) Aminoglycoside for gram-negative coverage

      (a) Gentamicin or tobramycin

      (b) Substitutions

         (i) Quinolones (e.g., ciprofloxacin)

           (a) Oral (PO) availability

           (b) Similar infection rates compared for type I and II open fractures compared with cefazolin and gentamicin

           (c) May inhibit fracture healing through effects on osteoblasts

         (ii) Aztreonam

         (iii) Third-generation cephalosporins (ceftriaxone)

   (5) Anaerobic coverage

      (a) Commonly farm injuries (organic contamination of wound) or vascular injuries

         (i) Low oxygen environments

      (b) Penicillin or ampicillin

   (6) Aquatic injury

      (a) Commonly *Vibrio, Pseudomonas, Aeromonas* species

(b) Brackish/salt water
  (i) Doxycycline and third-generation cephalosporin (e.g., ceftazidime)
  (ii) Fluoroquinolone (e.g., ciprofloxacin or levofloxacin)
(c) Freshwater
  (i) Fluoroquinolone (e.g., ciprofloxacin or levofloxacin)
  (ii) Third-generation cephalosporin (e.g., ceftazidime)
c. Bedside irrigation and debridement
  (1) High-volume normal saline (NS) irrigation
  (2) Removal of debris and contamination
d. Dressing of wounds
  (1) Saline-soaked gauze
  (2) Betadine-soaked gauze
    (a) May be cytotoxic to cells
e. Splint immobilization

4. Treatment

a. Formal irrigation and debridement
  (1) High-volume, low-flow irrigation
    (a) Bacitracin-added to the irrigation
    (b) Some advocate the use of 3 L for type I, 6 L for type II, and 9 L for type III open fractures.
    (c) Gravity cystoscopy tubing avoids the harmful effects of high-pressure pulsatile lavage.
  (2) Thorough debridement of all contaminants and devitalized and/or necrotic tissue
    (a) May require serial irrigation and debridements
  (3) Minimal use of tourniquet
    (a) Evaluate for soft tissue viability.
b. Definitive fracture fixation
  (1) External fixation versus definitive fixation
c. Wound management
  (1) Closure when soft tissue envelope allows
    (a) Use of monofilament, nonbraided suture
      (i) Polydioxanone (PDS) for deep layers
      (ii) Nylon for skin
    (b) Donati-Allgöwer suturing technique limits the degree of cutaneous vascular compromise.
  (2) Negative pressure wound vacuum therapy
    (a) Temporizing closure
    (b) Delayed wound closure prevents anaerobic environment and allows for drainage of wound.
  (3) Soft tissue reconstruction
    (a) Type IIIB wounds
    (b) Plastic surgery consultation early if anticipated need

C. COMPARTMENT SYNDROME

1. Overview
   a. Pressure in a fascial compartment exceeding capillary perfusion pressure creates an anoxic environment leading to irreversible tissue necrosis.
2. Causes
   a. Fractures—most common mechanism
      (1) Open fractures are not precluded.
         (a) Tibial diaphyseal fractures most common fracture (36%)
         (b) Distal radius (9.8%) and forearm diaphyseal fractures (7.9%)
   b. Gunshot wound
   c. Reperfusion/vascular injury
      (1) Prolonged tourniquet use
         (a) Often narcotic overdose
      (2) Patient found down
   d. Burns
      (1) Circumferential third-degree burns are highest risk
   e. Bleeding disorders
      (1) Genetic or iatrogenic (anticoagulants)
   f. Circumferential padding/casting
   g. Other
      (1) Epidural anesthesia can increase risk of compartment syndrome
         (a) Increases local blood flow through sympathetic blockade
3. Evaluation/diagnosis
   a. Predominantly a clinical diagnosis
      (1) Pain out of proportion to injury
      (2) Firmness of compartments
      (3) Pain with passive stretch of compartment
         (a) Reduces intracompartmental volume, thereby increasing pressure
      (4) Paresthesia
         (a) Eventually progress to hyperesthesia and anesthesia in untreated cases
      (5) Loss of pulses late findings
      (6) Serial examinations are imperative
   b. Intracompartmental pressure monitoring
      (1) Indications
         (a) Unreliable examination
         (b) Symptoms in confounding situations (neurologic injury, regional anesthesia, obtunded patient, etc.)
         (c) Prolonged hypotension in a firm extremity
      (2) Use of a Stryker Intra-Compartmental Pressure Monitor System (Stryker, Kalamazoo, MI)
         (a) Arterial line with a pressure transducer acts in a similar manner.
      (3) ΔP (intracompartmental pressure—diastolic blood pressure) less than 20 mm Hg

4. **Treatment**
   a. Release of circumferential bindings (e.g., casts)
   b. Complete fasciotomies of affected compartment
      (1) One- versus two-incision technique for leg fasciotomies
         (a) Long lateral incision
            (i) Release all four compartments
         (b) Versus medial and lateral incisions
            (i) Medial
               (a) Deep posterior and superficial posterior compartments
            (ii) Lateral
               (a) Anterior and lateral compartments
            (iii) Longer incisions better
               (a) Skin can still cause compression
      (2) Serial debridements may be necessary as zone of ischemic injury declares itself.
      (3) Closure only when swelling accommodates untensioned closure and no remaining necrotic tissue
      (4) Negative-pressure wound vacuum therapy versus open wounds in index fasciotomy
      (5) Split-thickness skin grafting may be necessary for final closure.
   c. Rhabdomyolysis/renal failure
      (1) Myoglobin from damaged muscle cells released into circulation
      (2) Close monitoring of plasma creatine kinase (CK)
      (3) Adequate high-dose hydration to prevent myoglobin nephrotoxicity

D. VASCULAR INJURY ASSOCIATED WITH EXTREMITY TRAUMA

1. **Overview**
   a. Less than 1% of extremity trauma associated with vascular injury
   b. Sixteen percent of knee dislocations have concurrent vascular injury.
2. **Associated injuries**
   a. Knee dislocations
   b. Comminuted tibial plateau fractures
   c. Open fractures
      (1) Especially open tibia fractures
   d. Segmental fractures
   e. Fractures with significant displacement
   f. Floating joints
      (1) Example: floating knee (femoral fracture with ipsilateral tibia fracture)
   g. Gunshot or penetrating trauma
3. **Evaluation**
   a. Multidisciplinary approach
      (1) Orthopedic surgeon, general surgeon, vascular surgeon, intervention radiologist
   b. Urgent reduction of injury

   c. Physical examination
     (1) Hard signs of vascular injury
       (a) Pulselessness
       (b) Pallor
       (c) Rapidly expanding hematoma
       (d) Massive bleeding
       (e) Palpable or audible bruit
     (2) Soft signs
       (a) History of bleeding in transit
       (b) Related bony injury in proximity to vessel
       (c) Neurologic findings from nerve adjacent to a named artery
       (d) Hematoma around a named artery
   d. Thorough vascular examination
     (1) Postreduction examination when appropriate
     (2) Use of Doppler ultrasonography when needed
     (3) Arterial pressure index less than 0.90 indicates potential vascular compromise.
       (a) Often ankle-brachial index measurement (lower extremity systolic pressure/upper extremity systolic pressure)
   e. Computed tomography (CT) angiography
   f. Duplex sonography
     (1) Quick
     (2) Noninvasive (compared with intravenous [IV] contrast)
     (3) Bedside evaluation
4. Treatment
   a. Treatment algorithm (Fig. 67.1)
   b. Orthopedic stabilization of bony injury to protect vascular repair
     (1) External fixation
       (a) Quicker
       (b) Need for subsequent procedure
     (2) Definitive fixation
       (a) Slower, potential delay in vascular intervention
   c. Vascular repair
     (1) Open techniques
     (2) Endovascular techniques
   d. Communication between teams is paramount.

E. TRAUMATIC ARTHROTOMIES
1. Overview
   a. Laceration over a joint with intraarticular communication
   b. Risk of intraarticular infection, septic arthritis, if missed diagnosis
2. Evaluation
   a. All deep lacerations over joint capsules merit further evaluation.
   b. Obtain radiographs of affected joint to rule out open fracture.
   c. Saline joint load is gold standard for evaluation.
     (1) Must have sufficient capsular distension

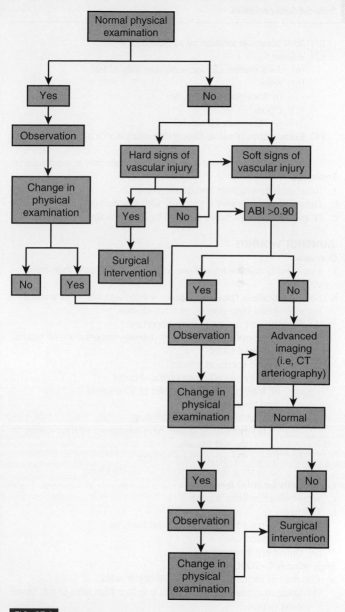

FIG. 67.1

Diagnostic algorithm for vascular injury associated with extremity trauma. *ABI*, Ankle-brachial index. (From Halvorson JJ, Anz A, Langfitt M, et al. Vascular injury associated with extremity trauma: initial diagnosis and management. *J Am Acad Orthop Surg*. 2011;19:495–504.)

(2) Joint access at location away from injury
(3) Volume
    (a) Joint motion can increase sensitivity of test
    (b) Knee
        (i) Minimum 150 mL NS
    (c) Elbow
        (i) Minimum 40 mL NS
(4) Extravasation of saline through the injury is indicative of traumatic arthrotomy
    (a) Use of methylene blue can aide in detection of extravasation

3. Treatment
a. Initial bedside irrigation and debridement
b. Definitive intraoperative arthrotomy with irrigation and debridement
c. IV antibiotics for 24 hours followed by PO antibiotics for 1 week

F. GUNSHOT WOUNDS
1. Overview
a. Low-velocity ballistic injuries are treated very differently than high velocity.
b. Some advocate to "treat the wound, not the weapon" in differentiating low- versus high-velocity gunshot injuries.
  (1) Effect on soft tissues is more important.
  (2) Multiple factors influence amount of energy imparted on soft tissues.
    (a) Caliber of bullet
    (b) Kinetic energy at impact
    (c) Stability and entrance profile of bullet
        (i) Maximum energy transfer at 90 degrees
    (d) Path through body
        (i) Penetrating versus perforating
           (a) Nonexiting bullets have transferred all their energy to the soft tissues.
    (e) Tissue disruption characteristics
        (i) Tearing versus crushing versus stretching

2. Low velocity (<2000 ft/sec)
a. Most civilian ballistic injuries
b. Fractures
  (1) Treated in same manner as closed fractures
  (2) Local wound care
  (3) Outpatient management

3. High velocity (>2000 ft/sec)
a. Common in military and hunting ballistic injuries
  (1) Shotgun injuries are included due to their high rates of soft tissue compromise.
b. Fractures
  (1) Treated in same manner as open fractures
    (a) Soft tissue management is paramount.

(2) Prophylactic antibiotics recommended
    (a) High incidence of subclinical contamination
(3) Thorough irrigation and debridement
    (a) Including debridement of necrotic skin edges

4. Complications
   a. Infection
      (1) Bullets are not sterilized on discharge (contrary to common belief).
      (2) Contamination
          (a) Bowel, skin flora, clothing
      (3) Need for bowel prophylactic antibiotics when contaminated bullet bony injury
   b. Vascular injury
      (1) See Section II.D
   c. Plumbism
      (1) Lead toxicity from retained bullet fragments
          (a) Worst in bones, joint spaces, intervertebral disc space
      (2) Chronic irritation, arthritis, rarely systemic effects

G. BITE INJURIES

1. Etiology
   a. Approximately 50% of people will experience an animal bite, often during childhood.
   b. More than 90% are from domesticated animals.
      (1) Dogs are responsible for 80%–90%.
      (2) Cats are responsible for 5%–15%.
      (3) Humans are responsible for 2%–3%.
   c. Most are hand injuries.

2. Bacteriology
   a. All bites
      (1) *Staphylococcus, Streptococcus*, anaerobic bacteria
   b. Human bites
      (1) *Eikenella*
      (2) Risk of human immunodeficiency virus (HIV), hepatitis B, hepatitis C transmission
   c. Dog/cat bites
      (1) *Pasteurella*
      (2) Risk of rabies transmission

3. Fight bites
   a. Clenched fist injuries from impact with teeth
   b. Often male, dominant hand
   c. Location is often proximal to the metacarpophalangeal (MCP) joint when fingers are extended secondary to soft tissue excursion.
      (1) Wound gets closed, creating an enclosed environment for infection.
   d. Tooth often penetrates extensor mechanism and MCP joint capsule.

4. Occlusive bites
   a. Teeth closing directly on skin
   b. Often in women, inflicted by men
   c. Multiple sites common
      (1) Breasts, genitalia, arms, legs in women
      (2) Shoulders, arms, hands in men
   d. Infection more common in distal extremities (hands, wrist)
      (1) Easier to penetrate joint capsules
5. Evaluation
   a. Radiographic evaluation
      (1) Rule out retained foreign body and bony injury.
   b. Ultrasonography
      (1) Evaluate for fluid collection.
   c. Inflammatory markers
      (1) Essential in all infectious cases, especially with concern for septic arthritis
      (2) May be normal in acute injuries
   d. Wound cultures
      (1) Allows for tailoring of antibiosis
      (2) Unreliable in acute injuries
6. Treatment
   a. Antibiotic prophylaxis
      (1) Antibiotic choices (Table 67.2)
   b. Open wound irrigation and debridement
      (1) Including arthrotomy and evaluation of joint if needed
      (2) Closure contraindicated in cases of heavy contamination
   c. Surgical repair of soft tissues as indicated
      (1) After thorough debridement of wounds
   d. Local wound management and close follow-up

TABLE 67.2

EMPIRIC ANTIBIOTIC PROPHYLAXIS FOR HUMAN, DOG, AND CAT BITES[a]

Route	Agents of Choice	Alternate Regimens
Oral	Amoxicillin-clavulanate	One of the following:[b] doxycycline, trimethoprim-sulfamethoxazole, penicillin VK, cefuroxime, fluoroquinolones (ciprofloxacin or moxifloxacin)
Intravenous	Ampicillin-sulbactam, piperacillin-tazobactam, ticarcillin-clavulanate, ceftriaxone plus metronidazole	Fluoroquinolones (e.g., ciprofloxacin) plus metronidazole, carbapenem monotherapy (e.g., imipenem, meropenem, ertapenem)

[a]Same for all three types of bites.
[b]Plus clindamycin or metronidazole.
From Kennedy SA, Stoll LE, Lauder AS. Human and other mammalian bite injuries of the hand: evaluation and management. *J Am Acad Orthop Surg.* 2015;23:47–57.

RECOMMENDED READINGS

Bartlett CS, Helfet DL, Hausman MR, Strauss E. Ballistics and gunshot wounds: effects on musculoskeletal tissues. *J Am Acad Orthop Surg.* 2000;8:21–36.

Bumbasirevic M, Lesic A, Mitkovic M, Bumbasirevic V. Treatment of blast injuries of the extremity. *J Am Acad Orthop Surg.* 2006;14:S77–S81.

Hak DJ, Smith WR, Suzuki T. Management of hemorrhage in life-threatening pelvic fracture. *J Am Acad Orthop Surg.* 2009;17:447–457.

Halvorson JJ, Anz A, Langfitt M, et al. Vascular injury associated with extremity trauma: initial diagnosis and management. *J Am Acad Orthop Surg.* 2011;19:495–504.

Kennedy SA, Stoll LE, Lauder AS. Human and other mammalian bite injuries of the hand: evaluation and management. *J Am Acad Orthop Surg.* 2015;23:47–57.

Melvin JS, Dombroski DG, Torbert JT, Kovach SJ, Esterhai JL, Mehta S. Open tibial shaft fractures: evaluation and initial wound management. *J Am Acad Orthop Surg.* 2010;18:10–19.

Noonburg GE. Management of extremity trauma and related infections occurring in the aquatic environment. *J Am Acad Orthop Surg.* 2005;13:243–253.

Olson SA, Glasgow RR. Acute compartment syndrome in lower extremity musculoskeletal trauma. *J Am Acad Orthop Surg.* 2005;13:436–444.

Prasarn ML, Ouellette EA. Acute compartment syndrome of the upper extremity. *J Am Acad Orthop Surg.* 2011;19:49–58.

Thakur NA, Czerwein JK, Butera JN, Palumbo MA. Perioperative management of chronic anticoagulation in orthopaedic surgery. *J Am Acad Orthop Surg.* 2010;18:729–738.

Tull F, Borrelli J. Soft-tissue injury associated with closed fractures: evaluation and management. *J Am Acad Orthop Surg.* 2003;11:431–438.

Webb LX, Dedmond B, Schlatterer D, Laverty D. The contaminated high-energy open fracture: a protocol to prevent and treat inflammatory mediator storm-induced soft-tissue compartment syndrome (IMSICS). *J Am Acad Orthop Surg.* 2006;14:S82–S86.

Weil YA, Mosheiff R, Liebergall M. Blast and penetrating fragment injuries to the extremities. *J Am Acad Orthop Surg.* 2006;14:S136–S139.

Zalavras CG, Patzakis MJ. Open fractures: evaluation and management. *J Am Acad Orthop Surg.* 2003;11:212–219.

67

ORTHOPEDIC SURGERY

Plastic Surgery: Breast Reconstruction

Fernando Ovalle Jr., MD

Plastic surgery is a perpetual battle of beauty versus blood supply.

—Sir Harold Gilles

I. INTRODUCTION

Surgical therapy of breast cancer remains not only an important therapeutic mainstay but has also evolved as common prophylactic intervention. Although the techniques of local excision and mastectomy have changed since Halsted's time, significant disfigurement may still occur. Breast reconstruction can profoundly help a woman's healing and self-image as she is treated for breast cancer. The Women's Health and Cancer Rights Act of 1988 mandates insurance coverage of breast reconstruction. Advancement in implant technology and autologous reconstruction techniques have vastly expanded the option breast cancer patients have for reconstruction. The surgeon should be familiar with the anatomy, indications, and contraindications for surgery and an overview of a variety of breast reconstruction options.

II. RELEVANT ANATOMY FOR RECONSTRUCTION

A. VASCULAR SUPPLY (FIG. 68.1)
1. Internal mammary vessels
2. Thoracoacromial trunk vessels
3. Lateral thoracic vessels
4. Thoracodorsal vessels
5. Intercostal perforators

B. INNERVATION
1. Supraclavicular nerve
2. Intercostobrachial nerve
3. Anteromedial intercostal nerves

III. PREOPERATIVE EVALUATION

A. GOALS OF RECONSTRUCTION
1. Desire for natural-appearing breast mound
   a. Ample breast volume
   b. Appropriate projection
2. Optimization of skin envelope reconstruction
   a. Skin-sparing mastectomy—conserving skin if it does not compromise the oncologic treatment will improve the ultimate aesthetic outcome.

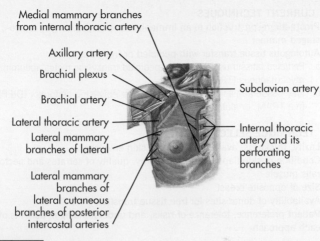

Medial mammary branches
from internal thoracic artery

Axillary artery

Brachial plexus

Brachial artery

Lateral thoracic artery

Lateral mammary
branches of lateral

Lateral mammary
branches of
lateral cutaneous
branches of posterior
intercostal arteries

Subclavian artery

Internal thoracic
artery and its
perforating
branches

FIG. 68.1
Arterial blood supply of the breast.

  b. Non–skin-sparing mastectomy—leads to techniques of expansion
    versus autologous tissue transfer
3. Symmetry
  a. Patient may need augmentation or reduction of contralateral
    breast.
  b. Some patients choose prophylactic mastectomy of disease-free con-
    tralateral breast to prevent new primary disease, which can improve
    symmetric outcome during reconstruction.
4. Nipple areolar complex reconstruction
  a. Matching pigmentation to contralateral breast
  b. Nipple projection corresponding to contralateral breast

B. TIMING
1. Immediate—occurring during initial breast resection procedure
  a. Allows inframammary fold to be preserved
  b. Provides psychological benefits to patients
2. Delayed reconstruction indications
  a. Postoperative radiation
    (1) Impaired wound healing
    (2) Induces fat necrosis of transposed tissue
    (3) Increases incidence and severity of prosthetic capsular con-
      tracture
  b. Chemotherapeutic agents
    (1) Impaired wound healing

C. CURRENT TECHNIQUES

1. Prosthetic reconstruction in an immediate or delayed, single- or two-staged manner
2. Autologous tissue transfer with pedicled or free flaps
   a. Pedicled latissimus dorsi flap or pedicled transverse rectus abdominis myocutaneous (TRAM) flap
   b. Free tissue transfer, such as deep inferior epigastric perforator (DIEP), free TRAM, or gluteal perforator flaps

D. TECHNIQUE SELECTION CRITERIA

1. Laxity, thickness, availability of chest skin envelope
2. Condition of skin flaps after mastectomy, quality of serratus and pectoralis muscle
3. Size of opposite breast
4. Availability of donor sites for free tissue transfer
5. Patient preference, tolerance of risks, and understanding of benefits of each approach

IV. TECHNIQUES

A. PROSTHETIC RECONSTRUCTION USING IMPLANTS AND EXPANDERS

1. Direct to implant reconstruction
   a. Placement
      (1) Subpectoral or subcutaneous
   b. Indications
      (1) Sufficient and viable skin envelope
      (2) Small- to medium-sized breasts, or planned contralateral procedure for symmetry
      (3) Patient's personal preference to avoid creation of additional donor site wound
   c. Contraindications
      (1) Lack of available/viable skin envelope
      (2) Postoperative radiation planned leading to common complications
         (a) Greater rate of capsular contracture and implant extrusion
         (b) Subsequent poor aesthetic outcome and poor patient satisfaction
      (3) Artificial implant unacceptable to patient
   d. Advantages
      (1) Decreased operative time
      (2) Single staged; additional procedures not necessary
      (3) No donor site morbidity
   e. Disadvantages
      (1) Implant complications: infection, capsular contracture, rupture

(2) Inability to expand existing pocket, unable to fill large mastectomy defects with sufficient volume

(3) Decreased durability/longevity/satisfaction of reconstruction compared with autologous

2. **Expander-based reconstruction**
   a. Type
      (1) Removable expander with indwelling injection port
   b. Stages of expansion
      (1) Expander is placed either during initial surgery (immediate) or at a later date (delayed).
      (2) Tissue is expanded with serial saline injections over approximately 6 weeks' time (overexpansion common to create skin envelope laxity), then maintained at final volume for approximately 3–6 months to allow capsule maturation before planned exchange.
   c. Positioning
      (1) Subpectoral (cover expander from thin mastectomy skin flaps, threat of extrusion), potentially also cover with serratus muscle inferiorly
   d. Indications
      (1) Skin envelope viable and sufficient
      (2) Planned postoperative radiation: partially filled expander will help preserve pocket from radiation contracture and help to induce laxity with expansion process.
      (3) Patient's personal preference to avoid creation of additional donor site wound
   e. Contraindications
      (1) Insufficient/nonviable skin envelope secondary to surgical procedure
      (2) Patient wishes reconstructed breast to match contralateral large or ptotic breast.
      (3) Permanent foreign body such as implants unacceptable to patient

B. AUTOLOGOUS TISSUE TRANSFER
1. Pedicled flaps (Fig. 68.2)
   a. Latissimus dorsi myocutaneous flap
      (1) Vascular supply—thoracodorsal artery and venae comitantes
      (2) In event of significant skin envelope loss secondary to mastectomy or radiation, it provides significant tissue for reconstruction. It may also be combined with an implant to provide further volume.
      (3) Versatile skin paddle design
   b. TRAM
      (1) Vascular supply—perforators from superior epigastric artery
      (2) Rectus abdominis muscle is disinserted from pubic symphysis, raised distally to proximally with its pedicle, and tunneled through subcutaneous tissue to transverse breast pocket.

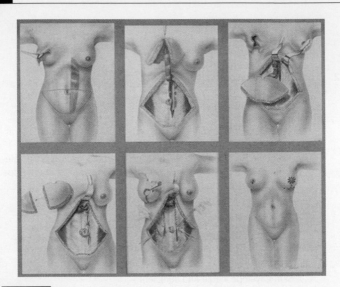

FIG. 68.2

Pedicled transverse rectus abdominis myocutaneous flap procedure. Flap is raised, then tunneled to the mastectomy. From Thorne CH. *Grabb and Smith's Plastic Surgery*. 6th ed. Philadelphia: Lippincott Williams & Wilkins; 2007:642.

      (3) May be performed in a delayed fashion to increase vascular perfusion. Delayed technique involves ligation of inferior epigastric vessels with a resulting increase in perfusion pressure three times reference levels.

  c. Pedicled flap common complications

      (1) Fat/skin necrosis at distal ends of pedicle—up to 20% of cases

      (2) Abdominal hernias (rectus muscle taken during TRAM flap)—up to 10% of cases. Mesh reinforcement of fascia often required

      (3) Wound dehiscence—6% of cases

2. Autologous free tissue transfer

  a. Free TRAM (Fig. 68.3) flap

      (1) Based on the more dominant inferior epigastric vascular pedicle

      (2) Advantages compared with pedicled flap: no pedicle bulge from tunneling, ease of breast-mound shaping, slightly lower risk of hernia due to smaller piece of muscle removed (up to 6%)

      (3) Disadvantages: microsurgical anastomosis increases risk of total flap loss (1%–3%).

  b. DIEP flap

      (1) Abdominal skin and soft tissue are raised based on its perforating blood supply from the deep inferior epigastric artery perforators (external iliac system).

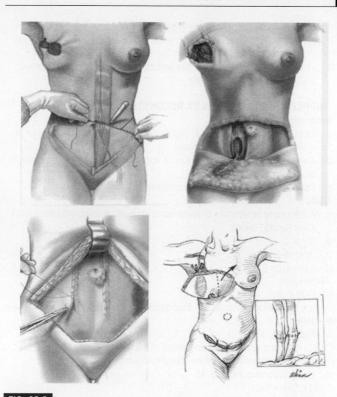

FIG. 68.3

Free transverse rectus abdominis myocutaneous flap. Flap is raised and then transposed to the mastectomy defect where microvascular anastomoses are performed. From Thorne CH. *Grabb and Smith's Plastic Surgery.* 6th ed. Philadelphia: Lippincott Williams & Wilkins; 2007:642.

(2) Perforators are dissected through the rectus muscle and no muscle is taken, sparing patients from potential morbidity of hernia.

(3) Disadvantages: meticulous dissection with increased operating time

c. Alternate free tissue transfer flaps

(1) Superficial inferior epigastric artery (SIEA) flap: minimal donor site morbidity and less difficult dissection than DIEP, but useable SIEA is present in less than 30% of cases

(2) Cutaneous gluteus maximus perforator flaps: superior gluteal artery perforator (SGAP) or inferior gluteal artery perforator (IGAP): usually less bulk than abdominally based flaps, must change patient position intraoperatively

(3) Transverse upper gracilis (TUG) myocutaneous flap: less soft tissue bulk than abdominal or gluteal-based flaps, vertical scar on medial thigh

d. Internal mammary artery is the recipient vessel of choice for blood supply to the free tissue flap.

C. NIPPLE AREOLAR COMPLEX RECONSTRUCTION (FIG. 68.4)

1. Anatomic considerations
   a. Ideal location is at the most prominent point of breast mound, or at or above inframammary crease.
   b. Areola has an average diameter of approximately 35–45 mm; nipple projects an average of 5 mm.
   c. Tattoo skin to match color of contralateral nipple.
2. Goals
   a. Appropriate position to provide symmetric result in comparison with contralateral breast
   b. Color
   c. Projection
   d. Sensitivity
3. Techniques
   a. Skin grafts
      (1) Best color/texture match found from contralateral areola or groin skin
   b. Tattoo
   c. Prosthesis
      (1) Silicone ectoprosthesis—mold of native breast created and silicone impression is then glued to the reconstructed breast.
   d. Local flaps (see Fig. 68.4)
      (1) Skate flap
      (2) Star flap
      (3) C-V flap

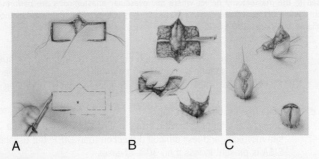

A   B   C

FIG. 68.4

Local flap for nipple reconstruction. (A) Flap design; (B) flap elevation; (C) flap formation. From Thorne CH. *Grabb and Smith's Plastic Surgery*. 6th ed. Philadelphia: Lippincott Williams & Wilkins; 2007:659.

V. ONCOPLASTIC SURGERY

A. DEFINITION

1. Combines several oncologic and plastic surgery goals and principles:
   a. Appropriate oncologic surgery to extirpate cancer with adequate margins
   b. Partial reconstruction to correct wide excision defects
   c. Immediate and delayed total reconstruction with access to a full range of plastic surgery techniques
   d. Correction of asymmetry of the reconstructed and the contralateral unaffected breast

B. CONSIDERATIONS

1. Indications: scenarios where adequate local excision cannot be achieved without significant risk of local deformity
   a. Resection of more than 20% of breast volume
   b. Central, medial, and/or lower pole resections
   c. Periareolar incisions in inferior quadrants
   d. Incomplete mobilization of breast parenchyma to allow reshaping of breast
2. Contraindications
   a. Clear margins cannot be ensured without performing a mastectomy
   b. T4 tumors
   c. Multicentric disease
   d. Extensive malignant microcalcification or inflammatory carcinoma
3. Location of tumor
4. Distribution of tumor
   a. Localized—involves only one major duct
   b. Segmental extension—involves more than one major duct

C. TECHNIQUES

1. Volume displacement
   a. Local glandular flaps and mobilized and transposed into the resection defect
   b. Overall net loss of breast volume and may necessitate contralateral breast balancing procedure for symmetry
   c. Batwing mastopexy (Fig. 68.5)
      (1) Centrally/upper pole–located tumor
      (2) Crescent mastopexy technique with wings on either side, allows mobilization of wide area of glandular tissue to advance into defect
   d. Donut mastopexy
      (1) Upper or lateral breast
      (2) Circumareolar incision allows access for tumor removal and subsequent nipple areolar complex elevation and advancement of local dermoglandular tissue into defect.

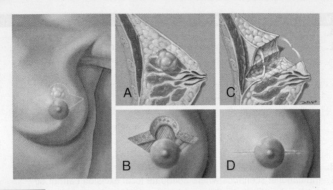

FIG. 68.5

Batwing mastopexy. (A) Preoperative view, (B) excision of mass, (C) flap advancement, and (D) final result. (From Anderson B, Masetti R, Silverstein M. Oncoplastic approaches to partial mastectomy: an overview of volume-displacement techniques. *Lancet Oncol.* 2005;6:145–157.)

    e. Wise pattern reduction
       (1) Inferior hemisphere of breast
       (2) Inverted "T" skin resection allows wide access to many areas of breast; able to remove large areas of glandular tissue and mobilize skin/glandular flaps to reduce breast and close wound, leaving inframammary fold and vertical scar

2. Volume replacement
    a. Autologous tissue harvested and transferred from local/distant site into resection defect to restore volume. See previous flap techniques section for examples and timing.

VI. POSTRECONSTRUCTION FOLLOW-UP

1. Serial evaluations of postoperative reconstruction to monitor wound healing and aesthetic outcome
2. Coordinated surveillance of reconstructed breasts for any signs of breast cancer recurrence (e.g., mammography)
3. Revision of reconstruction if necessary
    a. Poor implant position
    b. Implant capsular contracture
    c. Autologous tissue flaps requiring contouring with liposuction for better aesthetic appearance and symmetry with contralateral breast

RECOMMENDED READINGS

Association of Breast Surgery at BASO. BAPRAS and the Training Interface Group in Breast Surgery. Oncoplastic breast surgery—a guide to good practice. *EJSO*. 2007;33: S1–S23.

Beckenstein MS, Grotting JC. Breast reconstruction with free tissue transfer. *Plast Reconstr Surg*. 2001;108:1345–1353.

Hidalgo DA. Aesthetic refinement in breast reconstruction: complete skin sparing mastectomy with autogenous tissue transfer. *Plast Reconstr Surg*. 1998;102:63–70.

Mathes SJ. *Plastic Surgery*. Vol. 6. Philadelphia: Saunders; 2006:631–789.

Savalia ND, Silverstein MJ. Oncoplastic breast reconstruction: patient selection and surgical techniques. *Journal of Surg Oncol*. 2016;113:875–882.

Serletti JM, Fosnot J, Nelson JA, Disa JJ, Bucky LP. Breast reconstruction after breast cancer. *Plast Reconstr Surg*. 2011;127:124e–135e.

Spear SL, Spittler CJ. Breast reconstruction with implants and expanders. *Plast Reconstr Surg*. 2001;107:177–187.

Thorne CH. *Grabb and Smith's Plastic Surgery*. 6th ed. Philadelphia: Lippincott Williams & Wilkins; 2007:621–657.

Zhong T, McCarthy CM, Pusic AL. Evidence-based medicine: breast reconstruction. *Plast. Reconstr Surg*. 2013;132:1658–1669.

68

RECOMMENDED READINGS

PART XIII

Future of Surgery

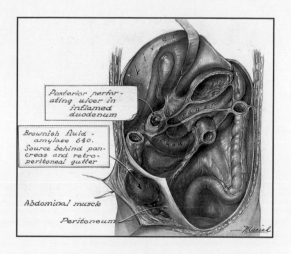

Posterior perforating ulcer in inflamed duodenum

Brownish fluid - amylase 640. Source behind pancreas and retroperitoneal gutter

Abdominal muscle

Peritoneum

Future of Surgery

Robotics and Newer Surgical Technologies

Leah Winer, MD

A robot may not injure a human being, or, through inaction, allow one to come to harm.

—Isaac Asimov

Minimally invasive surgery (MIS) describes an approach where major operations are performed through small incisions. MIS encompasses laparoscopy, robotic surgery, and natural orifice transluminal endoscopic surgery (NOTES), surgical techniques that promise to impact the way surgery is practiced. The goal of this chapter is to provide a basic overview of the aforementioned practices and their potential applications.

I. SINGLE-INCISION LAPAROSCOPIC SURGERY

1. Via an incision at the umbilicus, either several low-profile trocars or a single multilumen trocar is introduced.
2. It allows the use of conventional laparoscopic instruments while minimizing trauma and surgical scars.
3. Advantages include less pain, fewer wound complications, quicker return to activity, and better cosmesis.
4. Disadvantages include cost, ergonomic and technical difficulty, and lack of separate extraction site.
5. Studies show equivalency between single-incision laparoscopic surgery (SILS) and traditional laparoscopy in terms of complications.
6. Most common complications are intraabdominal abscess and wound infections.
7. Common applications include appendectomy, cholecystectomy, and nephrectomy.
8. In the future, combining SILS with a robotics platform may reduce the operative complexity and improve ergonomics.

II. ROBOTIC SURGERY

1. Perhaps more aptly called "computer-enhanced surgery," robotic surgery has experienced major growth over the past 2 decades. To date, more than 3 million robotic operations have been performed with the da Vinci system.
2. Robotic surgery was initially developed as a joint venture between the Stanford Research Institute and the Defense Advanced Research Projects Agency. Designed to allow US military surgeons to safely perform

TABLE 69.1

US FOOD AND DRUG ADMINISTRATION APPROVAL OF SPECIFIC PROCEDURES

Date of FDA Approval	Procedure
January 1997	Surgical assistance
July 2000	General laparoscopic surgery
March 2001	Internal mammary artery harvesting for coronary bypass and lung surgery
May 2001	Laparoscopic radical prostatectomy
November 2002	1. Laparoscopic assisted cardiotomy procedures
	2. Mitral valve repair
January 2003	Totally endoscopic atrial septal defect repair
April 2005	Gynecologic procedures

FDA, US Food and Drug Administration.

telesurgery, robotics uses laparoscopic methods, adding wristed instruments and enabling the surgeon to perform complex tasks in a more ergonomic fashion.

3. Using the robot platform, the surgeon can set up the working arms of the device over the patient and sit remotely at a console.

4. The evolution of robotic surgery can be traced through the US Food and Drug Administration (FDA) approval of specific procedures (Table 69.1).

5. The following are advantages of robotic surgery:
   a. Three-dimensional (3D), high-definition images
   b. Wristed instruments provide a wider range of movement
   c. Precision
   d. Reduced operator fatigue, particularly when operating on obese patients—the robot does the work instead of the surgeon leaning over the patient.
   e. Perfect ergonomic position
   f. Internal software filters out the natural tremor of a surgeon's hand.
   g. Alignment of the visual axis with the surgeon's hands further enhances hand-eye coordination.
   h. Single site procedures
   i. If used in military setting with threat of bioterrorism—infectious agents, toxins, and radiation—the surgeon can be in another room and/or protected from battlefield.
   j. Controlled pivot point and potential for less fascial pain
   k. Potential for reduced operating room personnel
   l. Operating surgeon does not have to remain sterile, improving comfort.
   m. Long-distance telesurgery for mentoring and proctoring

6. Disadvantages of robotic surgery include the following:
   a. No haptic feedback; tension is placed on tissues using visual cues only
      (1) Intuitive Surgical has developed robots with haptic feedback, but they are not currently commercially available.
   b. Cost—acquisition, training, ongoing maintenance, disposables

(1) Approximately \$3 million to buy; total \$4.5 million with installation and warranty

(2) Because of maintenance, it costs \$5.2 million total to purchase and operate in the first year.

(3) \$190,000 to train a surgeon and staff

c. Cannot move the operating room (OR) bed once docked

   (1) Exception: da Vinci Xi Surgical System uses Bluetooth so that the bed and robot can move in conjunction even after docking

d. Large machine with bulky footprint

e. Longer operative times with setup and docking (~10–35 extra minutes)

f. Bulk of literature consists of retrospective case reports and case series.

g. Best for one quadrant in abdomen; cumbersome for multiple quadrants

7. Although some would argue that robotics is the gold standard for selected urologic and gynecologic operations, its role in general and cardiothoracic surgery is yet to be determined. Critics question whether benefits are solely theoretical, adding cost without significant improvements in outcomes. Although it takes longer and is more expensive, the literature suggests that robotic surgery generally decreases hospital stay and blood loss. A variety of trials are under way to evaluate efficacy of robotics compared with standard laparoscopy.

8. Surgical and gynecologic training programs face the difficult task of determining how to best prepare residents for this newer wave of MIS.

9. Future directions include the following:

   a. Improved haptic feedback

   b. Increased cost effectiveness

   c. Integration of patient-centric data from computed tomography (CT) and magnetic resonance imaging (MRI) images into the 3D robotic interface. Overlaying radiologic imaging onto the operative visualization system, an augmented reality, will guide surgeon's dissection path by demonstrating vital anatomic structures beyond the visible surface. This union of image-guided therapy and robotic surgery may eventually lead to operative techniques that truly transcend human capability.

III. NATURAL ORIFICE TRANSLUMINAL ENDOSCOPIC SURGERY

1. Next phase of MIS that involves the use of flexible endoscopy to enter natural orifices (i.e., the mouth, vagina, and anus) as a means of accessing the peritoneum, mediastinum, or chest

2. Proposed benefits include the following:

   a. Reduced recovery time

   b. Reduced pain or physical discomfort

   c. Avoidance of visible scars and wound complications, such as hernias and infection

69

ROBOTICS AND NEWER SURGICAL TECHNOLOGIES

3. Limitations include the following:
   a. Challenges to accessing peritoneal cavity
   b. Technique of gastric closure
   c. Prevention of infection
   d. Development of suturing device
   e. Stability of the platform and maintenance of spatial orientation, and thus difficulty with maneuverability and exposure
   f. Management of iatrogenic intraperitoneal injuries
   g. Safety concerns and limited access to instruments present barriers to wide adoption of this technique.
4. In practice, NOTES is still typically a hybrid operation, combining the natural orifice approach with a laparoscopic port to ensure proper visualization and retraction.
5. Examples
   a. Transvaginal cholecystectomy
   b. Transanal endoscopic microsurgery
6. Future applications
   a. Intensive care unit (ICU)
      (1) Transgastric endoscopic approach would provide access to the peritoneal cavity (peritoneoscopy) to evaluate for abdominal sepsis.
      (2) Would allow visualization of all four quadrants of abdomen, as well as allow for therapeutic procedures, such as biopsy and aspiration of fluid.
      (3) The aims of NOTES in the ICU would be to decide whether critically ill or unstable patients need the OR and to reduce risk of negative laparotomy.
   b. Developing world and military setting—in resource-poor areas, NOTES could eliminate need for sterile facilities and, potentially, general anesthesia.

IV. ENDOLUMINAL AND ENDOVASCULAR SURGERY

1. This involves use of access devices, catheters, guidewires, balloon dilators, and stents to dilate stenoses.
2. It can be inserted endoscopically or endovascularly under fluoroscopic guidance.
3. A set of fundamental techniques are applicable across a wide variety of disciplines and settings.
4. Applications include self-expanding metal stents for obstructive gastrointestinal malignancies, endovascular stenting of aneurysmal disease, and esophageal balloon dilation.

RECOMMENDED READINGS

Anderson JE, Chang DC, Parsons JK, Talamini MA. The first national examination of outcomes and trends in robotic surgery in the United States. *J Am Coll Surg*. 2012;215:107–114.

Higgins RM, Frelich MJ, Bosier ME, Gould JC. Cost analysis of robotic versus laparoscopic general surgery procedures. *Surg Endosc*. 2016;31:185–192. http://dx.doi.org/10.1007/s00464-016-4954-2.

Nikfarjam M, Marks JM. Notes: what the future holds. In: Cameron JL, Cameron AM. eds. *Current Surgical Therapy*. 10th ed. Philadelphia: Elsevier; 2011:1323–1326.

Onders RP. Notes in the intensive care unit. In: Cameron JL, Cameron AM, eds. *Current Surgical Therapy*. 10th ed. Philadelphia: Elsevier; 2011:1321–1323.

Rieder E, Swanstrom LL. Notes: what is currently possible?. In: Cameron JL, Cameron AM, eds. *Current Surgical Therapy*. 10th ed. Philadelphia: Elsevier; 2011:1317–1320.

Spight DH, Hunter JG, Jobe BA. Minimally invasive surgery, robotics, natural orifice transluminal endoscopic surgery, and single-incision laparoscopic surgery. In: Brunicardi FC, Andersen DK, Billiar TR, et al., eds. *Schwartz's Principles of Surgery*. 10th ed. New York: McGraw-Hill; 2010:415–442.

ROBOTICS AND NEWER SURGICAL TECHNOLOGIES

RECOMMENDED READING

PART XIV

Procedures

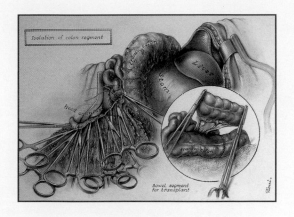

Isolation of colon segment

freed colon

transverse colon

liver

jejunum

transplant

Bowel segment
for transplant

Procedures

Jeffrey M. Sutton, MD

I. INDICATIONS FOR AN ARTIFICIAL AIRWAY

A. ABSOLUTE

1. Hypoxia—inadequate tissue oxygenation (partial pressure of oxygen [Po_2] <55 mm Hg), unresponsive to supplemental O_2
2. Hypoventilation—increasing partial pressure of carbon dioxide (Pco_2; >50 mm Hg) indicates inability to clear CO_2
3. Acute airway obstruction—refractory to oropharyngeal "finger sweep" or Heimlich maneuver
4. Penetrating neck trauma
   a. Direct tracheal injury
   b. Lateral neck injuries with associated expanding hematoma
5. Central nervous system disorder—accompanying Glasgow Coma Scale score ≤8

B. RELATIVE

1. Central nervous system disorders
   a. Status epilepticus/seizure disorder
   b. Severe alcohol/drug intoxication
   c. Severe head injury/combative patient
2. Chest wall injury
   a. Flail chest
   b. Multiple rib fractures with inadequate pain control ("splinting")
   c. Open pneumothorax
3. Inadequate pulmonary toilet
   a. Assists with airway suctioning and clearing of secretions
   b. Allows for diagnostic procedures (i.e., bronchoscopic alveolar lavage)
4. Shock
5. Trauma
   a. Burns with documented inhalational injury
   b. Maxillofacial injuries

II. NONSURGICAL TECHNIQUES

A. INITIAL/TEMPORIZING MANEUVERS

1. Foreign body removal (for acute airway obstruction)
   a. Performed via finger sweep of oropharynx, Heimlich maneuver, or under direct visualization (i.e., bronchoscopy)
2. Supplemental oxygen
   a. Via nasal cannula or face mask
      (1) For every 1 L/min oxygen delivered via nasal cannula, the fraction of inspired oxygen (FiO_2) increases by 4% up to 6 L/min (~45%).

   b. Continuous positive airway pressure mask may decrease patient's
      work of breathing and circumvent need for invasive airway.
3. **Chin lift/jaw thrust**
   a. Maintains inline cervical immobilization for trauma patients
   b. Helps to relieve partial airway obstructions
4. **Oropharyngeal airway**
   a. This is useful in obtunded patient but not tolerated in an alert individual.
   b. It relieves partial obstruction by moving tongue away from pharyn-
      geal wall.
   c. Correct size chosen by measuring from oral commissure to earlobe.
      Insert with curve aimed toward oral palate, and rotate 180 degrees
      into anatomic position to rest along base of the tongue.
5. **Nasopharyngeal airway (nasal "trumpet")**
   a. This is useful in awake patient because it is better tolerated than
      oropharyngeal and as adjunct for nasal suctioning.
   b. It also relieves partial obstruction by moving soft palate away from
      pharyngeal wall.
   c. Lubricate it well and insert into nares with bevel toward septum, and
      rotate it 90 degrees so that it lies in anatomic position.
6. **Algorithm for airway management (Fig. 70.1)**

B. OROTRACHEAL INTUBATION
1. Basics
   a. Most common definitive airway, used in unconscious or anesthetized
      patients
   b. Performed under direct visualization or fiberoptic guidance
2. Procedure
   a. Preparation
      (1) Obtain consent if possible and/or notify family.
      (2) Obtain and position necessary equipment—Ambu bag, O_2 satu-
          ration monitor, suction setup, laryngoscope (straight or curved
          blade depending on preference) with functioning light, and a
          variety of endotracheal tubes (ETs); stylet is placed in tube of
          choice, 10-mL syringe to inflate balloon at the end of the proce-
          dure
      (3) Tube choice—diameter of ring finger approximates ET size in
          adults; male individuals = 8, female individuals = 7–7.5; ET
          size ≥8 allows for bronchoscopy; for children, ET size estimated
          by fifth digit or ET size = (16 + age in years)/4.
   b. Technique
      (1) Preoxygenate patient with 100% oxygen via Ambu bag and
          monitor O_2 saturation; this ensures optimal tissue delivery of
          oxygen during the procedure.
      (2) Time permitting and in conscious patient, sedate and induce
          anesthesia (short- and quick-acting agents such as midazolam
          and succinylcholine are ideal).

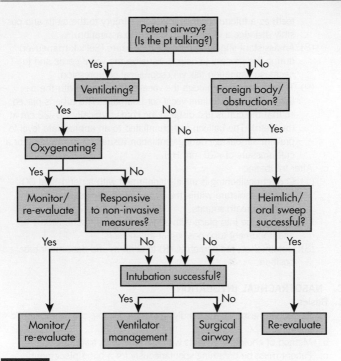

FIG. 70.1

Algorithm for airway management.

Inside the figure:

Patent airway?
(Is the pt talking?)

Yes / No

Ventilating?

Foreign body/
obstruction?

Yes / No

Oxygenating?

No

Yes / No

Monitor/
re-evaluate

Responsive
to non-invasive
measures?

Heimlich/
oral sweep
successful?

Yes / No

No / Yes

Intubation successful?

Yes / No

Monitor/
re-evaluate

Ventilator
management

Surgical
airway

Re-evaluate

(3) Unless contraindicated (neck injury), place patient in "sniffing" position with neck gently extended and crown of head touching the bed.

(4) Open mouth widely with right hand using cross-finger or "scissor" technique (thumb pushes down on lower incisors and index finger presses up on upper incisors).

(5) With the left hand holding the laryngoscope, place it in the right side of the mouth, moving to the left and posterior to sweep the tongue out of the way and visualize the epiglottis.

(6) For curved (Macintosh) blades, the tip of the blade is placed anterior to the epiglottis and should not touch the epiglottis itself. For straight (Miller) blades, the tip of the blade will be placed gently below (posterior) the epiglottis to retract it. Special attention should be made not to traumatize the epiglottis, especially when using a straight blade.

(7) After blade is in correct position, lift handle toward the ceiling to visual cords. Special attention should be made not to use the

teeth as a fulcrum, which may cause injury to the teeth and possibly dislodge a loose tooth, leading to aspiration.

(8) An assistant should apply cricoid pressure (Sellick maneuver) during the process to help to visualize the vocal cords and to decrease aspiration risk via esophageal compression.

(9) The ET is placed through the vocal cords, timed with the patient's breathing to limit vocal cord damage. The tube is placed so that the cuff is just distal to the cords (typically 20–22 cm at the teeth). The balloon is then inflated to an appropriate level to prevent air leakage during ventilation (usually 3–5 mL of air or a cuff pressure of ≤20 mm Hg).

c. After intubation
   (1) Correct positioning is initially confirmed with an end-tidal CO_2 monitor, moisture within the ET, equal chest rise, and equal, bilateral breath sounds.
   (2) Secure tube into place with adhesive tape or tracheostomy tie and document tube position at the incisors.
   (3) Obtain chest radiograph (CXR) to confirm and document tube position.

C. NASOTRACHEAL INTUBATION

1. Basics
   a. Placed via nasopharynx blindly, via laryngoscope, or with fiberoptic guidance
   b. Method of choice in patients with possible neck trauma
   c. Patient must be breathing spontaneously for a blind placement.
   d. Contraindicated in patients with suspected basilar skull fractures—intubation of the cranium has occurred with catastrophic consequences.
   e. Advantages—more comfortable for patient than orotracheal, easier oral care by nursing staff
   f. Disadvantages—more difficult to place; can take more time to place appropriately; smaller tube size needed, and thus may preclude future bronchoscopy

2. Technique
   a. Preprocedure setup and patient positioning are identical to the orotracheal route of intubation.
   b. For patient comfort, anesthetize oropharynx and nasal mucosa (benzocaine/butamben/tetracaine [Cetacaine spray] or viscous lidocaine work well).
   c. Preoxygenate patient as for orotracheal intubation.
   d. With well-lubricated tube, gently advance appropriate-sized tube cephalad into nostril (this avoids the large inferior nasal turbinate) and then posterior and caudad into nasopharynx. Slight rotation of the tube will facilitate passage, and the natural curve of the nasopharynx will aid the passage of the ET.

e. Look for moisture collecting in the ET during the patient's exhalation, and time the passage of the tube into the trachea during inhalation, when the patient's vocal cords will be open.

f. If unable to pass the ET blindly, use a laryngoscope and McGill forceps to visualize the tube position and guide the tube into the trachea.

3. After intubation—identical to orotracheal intubation

D. COMPLICATIONS
1. Aspiration during attempted intubation
2. Airway trauma from multiple failed attempts or malposition of the laryngoscope that prevents placement of a nonsurgical airway
3. Malposition—esophageal intubation, right mainstem bronchial intubation
4. Trauma to teeth
5. Tube obstruction—mucous plug, tube kinking, or compression

III. SURGICAL AIRWAY OPTIONS AND METHODS
A. CRICOTHYROIDOTOMY
1. Basics
   a. Surgical airway through the cricothyroid membrane in emergent situations when orotracheal or nasotracheal intubation cannot be performed
2. Technique
   a. Ensure presence of all necessary equipment as for endotracheal intubation, including size 6 or 7 tracheostomy (in truly emergent setting, ET can be used and trimmed at the end of the procedure).
   b. Position head with the neck extended and palpate thyroid cartilage and cricothyroid membrane.
      (1) If time permits, quickly prep neck with Betadine or chlorhexidine, but this should never take precedence to securing an airway.
   c. With a #15 blade scalpel, make a vertical midline incision, which is large enough to allow palpation of the membrane with a fingertip, over the cricothyroid membrane.
      (1) Vertical incision reduces the chance of transecting the anterior jugular vein.
   d. Visualize cricothyroid membrane, incise membrane in a horizontal direction, insert handle through the incised membrane, and turn 90 degrees to enlarge the ostomy. Alternatively, a tracheal spreader can be used to enlarge the ostomy. Ensure that the ostomy is large enough to accommodate tracheostomy.
   e. Insert appropriate tracheostomy, following the curve of the tracheostomy in a caudad direction. Inflate tracheostomy cuff, attach to oxygen supply, and confirm appropriate placement with auscultation and end-tidal CO_2 monitor as before. Secure airway with sutures, adhesive tape, or tracheostomy tape.
      (1) If appropriate placement cannot be confirmed, remove tracheostomy and ensure ostomy is large enough. On occasion, the

70

PROCEDURES

tracheostomy/ET can track anterior to the trachea in the subcutaneous tissue (especially in obese individuals).

   (2) If a tracheostomy tube is not available, an ET can be used—insert ET through ostomy just past the balloon, inflate the balloon, and gently pull the ET back so that the balloon abuts the ostomy. This will prevent placement of the ET in the right mainstem bronchus.

3. After the procedure
  a. Obtain radiograph to confirm and document tube position.
  b. Convert cricothyrotomy to formal tracheostomy or orotracheal intubation when the patient's condition stabilizes.

B. TRACHEOSTOMY
1. Basics
  a. Surgical airway placed through the second or third tracheal rings
  b. Considered an elective procedure—emergent airway needs are better served by a cricothyrotomy.
  c. Performed for those with prolonged or anticipated prolonged intubation
  d. Often used before elective head/neck operations when airway compromise may occur during the procedure
  e. Less dead space, better patient comfort, and easier for nursing staff to care for the airway than endotracheal intubation

2. Technique
  a. Place rolls under patient's shoulders to allow neck hyperextension.
  b. Palpate thyroid cartilage, cricothyroid membrane, and mark landmarks (e.g., thyroid notch, suprasternal notch, borders of trachea) with a surgical pen.
  c. Sterilely prep and drape patient from chin to upper chest.
  d. Ensure tracheostomy of appropriate size is available, inner cannula is in place, cuff functions appropriately, and tracheostomy is lubricated.
  e. Make a horizontal or vertical incision, approximately 3–5 cm, over the second to third tracheal rings and continue dissection through platysmas.
  f. Strap muscles can be bluntly separated at the midline along their vertical plane.
  g. The thyroid, thyroid isthmus, or both are encountered and can be retracted cranially with gentle dissection.
  h. Tracheal rings are encountered and must be counted exactly to ensure preservation of the first tracheal cartilage, so that the tracheostomy tube does not erode into the first tracheal ring or cricothyroid cartilage.
  i. Stay sutures with 3–0 or 4–0 monofilament placed laterally at the level where the tracheostomy will be created; these can be used for traction during the procedure as well if the tracheostomy tube becomes inadvertently dislodged after the procedure to relocate the tracheostomy site. A tracheal hook can be used at this time to elevate the trachea into the operative field to facilitate placement of the sutures and creation of the ostomy site.

    j. The midline trachea is incised at the second and third tracheal rings. Care should be taken not to puncture the cuff of the ET. A small portion may be excised, or a simple incision can be created.

    k. The ET will now be seen through the ostomy, and the anesthesia team can deflate the cuff and withdraw the ET just proximal to the ostomy.

    l. Use tracheal spreader to gently enlarge the ostomy to accommodate the tube and place the previously lubricated tube into the ostomy following the curve of the tube into the trachea. Ensure that the tube enters the ostomy and does not track anterior to the trachea.

    m. Remove inner tracheostomy cannula, attach tracheostomy to ventilator circuit, and confirm proper position with end-tidal CO_2 monitor, symmetric chest rise, and auscultation.

    n. Only after intratracheal position is confirmed should the anesthesia team remove the previously placed ET.

3. After the procedure

    a. Suture tracheostomy to the skin.

    b. Obtain postprocedure radiograph to confirm and document tube position.

C. PERCUTANEOUS TRACHEOSTOMY

1. Basics

    a. Minimally invasive tracheostomy that can be done at the bedside

    b. Uses Seldinger technique to gain access to the trachea and series of dilatations of the soft tissue and ostomy site

    c. Used with bronchoscopy to ensure safest procedure to visualize location of the needle used to access the airway

    d. Complications similar to open tracheostomy

    e. Contraindicated in emergency airway situations, pediatrics, midline neck mass, and nonintubated patients

2. After the procedure

    a. Suture tracheostomy to skin.

    b. Obtain postprocedure radiograph to confirm and document tube position.

D. COMPLICATIONS

1. Bleeding
2. Wound infection
3. Tube dislodgement or malposition
4. Pneumothorax, pneumomediastinum, subcutaneous emphysema
5. Esophageal perforation
6. Tracheal malacia
7. Tracheal stenosis
8. Fistulas—tracheoesophageal, tracheoinnominate artery

70

PROCEDURES

IV. ALTERNATE AIRWAY METHODS

A. COMBITUBE
1. Dual lumen tube inserted blindly into oropharynx in which the distal lumen usually intubates the esophagus. This distal lumen is occluded and ventilation of the second lumen is undertaken to ventilate the lungs. If the distal lumen enters the trachea, then this lumen is used to ventilate the patient.

B. FIBEROPTIC BRONCHOSCOPY
1. ET of choice is placed over a bronchoscope, and the patient is scoped. After the tube is in correct position, the bronchoscope is withdrawn while leaving the ET in position. This technique is useful for difficult intubations or those with airway trauma.

C. LARYNGEAL MASK AIRWAY
1. Mask ventilation in which a seal is made against the glottis to ventilate and oxygenate. A laryngeal mask airway does not protect the patient from aspiration.

V. ARTERIAL CATHETERIZATION

A. INDICATIONS
1. Continuous real-time-blood pressure monitoring
   a. Examples include predictable or ongoing hemodynamic instability, titration of vasopressors, unreliable noninvasive measurements.

B. TECHNIQUES
1. Radial artery catheterization—considered the gold standard technique in most controlled settings
   a. Perform Allen test.
      (1) Exsanguinate the hand by squeezing the patient's hand in a fist. Hold firm digital pressure over the radial pulse, and open the hand to observe rapid vascular refill throughout the hand. If abnormal, abort radial artery catheterization.
      (2) The test can also be completed using a pulse oximeter on the index finger or thumb when occluding the radial artery. A decreased reading suggests poor ulnar contribution and should deter the surgeon from catheterizing the radial artery.
   b. Prepare the room.
      (1) Ensure nursing available with pressure transduction setup and a sterile line to connect.
      (2) Prepare yourself with universal precautions (gown, gloves, mask, eye protection).
      (3) Place the patient's wrist in slight extension using a gauze roll and an armboard. It is helpful to tape the patient's hand over the roll and armboard to a Mayo stand or procedure table.

(4) Prep along the radial pulse from the wrist crease to several centimeters proximal and use sterile towels to create a large sterile field to prevent contaminating the wire.

c. Choose the catheter. Several devices exist to assist with arterial access; become familiar with all of them and select the technique that works best for you.

(1) Large-bore needle (size varies by kit)

(a) Inject local anesthesia adjacent to artery to help with vasodilatation.

(b) Insert the needle at a 30-degree angle to the skin, bevel up. Pulsatile red blood will be noted on entry to the artery.

(c) While stabilizing the needle, advance the wire through the needle. If there is good pulsatile blood return but the wire does not advance, lower the needle to a more acute angle (more parallel with the course of the artery) and try again.

(d) Remove the needle while controlling the wire.

(e) Guide the short catheter over the wire. Remove the wire and place your thumb over the catheter while you ask for the transduction tubing. Connect the tubing.

(f) Confirm an arterial tracing on the monitor and secure your line at three points.

(2) Needle with catheter (most central line kits have the short catheter preloaded onto this needle):

(a) Insert the needle and catheter as described earlier.

(b) Upon encountering pulsatile return, advance the needle and catheter a few millimeters. Blood return stops as you exit the lumen.

(c) Remove the needle.

(d) With the wire prepared for insertion in your dominant hand, slowly withdraw the catheter with your nondominant hand. When pulsatile return is encountered, again advance the wire.

(e) After the wire freely advances into the artery, the catheter can be advanced and the wire removed.

(f) Connect, confirm, and secure as described earlier.

(3) Self-contained device (e.g., "Dart"): These devices have the advantage of a needle, wire, and catheter in one unit.

(a) Holding the device like a pencil, enter the artery as described earlier.

(b) Once red blood begins filling the device, lower your hand to create a more acute angle between the skin and device. Advance the wire; it should meet little to no resistance.

(c) Once the wire is fully advanced, slide the catheter over the wire into the artery.

(d) Remove the device while holding the catheter at the skin. If there is no return after the device is removed, slowly

70

PROCEDURES

withdraw the catheter until pulsatile return is present. At this point the wire can be introduced and the catheter advanced again over the wire.

    (e) Connect, confirm, and secure the catheter in place as explained earlier.

2. Femoral artery catheterization

a. Perform expedient femoral ultrasound if available.

    (1) The femoral artery lies lateral to the femoral vein.

b. Prepare the room.

    (1) Ensure nursing available with pressure transduction setup and a sterile line to connect.

    (2) Prepare yourself with universal precautions (gown, gloves, mask, eye protection).

    (3) Prep widely, including visual or palpable access to anterior superior iliac spine.

        (a) The groin crease is an approximation of the inguinal ligament in a thin person; however, increased abdominal fat or pannus can be deceiving. In these patients, an assistant with sterile garb can assist by providing superior traction on the pannus.

c. Appreciate the pulse below the groin crease.

    (1) A pulseless patient can be catheterized by noting the position of the lateral aspect of the pubis and the anterior superior iliac spine; the artery is exactly at the midpoint of these two structures.

d. Enter the artery with a large-bore needle from the arterial line kit with a readied wire and guide.

    (1) When pulsatile flow is encountered, advance the wire. Lowering to a more acute angle assists with wire advancement.

    (2) Remove the needle while controlling the wire and advance the long catheter over the wire.

    (3) Connect, confirm, and secure the catheter as described earlier.

3. Alternative arterial options for catheterization

a. Examples include brachial, axillary, and dorsalis pedis arteries.

b. Typically considered "third line" options when attempts at radial and femoral access have failed

C. COMPLICATIONS

1. Hematoma
2. Arteriovenous fistula
3. Thrombosis/embolus
4. Infection

VI. BLADDER CATHETERIZATION

A. INDICATIONS FOR INDWELLING URETHRAL CATHETER

1. Continuous urine output monitoring
2. Relief of bladder obstruction (benign prostatic hypertrophy, acute urinary retention)

3. Used after genitourinary procedure—a stent to guide healing to reduce incidence of stricture
4. Provide continuous decompression after bladder and/or urethral repair
5. Prevent contamination of perineal wounds
6. Short-term management of incontinence
7. Short-term management of neurogenic bladder
8. Urologic study of the lower urinary tract
9. Use to monitor for abdominal compartment syndrome (pressure >25–30 mm Hg)

B. COMPLICATIONS OF INDWELLING URINARY CATHETER
1. Urinary tract infection
   a. Most common nosocomial infection—occurs in 40% of hospital inpatients
      (1) Comprises 80% of all nosocomial infections
   b. Incidence rate—30%–40% if left in place more than 4 days; 70%–80% if left in place more than 2 weeks
2. False passage/urethral disruption
   a. Can be caused by balloon inflation in urethra
   b. If suspected, urgent urologic consultation is indicated
3. Hematuria—may be transient because of mucosal trauma of the procedure
4. Traumatic discontinuation
   a. Treatment is to place a new Foley to tamponade bleeding.
5. Erosion of bladder neck
6. Postcatheter stricture

C. CONTRAINDICATIONS OF BLADDER CATHETERIZATION
1. Suspected urethral disruption in the setting of trauma
   a. Signs
      (1) Blood at urethral meatus
      (2) Scrotal hematoma
      (3) High-riding prostate on rectal examination
   b. Management
      (1) Urologic consultation
      (2) Retrograde urethrogram
2. Prostatitis

D. TECHNIQUES
1. Materials (Figs. 70.2 and 70.3)
   a. Robinson catheter (also known as "straight cath" or "red rubber")
      (1) Used for intermittent bladder catheterization
   b. Coudé catheter
      (1) Designed to bypass the S-shaped male bulbar urethra and often narrowed urethral angle of the prostatic urethra
      (2) Curved, firm rubber tip
      (3) Always insert with tip pointing up (12 o'clock position).

70

PROCEDURES

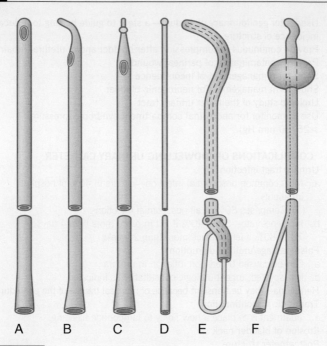

FIG. 70.2
Urethral catheters, including soft rubber (A), coudé (B), and Phillips (C), which attaches to filiform (D), which may be threaded over wire stylet (E). (F) Foley self-retaining urethral catheter.

   c. Foley catheter
      (1) Double-lumen catheter—small balloon lumen and large drainage lumen. Typically use 16 French (Fr).
         (a) 1 Fr = 0.33 mm external diameter.
      (2) Use silicone Foley if patient is expected to leave in more than 1 week.
   d. Filiform catheter—serially inserted to find true urethral passage around stricture
   e. Phillips catheter—used to follow filiform to dilate urethral stricture
   f. Malecot
      (1) Self-retaining catheter with wide outlet
      (2) Useful for draining clots
   g. Pezzer
      (1) Self-retaining catheter with wide outlet
      (2) Used for cystostomy drainage

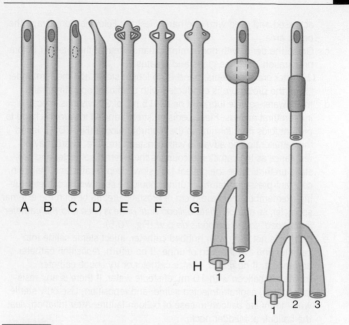

FIG. 70.3

Large-diameter catheters. (A) Conical-tip urethral catheter. (B) Robinson urethral catheter. (C) Whistle-tip urethral catheter. (D) Coudé hollow olive-tip catheter. (E) Malecot self-retaining, four-wing urethral catheter. (F) Malecot self-retaining, two-wing urethral catheter. (G) Pezzer self-retaining drain, open-end head, used for cystostomy drainage. (H) Foley-type balloon catheter. (I) Foley-type, three-way balloon catheter, one limb of distal end for balloon inflation *(1)*, one for drainage *(2)*, and one to infuse irrigating solution to prevent clot formation within the bladder *(3)*.

   h. Three-way irrigation catheter
      (1) Three-lumen design—small balloon lumen, small irrigation lumen, large drainage lumen
   i. Pediatric feeding tube
      (1) Five to 8 Fr may be used in infants. Catheter may be held in place with tape.
      (2) Do not use in adults because of coiling in the urethra.
2. Male procedure
   a. Assemble all necessary equipment. Items usually in tray are sterile gloves, drapes, Foley catheter, 10 mL of sterile saline in syringe, collection bag, cotton swabs, povidone-iodine or chlorhexidine prep, prep forceps, sterile water, and soluble lubricant or 2% viscous lidocaine.
   b. Place patient in supine position. Open Foley tray in sterile fashion, then put on sterile gloves. Arrange all items so they are easily

accessed and used with one hand. Test the Foley balloon. Drape the pelvic area.

c. Grasp the penis with nondominant hand. Retract the foreskin before preparation. Prep the glans and meatus.

(1) After grasping penis, hand is no longer sterile and the remainder of the procedure is conducted with dominant operating hand.

d. Inject water-soluble lubricant or 10–15 mL of 2% viscous lidocaine into urethral meatus. Place penis on stretch angled toward the head to prevent folds from forming in the urethral mucosa (Fig. 70.4). Insert the catheter tip and advance with constant pressure. There may be resistance as the catheter encounters the external sphincter and pro-static urethra. Have the patient take slow, deep breaths and maintain constant pressure. Return of urine should be seen within catheter tubing. Remember, there are 3 cm of prostatic urethra beyond the external sphincter, so *do not inflate balloon until urine is seen and the catheter is "hubbed" to the balloon side port* (Fig. 70.5).

e. If urine is not seen with hubbed catheter, inject sterile saline into catheter and await return of urine. If no return, reposition catheter and repeat. If no return, upsize catheter or try coudé catheter.

f. Inflate the balloon with 10 mL of sterile water. If there is any resistance, stop, aspirate injected saline, and reposition. Use only sterile water to inflate balloon in case of balloon failure. After inflation, seat the balloon at bladder neck.

g. Secure catheter to thigh with umbilical tape in correct position to prevent traumatic withdrawal. *Advance foreskin to prevent paraphimosis* (most common cause of paraphimosis is forgetting to replace after bladder catheterization).

3. **Female procedure (Fig. 70.6)**

a. Prepare equipment as outlined.

b. Patient is positioned supine and "frog-legged."

c. Retract labia with first finger and thumb of nondominant hand to expose urethra. Nondominant hand is now contaminated, and the remainder of the procedure must be done with sterile dominant hand. Urethra may be difficult to visualize at this point. Using povidone-iodine (Betadine) or chlorhexidine-soaked cotton swabs, prep the urethra, superior vagina, and labia using downward swipes, one swipe per cotton swab. At this point, a difficult to visualize urethra may be seen with a slight pool of Betadine or a "wink" seen at urethral meatus.

d. Generously coat catheter tip with water-soluble lubricant or 10–15 mL of 2% viscous lidocaine. With dominant operating hand, insert catheter into urethral meatus and await return of urine.

e. Inflate balloon with 10 mL sterile water. Retract catheter to seat balloon at bladder neck.

f. Secure catheter to leg with umbilical tape to prevent traumatic withdrawal.

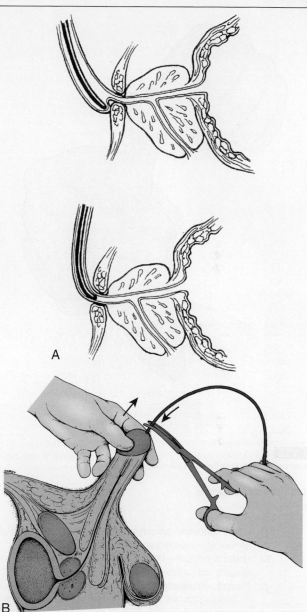

A

B

FIG. 70.4
The importance of stretch in male catheterization.

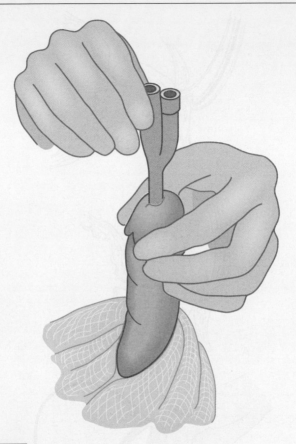

FIG. 70.5
Urethral catheterization in the male patient.

4. **Difficult catheterizations**
   a. Male patients
      (1) Causes
         (a) Meatal stricture—balanitis xerotica obliterans, congenital narrowing, sexually transmitted disease
         (b) Urethral stricture—fibrosis after trauma, instrumentation, sexually transmitted disease
         (c) Prostatic enlargement
            (i) Benign prostatic hypertrophy affects one-third of men older than 50 years, 90% of men older than 80 years.
            (ii) It affects periurethral prostate tissue, causing impaired voiding symptoms and difficult catheterizations.

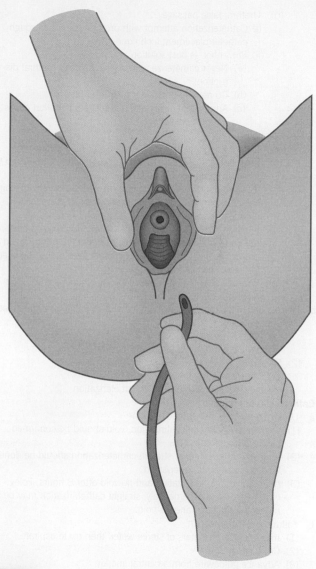

FIG. 70.6
Urethral catheterization in the female patient.

(d) Urethral false passage
  (i) Catheterization attempt with urethral trauma or rough catheter placement technique
  (ii) Prevention is best solution.
    (a) Never catheterize with classic signs of urethral disruption.
    (b) Do not use unfamiliar instrumentation.
    (c) Any patient suspected of urethral disruption needs urologic consultation.
(2) Solutions
  (a) Ensure adequate lubrication and traction on penis.
  (b) If patient is anxious, lorazepam or morphine can be used to facilitate sphincter relaxation.
  (c) If failure at first attempt, 10–15 mL of 2% viscous lidocaine should be injected into meatus and kept in place for 5 minutes before next attempt.
  (d) If resistance is still met, catheter should be upsized (yes, upsized) to 20–24 Fr to be able to maintain pressure and prevent coiling. If available, coudé catheter should be used to help to navigate prostatic urethra.
  (e) If failure after two attempts, a urologic consultation is warranted.
b. Female patients—mostly stem from inability to locate urethral meatus
  (1) Causes
    (a) Obesity
    (b) Vulvar atrophy
  (2) Solutions
    (a) Assistance in retraction
    (b) Vaginal speculum-assisted catheterization
5. **Catheter discontinuation**
  a. Urinary retention after catheterization
    (1) Void check—after discontinuation, void should be confirmed within 8 hours.
    (2) If no void after 8 hours, straight catheterization should be done. Void check should be repeated.
    (3) After straight catheterization and no void after 8 hours, Foley may be replaced. Alternatively, straight catheterization may be repeated until spontaneous void.
  b. Failure to deflate balloon
    (1) Inject several milliliters of sterile water, then try to aspirate.
    (2) Cut balloon port.
    (3) Advance guidewire from a central line kit.
      (a) This may dislodge occluding material.
      (b) Central line catheter may be advanced over wire into balloon to deflate once guidewire is withdrawn.
        (i) Limited by length—male urethra is approximately 20 cm.

(4) Balloon rupture (second choice)
  (a) Hyperinflation of balloon followed by firm end of guidewire insertion to pop balloon
  (b) External needle puncture with ultrasound guidance
  (c) Inspection of balloon after removal to ensure all portions were removed
    (i) If fragments left in bladder, removal with cystoscopy

E. ALTERNATIVES
1. Suprapubic catheter
2. Condom (also known as Texas) catheter
   a. Good alternative for immobilized male patients with normal voiding function
   b. Often used in critically ill patients to avoid infectious risk of an indwelling catheter but provide accurate output recording

VII. CENTRAL VENOUS LINES
A. INDICATIONS
1. Large-volume resuscitation
2. Total parenteral nutrition infusion
3. Invasive monitoring (pulmonary artery catheters)
4. Infusion of inotropic agents
5. Hemodialysis
6. Chemotherapy delivery
7. Poor venous access

B. CONTRAINDICATIONS (ALL ARE RELATIVE IN A LIFE-THREATENING SITUATION)
1. Presence of a deep venous thrombosis in site of choice
2. Presence of a coagulopathy or significantly depressed platelet count (i.e., $<50,000/mm^3$)
3. Subclavian vein approach in a patient on hemodialysis or expected to require hemodialysis in the future because of the increased rate of subclavian vein stenosis after central venous catheter (CVC) placement
4. Untreated sepsis/bloodstream infections
5. Previous femoral vascular surgery (for femoral approach)

C. TECHNIQUES
1. Patient evaluation
   a. Evaluate the patient's prothrombin time/international normalized ratio/partial thromboplastin time, platelet count, hemoglobin and hematocrit, and history of bleeding disorders.
   b. History of deep venous thrombosis
   c. Physical examination for deformities or scars from previous CVC placement

70

PROCEDURES

2. **Preparation**
   a. Cardiac monitoring
   b. Collection of necessary supplies
      (1) CVC kit
      (2) Obtaining ultrasound device if available
      (3) Sterile gown, sterile gloves, face mask, head protection, 0.9% normal saline for flush, sterile towels, sterile drape, sterilization/prepping agent (i.e., chlorhexidine), sterile dressing kit, 1% lidocaine, shoulder roll, sterile intravenous tubing, ultrasound with sterile covering and gel
   c. Correct patient positioning
      (1) Subclavian/internal jugular (IJ): Place patient in supine Trendelenburg position (head down) with a shoulder roll placed under the patient (longitudinally for subclavian and transversely for IJ). Allow patient's ipsilateral shoulder and arm to fall to the side and be as relaxed as possible; gentle retraction may need to be applied by an assistant. Turn patient's head toward the contralateral shoulder for an IJ approach. For patients with large pendulous breasts, gentle retraction is beneficial in the subclavian approach.
      (2) Femoral: Place patient in supine reverse Trendelenburg position, retract any significant panus, and make sure leg is not maximally externally or internally rotated.
   d. Flush the proximal and middle ports before insertion.
3. **Placement**
   a. Depth of CVC placement depends on patient body habitus, type of catheter used, and site of insertion
   b. On CXR, the catheter tip of a CVC should at least make a bend into the superior vena cava; extension into the right atrium is tolerable as long as it does not cause ectopy but ideally should be pulled back into the superior vena cava.
4. **Seldinger technique**
   a. After insertion site is selected, create a weal with 1% lidocaine, as well as infusing some along the subcutaneous track in the direction of planned needle insertion.
   b. Insert an 18-gauge needle according to the technique unique to the selected site, aspirating while probing.
   c. If blood is encountered and it can be easily aspirated, remove the syringe.
   d. Without the slightest movement of the needle, insert the J-wire, J-tip first; it should pass with little resistance. Advance the wire at least 20 cm into the patient; if cardiac ectopy on the cardiac monitor is encountered, this confirms that the wire is within the heart (for nonfemoral lines).
   e. Make at least a 3-mm nick in the skin with the scalpel and then remove the needle.
   f. Always keep a hand on the wire so as not to lose it in the patient.

g. Insert the dilator only 3–4 cm to dilate the subcutaneous tissues, and remove while maintaining control of the wire.

h. Slide the CVC over the wire keeping the wire still in space.

i. Advance the CVC to desired depth and then remove the wire.

j. Withdraw and flush all ports with normal saline.

k. Suture the CVC onto the skin in at least three locations and place a sterile dressing.

l. Obtain CXR to verify correct position and rule out pneumothorax.

5. **Infraclavicular subclavian vein approach**

a. Technique

(1) Palpate the deltopectoral groove and infiltrate 1% lidocaine, two fingerbreadths inferior to the clavicle along the deltopectoral groove, creating a weal. Place index finger of the nondominant hand in the sternal notch and the thumb between the weal of lidocaine and the clavicle along an imaginary line between the weal of lidocaine and the tip of the index finger in the sternal notch. While aspirating, advance the needle down to the clavicle, and infuse lidocaine onto the periosteum and inject lidocaine while withdrawing the needle.

(2) With an 18-gauge needle, and the bevel facing either toward the ceiling or the patient's feet, advance the needle while aspirating toward the center of the sternal notch/tip of the index finder, always keeping it parallcl to thc floor, and sliding it under the clavicle. Transcutaneous pressure from the infraclavicular thumb assists driving the needle under the clavicle.

6. **Anterior internal jugular vein approach**

a. Positioning

(1) Position the patient with the head rotated toward the contralateral side and in the Trendelenburg position.

b. Identification of landmarks

(1) Identify the SCM muscle and the insertion of the sternal and clavicular heads, and trace them back to their point of convergence. This point forms the superior apex of a triangle formed by the clavicle and the sternal and clavicular heads of the SCM. Palpate the carotid pulse as it courses through the neck.

c. Technique

(1) Infuse 1% lidocaine at the superior apex of the two heads of the SCM superficially.

(2) Under ultrasound guidance, advance the needle while aspirating at 45–60 degrees to the skin.

(3) Insert the CVC using the Seldinger technique as described in the previous section.

7. **Femoral vein approach**

a. Positioning

(1) Position the patient on a flat bed in reverse Trendelenburg position with the leg slightly abducted. Avoid allowing the leg to

be maximally rotated either internally or externally. Retract any panus up and away from the groin.

b. Identification of landmarks
   (1) Identify the pubic tubercle, anterior superior iliac spine, and inguinal ligament, and palpate the femoral pulse. Remember "venous toward the penis."

c. Technique
   (1) Administer 1% lidocaine inferior to the inguinal ligament, medial to the femoral pulse.
   (2) Retract the femoral artery laterally and insert the 18-gauge introducer needle, while aspirating, at a 45-degree angle to the skin in a direction parallel to the palpated pulse, 1 cm medial to the palpated femoral pulse. Ultrasound guidance may be used to assist in localizing the femoral vein.
   (3) If there is no blood return, slowly withdraw the needle to the level of the skin and redirect it just medially. If further attempts are unsuccessful, insert the introducer needle just medial to the palpated pulse.
   (4) After good blood return has been demonstrated, place CVC via Seldinger technique as described earlier. If arterial blood is seen, stop and hold pressure for at least 5 minutes before reattempting to find the vein just medial to where the femoral artery is encountered.

D. COMPLICATIONS

1. Arterial puncture
   a. Withdraw needle, and hold pressure for 10 minutes.
   b. Monitor vitals and breath sounds for possible hemothorax.
   c. Catheterization can be resumed, assuming no signs of bleeding are present (hematoma).
   d. Uncertain arterial versus venous puncture
      (1) Obtain sterile intravenous extension tubing and attach on end to the needle; withdraw blood into the tubing and hold the tubing up toward the ceiling; arterial pressure will maintain the blood at the level to which it is withdrawn, whereas venous pressure is not sufficient to maintain the blood at the level to which it is withdrawn and will fall back down the intravenous tubing.
      (2) If the catheter has been placed, it can be hooked up to a pressure transducer, and if arterial pressure and waveform are seen, arterial placement is confirmed. Alternatively, an arterial blood gas can be sent.
   e. Arterial cannulization
      (1) After the artery is dilated with either the dilator or placement of CVC, the safest course of action is to place the CVC into the artery to control the bleeding by plugging the hole with the catheter. Notify upper-level resident and staff.

2. Pneumothorax
   a. Tension pneumothorax
      (1) If suspected, place a 16-gauge Angiocath needle in the second intercostal space along the midclavicular line, with subsequent chest tube placement.
   b. Simple pneumothorax
      (1) If small (<10% or <2 rib spaces on CXR), nonexpanding, and asymptomatic, chest tube placement is not necessary. Follow the patient with serial examinations and place him or her on a cardiopulmonary monitor.
      (2) If more than 10%, expanding, or symptomatic, place a chest tube to evacuate the pneumothorax.

3. Air embolus
   a. Management
      (1) Attempt to withdraw air through the CVC if possible.
      (2) Place patient into Trendelenburg position, rotated to the patient's left to trap the air in the apex of the right ventricle.
      (3) Maintain supportive care if the patient becomes symptomatic, and transfer patient to appropriate level of care (intensive care unit). Initiate Advanced Cardiac Life Support if cardiac or pulmonary arrest develops.

VIII. ENTERAL ACCESS

A. NASOGASTRIC TUBES

1. Indications
   a. Decompression of stomach and small bowel
   b. Analysis of gastric contents
   c. Gastric lavage
   d. Introduction of fluids (e.g., oral contrast material)

2. Contraindications
   a. Head trauma and/or maxillofacial fractures (risk for intracranial penetration)
   b. Known presence of esophageal stricture or varices
   c. Recent esophageal or gastric surgery
   d. History of alkaline reflux (risk for perforation)
   e. Unsecured airway in neurologically impaired (risk for aspiration)

3. Types of tubes
   a. Salem sump tube—dual-lumen tube. The main lumen (clear/white) should be placed to continuous low suction; the second port (blue) vents the tube to allow continuous sump suction without mucosal injury. The venting port should NEVER be flushed with fluid. Instead, flush with 15 mL of air every 3–4 hours to ensure patency. The main lumen may also be flushed with 30 mL water as needed. The vent is patent when it "whistles" continuously.
   b. Levin tube—a soft, single-lumen tube. Connect to low intermittent suction to prevent occlusion by gastric mucosa.

70

PROCEDURES

4. **Technique**
   a. Position patient: If awake, patient should be sitting with neck flexed. If patient is unconscious, elevate the head of bed at least 30 degrees.
   b. Estimate the distance required to reach the stomach by measuring the length from the nose to the earlobe and from the earlobe to the xiphoid process. Add the measurements together for the total distance.
   c. Lubricate the tube with water-soluble lubricant or viscous lidocaine. Viscous lidocaine may also be inserted into the nostril with cotton-tip applicators or syringe.
   d. Insert the tube into a nostril, and pass it into the nasopharynx (a small bend in the tip of the tube aids passage).
   e. Instruct the patient to swallow when the tube is felt in the back of the throat. Sips of water through a straw can help to facilitate easy passage of the tube into the esophagus in an awake patient.
   f. Advance into the stomach.
   g. Ask the awake patient to say his or her name. Phonation is a good indicator that the vocal cords (and hence the trachea) are not occluded. Coughing, gasping for air, or inability to speak may be an early sign of tracheal intubation. Condensation may be visible in the tube. Immediately pull back the tube.
   h. Confirm the tube position by instilling 20–30 mL of air while listening over the stomach with a stethoscope and by aspirating gastric contents. Aspiration of gastric contents is a more reliable method. Always confirm with a radiograph if the tube is to be used for feeding.

B. OROGASTRIC TUBES

1. **Indications**
   a. Nasogastric (NG) intubation contraindicated (anterior basilar skull fracture, nasopharyngeal trauma)
2. **Types of tubes**
   a. Ewald tube—most commonly used. Especially suited for lavage of the stomach and emergency evacuation of blood, toxic agents, medications, or other substances. It is a large (18/36-Fr) double-lumen tube. The 36-Fr lumen is connected to continuous suction; the 18-Fr lumen is used for irrigation.
3. **Technique**
   a. It is similar to NG tube insertion described earlier, except the tube is introduced into the mouth and down the esophagus into the stomach.
   b. In patients with loss of consciousness or loss of the gag reflex, insertion of a cuffed ET before orogastric tube insertion is preferred.
   c. Verify the position of the tube by aspiration of gastric contents and by auscultation.

C. FEEDING TUBES
1. Need for supplemental enteric feeding. Indications include:
   a. Inadequate caloric intake (prematurity/failure to thrive)
   b. Central nervous system dysfunction
   c. Burns/trauma
   d. Esophageal anomalies/dysmotility
   e. Malignancy
   f. Eating disorders
2. Short-term enteric feeding
   a. These tubes are smaller in diameter, softer, and more flexible than NG tubes.
      (1) Corpak—nonweighted; a wire stylet may be used to pass the tube into the duodenum under fluoroscopic guidance.
      (2) Frederick–Miller—has a stylet that allows for improved manipulation.
      (3) pH-guided nasointestinal feeding tubes—rapid, easy placement of feeding tube with elimination of endoscopic/fluoroscopic requirement. Placement is similar to that for standard bedside feeding tube. The pH monitor allows for continuous readings. A pH of 3.5–5 confirms placement of tube in stomach. The tube is advanced until a sudden, rapid increase in pH readings is encountered, signifying transpyloric passage. If the rate of pH increase is gradual, the tube is likely to be curled in the stomach with the tip at the gastroesophageal junction.
   b. Tubes may be placed blindly in a similar fashion as outlined earlier for NG tubes or under fluoroscopic guidance.
   c. Placement must be confirmed radiographically before initiation of tube feedings.
   d. Placement of the tube past the ligament of Treitz eliminates most of the potential for aspiration.
3. Long-term enteric feedings
   a. Percutaneous endoscopic gastrostomy (PEG) tube—provides long-term enteric access
      (1) Advantages—fast, safe placement of gastrostomy tube. May be placed under sedation versus general anesthesia.
      (2) Contraindications are relative. Prior abdominal surgery makes this procedure higher risk.
      (3) Technique: An endoscope is passed through the mouth and into the stomach. A site on the anterior gastric wall is identified and a needle introduced into the stomach percutaneously under direct visualization. A wire is then passed through the needle into the stomach and out through the oral pharynx. The gastrostomy tube is then attached to the wire and guided through the stomach, exiting the skin at the site of the previous needle puncture. The distance of the PEG tube at the skin level should be noted and documented after surgery and on daily rounds.

70

PROCEDURES

b. Open (Stamm) gastrostomy tube (G-tube)
   (1) Advantages: Allows for safe placement of gastrostomy tube even in the most difficult abdomen
   (2) Technique: A small upper midline incision is made through the abdominal wall. Clamps are used to elevate the anterior gastric wall approximately 6–10 cm from the gastroduodenal junction. Two silk purse-string sutures are placed on the anterior wall of the stomach, and a small incision is made at the center of the purse-string sutures. A large-bore (18–22-Fr) Foley catheter is then passed into the stomach, and the balloon is inflated. The catheter is secured in place with the purse-string sutures, and the open is end passed through the anterior abdominal wall through a separate site. The anterior gastric wall is fixed to the anterior abdominal wall with silk sutures to minimize dead space; care should be taken to ensure that the balloon of the catheter is pulled up against the stomach and up to the abdominal wall. With time, the tract epithelializes to facilitate frequent exchanges of tubes as needed for optimal feeding.

IX. FOCUSED ASSESSMENT WITH SONOGRAPHY IN TRAUMA (FAST EXAMINATION)

1. Evaluation of trauma patients or coagulopathic patients suspected of having intraperitoneal hemorrhage
2. Rapid, inexpensive, and accurate test when performed in appropriately selected patients suspected to have intraperitoneal hemorrhage after abdominal trauma
   a. Has replaced diagnostic peritoneal lavage (DPL) as an efficient bedside evaluation of blunt trauma patients
   b. Usually performed early in the evaluation of the trauma patient, typically during the secondary survey
   c. Depends on the familiarity of the diagnosing physician with the use of ultrasound and interpretation of images (Table 70.1)
   d. Learning curve is steep, with expertise gained between 50 and 200 examinations.

TABLE 70.1

DIAGNOSTIC PERITONEAL LAVAGE VERSUS ULTRASOUND VERSUS COMPUTED TOMOGRAPHY IN BLUNT ABDOMINAL TRAUMA

	Ultrasound	Computed Tomography Scan
Indications	Document fluid if decreased blood pressure	Document organ injury if blood pressure stable
Advantages	Early diagnosis; noninvasive and repeatable; 86%–97% accurate	Most specific for solid organ injury; 92%–98% accurate
Disadvantages	Operator dependent; bowel gas and subcutaneous air distortion; misses diaphragm, bowel, and some pancreatic injuries	Cost and time; misses some diaphragm, bowel tract, and pancreatic injuries

Data from Advanced Trauma Life Support. Chicago, American College of Surgeons, 1997.

3. Advantages
   a. Rapid, noninvasive means to diagnose intraabdominal injuries during ongoing primary and secondary survey
   b. May be repeated quickly at the bedside, allowing ongoing investigation
   c. Accurate means of diagnosing hemoperitoneum
   d. Useful in diagnosing cardiac injuries with pericardial fluid through the subxiphoid window
      (1) Could aid in deciding which organ cavity to explore first in a patient with multisystem injuries
   e. Safe in pregnant and pediatric patient populations
4. Disadvantages
   a. Operator dependence and experience
5. Complicating factors
   a. Obesity
   b. Subcutaneous air
6. Technique
   a. Includes visualization of the following:
      (1) Hepatorenal recess (Morison pouch)
         (a) Most dependent space within the supramesocolic region
         (b) Place the transducer probe along the right upper quadrant or laterally along the costal margin.
      (2) Splenorenal fossa
         (a) Place the transducer probe over the left flank along the posterior axillary line and move cephalad and caudally.
      (3) Subxiphoid pericardial window
         (a) Place the transducer probe in the epigastrium, angle parallel to the skin, and aim toward the left shoulder.
      (4) Suprapubic window (Douglas pouch)
         (a) This is the most dependent space within the inframesocolic region.
         (b) Place the transducer probe cephalad to the pubic symphysis and aim caudally toward the pelvis
      (5) E-FAST (Extended Focused Assessment with Sonography for Trauma) includes the previously described four windows plus views of bilateral pneumothoraces and upper anterior chest wall.
   b. Intraperitoneal fluid appears as an anechoic stripe.

X. PULMONARY ARTERY (SWAN-GANZ) CATHETERIZATION
A. INDICATIONS
1. Invasive cardiac monitoring
   a. Pulmonary artery catheter—CVP, pulmonary artery systolic and diastolic pressures, pulmonary capillary wedge pressure (PCWP), cardiac output, systemic venous resistance
2. Complex surgical procedures with associated intravascular volume shifts

70

PROCEDURES

3. Hemodynamic instability
4. Difficulty with fluid management/inappropriate response to volume challenge
5. Deteriorating cardiopulmonary function
6. Severe head injury
7. Surgical procedures in patients with baseline poor cardiac, respiratory, or renal function

B. DESIGN

1. Catheter tip with balloon (1.5-mL capacity) allowing placement of the tip into the pulmonary artery and measurement of pulmonary artery systolic and diastolic pressures, as well as capillary wedge pressures
2. Proximal port allowing measurement of CVP
3. Thermistor 4 cm from tip senses changes in temperature.
   a. Measures the flow of cold fluid injected via the proximal port, allowing calculation of cardiac output/index

C. MEASUREMENT

1. Measurement of pulmonary arterial diastolic and wedge pressures, thus approximating left atrial filling pressure (preload)
2. Continuous monitoring of pulmonary artery systolic and mean pressures reflects changes in pulmonary vascular resistance secondary to hypoxemia, pulmonary edema, pulmonary emboli, and pulmonary insufficiency; helps to distinguish cardiogenic from noncardiogenic pulmonary edema
3. Sampling of global mixed venous blood
   a. Global mixed venous blood saturations (SvO_2) provide an index of tissue perfusion and oxygenation. Increasing SvO_2 correlates with increasing cardiac output and tissue perfusion or decreased oxygen extraction (in sepsis or liver failure). Decreasing SvO_2 signifies decreasing cardiac output or tissue perfusion with increased oxygen extraction. However, SvO_2 cannot reflect the changes in regional perfusion, which are often present in critically ill patients.
4. Accurate, reproducible measurement of cardiac output by thermodilution technique
5. Monitoring of RV filling pressure through the CVP access port
6. Evaluation of myocardial function—preload, contractility, and afterload (Table 70.2)
   a. Myocardial perfusion pressure can be estimated from the difference between systemic diastolic pressure and PCWP.
   b. Heart rate and systolic pressure can be combined to provide a "time tension index."
   c. Systemic vascular resistance as an estimate of aortic impedance (afterload) can be calculated.
   d. Effect of therapeutic interventions can be quantified in terms of physiologic cost.

TABLE 70.2
DETERMINANTS OF CARDIAC OUTPUT

Determinant	Definition	Effect on Cardiac Output	Measurement	Treatment
Preload	Length of myocardial fibers at end diastole, which is the result of ventricular filling pressure	Direct, up to physiologic limit	End-diastolic volume and pressure of the ventricles Pulmonary diastolic pressure Pulmonary capillary wedge pressure Direct left atrial pressure measurements CVP (right atrial)	Volume expansion Pericardiocentesis Reduction of PEEP
Contractility	The inotropic state of the myocardium; length/tension/ velocity relationship of the myocardium independent of initial length and afterload	Direct	Ventricular function curves Ejection fraction V_{max} V_{cf} PEP/LVET dP/dt	Dopamine Norepinephrine Epinephrine Isoproterenol Dobutamine Digitalis Glucagon GKI Milrinone
Afterload	Systolic ventricular wall stress, which is produced by the force against which the myocardial fibers must contract	Inverse, as long as coronary flow is maintained	Aortic pressure for left ventricle Pulmonary artery pressure for right ventricle	Diuretics Phentolamine Sodium nitroprusside Nitroglycerin Intraaortic balloon pumping External counterpulsation
Pulse rate	The number of cardiac systoles per minute	Direct, >60 and <180 beats/min	Electrocardiogram Count pulse	Bradycardia Atropine Pacemaker Epinephrine Tachycardia Digitalis Lidocaine Electroversion

CVP, Central venous pressure; *dP/dt,* rate of change of left ventricular pressure; *GKI,* glucose-potassium-insulin; *LVET,* left ventricular ejection time; *PEP,* preejection period; *PEEP,* positive end-expiratory pressure; V_{cf}, velocity of circumferential fiber shortening; V_{max}, peak velocity.
Data from Hardy JD: *Textbook of Surgery.* Philadelphia: JB Lippincott; 1983:54.

70

PROCEDURES

7. Specialized pulmonary artery catheters permit (1) atrial, ventricular, or sequential atrioventricular pacing simultaneously; (2) continuous measurement of mixed venous oxygen saturations; (3) continuous cardiac output measurements; or (4) measurement of end-diastolic volumes.

D. PITFALLS
1. PCWP is at best an estimation of LV filling pressures. The gold standard for measuring preload is LV end-diastolic volume, which is not practical clinically. PCWP is an extrapolation of left atrial pressure, which, in turn, is an estimate of LV end-diastolic pressure. Thus in cardiac disease states with changes in myocardial compliance or valvular function, PCWP may be an inaccurate estimation of preload. Specialized catheters with the ability to measure end-diastolic volume provide more accurate estimations of LV filling pressures.
2. Catheter artifact (whip) and high positive end-expiratory pressures may produce inaccurate measurements.
3. Catheters may be difficult to "float" in patients with cardiomegaly or low cardiac output. Placing the patient upright and with the left side down may alleviate this problem. Fluoroscopy may also be helpful.
4. Arrhythmias during insertion include ventricular irritability (premature ventricular complexes and ventricular tachycardia) and right bundle branch block. Catheter placement in a patient with previous left bundle branch block may produce complete heart block. If pulmonary artery monitoring is essential, preparation for emergency pacing should be made.
5. Pulmonary artery rupture
   a. More common in elderly adults and those with pulmonary hypertension
   b. Avoid overwedging the balloon and prolonged balloon inflation.
   c. Continuous monitoring of pulmonary artery tracing—balloon inflation must be stopped once the waveform changes. If the tip has migrated distally, less than 1.5 mL will cause the balloon to wedge.
   d. Daily CXRs should be reviewed to ensure proximal catheter positioning.
   e. Signs of rupture—hemoptysis or bleeding from ET
   f. Treatment
      (1) Deflate balloon and remove Swan-Ganz catheter.
      (2) Supportive care
         (a) Given low pressure within pulmonary vascular system, some patients will spontaneously cease bleeding.
      (3) If patient continues to bleed or becomes unstable, operative intervention (wedge resection, pneumonectomy) may be required. Endotracheal intubation with either single- or double-lumen tube should protect the uninjured lung (most ruptures occur in the right lower lobe).
         (a) Position patient with uninjured side up.

XI. ABSCESS DRAINAGE

A. TECHNIQUE

    a. Obtain a history and perform a focused physical examination.

        (1) Individuals with prior abscesses, diabetes, history of intravenous drug abuse, recent trauma, dialysis dependence, prior solid organ transplantation, or additional immunocompromised states are prone to recurrent abscess development.

        (2) Localize the abscess, typically clinically evidenced by a fluctuant mass in an area of erythema, induration, and tenderness.

           (a) Ultrasound may be used to identify an abscess located deeper within the subcutaneous tissue.

    b. Consider intravenous pain control and sedation (see Chapters 7 and 8) when possible.

    c. Prep and drape the area in a sterile manner.

    d. Use a local anesthetic to perform a field block of area (e.g., 1% lidocaine with epinephrine).

        (1) Local anesthesia in the abscess can be difficult to obtain secondary to the low pH of the abscess cavity, but anesthesia of the superficial overlying skin should not be affected.

        (2) The addition of 8.4% sodium bicarbonate at a ratio of 1 mL bicarbonate to 5 mL of lidocaine may help to offset the low pH and reduce burning caused by lidocaine injection.

    e. Consider using an 18- or 20-gauge needle to collect a sample for Gram stain as well as aerobic and anaerobic cultures.

        (1) In addition to ultrasonography, this may also help to localize the fluid collection.

    f. Using a #11 or #15 scalpel blade, make an incision over the most fluctuant area overlying the abscess cavity.

        (1) A linear incision is preferred, but some providers use an elliptical or cruciate incision to ensure adequate and ongoing drainage.

        (2) Use the skin creases when possible to minimize scarring. It is possible to use a smaller incision in cosmetically important areas, but it is essential that the abscess be fully drained.

        (3) If the initial incision only yielded sanguineous (but not purulent) effluent, an additional deeper incision may be required.

    g. Use a curved hemostat or Kelly clamp to gently disrupt all loculations to ensure adequate drainage.

    h. Irrigate the cavity liberally with saline.

    i. Pack the cavity completely but loosely with thin-strip packing gauze and cover with a gauze dressing.

XII. THORACENTESIS

A. INDICATIONS

1. Diagnostic evaluation of pleural fluid

2. Therapeutic aspiration of fluid or air to improve lung expansion

B. TECHNIQUE
1. Materials and preparation
   a. Become familiar with the thoracentesis kit available at your institution. All are based on a Seldinger catheter-over-needle design.

C. POSITIONING
1. Have the patient in a comfortable position, sitting erect, leaning forward, with extended arms resting on a table. If patient is critically ill, the lateral decubitus position may be used.
2. Locate the effusion and determine its extent, both clinically by percussion and auscultation, as well as by CXR or ultrasound. Do not attempt unguided thoracentesis on loculated fluid.
3. Ultrasound is ideal for locating proper needle insertion site in high-risk patients, as well as locating fluid in small effusions, assessing the depth of fluid from the skin to the pleura, and for needle guidance during the procedure.
4. Needle insertion site
   a. Perform along midscapular line or posterior axillary line from the back.
   b. Correct site is one or two interspaces below the fluid level and 5–10 cm lateral to the spine. Never insert the needle below the eighth posterior intercostal space.

D. PROCEDURE
1. Using sterile technique and observing universal blood and body fluid precautions, prep and drape the previously chosen area.
2. Infiltrate anesthetic intradermally over the superior margin of the rib (to avoid the neurovascular bundle) below the chosen interspace. Continue through the subcutaneous tissue and down to the periosteum of the rib. After making contact with the superior boarder of the rib, "walk the needle" over the border and continue to inject into the intercostal muscle layer. Remember to aspirate and inject small aliquots of anesthetic as the needle is advanced. Continue until pleural fluid is aspirated, and note the depth of the needle by attaching a clamp at the level of the skin. At this point, withdraw the needle 0.5 cm and infiltrate the pleura, then remove the needle.
3. After the needle is removed, access the same site using a 16–18-gauge Angiocath and advance to the previously measured depth. When fluid returns, carefully slide the Angiocath over the needle and remove the needle.
4. Fluid is collected in a closed system with one-way valves. Most systems have a 60-mL Luer-Lok syringe attached to a limb of tubing that allows aspiration of fluid from the Angiocath. Another limb of tubing in turn connects the Luer-Lok syringe to the collection bag.

Aspiration and collection of fluid occurs by moving the piston on the Luer-Lok syringe in and out in a pumping motion. The valve in the tubing automatically directs fluid from the Angiocath into the collection bag. Note that most systems have a side port where chemotherapeutic or sclerosing agents may be instilled, such as in a chemical pleurodesis.

5. For diagnostic purposes, removal of between 50 and 100 mL of fluid is adequate. For therapeutic purposes, fluid removal is continued until patient reports relief of dyspnea, or until 1000 mL fluid has been withdrawn. Note that after removal of 1000 mL fluid, it becomes necessary to monitor pleural pressures because of the risk for reexpansion pulmonary edema; at this point, terminate the procedure when the pleural pressure exceeds –20 mm Hg.

6. Remove the angiocatheter and apply a sterile dressing.

7. Send pleural fluid for the following studies:
   a. Hematology—cell count and differential
   b. Chemistry—specific gravity, pH, lactate dehydrogenase, amylase, glucose, and protein
   c. Microbiology—Gram stain, bacterial/fungal and acid fast bacillus cultures
   d. Pathology—cell cytology

8. Obtain CXR to confirm efficacy of aspiration and to rule out pneumothorax.

E. INTERPRETATION OF RESULTS (TABLE 70.3)

1. Transudative—cirrhosis, nephritic syndrome, congestive heart failure, lobar atelectasis, viral infection
2. Exudative—empyema, malignant effusion, intraabdominal infection, pancreatitis, tuberculosis, trauma, pulmonary infection, chylothorax
3. Grossly bloody—iatrogenic injury, pulmonary infection, trauma, tumor, hepatic or splenic puncture
4. Extremely low glucose is consistent with rheumatoid process.

TABLE 70.3

DIAGNOSIS OF EXUDATE VERSUS TRANSUDATE

Lab Studies	Transudate	Exudate
Protein	<3 g/dL	>3 g/dL
Protein ratio (effusion:serum)	<0.6	>0.6
Specific gravity	<1.016 g/mL	>1.016 g/mL
LDH	Low	High
LDH ratio	<0.6	>0.6
Glucose	2/3 serum glucose	Low
Amylase	<200 IU/mL	>500 IU/mL
RBC	<10,000/mm^3	>100,000/mm^3
WBC	<1000/mm^3	>1000/mm^3

LDH, Lactate dehydrogenase; *RBC,* red blood cell; *WBC,* white blood cell.

F. COMPLICATIONS
1. Pneumothorax
2. Hemothorax
3. Hepatic or splenic puncture
4. Parenchymal tear
5. Empyema

RECOMMENDED READINGS

Marino P. *Marino's The ICU Book*. 4th ed. Philadelphia: Wolters Kluwer; 2013.

PART XV

Rapid References

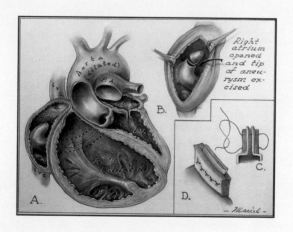

Rapid References

Jeffrey M. Sutton, MD

CLINICAL LABORATORY REFERENCE RANGES AT THE UNIVERSITY OF CINCINNATI MEDICAL CENTER

Test[a]	Normal Values	Units
Hematology		
Complete Blood Count (CBC)		
Leukocyte count (WBC)	3.8–10.8	$10^3/\mu L$
Hemoglobin (Hg)	Male: 13.2–17.1	g/dL
	Female: 11.7–15.5	
Hematocrit (Hct)	Male: 38.5–50.0	%
	Female: 35.0–45.0	
Platelet count (Plt)	140–400	$10^3/\mu L$
Renal Panel		
Sodium (Na)	135–146	mmol/L
Potassium (K)	3.5–5.3	mmol/L
Chloride (Cl)	98–110	mmol/L
Bicarbonate (CO_2)	21–33	mmol/L
Anion gap	3–16	mmol/L
Blood urea nitrogen (BUN)	7 25	mg/dL
Creatinine (Cr)	0.60–1.30	mg/dL
Glucose (Glu)	70–100	mg/dL
Calcium (Ca)	8.6–10.3	mg/dL
Magnesium (Mg)	1.5–2.5	mg/dL
Phosphorus (Phos)	2.1–4.7	mg/dL
Liver Profile		
Aspartate aminotransferase (AST)	13–39	U/L
Alanine aminotransferase (ALT)	7–52	U/L
Bilirubin, total	0.0–1.5	mg/dL
Bilirubin, direct	0.0–0.4	mg/dL
Bilirubin, indirect	0.0–1.1	mg/dL
Alkaline phosphatase	36–125	U/L
Albumin	3.5–5.7	g/dL
Protein, total	6.4–8.9	g/dL
Coagulation		
Prothrombin time (PT)	11.6–14.4	s
Activated partial thromboplastin time (aPTT)	24.3–33.1	s
Heparinized partial thromboplastin time (hPTT)	90.0–130.0	s
International normalized ratio (INR)	0.9–1.1	—

71

Test[a]	Normal Values	Units
Bleeding time	<9.5	min
Fibrinogen	239–419	mg/dL
Anti-Xa—low-molecular-weight heparin	0.50–1.10	U/mL
Thromboelastography (TEG)		
R	22–44	seconds
K	34–138	seconds
α (angle)	64–80	degrees
Maximum amplitude (MA)	52–71	mm
Lysis 30	—	%
Activated clotting time (ACT)	86.0–118.0	sec
Hemolysis/Iron Studies		
Ferritin	Male: 23.9–336.2	ng/mL
	Female: 11–306.8	
Fibrin degradation	<16	Pμg/mL
Fibrinogen	150–400	mg/dL
Haptoglobin	44–215	mg/dL
Lactate dehydrogenase (LDH)	110–270	U/L
Iron	50–212	μg/dL
Folate	5.9–24.8	ng/mL
B12	180–914	pg/mL
Total iron-binding capacity (TIBC)	Male: 261–462	μg/dL
	Female: 265–497	

Cardiac

Creatinine kinase (CK)	30–233	U/L
Creatinine kinase, myocardial b fraction (CKMB)	0.6–6.3	ng/mL
Troponin I	<0.04	ng/mL
Cholesterol	<200	mg/dL
High-density lipoprotein (HDL)	≥60	mg/dL
Low-density lipoprotein (LDL), calculated	<100	mg/dL
LDL, direct	75–193	mg/dL
Triglycerides	<150	mg/dL

Critical Care

Arterial Blood Gas (ABG)		
pH	7.35–7.45	—
Partial pressure of carbon dioxide (P_{CO_2})	35–45	mm Hg
Partial pressure of oxygen (P_{O_2})	80–100	mm Hg
HCO_3	22–26	mmol/L
TCO_2	23–27	mmol/L
Base excess	−2.0 to 3.0	mmol/L
O_2 saturation	95.0–98.0	%
Carboxyhemoglobin	Nonsmoker: 0%–2%	%
	Smoker: 0%–8%	

Test[a]	Normal Values	Units
Nutrition		
Albumin	3.5–5.7	g/dL
Prealbumin	17–34	mg/dL
Retinol-binding protein	3.0–6.0	mg/dL
Transferrin	203–362	mg/dL
Miscellaneous		
Ammonia	27–90	μg/dL
Calcium, free	4.5–5.3	mg/dL
Calcium	1.0–1.4	mg/dL
Cortisol, serum, AM	6.7–22.6	μg/dL
Cortisol, serum, PM	<10	μg/dL
Cortisol, adrenocortico-tropic hormone (ACTH) stimulation	>2× basal values	μg/dL
Cortisol, dexamethasone suppression	Below basal values for screening, low-dose, and high-dose tests	μg/dL
Cortisol, urine	29–140	μg/24 h
C-reactive protein (CRP)	1.0–10.0	mg/L
Erythrocyte sedimentation rate (ESR)	0–15	mm/h
Lactic acid	0.5–2.2	mmol/L
Osmolality, serum	278–305	mOsm/kg
Osmolality, urine	50–1200	mOsm/kg
Pancreatitis		
Amylase, serum	16–117	U/L
C-peptide	0.9–7.10	ng/mL
Fecal fat	<15.0	g/72 h
Lipase, serum	4–82	U/L
Insulin	2.00–29.10	mIU/mL
(Para)Thyroid Studies		
Calcitonin	Male: 4.4–31.6 Female: 3.0–14.8	pg/mL
Parathyroid hormone (PTH), intact	6.6–55.8	ng/mL
Parathyroid hormone (PTH), mid-molecule	0.3–1.08	ng/mL
T3	0.6–2.2	ng/mL
T4	4.6–11.5	μg/dL
T3, free	2.0–3.6	pg/mL
T4, free	0.61–1.76	ng/dL
Thyroglobulin	1.6–59.9	ng/mL
Thyroxine binding globulin	11.0–27.0	μg T4/dL
Thyroid-stimulating hormone (TSH)	0.34–5.60	μIU/mL
Antithyroglobulin	0.0–39.0	IU/mL

71

RAPID REFERENCES

Test[a]	Normal Values	Units
Tumor Markers		
α-Fetoprotein (AFP)	<9	ng/mL
Cancer antigen 15-3 (CA 15-3)	0.7–35.0	U/mL
Carbohydrate antigen 19-9 (CA 19-9)	1.4–37.0	U/mL
Carbohydrate antigen 125 (CA 125)	5.5–35.0	U/mL
Carcinoembryonic antigen (CEA)	Nonsmoker: 0–3 Smoker: 0–5	ng/mL
Gastrin	<97.0 (fasting)	pg/mL
Prolactin	Males: 2.6–13.1 Female <50: 3.3–26.7 Female ≥50: 2.7–19.6	ng/mL
Prostate-specific antigen (PSA)	0.0–4.0	ng/mL
Miscellaneous		
α1-Antitrypsin	84–218	mg/dL
Amylase, fluid (e.g., Jackson-Pratt drain)	0–400	U/Tvol
Clostridium difficile, stool	Negative	n/a
Creatinine, urine/fluid	1.0–1.8	g/Tvol
Hemoglobin A1C (glycohemoglobin)	4.8–6.4	%
Phosphate, urine	0.0–1600.0	mg/Tvol
Potassium, urine	25–125	mEq/Tvol
Protein, urine	0–150	mg/Tvol per 24 h
Sodium, urine/fluid	40–220	mEq/Tvol
Urea, urine/fluid	7.0–16.0	g/vol
Uric acid	3.8–8.7	mg/dL
Gamma-glutamyl transpeptidase (GGT)	9–64	U/L
Glucose, cerebrospinal fluid (CSF)	40–70	mg/dL
Protein, CSF	15–45	mg/dL

[a]Specimen source is blood/serum unless otherwise specified.

n/a, Not applicable.

Index

Page numbers followed by *f* indicate figures; *t,* tables.

INDEX

INDEX

INDEX